Exam Oriented Anatomy
Regional and Applied

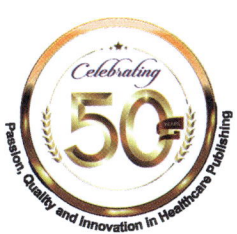

Volume 1

Exam Oriented Anatomy
Regional and Applied

Samar Deb MS

Fellow, The Academy of Anatomical Society of India
Academic Director and Emeritus Professor
Department of Anatomy, MGM Medical College
Kishanganj, Bihar, India

Formerly
Dean and Professor, Department of Anatomy
North Bengal Medical College
Darjeeling, West Bengal, India

Academic Director
Principal and Professor, Department of Anatomy
Katihar Medical College
Katihar, Bihar, India

Principal and Professor, Department of Anatomy
College of Medicine and JNM Hospital
Kalyani, West Bengal, India

Professor, Department of Anatomy
Agartala Government Medical College
Tripura, India
IQ City Medical College, Durgapur
West Bengal, India

Principal and Professor, Department of Anatomy
MGM Medical College
Kishanganj, Bihar, India

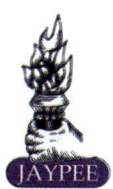

JAYPEE BROTHERS MEDICAL PUBLISHERS
The Health Sciences Publisher
New Delhi | London

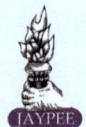
Jaypee Brothers Medical Publishers (P) Ltd

Headquarters
Jaypee Brothers Medical Publishers (P) Ltd
4838/24, Ansari Road, Daryaganj
New Delhi 110 002, India
Phone: +91-11-43574357
Fax: +91-11-43574314
Email: jaypee@jaypeebrothers.com

Overseas Office
J.P. Medical Ltd
83 Victoria Street, London
SW1H 0HW (UK)
Phone: +44 20 3170 8910
Fax: +44 (0)20 3008 6180
Email: info@jpmedpub.com

Website: www.jaypeebrothers.com
Website: www.jaypeedigital.com

© 2020, Jaypee Brothers Medical Publishers

The views and opinions expressed in this book are solely those of the original contributor(s)/author(s) and do not necessarily represent those of editor(s) of the book.

All rights reserved. No part of this publication may be reproduced, stored or transmitted in any form or by any means, electronic, mechanical, photocopying, recording or otherwise, without the prior permission in writing of the publishers.

All brand names and product names used in this book are trade names, service marks, trademarks or registered trademarks of their respective owners. the publisher is not associated with any product or vendor mentioned in this book.

Medical knowledge and practice change constantly. This book is designed to provide accurate, authoritative information about the subject matter in question. However, readers are advised to check the most current information available on procedures included and check information from the manufacturer of each product to be administered, to verify the recommended dose, formula, method and duration of administration, adverse effects and contraindications. It is the responsibility of the practitioner to take all appropriate safety precautions. Neither the publisher nor the author(s)/editor(s) assume any liability for any injury and/or damage to persons or property arising from or related to use of material in this book.

This book is sold on the understanding that the publisher is not engaged in providing professional medical services. If such advice or services are required, the services of a competent medical professional should be sought.

Every effort has been made where necessary to contact holders of copyright to obtain permission to reproduce copyright material. If any have been inadvertently overlooked, the publisher will be pleased to make the necessary arrangements at the first opportunity. The **CD/DVD-ROM** (if any) provided in the sealed envelope with this book is complimentary and free of cost. **Not meant for sale**.

Inquiries for bulk sales may be solicited at: jaypee@jaypeebrothers.com

Exam Oriented Anatomy—Regional and Applied (Volume 1)

First Edition: **2020**

ISBN 978-93-89188-77-6

Printed at Sanat Printers

Dedicated to

My wife late Paroma (Gita)

PREFACE

Immense importance of the knowledge of anatomy can never be ignored by anyone of any branch of medical science. Undergraduate students face a great difficulty to develop a crystal clear concept on this subject during their very limited duration of one year first professional course. That is why they do not become satisfied with their performance nowadays, while they appear in anatomy examination. It is ensured that this book titled *Exam Oriented Anatomy—Regional and Applied* will help them to develop full confidence on this subject. Moreover, if the students go through the questions–answers thoroughly and sequentially in every chapter, they will definitely develop a command on the knowledge of this subject. Questions and answers are 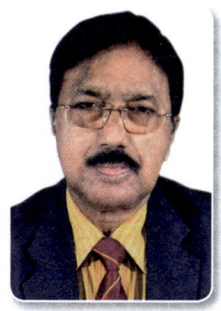 placed in such a manner that this book will be useful for the students as a precise textbook. The book will also be very helpful for a teacher before taking a class on a particular topic. The presentation of the answers has been made student-friendly to make it easy for self-learning. The text has been written with optimum integration of clinical anatomy. All the areas of the subject have been covered in such a fashion that the postgraduate students as well as the readers of other disciplines will also be benefited.

Samar Deb

ACKNOWLEDGMENTS

For preparation of this book as I received the assistance and/or inspiration, I express my sincere thanks and gratefulness, and deep gratitude to:

- My beloved students, undergraduates as well as postgraduates, of all the times and all the places, for taking keen interest for my classes, which always encouraged and enabled me to present any topic in a most palatable and interesting manner.
- My honorable teachers of all the times from whom I gathered many stones to build the approach road through which I have been able to reach the destination of art and quality of a good teacher.
- My parents who gave me direction to achieve the success in life.
- My cordial colleagues, senior and junior, and my professional friends, of all the times and all the places, who have always been kind enough to share their knowledge with me.
- All the eminent personalities in the field of anatomy of the country from whom I have been able to enrich my knowledge.
- All the experts of Medical Council of India, National Medical Commission and Anatomical Society of India who brought the revolution in anatomy teaching to make it more interesting and integrated.
- Dr Hironmoy Roy, one of my brilliant postgraduate students for his time to time suggestions to make the book more acceptable to the readers.
- Dr Ritonik Choudhury, my nephew, for his proposal to make this book more student-friendly.
- All the dignitaries, officials and staff of M/s Jaypee Brothers Medical Publishers (P) Ltd, New Delhi, India especially Shri Jitendar P Vij (Group Chairman), Mr Ankit Vij (Managing Director), Mr MS Mani (Group President), Dr Madhu Choudhary (Publishing Head–Education), Ms Pooja Bhandari (Production Head), Ms Sunita Katla (Executive Assistant to Group Chairman and Publishing Manager), and Dr Sneha Kashyap (Development Editor), for giving valuable opportunity for publication of the book.
- Shams Jamal Hashmi, for his untiring meticulous and neat computer preparation of the manuscript.
- Sukho Ranjan De Sarkar, for beautiful art work of the book.
- Rita Sarkar, Sudipto Saha and Arijit Ganguli, for their valuable technical assistance with the help of their computer works.
- Madhubanti my daughter, as she used to admire me whenever she came close to my working table during the late hours of all the days while at home.

CONTENTS

Section 1: Upper Limb

1. **Pectoral Region and Breast**   1
   Pectoralis Major Muscle 1
   Deltopectoral Groove 1
   Pectoralis Minor 1
   Clavipectoral Fascia 3
   Axillary Tail of Spence 4
   Breast 4
   Soft Tissue Architecture of Breast 5
   Blood Supply of Breast 6
   Lymphatic Drainage of Breast 7

2. **Axilla and Scapular Region**   11
   Axilla 11
   Serratus Anterior Muscle 13
   Axillary Artery 14
   Axillary Lymph Nodes 16
   Brachial Plexus 18
   Deltoid Muscle 23
   Triangular and Quadrangular Spaces 24

3. **Anterior Compartment of Arm and Cubital Fossa**   26
   Muscles of Anterior Compartment of the Arm 26
   Nerve Supply of the Muscles 27
   Action of the Muscles 28
   Brachial Artery 28
   Cubital Fossa 30

4. **Posterior Compartment of Arm**   32
   Triceps Brachii Muscle 32
   Anconeus 33
   Profunda Brachii Artery 34

5. **Shoulder Girdle and Shoulder Joint**   35
   Shoulder Girdle 35
   Sternoclavicular Joint 36
   Acromioclavicular Joint 37
   Shoulder (Glenohumeral) Joint 40

6. **Anterior Compartment of Forearm**   48
   Muscles of the Front of Forearm 48
   Anterior Interosseous Nerve 54
   Radial Artery 55
   Arterial Anastomosis Around Elbow Joint 56

7. **Posterior Compartment of Forearm**   58
   Muscles of the Posterior Compartment of Forearm 58
   Posterior Interosseous Nerve 65

8. **Elbow Joint and Radioulnar Joints**   67
   Elbow Joint 67
   Proximal (Superior) Radioulnar Joint 71
   Interosseous Membrane 72
   Pronation and Supination 73

9. **Hand**   75
   Flexor Retinaculum of Hand 75
   Palmar Aponeurosis 77
   Fibrous Flexor Sheath of Fingers 78
   Intrinsic Muscles of the Hand 79
   Synovial Sheath of Flexor Tendons 81
   Lumbrical Muscles 82
   Superficial Palmar Arch 84
   Interossei Muscles of Hand 85
   Median Nerve in the Palm 86
   Ulnar Nerve in the Palm 87
   Fascial Spaces of Hand 89
   Cutaneous Nerves of Dorsum of Hand 94
   Extensor Retinaculum of Hand 95
   Dorsal Digital Expansion (Extensor Expansion) 96
   Anatomical Snuff Box 98

10. **Joints of the Wrist and Hand**   99
    Radiocarpal (Wrist) Joint 99
    First Carpometacarpal Joint 102

11. **Major Nerves of the Upper Limb**   105
    Axillary Nerve 105
    Musculocutaneous Nerve 107

Median Nerve 108
Carpal Tunnel Syndrome 111
Ulnar Nerve 111
Radial Nerve 115

12. **Explanatory Notes (Clinical/ Embryological/Morphological)** 119
    Radial Nerve Injury at the Axilla 123
    Radial Nerve Injury at the Spiral Groove 123
    Full Claw Hand 124
    Ulnar Claw Hand 124

Section 2: Lower Limb

13. **Front of Thigh** 131
    Inguinal Lymph Nodes 131
    Saphenous Opening 132
    Iliotibial Tract 133
    Femoral Triangle 134
    Femoral Sheath 136
    Sartorius 138
    Pectineus 139
    Quadriceps Femoris 140
    Articularis Genu 142
    Adductor Canal 142
    Femoral Artery 144
    Femoral Nerve 146

14. **Medial Side of the Thigh** 149
    Muscles of Medial Compartment of Thigh 149
    Obturator Nerve 152
    Profunda Femoris Artery 153

15. **Gluteal Region, Back of Thigh and Popliteal Fossa** 155
    Sacrotuberous Ligament 155
    Sacrospinous Ligament 155
    Gluteus Medius and Gluteus Minimus 155
    Tensor Fasciae Latae 156
    Structures Under Gluteus Maximus 157
    Hamstring Muscles 160
    Arteries of Back of Thigh 162
    Boundaries of Popliteal Fossa 164
    Muscles of the Popliteal Fossa 165
    Neurovascular Structures of Popliteal Fossa 165
    Genicular Anastomosis 168
    Popliteus 169

16. **Anterolateral Compartment of Leg and Dorsum of Foot** 171
    Muscles of Anterior Compartment of Leg 171
    Cutaneous Nerve Supply of Dorsum of Foot 174
    Extensor Retinacula of the Foot 175
    Extensor Digitorum Brevis 176
    Deep Fibular (Deep Peroneal) Nerve 177
    Anterior Tibial Artery 178
    Muscles of Lateral (Peroneal) Compartment 179
    Fibular (Peroneal) Retinacula 181
    Superficial Fibular (Peroneal) Nerve 182

17. **Back of the Leg and Sole of the Foot** 183
    Flexor Retinaculum of Ankle 183
    Soleus Muscle 184
    Posterior Tibial Artery 184
    Second Layer 186
    Interosseous Muscles 187
    Blood Vessels and Nerves of Sole of Foot 188

18. **Joints of Lower Limb** 190
    Hip Joint 190
    Knee Joint 196
    Ankle (Talocrural) Joint 209
    Tarsal Joints 214
    Inversion and Eversion of the Foot 216

19. **Miscellaneous Topics** 218
    Arches of Foot 218
    Venous Drainage of Lower Limb 223
    Great Saphenous Vein 224
    Short Saphenous Vein 225
    Deep Veins 227

20. **Explanatory Notes (Clinical/ Embryological/Morphological)** 229
    Flat Foot (Pes Planus) 237
    Clubfoot (Talipes) 237

Section 3: Abdomen and Pelvis

21. **Anterior Abdominal Wall** 239
    Umbilicus 239
    External Oblique Abdominis 240
    Linea Alba
    Rectus Abdominis Muscle 243
    Pyramidalis Muscle 244
    Rectus Sheath 244
    Inguinal Canal 246

22. Peritoneum — 255
Primitive Ventral and Dorsal Mesenteries of Gut 255
Functions of Peritoneum 257
Changes in the Foregut Making Peritoneal Cavity Complex 257
Disposition of Peritoneal Membrane in Abdominal Cavity 261
Important Peritoneal Spaces 265

23. Stomach and Small Intestine — 268
Stomach 268
Arterial Supply of Stomach 273
Venous Drainage of Stomach 273
Lymphatic Drainage of Stomach 274
Duodenum 274
First Part of Duodenum 276
Second Part of Duodenum 277
Suspensory Muscle of Duodenum (Ligament of Treitz) 279
Jejunum and Ileum 280
Arterial Supply of Jejunum and Ileum 282
The Mesentery (Mesentery of Small Intestine) 283
Differences Between Jejunum and Ileum 284
Meckel's Diverticulum 285

24. Liver and Biliary Apparatus — 287
Liver 287
Basic Architecture of Liver 297
Biliary Apparatus 299

25. Pancreas, Spleen and Celiac Trunk — 306
Pancreas 306
Spleen 315
Splenic Circulation 319
Celiac Trunk 320
Branches 321

26. Abdominal Part of Large Gut, Mesenteric Arteries and Portal Vein — 323
Large Intestine 323
Cecum 324
Vermiform Appendix 329
Transverse Colon 332
Superior Mesenteric Artery 335
Inferior Mesenteric Artery 337
Portal Vein 338

27. Posterior Abdominal Wall — 342
Cisterna Chyli 342
Psoas Major Muscle 342
Iliacus Muscle 343
Psoas Minor Muscle 343
Quadratus Lumborum Muscle 344
Psoas Sheath 345
Thoracolumbar Fascia 345
Abdominal Aorta 347
Inferior Vena Cava 350
Lumbar Plexus of Nerves 352
Autonomic Nervous System in Posterior Abdominal Wall 354

28. Thoracoabdominal Diaphragm — 358
Thoracoabdominal Diaphragm 358
Lymphatic Drainage 363

29. Kidney and Suprarenal Gland — 367
Kidney 367
Suprarenal Gland 374
Chromaffin System 378

30. Pelvis — 379
Bony Pelvis 379
False Pelvis 379
True Pelvis 380
Pelvic Inlet (Pelvic Brim) 380
Pelvic Outlet 380
Pelvic Cavity 380
Axis of the Pelvis 380
Pelvic Parameters 381
Sex Differences of Pelvis 381
Types of Female Pelvis 382
Clinical Anatomy 382
Piriformis 382
Obturator Internus 383
Pelvic Diaphragm 384
Internal Iliac Artery 389
Sacral Plexus 391
Autonomic Nerves of the Pelvis 393

31. Pelvic Part of the Large Gut — 395
Rectum 395
Anal Canal 399

32. Urinary Bladder and Ureter — 407
Urinary Bladder 407
Pelvic Part of Ureter 416

33. **Organs of Male Reproductive System** 417
    Prostate Gland 417
    Microstructure 422
    Vas Deferens 426
    Scrotum 427
    Testis 429
    Structure of the Testis 431
    Arterial Supply 431
    Venous Drainage 432
    Lymphatic Drainage 432
    Nerve Supply 432
    Descent of Testis 432

34. **Organs of Female Reproductive System** 435
    Uterus 435
    Uterine (Fallopian) Tubes 446
    Ovaries 449

35. **Perineum and Urethra** 453
    Perineal Body 453
    Ischiorectal Fossa 454
    Pudendal Canal 455
    Superficial Perineal Pouch 457
    Deep Perineal Pouch 459
    Urogenital Diaphragm 460
    Male Urethra 461

36. **Explanatory Notes (Clinical/Embryological/Morphological)** 466

Index *479*

SECTION 1: UPPER LIMB

Chapter 1

Pectoral Region and Breast

SA 1.1 Write a brief note on pectoralis major and pectoralis minor muscles.

PECTORALIS MAJOR MUSCLE (FIG. 1.1)

It is the largest muscle of pectoral region. It forms anterior wall of axilla. Lower border of the muscle forms anterior axillary fold.

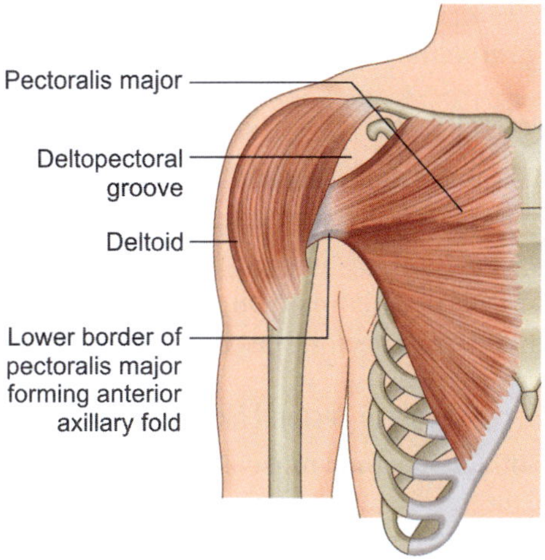

Origin
- **Clavicular head:** From anterior surface of medial half of clavicle.
- **Sternocostal head**: It is wide, flat and triangular. This head takes origin from the following sources:
  - Respective half of anterior surface of **manubrium** and **body of sternum**
  - Anterior surface of **2nd to 6th costal cartilage**
  - Lower most aponeurotic fibers arise from **aponeurosis of external oblique muscle.**

DELTOPECTORAL GROOVE (FIG. 1.1)

It is a furrow between adjacent borders of the deltoid and the clavicular head of pectoralis major muscles.

The groove is important because it lodges:
- Terminal part of **cephalic vein** before it passes deeper to drain into axillary vein.
- **Deltopectoral group of lymph nodes** which are clinically important as they receive some lymph vessels from the breast.

Fig. 1.1: Pectoralis major and deltopectoral groove.

Insertion
Two heads of pectoralis major muscle are inserted into **lateral lip of intertubercular sulcus** of humerus **in bilaminar fashion** as follows:
- **Clavicular head**: Anterior, shorter and lower lamina.
- **Sternocostal head**: Posterior and longer lamina extending up to higher level.

PECTORALIS MINOR (FIG. 1.2)

Pectoralis minor is the smaller of the two pectoral muscles. It is triangular in outline with its apex directed upwards and laterally towards the coracoid process. So the two margins of the muscle are superomedial and inferolateral. The pectoralis minor lies under cover of pectoralis major.

Origin

Pectoralis minor muscle takes origin from anterior end of outer surface of **3rd, 4th and 5th ribs** and adjacent parts of their costal cartilage.

Insertion

The muscle is inserted into medial border and adjacent part of superior surface of horizontal part of coracoid process of scapula.

Extension of tendinous insertion: Tendon of insertion of pectoralis minor may extend beyond coracoid process and shoulder joint to be attached to greater tuberosity of humerus.

Normally these fibers are represented as *coracohumeral ligament* of shoulder joint.

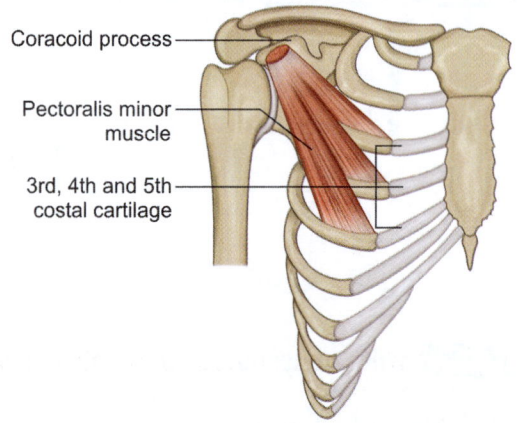

Fig. 1.2: Pectoralis minor muscle.

Pectoral Fascia

This is the **deep fascia of pectoral region wraping the pectoral muscles**. Prominent component of this fascia covers the surface of pectoralis major muscle.

Pectoral fascia is separated from superficial fascia by a plane containing mammary gland or breast which is well developed in child-bearing period of life of female. Breast is freely mobile over pectoral fascia by a space of loose fibrous connective tissue called retromammary space.

Nerve Supply of Pectoral Muscles

Both the pectoral muscles are supplied by both **lateral as well as medial pectoral nerves**.

Actions of Pectoral Muscles

Pectoralis Major

- Pectoralis major, as inserted beyond shoulder joint, acts on the same joint (it is better understood after shoulder joint is studied).
- **Acting as a whole**, pectoralis major causes **adduction** and **medial rotation** of arm
- **Clavicular head** causes **flexion** of arm
- **Sternocostal head** alone, causes **extension** of arm (shoulder) **against the resistance**. This action is well demonstrated during **climbing**.

Pectoralis Minor

As the muscle is inserted into coracoid process of scapula, proximal to shoulder joint, it **does not have any action on shoulder joint**. The muscle acts on movement of scapula (its action is better understood after study of shoulder girdle).

- **Acting with serratus anterior**, the pectoralis minor causes forward movement or **protraction of scapula** along the chest wall.
- Acting **with lower fibers of trapezius**, the muscle helps in downward movement or **depression of scapula**.

SN 1.2 Write a short note on clavipectoral fascia.

CLAVIPECTORAL FASCIA (FIG. 1.3)

Introduction

Clavipectoral fascia is a strong fascial sheet which extends between **clavicle** and **pectoralis minor muscle**.

The fascia **splits** in two levels **to enclose two muscles:**

1. Above—subclavius
2. Below—pectoralis minor.

The fascia **forms two ligaments:**

1. Upper end—costocoracoid ligament
2. Lower end—suspensory ligament of axilla.

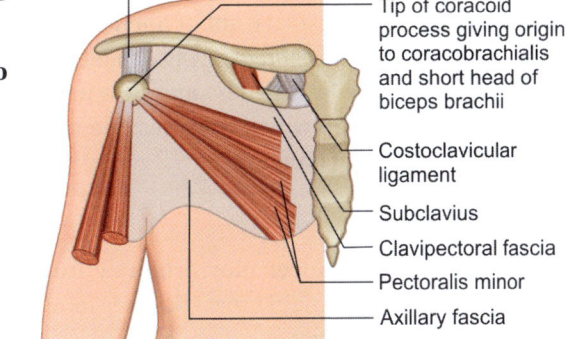

Fig. 1.3: Clavipectoral fascia.

Vertical Extent

Above

Below the clavicle, the clavipectoral fascia splits to enclose the subclavius muscle and two split-up layers are attached to anterior and posterior lips of groove for subclavius on inferior aspect of the clavicle. Further upwards, beyond clavicle, posterior lamina is continuous with investing layer of deep fascia of the neck.

Below

Along the line of upper border of pectoralis minor, the fascia splits to enclose the muscle. At the lower border of the muscle, the split-up layers unite to form single layer which is attached to the convex superior surface of dome shaped deep fascia of the floor of axilla. This downward extension of clavipectoral fascia is called **suspensory ligament of axilla**.

Mediolateral Extent

- **Laterally**: Between subclavius and pectoralis minor, the clavipectoral fascia extends laterally up to horizontal part of **coracoid process of scapula**.
- **Medially**: It blends with fascia of first two intercostal spaces.
- **Costocoracoid ligament**: It is the condensed upper margin of the fascia which extends from first costal cartilage to coracoid process of scapula.

Structures Piercing Clavipectoral Fascia

- Terminal end of cephalic vein, to drain into axillary vein.
- Thoracoacromial artery which is a branch of second part of axillary artery.
- Lateral pectoral nerve—to supply pectoralis major muscle from its deep surface.
- Some lymph vessels which includes vessels draining from deeper half of breast tissue to apical group of axillary lymph nodes.

SN 1.3 Write a short note on axillary tail of Spence.

AXILLARY TAIL OF SPENCE (FIG. 1.4)

From superolateral quadrant of breast a narrow prolongation extends upwards and laterlly along the lower border of pectoralis major towards the base of axilla, called axillary tail of Spence **(Fig. 1.4)**. It is the *only part of breast lying beneath the deep fascia* (axillary fascia). The aperture in the axillary fascia through which it passes deeper is known as **foramen of Langer**.

Clinical Importance

Initially the breast cancer may originate from axillary tail, when the main breast tissue is found to be normal and healthy.

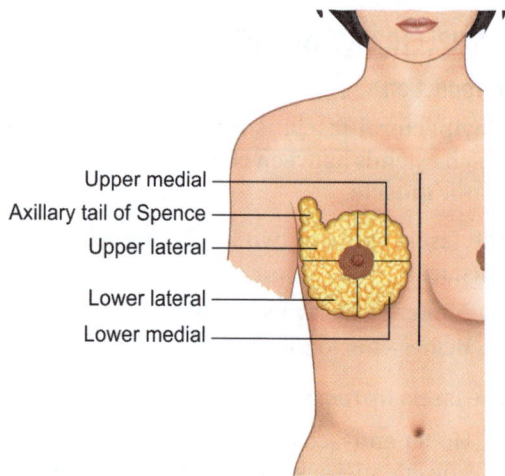

Fig. 1.4: Location and quadrants of the breast.

SA 1.4 Write a brief note on the location, extent and deep relations of the breast.

BREAST

Introduction

- Breast is *accessory gland of female reproductive system*. It is present in male in rudimentary form.
- It is considered to be *organ of secondary sexual features in female*.
- Following puberty, breast is *fully developed in young adult female*.
- It is *source of nutrition for neonates* (newborn) through secretion of milk from its glandular element following childbirth.
- Breast is *one of the commonest sites of malignant disease*.
- Breast is present in the form of rounded eminence *within the superficial fascia in upper part (pectoral region) of anterior chest wall*, extending laterally to a variable extent, even up to the plane of midaxillary line.

Extent

In female, the base or posterior surface of breast extends as follows.
- **Vertically:** From the level of 2nd to 6th rib, upper limit may be up to 3rd rib.
- **Horizontally:** From lateral margin of sternum to almost midaxillary line.

Axillary Tail of Spence

Axillary tail of Spence: From superolateral quadrant of breast a narrow prolongation extends upwards and laterally along the lower border of pectoralis major towards the base of axilla, called axillary tail of Spence **(Fig. 1.4)**. It is the *only part of breast lying beneath the deep fascia* (axillary fascia). The aperture in the axillary fascia through which it passes deeper is known as foramen of Langer.

Breast—Positioned in Superficial Fascia System (Fig. 1.5)

Superficial fascia system of pectoral region, below the clavicle and in front of pectoralis major muscle, splits into two layers. Breast or mammary gland is enclosed in between these two split-up layers, in front of deeper pectoral fascia. Enclosing the breast tissue both the layers of superficial fascia system fuse along the curved inferior outline of breast which is known as **inferior crescent of the breast**.

Deep Relations (Fig. 1.5)

Breast lies upon a fascia called *pectoral fascia*. Though it is called pectoral fascia, it separates breast from pectoralis major and serratus anterior seperiorly and upper part of external oblique with its aponeurosis inferiorly. Further deeper, beneath pectoralis major lie pectoralis minor and clavipectoral fascia.

Between the base or deeper surface of breast and pectoral fascia, a plane of loose connective tissue form 'retromammary space' or 'submammary space'. Layer of loose connective tissue in the space allow free mobility of healthy normal breast on deep pectoral fascia. In case of advanced carcinoma of breast, the gland may be fixed to the pectoral fascia and also the muscles.

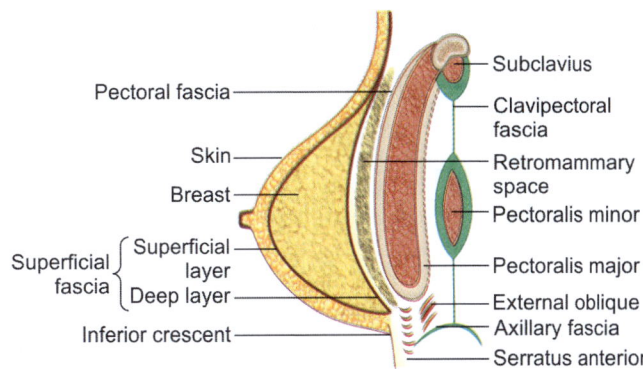

Fig. 1.5: Breast positioned in superficial fascia with deep relations.

SA 1.5 Discuss briefly the soft tissue architecture of the breast.

SOFT TISSUE ARCHITECTURE OF BREAST (FIG. 1.6)

Fundamentally the breast tissue is made up of two gross components:
1. **Glandular parenchyma**—which is an example of modified sebaceous gland.
2. **Connective tissue stroma**—which is the supporting element for glandular component.

Glandular Parenchyma

This is made up of groups of exocrine glands. Three-dimensional basic glandular elements form units known as **lobes of the breast** which are broader towards the pectoral fascia and converging narrower ends are directed towards nipple and areola **(Fig. 1.6)**. Although the lobes are considered to be very discrete and adjacent lobes are separated by connective tissue septa, during surgery they cannot be distinguished.

Each of the lobes contains one **lactiferous duct** which shows

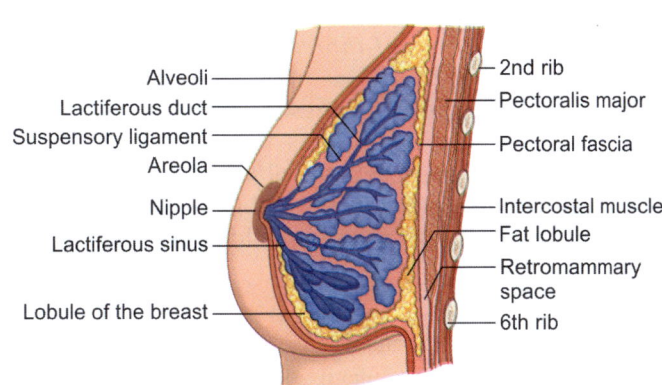

Fig. 1.6: Soft tissue architecture of breast.

terminal branching each of which end in glandular unit known as **lobules of the breast**. The lobular unit from terminal duct possesses following importance.
- **Physiological:** It is the functional milk secretory component.
- **Pathological:** Primary malignant lesion starts from this unit.

Connective Tissue Stroma

- **Interlobar stroma**: It is made up of **connective tissue septa**, which are of course, as already stated, not clinically definable during surgery. Interlobar stroma also contains variable amount of **adipose tissue** which is responsible for increase in size of breast beyond puberty.
- **Interlobular stroma**: It is of loose texture which allows expansion of secretory unit of the lobes during pregnancy.

Support of the Breast

Fully developed breast, particularly in its upper part, presents **connective tissue septa**. These fibrous tissue sheets extending from deep muscular fascia covering muscles of pectoral region to the deep surface of dermis of skin, are also adherent to glandular element of lobes. These are known as **suspensory ligament of Astley Cooper**. These act as mechanical support of the breast, especially in upper part of breast. These ligaments maintain *non-ptotic condition* of breast and prevent its dropping.

SA 1.6 Write a brief note on the blood supply of breast.

BLOOD SUPPLY OF BREAST (FIG. 1.7)

Arteries

Arterial supply of breast is derived from following sources:
- *Branches of axillary artery:* From above
  - Branches of *superior thoracic artery*
  - Pectoral branches of *acromio-thoracic artery*
  - Along lateral border of pectoralis minor, branches of *lateral thoracic artery.*
- *Branches of internal thoracic artery*
  - Direct medial branches— supply medial part of breast perforating anterior chest wall
  - Lateral branches from posterior *intercostal branches* of 2nd, 3rd and 4th space. One perforating branch of second space is usually largest to supply nipple and areola.

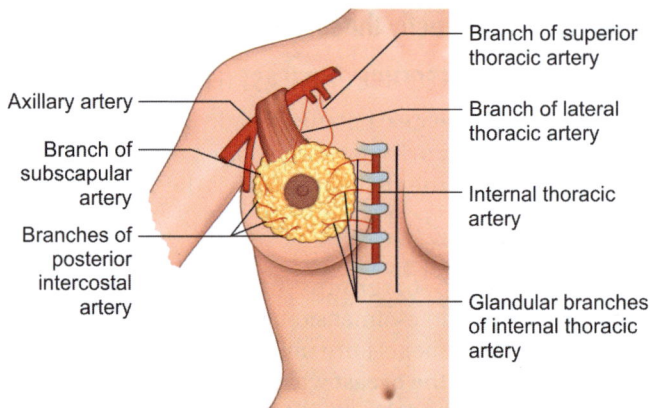

Fig. 1.7: Arterial supply of the breast.

Veins

Like lymphatics, superficial veins form a plexus beneath the skin of areola. Veins from this plexus, along with tributaries from glandular tissue drain into veins which correspond to the arteries. These are:
- Superior thoracic, lateral thoracic and acromiothoracic veins which are tributaries of axillary vein.

- From medial side of breast veins perforate anterior chest wall and drain into the internal thoracic vein.
- Intercostal veins drain the lateral part of breast. *Veins of the breast draining into posterior intercostal veins are important because, metastasis of cancer cells of breast may pass through this venous route to posterior mediastinal lymph nodes.*

LA 1.7 Give a brief account of the lymphatic drainage and clinical anatomy of the breast.

LYMPHATIC DRAINAGE OF BREAST

General Consideration
- Lymphatic drainage of breast is of immense clinical importance because metastasis or dissemination of cancer cells from the breast takes place principally through lymphatic route.
- Major part of lymphatic drainage occurs through extensive dermal network.
- Dermal lymphatic network beneath the skin of nipple and areola follows the route of lymph vessels from glandular parenchyma.
- Breast lymphatics show extensive branching and possess no valves. So, in case of occlusion of lymph channels due to tumors, lymphatic flow show reverse direction opposite to direction of venous flow.

Surrounding Lymph Nodes to Receive Lymph Vessels from Breast

Lymph vessels from different quadrants of breast (either from dermal plexus or from glandular parenchyma) drain into regional lymph nodes around breast.

Axillary Lymph Nodes
- **Anterior set:** These are main lymph nodes for the breast which lie along lateral thoracic vein under lower border of pectoralis major forming anterior axillary fold. Axillary tail of Spence is in actual contact with these glands. Initially growth appearing in this prolongation of gland may be mistaken as enlarged anterior or pectoral set of glands.
- **Posterior set:** These are along posterior axillary fold in relation to subscapular vessels.
- **Lateral set:** In relation to axillary vein, at the upper end of medial side of arm.
- **Central set:** This group of glands are embedded in the fat deep to axillary fascia. Intercostobrachial nerve passes in mediolateral direction in relation to these glands. Metastatic infiltration of these glands causes intense pain in the distribution of the nerve along medial border of arm.
- **Apical set:** These are also called infraclavicular set in reference to supraclavicular group of cervical lymph nodes. They are situated deep to clavipectoral fascia and in front of axillary vein.

Groups of Lymph Vessels of Breast and their Destination

Lymph vessels draining breast are divided into following three groups for three different destinations:
1. Lymph vessels from *skin of nipple and areola.*
2. Lymph vessels from *skin* (dermal plexus) of breast *except nipple and areola.*
3. Lymph vessel from *parenchyma of breast.*

Lymph Vessels from Skin Except Nipple and Areola (Fig. 1.8)

These lymph vessels *drain the integuments* over the breast, but not the skin of nipple and areola. The vessels form initially *dermal plexus* beneath the skin and finally *run radially to end in surrounding glands.*

Lymph vessels from **outer quadrants (upper lateral and lower lateral)** drain mostly in *pectoral or anterior group* of lymph nodes. Some of these particularly from lower lateral quadrant drain in *subscapular or posterior group.*

Skin over upper marginal part of breast is drained by vessels which go to *supraclavicular (lower deep cervical)* group of lymph nodes. Some of these vessels end in *deltopectoral group* which lie in relation to cephalic vein lying in the deltopectoral groove.

Lymph vessels from **inner quadrants (upper medial and lower medial)** drain in *internal thoracic group of lymph nodes* piercing the anterior thoracic wall along the direction of perforating vessels. Some vessels *cross the midline to drain into lymph nodes of same group of opposite side*. Some lymph vessels from skin of outer (lateral) quadrants may also drain in internal thoracic lymph nodes.

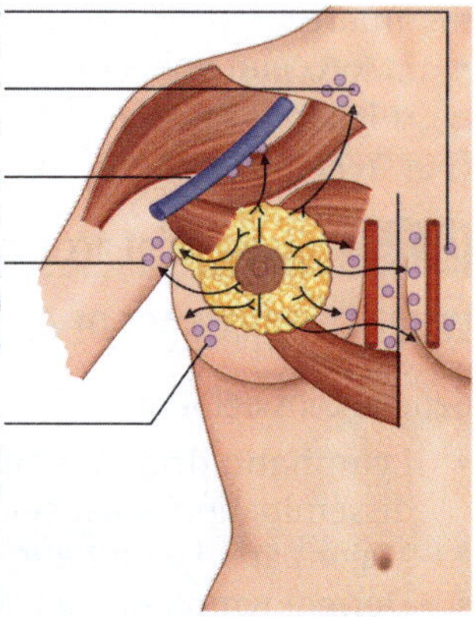

Lymph Vessels from Nipple and Areola (Fig. 1.9)

Lymph vessels beneath the nipple and areola form a plexus of larger vessels. This is known as **subareolar lymphatic plexus of Sappey**. From this plexus, lymph vessels pass upward and laterally below and parallel to lower border of pectoralis major along the direction of axillary tail of Spence to drain into pectoral group of lymph nodes.

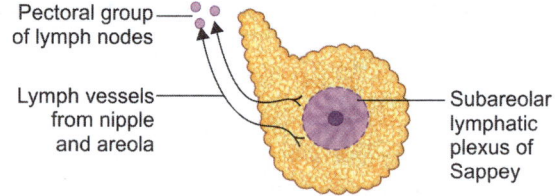

Fig. 1.8: Lymphatic drainage of breast in the surrounding lymph nodes.

Lymph Vessels from the Parenchyma

Lymph vessels from the parenchyma of breast form initially, *periductular* and *perilobular plexuses*. From this plexuses, lymph vessels run in three different directions.

Central (Fig. 1.10)

Lymph vessels from deeper part of parenchyma of breast pierce pectoralis major muscle and clavipectoral fascia to drain into *apical group of axillary lymph nodes*. Earlier it was thought that these lymph vessels initially drain into the retromammary lymphatic space which was used to be called *lymphatic lake of Haller*. But lymph vessels of parenchyma of breast do not actually have any relation with this space.

From the apical group of axillary lymph nodes, efferent pass to *supraclavicular group* of deep cervical lymph nodes.

Fig. 1.9: Lymphatic drainage of nipple and areola.

Medial

Lymph vessels from parenchyma of both medial as well as lateral halves of breast pass to *internal thoracic group* of lymph nodes which are parasternal deep to anterior chest wall. The lymph vessels follow the route of perforating branches of internal thoracic arteries **(Fig. 1.11)**.

Lateral

A few lymph vessels from parenchyma of lateral half of breast follow the path of lateral perforating branches of posterior intercostal arteries and finally pass along

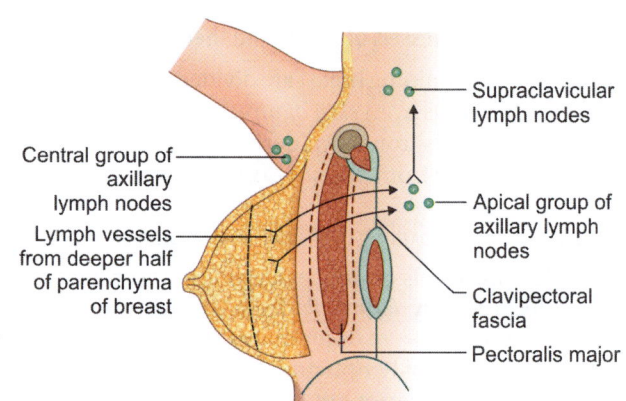

Fig. 1.10: Lymphatic drainage from deeper half of parenchyma of the breast.

the intercostal vessels backwards to drain into *posterior intercostal lymph node* lying in relation to head of ribs (**Fig. 1.11**).

Highly Clinically Significant Lymph Vessels Draining Lower and Medial Quadrant

Lower and medial quadrant of breast is only 2.5 cm away from xiphoid process. Some of the lymph vessels pass down from lower and medial quadrant of breast to the **subperitoneal lymph plexus** piercing

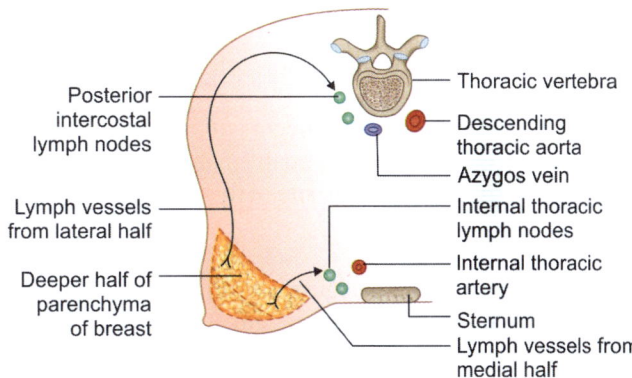

Fig. 1.11: Lymphatic drainage of deeper half of the breast through lateral and medial sets of vessels.

upper part of linea alba. This is the shortest route along which cancer cells may **spread from breast to peritoneum**. From this site a **secondary deposit of malignant cells** may be **in liver**. Furthermore, cancer cells **may drop** by gravity **into the pelvis**, causing metastasis of pelvic viscera including **ovary (Kruckenberg's tumor)**. That is why, clinical examination of abdomen and pelvis with per vaginal and per rectal digital examination is mandatory in a patient suffering from carcinoma of breast.

Clinical Anatomy

Knowledge of embryology, architecture and lymphatic drainage of breast is important for clinicians as the breast is common site for cancer in case of women. In addition, benign tumor, cyst formation and incidence of breast abscess following inflammation are also very often found.

Breast Abscess

Breast abscess is the complication of inflammatory changes in the breast which usually occurs during the phase of lactation. It occurs due to *crack in the nipple*, in which condition pathogen get entry to breast tissue through lactiferous ducts in cracked nipple.

Line of Incision for Drainage

Line of incision for drainage: If detected in time, breast abscess is confined in one lobule or compartment demarcated by fibrous septa. The abscess is drained by radial incision on the skin, as it is parallel to the line of lactiferous duct which is prevented from injury. Radial incision also prevents spread of infection to the adjacent compartments.

Congenital Anomalies

- **Supernumerary nipple**: This is also known as **polythelia**. Existence of additional nipple may be found to be present anywhere along the line of milk ridge. Milk ridge is the line extending from axilla to groin. Very often they are liable to be mistaken for moles.
- **Miromastia:** An excessive small breast may occur on one side as a result of lack of development.
- **Macromastia:** It is a condition characterized by diffuse hypertrophy of one or both breast which occurs in otherwise normal girls at the age of puberty.
- **Gynecomastia**: Unilateral or bilateral enlargement of male breast at the age of puberty is known as gynecomastia. Exact cause of this condition is unknown, but probably it occurs due to hormonal imbalance.

Rectracted Nipple
- **Congenital retraction** of nipple is found due to failure of evagination of lactiferous duct, during development.
- **Inflammatory retraction** occurs following burst of abscess in the nipple.
- **Cancerous retraction:** When the malignant growth infiltrates lactiferous duct opening at nipple, subsequent fibrosis at the site of the duct will pull the nipple inwards to cause its retraction.

Advantage of Mammography

Mammography is a radiological investigation for screening the breast for benign and malignant tumors or for cysts. A very low strength of X-ray is used and that is why investigation can be repeated if necessary. An advantage is enjoyed through this investigation, a tiny size of growth of a few millimeter can be diagnosed, which is difficult to be detected by clinical examination of breast.

Lymphatic Drainage and Carcinoma of Breast

More than 75% of lymph from the breast drain into axillary lymph nodes, most of which are of pectoral group. Other groups are subscapular, central and apical. In reference to their primary, secondary and tertiary stage of drainage, they are classified as level I, level II and level III as follows:
- **Level I:** Primary set, in relation to **lower border of pectoralis minor.**
- **Level II:** Secondary set, in relation to **posterior aspect of pectoralis minor.**
- **Level III:** Tertiary set, in relation to **upper border of pectoralis minor** and **deep to clavipectoral fascia.**

Prognosis of cancer of breast in reference to lymphatic drainage

Cancer arising from different quadrants of breast has different of degree of prognosis depending upon the group of lymph node of corresponding quadrants.
- **Upper and outer quadrant:** Favorable prognosis. Incidence of cancer is commonest, lymph vessels drain mostly in pectoral group.
- **Lower and outer quadrant:** Less dangerous.
- **Upper and inner quadrant:** More dangerous because of its proximity to the mediastinum.
- **Lower and inner quadrant:** Also more dangerous because of its proximity to the peritoneal cavity. Disseminated cancer cells from lower and medial quadrant follow the route of superior epigastric vein, pierce the linea alba to reach peritoneal cavity and may infiltrate the liver. From upper abdomen cancer cells may drop in pelvic cavity causing metastasis of pelvic viscera including ovary.

Importance of Fibrous Septa

Glandular parenchyma of breast is divided into 15 to 20 compartments by fibrous septa extending to the depth from deep surface of skin. Each of the compartments contains a glandular unit called lobule of the gland. These septa are also known as suspensory ligament of breast. It is true that, in initial stage of breast abscess these septa acts as line of barrier against spread of infection. But due to subsequent fibrosis of the septa during healing process of abscess and infiltration of the septa in carcinoma, the contracture of the septum pulls the skin inwards producing dimple of the skin surface.

Blockage of Lymphatics Draining the Skin

Sometimes due to growth (cancer) appearing beneath the skin, there may be blockage of lymph vessels draining from the root of hair follicles of the skin. Blockage of lymph vessels may lead to edematous appearance of the skin over the breast with number of pits on the surface due to traction of root of hair follicles. This condition is known as *peau d'orange* as it looks like the swollen and pitted orange peels.

Chapter 2

Axilla and Scapular Region

SA 2.1 Discuss the boundaries and contents of axilla.

AXILLA

Boundaries

Boundaries of axilla is better understood in abducted position of arm. Axilla is the site of armpit. It possesses anterior, posterior, medial and lateral walls with apex and base.

Anterior wall is formed by:
- **Pectoralis major muscle**: It extends through the whole anterior wall and is in front of following structures from above downwards
- **Subclavius muscle**
- **Clavipectoral fascia**
- **Pectoralis minor muscle.**

(Structures of anterior wall of axilla are illustrated in the figures of *pectoral region*)

Posterior wall is formed by following muscles **(Fig. 2.1)**:
- Subscapularis
- Teres major
- Latissimus dorsi

Tendinous insertion of latissimus dorsi is twisted to spiral round the lower border of tendon of teres major, as it comes from behind forwards **(Fig. 2.2)**.

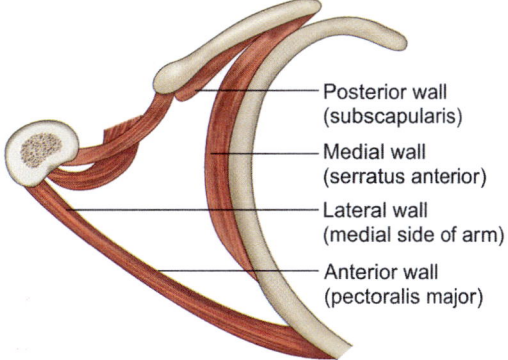

Fig. 2.1: Cross section through axilla to show its walls.

Medidal wall is formed by following **(Fig. 2.3)**:
- **Upper four ribs** and corresponding **intercostal spaces** with **intercostal muscles**
- Upper four digitations of **serratus anterior muscle**.

Lateral wall is narrow and linear as anterior and posterior walls of axilla converge here. It is formed by following **(Fig. 2.4)**:
- Upper end of shaft of humerus at the level of **bicipital groove** lodging the tendon of long head of **biceps brachii muscle**.
- **Coracobrachialis** and **short head of biceps brachii muscles**.

Apex of Axilla

Apex of axilla is a **truncated aperture** having **bony outlines**. It is called **cervicoaxillary canal**. It is so called because neurovascular bundle containing bunch of nerves and vessels passes through this canal from cervical region (neck) to axilla.

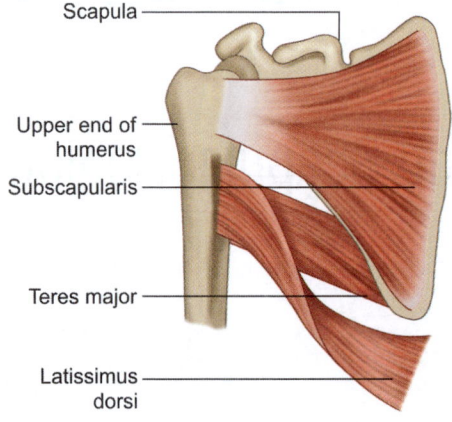

Fig. 2.2: Muscles of posterior wall of axilla.

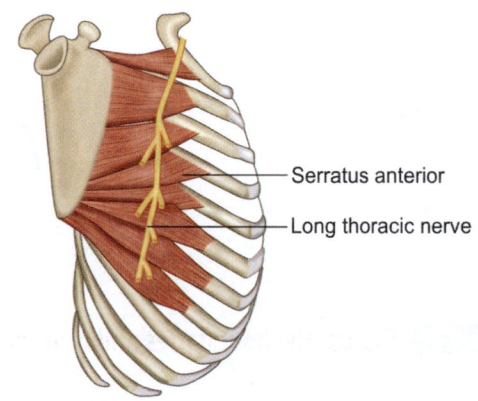

Fig. 2.3: Serratus anterior forming medial wall of axilla.

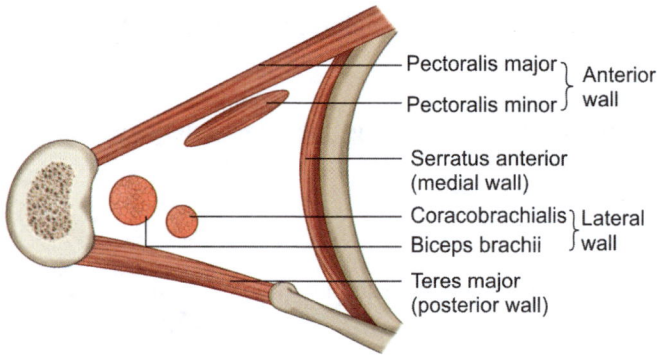

Fig. 2.4: Muscles of different walls of axilla.

Outlines of Cervicoaxillary Canal (Fig. 2.5)
- **Medially** : Outer border of 1st rib
- **Anteriorly** : Clavicle
- **Posteriorly** : Upper border of body of scapula

Base of Axilla (Fig. 2.6)

It is the floor of axilla formed by the deep fascia bridging the chest wall and the arm. It is called **axillary fascia** which is dome shaped with convexity upwards due to pull by the fascia attached to it from lower border of pectoralis minor muscle.

Beneath the axillary fascia, **axillary pad of fat** contains some of the **axillary lymph nodes**. The lateral cutaneous branch of second intercostal nerve runs along the base of axilla. It is called **intercostobrachial nerve.** The nerve passes from second intercostal space to medial side of arm.

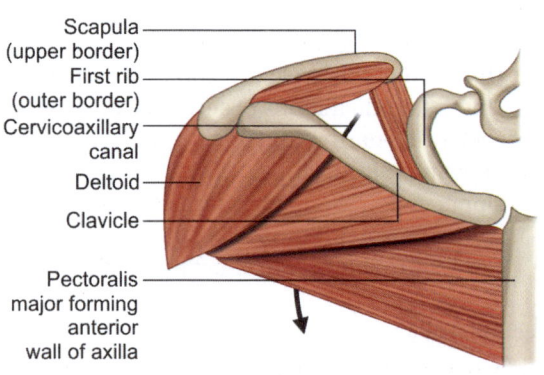

Fig. 2.5: Cervicoaxillary canal connecting root of neck with axilla.

Contents of Axilla

- Axillary artery and the branches from its three parts
- Axillary vein and its tributaries
- Brachial plexus giving rise to all the nerves for the upper limb
- Axillary lymph nodes embedded in axillary fascia.

SA 2.2 Write a note on serratus anterior muscle.

SERRATUS ANTERIOR MUSCLE (FIG. 2.3)

Introduction

- Serratus anterior is actually the muscle of lateral chest wall
- It is so called because in posterior chest wall there are two serratus posterior (superior and inferior) muscles. Their origin ends are serrated or denticulate
- Serratus anterior muscle slips related to upper four ribs form medial wall of axilla
- The muscle, as inserted to scapula, is concerned with movements of shoulder girdle.

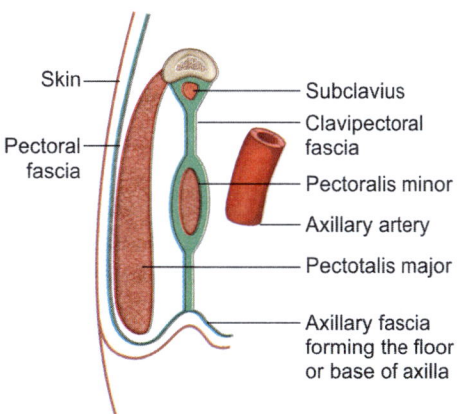

Fig. 2.6: Structures of anterior wall of axilla.

Origin

- Outer surface of upper eight ribs close to their upper border in lateral chest wall
- Fascia covering the intervening external intercostal muscles.

Insertion

The muscle wraps over the lateral chest wall and its fibers are directed backwards and slightly upwards and medially.

Eight digitations of the muscle arising from upper eight ribs are inserted as follows:
- *First digitation* is inserted into the costal surface of vertebral (medial) border of scapula from superior angle to root of spinous process.
- *Second and third digitations* are inserted into rest of costal surface of vertebral border of scapula.
- *Fourth to eight digitations* are inserted into costal surface of inferior angle of scapula.

Nerve Supply

Nerve to serratus anterior is called long thoracic nerve (C_5, C_6, C_7) as it presents a long course in lateral thoracic wall and gives separate branches to all the slips of the muscle.

Actions

Main action of serratus anterior is **protraction of scapula** when scapula glides in forward direction over the lateral chest wall. This movement is done by the muscle along with pectoralis minor. *Punching* or *pushing movement* of the hand forwards in day to day life is the manifestation. That is why serratus anterior is called *boxer's muscle*.

Serratus anterior also *depresses the scapula* when acting in combination with the lower fibers of trapezius.

Clinical Test for Serratus Anterior Function

With arm stretched, one is asked to push the hand placed on a wall. Protraction of scapula in normal person, will further fix the scapula on the chest wall. In case of weakness or paralysis of serratus anterior, vertebral border of scapula will be raised to become prominent through the skin. The clinical condition is called **winging of scapula**.

SA 2.3 Discuss briefly the axillary artery.

AXILLARY ARTERY

Introduction
Axillary artery is the artery of the upper limb. It is so called because the artery is contained in the axilla. Lower down the same artery is known as brachial artery.

Extent
- **Beginning:** Axillary artery starts as a continuation of **subclavian artery** at **outer border of 1st rib**.
- **Termination:** The artery ends at **lower border of teres major** where it is continued as **brachial artery**.

Parts
Axillary artery, running from medial to lateral wall of axilla, with slight convexity upwards and laterally, is crossed by pectoralis minor in front at its middle. So the artery is divided by the muscle into three parts as follows.
1. 1st part: Proximal to pectoralis minor
2. 2nd part: Behind pectoralis minor
3. 3rd part: Distal to pectoralis minor.

Axillary Sheath
Axillary artery, while entering axilla through cervicoaxillary canal, prolongation of deep fascia of neck encloses the artery with the axillary vein and a bunch of nerves of brachial plexus. This fascial sleeve is known as axillary sheath.

Important Relations
- **Pectoralis major** muscle covers all the three parts of axillary artery from the front. In addition, **pectoralis minor** covers the second part of the artery.
- **Muscles related posteriorly** are the following:
  1st part: First two digitations of **serratus anterior**
  2nd part: Subscapularis
  3rd part: Subscapularis, teres major and **latissimus dorsi**
- **Medially** axillary artery is related to **axillary vein**.
- **Nerves of brachial plexus** are related to all the three parts of axillary artery. First two parts of the artery are related to the cords of brachial plexus. Third part is related to the nerves arising from the cords. The relations are as follows.
  First part: Posteriorly: Medial cord
                 Laterally: Posterior and lateral cords
  Second part: Medially: Medial cord (lying between artery and vein)
                 Posteriorly: Posterior cord
                 Laterally: Lateral cord

Third part:	**Medially:**	Ulnar nerve and medial cutaneous nerve of forearm (lying between artery and vein)
		Medial cutaneous nerve of arm (lying medial to vein)
	Posteriorly:	Radial nerve and axillary nerve
	Laterally:	Musculocutaneous nerve and median nerve

Branches of Axillary Artery (Fig. 2.7)

The branches of three parts of axillary artery are the following:

First part:	1 branch	=	Superior thoracic artery
Second part:	2 branches	=	Lateral thoracic artery
			Acromiothoracic (thoracoacromial) artery
Third part:	3 branches	=	Subscapular artery
			Anterior circumflex humeral artery
			Posterior circumflex humeral artery

Superior thoracic artery arises from 1st part of axillary artery, below the clavicle near subclavius. The artery runs *along the superomedial border of pectoralis minor* muscle. It supplies pectoral muscles and anterior part of intercostal muscles of 1st and 2nd spaces.

Acromiothoracic artery is also known as thoracoacromial artery. It arises from second part of axillary artery behind pectoralis minor muscle. The artery then turns around upper border of pectoralis minor and *pierces clavipectoral fascia*. Appearing superficial to the fascia, it divides into following four branches.

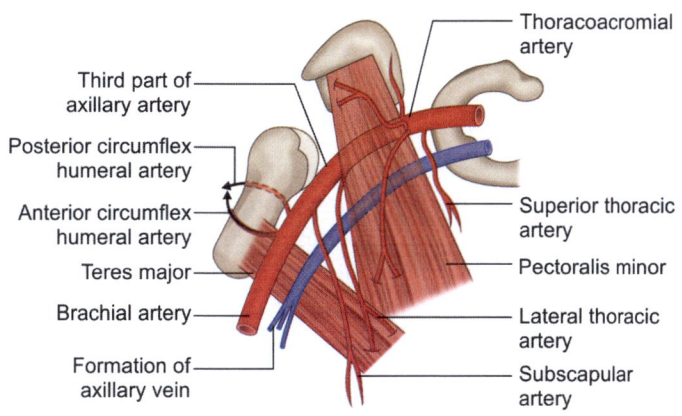

Fig. 2.7: Axillary artery (with branches) and axillary vein.

1. **Pectoral branch** runs between pectoral muscles. It supplies both the muscles and the breast.
2. **Clavicular branch** passes superomedially towards the clavicle to supply subclavius muscle and sternoclavicular joint.
3. **Deltoid branch** approaches the deltopectoral groove to supply deltoid muscle.
4. **Acromial branch** runs superolaterally towards the acromion process of scapula for anastomosis with other arteries.

Lateral Thoracic Artery

It emerges below the pectoralis minor and runs *along the lower border of the* muscle. The artery has an important relation with anterior (pectoral) group of axillary lymph node.

In female, lateral mammary branches of lateral thoracic artery are important as these branches supply the breast.

Subscapular Artery

It is the largest branch of the third part of axillary artery. Subscapular artery runs downward along the lateral border of scapula in front of subscapularis muscle on the posterior wall of axilla. It gives branches to muscles of posterior wall of axilla, which are subscapularis, teres major and latissimus dorsi.

Subscapular artery gives rise to a branch named **circumflex scapular artery** which winds round the lateral border of scapula to pass through the interval between teres major and teres minor. The artery passes dorsally to the infraspinous fossa to anastomose with other arteries of scapular region.

Anterior Circumflex Humeral Artery

This artery is a small branch arising from third part of axillary artery. It is found to arise at the lateral border of subscapularis and it runs laterally in front of surgical neck of humerus to anastomose with posterior circumflex humeral artery which comes from behind.

Ascending branch of anterior circumflex humeral artery runs upwards along intertubercular sulcus to supply the shoulder joint.

Posterior Circumflex Humeral Artery

- This artery is wider than the anterior circumflex humeral artery.
- It also arises at the level of lower border of subscapularis muscle.
- It curves round the medial, posterior and finally the lateral aspects of surgical neck of humerus and is under cover of deltoid muscle.
- During this course, it passes through the quadrangular space of scapular region and is accompanied by circumflex (axillary) nerve.
- It ends by anastomosing with anterior circumflex humeral artery on the anterior aspect of surgical neck of humerus.
- It gives a descending branch which anastomoses with ascending branch of the profunda branchii artery.

SA 2.4 Write a brief note on the axillary lymph nodes.

AXILLARY LYMPH NODES (FIG. 2.8)

Axillary lymph nodes are embedded in fibrofatty tissue of axilla. Some are related to the walls of axilla.

Area of Drainage

Axillary lymph nodes receive lymph vessels from:
- Whole of upper limb
- Ventral body wall up to the level of umbilicus
- Dorsal body wall up to the level of iliac crest
- About 75% of breast tissue.

Direction of Lymphatic Flow

Lymphatics flow according to following route through different groups of axillary lymph nodes.

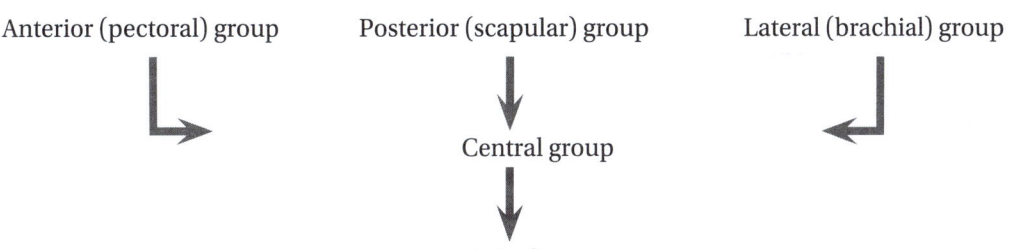

Lymph Node Groups

Axillary lymph nodes are arranged in following five groups:
1. Anterior or pectoral
2. Posterior or scapular
3. Lateral or brachial
4. Central
5. Apical

Anterior (Pectoral) Group

This group of lymph nodes is situated in relation to anterior wall of axilla along the lower border of pectoralis minor so also the lateral thoracic vessels. It receives *afferent* lymph vessels from:
- Anterior thoracic wall with pectoral region
- Anterior abdominal wall up to umbilicus
- Major portion of breast tissue.

Efferent vessels go mainly to the *central group* of axillary nodes.

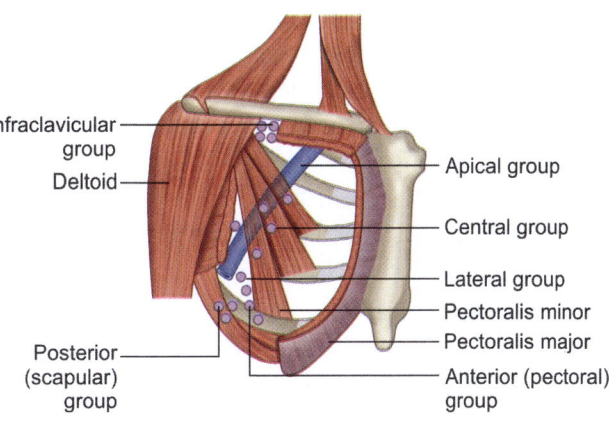

Fig. 2.8: Axillary lymph nodes.

Posterior (Scapular) Group

This group of lymph node is situated:
- In posterior wall of axilla
- In front of subscapularis muscle
- Along the course of subscapular artery.

Afferent lymph vessels draining into this group are from:
- Posterior wall of axilla
- Posterior thoracic wall
- Posterior abdominal wall up to the level of *iliac crest*.

Efferent vessels go to *central* group.

Lateral (Brachial) Group

This group of lymph nodes are situated:
- In lateral wall of axilla
- In relation to the axillary vein.

Afferent lymph vessels draining into this group are from:
- *Whole upper limb except* some vessels running along the cephalic vein which drain either into deltopectoral lymph nodes or apical group of axillary lymph node.
- *Supratrochlear lymph nodes* close to medial aspect of elbow which receive lymph vessels along the course of basilic vein.

Central Group

Central group of lymph nodes are well defined 3–4 prominent nodes embedded *in fibrofatty tissue of axilla*.

Afferent lymph vessels to central group come from:
- Anterior (pectoral) group
- Posterior (scapular) group
- Lateral (brachial) group
- Direct lymph vessels from the floor of axilla.

Efferent vessels drain into apical group of lymph nodes.

Central group of axillary lymph nodes is related to intercostobrachial nerve as it passes from lateral chest wall to medial side of arm. Inflamed condition (lymphadenitis) of central nodes may cause pain along the medial side of arm and the base of axilla.

Apical Group

Apical group of axillary lymph nodes, 6 to 8 in number, is situated:
- At the apex of axilla
- In the triangular interval bounded by outer border of 1st rib, superomedial margin of pectoralis minor and axillary vein
- In relation to distal part of axillary vein
- Deep to clavipectoral fascia.

Afferent vessels are received from *central group of axillary lymph nodes* and *deeper half of breast tissue*.

Efferent vessels go to *supraclavicular group of lymph nodes*.

Clinical Anatomy

Enlargement of lymph nodes is known as lymphadenopathy. When axillary lymph nodes are involved, it is known as **axillary lymphadenopathy**. Cause of enlargement may be inflammatory or non-inflammatory. Inflammatory condition is known as **lymphadenitis**. Non-inflammatory enlargement of axillary lymph nodes occurs mostly due to secondary spread of cancer cells through lymphatic channel from breast cancer.

LA 2.5 Give a brief account of the brachial plexus.

BRACHIAL PLEXUS (FIG. 2.9)

Introduction

Upper limb develops from the upper limb bud which grows from **ventrolateral aspect** of **cervicothoracic junction of trunk**. That is why, nerve supply of upper limb bud is derived from ventral (anterior) division of lower cervical and upper thoracic spinal nerves. Ventral divisions of 5th, 6th, 7th and 8th cervical nerves and one ascending branch of 1st thoracic nerve are outstretched to the upper limb bud. After origin of ascending branch, 1st thoracic nerve will be continued as 1st intercostal nerve of thoracic wall. 5th to 8th cervical nerves and ascending branch of 1st thoracic nerve, as pulled toward the upper limb bud, will form a network (plexus) by intercommunicating and branching which is called **brachial plexus**. But ultimately from plexus of these nerves, individual nerves will arise for innervation of the upper limb.

Peripheral Distribution from Brachial Plexus

Through various nerves, distribution of brachial plexus to the upper limb are as follows:
- **Sensory branches** to:
  - Skin = Cutaneous branches = Superficial sensory branches
  - Joint = Articular branches = Deep sensory branches
  - Tendon and muscles = Proprioceptive deep sensory branches
- **Motor branches** to muscles of upper limb
- **Secretomotor branches** to sweat glands
- **Vasomotor branches** to regulate the diameter of blood vessels, thereby amount of blood flow.

Formation

Brachial plexus is formed by:
- Whole of ventral rami (divisions) of 5th, 6th, 7th and 8th cervical nerves (C_5 to C_8)
- An ascending branch from ventral ramus (division) of 1st thoracic nerve (T_1).

Variation in Formation

- **Prefixed plexus**: Brachial plexus is called prefixed when the plexus is contributed by a small branch from *4th cervical nerve (C_4)*.
- **Postfixed plexus**: In this variety, brachial plexus receives a small branch from *2nd thoracic nerve (T_2)*.

Stages of Plexus Formation (Fig. 2.9)

1. **Root stage**: Ventral division of C_5 to C_8 nerves and ascending branch of ventral division of T_1 nerve are known as **roots of brachial plexus**.
2. **Trunk stage**: 5 roots take part in formation of 3 trunks as follows:
   - **Upper trunk**: Formed by union of C_5 and C_6 nerve roots
   - **Middle trunk**: Formed by continuation of root of C_7 nerve root
   - **Lower trunk**: Formed by union of C_8 and T_1 nerve roots
3. **Trunk division stage**: Each of the three trunks, upper, middle and lower, divides into **anterior and posterior divisions.**
4. **Cord stage**: Trunk divisions form three cords as follows:
       Posterior cord: Formed by union of **posterior divisions** of *all the three trunks*
       Lateral cord: Formed by union of **anterior divisions** of *upper and middle trunks*
       Medial cord: Formed by continuation of **anterior division** of *lower trunk.*

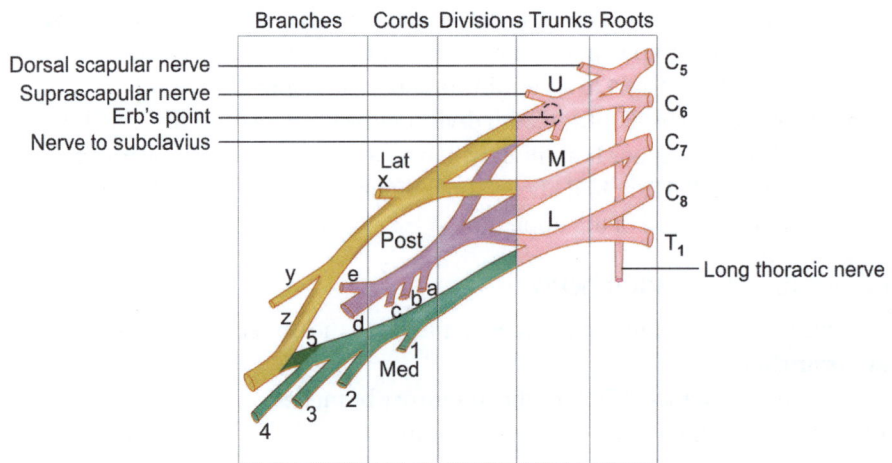

Nerves of lateral cord
x. Lateral pectoral nerve
y. Musculocutaneous nerve
z. Lateral root of median nerve

Nerves of medial cord
1. Medial pectoral nerve
2. Medial cutaneous nerve of arm
3. Medial cutaneous nerve of forearm
4. Ulnar nerve
5. Medial root of median nerve

Nerves of posterior cord
a. Upper subscapular nerve
b. Nerve to latissimus dorsi
c. Lower subscapular nerve
d. Radial nerve
e. Axillary nerve

Fig. 2.9: Formation of brachial plexus (U: upper; M: middle; L: lower; Lat: lateral; Post: posterior; Ked: medial).

5. **Main branching stage:** Three parts of axillary artery are related to cords of brachial plexus and ultimately their main branches in axilla as follows:
   1st part : Posteriorly = Medial cord
   Laterally = Posterior and lateral cords
   2nd part: Medially = Medial cord
   Posteriorly = Posterior cord
   Laterally = Lateral cord
   3rd part: Medially, posteriorly and laterally = Main branches of respective cords.

Location of Brachial Plexus

Brachial plexus is well visualized in dissection of axilla. But the plexus is divided into following two parts.
1. **Supraclavicular part:** This part is above the clavicle in the root or lower end of neck. Supraclavicular part consists of **roots, trunks** and their **anterior and posterior divisions.**
2. **Infraclavicular part:** This part is below the clavicle and so beyond the cervicoaxillary canal. This part is visualized in axilla. Infraclavicular part is present in the form of cords of brachial plexus and their branches in relation to the three parts of axillary artery.

Branches from Brachial Plexus

- **Branches from supraclavicular part**
  1. **Branches from the roots: Long thoracic nerve** arises from roots of 5th, 6th and 7th cervical nerves. It runs downwards with an elongated course over *serratus anterior* muscle in lateral chest wall and sends branches to each digitation of the muscle.
     Dorsal scapular nerve (C_5), arising from C_5 roots only, supplies *levator scapulae, romboideus major* and *rhomboideus minor*.

2. **Branches from the trunk:** These are **suprascapular nerve** and **nerve to subclavius** which arise from a point of **upper trunk** called **Erb's point**. Erb's point is the point at upper trunk where C_5 and C_6 nerves join to form the upper trunk and the trunk divides into anterior and posterior divisions. The same point is the site of origin of suprascapular nerve and nerve to subclavius.
- **Branches from infraclavicular part**
  These are the named nerves which **arise from three cords**.

Lateral Cord Branches
- **Lateral pectoral nerve**: It supplies pectoralis major muscle after piercing clavipectoral fascia. It may supply also the pectoralis minor.
- **Musculocutaneous nerve**: This nerve supplies all the three muscles of the anterior (flexor) compartment of arm and is continued as *lateral cutaneous nerve of forearm.*
- **Lateral root of median nerve**, uniting with the medial root, forms the trunk of median nerve. The median nerve is for innervation of many of the muscles of front of forearm and palm of hand.

Medial Cord Branches
- **Medial pectoral nerve**: It supplies both the pectoralis muscles of anterior wall of axilla
- **Medial cutaneous nerve of the arm** is the sensory branch for medial side of the arm
- **Medial cutaneous nerve of the forearm** supplies skin of medial side of ventral aspect of the forearm
- **The ulnar nerve,** shared with the median nerve, supplies the muscles of front of the forearm and palm of hand as follows:
  In the forearm, major share of nerve supply is by the median nerve. The ulnar nerve supplies only one and a half muscles in the forearm, but it supplies 15 out of 20 muscles of the palm of the hand. Remaining 5 muscles of the palm are supplied by the median nerve.
- **Medial root of median nerve**, arising from medial cord, crosses in front of axillary artery and joins with lateral root to form the trunk of the nerve.

Posterior Cord Branches
- **Upper subscapular nerve** arises from posterior cord of brachial plexus proximal to origin of the nerve to latissimus dorsi (thoracodorsal nerve) and supplies subscapularis.
- **Thoracodorsal nerve** is longer than subscapular nerve, runs along posterior wall of axilla and supplies latissimus dorsi.
- **Lower subscapular nerve** arises distal to the abovementioned nerves and supplies not only the subscapularis muscle but also the teres major which are the muscles of posterior wall of axilla.
- **Axillary nerve** follows the course backwards from axilla to supply the muscles of posterolateral aspect of arm, i.e. deltoid and teres minor.
- **Radial nerve** is longest nerve of the posterior cord. It is the nerve for most of the innervation of back of upper limb. It supplies all muscles of posterior compartments of arm and forearm. Radial nerve is the nerve for sensory innervation of almost whole of the skin of the back of upper limb.

It is to be noted here that, among the nerves of posterior cord, upper and lower subscapular, and thoroacodorsal nerves supply muscles of posterior wall of axilla. Axillary nerve supplies the muscles on posterolateral aspect of shoulder. Radial nerve is the nerve for innervation of extensor (posterior) compartments of arm and forearm.

Clinical Anatomy

Trunk Lesion

Incomplete injury of the trunks of the brachial plexus at the root of neck or the axilla is found in the following two types:

Upper lesion (Erb-Duchenne palsy)

Upper lesion of the brachial plexus results from violent forceful increase of the angle between the side of the neck and the top of the shoulder. It causes displacement of the head to the opposite side and depression of the shoulder to the same side. It results excessive traction or even tearing of the upper trunk (C_5 and C_6 roots). As C_5 and C_6 roots are lesioned, the motor functions will be affected due to less of functions of suprascapular nerve (C_5, C_6), axillary nerve (C_5, C_6) and musculocutaneous nerve (C_5, C_6, C_7). So following muscles will be paralyzed.

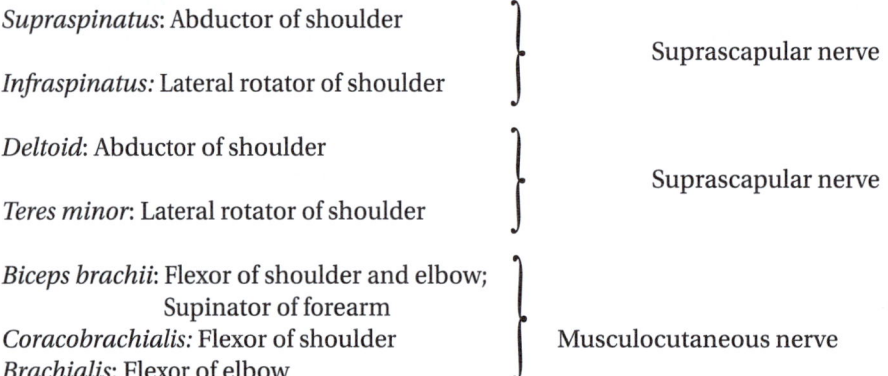

So the **deformity** in Erb-Duchenne Palsy will be manifested as follows:
- The upper limb will hang freely by the side of the body with extension of elbow.
- The arm will be medially rotated and the forearm will be in pronatated condition.
- The position of the upper limb will look like that of a porter or waiter hinting for a tip.

Sensory loss

Loss of cutaneous sensation on the lateral aspect of the arm (C_5) and forearm (C_6).

Lower lesion (Klumpke palsy)

It results due to sudden hyperabduction of the shoulder leading to widening of the angle between the medial side of the arm and the lateral thoracic wall. In this injury, C_8 and T_1 nerve roots forming the lower trunk will be subjected to traction or tear. Motor fibers of C_8 and T_1 roots mostly travelling through the median and ulnar nerves to supply all the small muscles of the hand are affected.

The **deformity** will be as follow:
- Due to paralysis of the lumbricals and interossei, there will be loss of flexion of the metacarpophalangeal joints and extension of the interphalangeal joints. The hand will show the deformity with extension of the metacarpophalangeal joints and flexion of the interphalangeal joints due to unopposed action of extensor digitorum and flexor digitorum (superficial as well as deep) respectively. The deformity is known as **Claw hand.**
- Chronic lesion will show wasting of the thenar and hypothenar muscles.

Sensory loss

Loss of cutaneous sensation along the medial side of the forearm (C_8) and arm (T_1).

Root Lesion

The long thoracic nerve, arising from C_5, C_6 and C_7 roots and supplying the serratus anterior, can be injured by blows to or pressure on the side of the root of the neck. However, the nerve may also be peripherally injured following radial mastectomy operation in carcinoma of breast.

Effect

- Inability to raise the arm above the shoulder for loss of power of elevation of the shoulder with upward and forward rotation.
- Due to loss of tone of the serratus anterior, the vertebral border and the inferior angle of scapula is raised from the chest wall contact, leading to a deformity called 'winging of scapula'.

SN 2.6 Write a short note on the deltoid muscle.

DELTOID MUSCLE (FIG. 2.10)

Introduction

- Deltoid is the muscle which is responsible for rounded curve or contour of the shoulder
- It is triangular in outline but presents a curved shape covering anterior, lateral and posterior aspects of shoulder
- It overhangs many of the short muscles around shoulder.

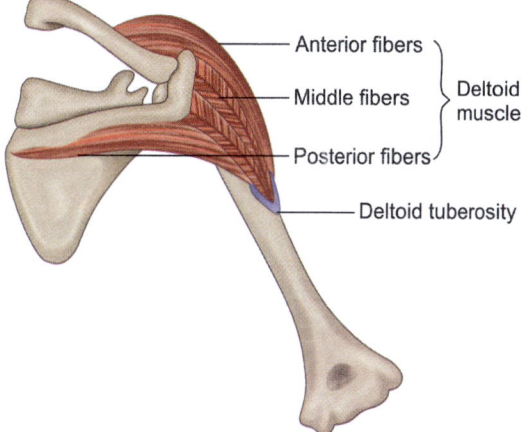

Fig. 2.10: Deltoid muscle seen from behind.

Origin

- **Anterior fibers**: From anterior margin and adjacent part of superior surface of lateral one third of **clavicle**.
- **Middle fibers**: Through tendinous bands attached to lateral margin of **acromion process**. The fibers are **multipennate** in origin (Fig. 2.10).
- **Posterior fibers**: From lower lip of **crest of spine of scapula** and also from **posterior margin of acromion process**.

Insertion

To a 'V' shaped rough area called **deltoid tuberosity** on anterolateral surface of humerus.

Nerve Supply

Deltoid is supplied by both anterior as well as posterior divisions of axillary nerve (C_5, C_6).

Actions

Three different groups of fibers of deltoid have three different actions:
1. **Anterior fiber** causes *flexion* and *medial rotation* of shoulder along with other muscles, like pectoralis major

2. **Middle fibers** causes *abduction* of shoulder from the range of 15°–90°.
3. **Posterior fibers** causes *extension* and *lateral rotation* of shoulder along with latissimus dorsi, infraspinatus and teres minor.

SA 2.7 Discuss the boundaries and contents of the triangular and quadrangular spaces.

TRIANGULAR AND QUADRANGULAR SPACES (FIG. 2.11)

There are *three intermuscular spaces* bounded by muscles of the scapular region.
These spaces are *under cover of deltoid* muscles.
The spaces are *traversed by some nerves and blood vessels*.

These spaces are:
1. Upper triangular space = *Medial to long head of triceps*
2. Quadrangular space
3. Lower triangular space } *Lateral to long head of triceps*

Upper Triangular Space (Fig. 2.11)

Location

While dissecting out, this space is to be searched between adjacent margins of teres minor and major, close to lateral border of scapula but medial to long head of triceps brachii arising from infraglenoid tuberosity of scapula.

Communication

This upper triangular space establishes communication between axilla and scapular region.

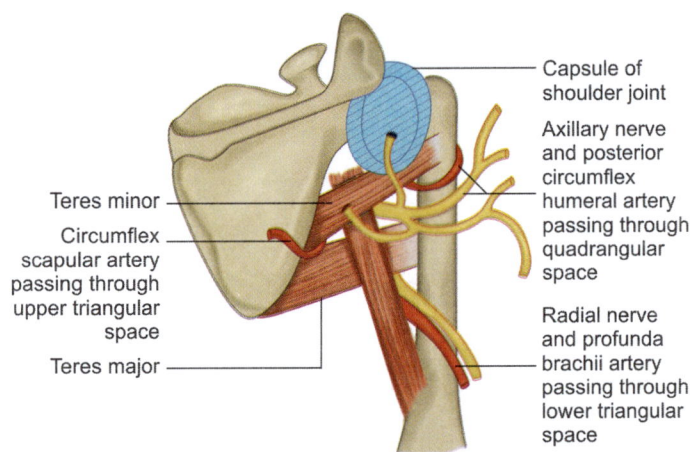

Fig. 2.11: Quadrangular and triangular spaces.

Boundaries

This triangular space present following boundaries
- *Above:* Lower margin of teres minor
- *Below:* Upper margin of teres major
- *Medially (apex):* Meeting point of above two muscles at lateral border of scapula
- *Laterally (base):* Long head of triceps brachii.

Structures Passing Through

Circumflex scapular artery with corresponding vein winds round the lateral border of scapula to reach infraspinous fossa from axilla. The artery supplies muscles in scapular region and takes part in **scapular anastomosis**. Circumflex scapular artery is a branch of subscapular artery.

Quadrangular Space (Fig. 2.11)

Location

- Quadrangular space is also between adjacent margins of teres minor and major, *but lateral to long head of triceps.*
- Through this space, axillary nerve, arising from posterior cord of brachial plexus, enters backwards in the scapular region.

Communication

Quadrangular space is an window between axilla in front and scapular region behind. It transmits neurovascular bundle from before backwards.

Boundaries

- *Above*: From before backwards:
  - Subscapularis
  - Capsule of shoulder joint
  - Teres minor
- *Below*: Teres major
- *Medially*: Long head of triceps brachii
- *Laterally*: Surgical neck or humerus

Structures Passing Through

- Axillary nerve
- Posterior circumflex humeral vessels.

Lower Triangular Space (Fig. 2.11)

Location

It is the space below quadrangular space, lateral to triceps.

Communication

It communicates axilla with the back of the arm.

Boundaries

- **Base (upper boundary)**: Lower margin of teres major
- **Medial side**: Long head of triceps brachii
- **Lateral side**: Shaft of humerus.

Structures Passing Through

- Radial nerve
- Arteria profunda brachii.

These two structures approach radial groove.

Note: Axillary nerve has been described in Chapter 11: Major Nerves of the Upper Limb.

Chapter 3

Anterior Compartment of Arm and Cubital Fossa

SA 3.1 Write a brief note on the muscles of anterior compartment of the arm.

Individual muscle may be asked in the form of short note.

MUSCLES OF ANTERIOR COMPARTMENT OF THE ARM

Biceps Brachii (Fig. 3.1A)

The biceps brachii is so named because it has two heads of origin called short head and long head. *Origin of both the heads are tendinous in nature.*

Origin
- **Short head** takes origin by a thick flat tendon from the tip of coracoid process along with origin of coracobrachialis muscle.
- **Long head** arises in the form of long narrow tendon. Origin of the tendon is within the capsule of shoulder joint from supraglenoid tuberosity of scapula just above the glenoid cavity. The intracapsular tendon of long head of biceps arches over the humeral head and comes out of capsule taking a double layer sleeve of synovial membrane in the form of its synovial sheath. The tendon runs down over the intertubercular sulcus (bicipital groove) of humerus retained in position by the transverse humeral ligament.

Both the tendons end in fleshy bellies which are very closely applied to each other till a little above the elbow.

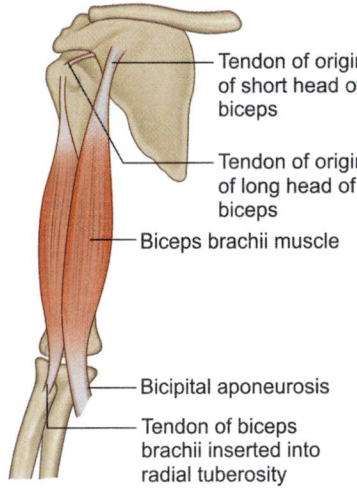

Fig. 3.1A: Biceps brachii muscle.

Insertion

The flattened tendon, before its insertion beyond elbow joint *shows a twist* or spiral turn, so that *its anterior surface faces laterally*. Then it is inserted into the rough posterior part of radial tuberosity, whose smooth anterior part is related to a bursa.

Bicipital aponeurosis

A thin, flat and strong expansion of tendon of biceps in front of elbow passes downwards medially. It is called bicipital aponeurosis. It blends with the deep fascia in upper and medial end of front of forearm. It crosses in front of brachial artery.

Additional third head of biceps brachii

In 10% of cases, a third head of biceps arises from medial aspect of brachialis and is inserted through the fibers of bicipital aponeurosis and also to the medial aspect of biceps tendon.

Coracobrachialis (Fig. 3.1B)

Coracobrachialis is the muscle of anterior compartment of arm which crosses only front of shoulder joint.

Origin
- Coracobrachialis arises from tip of coracoid process of scapula jointly with the tendon of short head of biceps brachii.
- It also arises in the form of muscular slips from proximal end of the tendon of short head of biceps. Musculocutaneous nerve passes between the two components of muscle.

Insertion
- Coracobrachialis is inserted at the middle of medial border of shaft of humerus on a rough linear impression which is 3 to 5 cm long.
- Accessory slips of the muscle may be attached to *the lesser tubercle, medial epicondyle* and *medial intermuscular septum*.

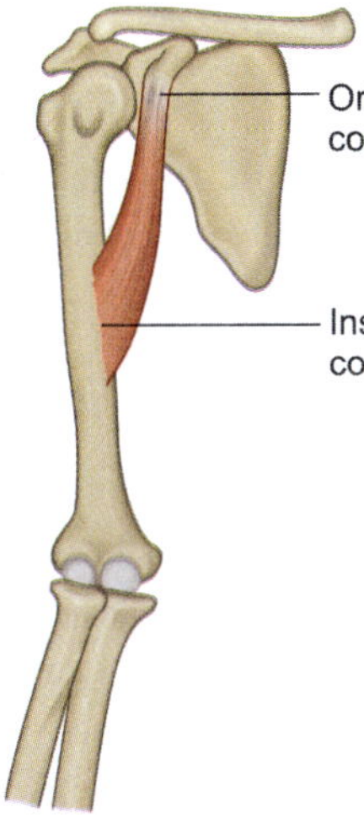

Fig. 3.1B: Coracobrachialis muscle.

Brachialis (Fig. 3.1C)

Brachialis is the muscle of anterior compartment of arm which crosses over only the front of elbow joint. This muscle wraps the lower half of shaft of humerus.

Origin
Brachialis takes origin as muscular ships from:
- Lower half of front of shaft of humerus. Highest fibers arises from the bone on either side of insertion of deltoid.
- Anterior aspect of both intermuscular septa.

Insertion
Brachialis muscle ends in a thick broad tendon which is inserted into ulnar tuberosity on anterior aspect of coronoid process of ulna.

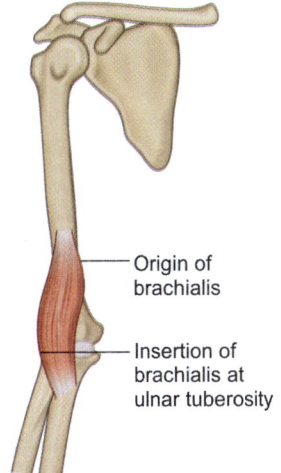

Fig. 3.1C: Brachialis muscle.

Variations
- Brachialis may be divided into two or more parts
- It may be fused with brachioradialis, pronator teres or biceps brachii
- In some cases, it sends a tendinous slip to radius or bicipital aponeurosis.

NERVE SUPPLY OF THE MUSCLES

Muscles of anterior compartment of arm, namely the biceps brachii, coracobrachialis and brachialis (except its lateral part) are supplied by *the musculocutaneous nerve (C_5, C_6, C_7)* which is the nerve of this compartment and arises from lateral cord of brachial plexus.

Supplying these three muscles, the nerve is continuous as sensory branch called lateral cutaneous nerve of forearm beyond elbow.

Small lateral part of brachialis is supplied by radial nerve, as it is a hybrid or composite muscle.

ACTION OF THE MUSCLES

Coracobrachialis

It flexes the shoulder joint moving the arm forwards and medially. This action is more clearly observed when the arm is flexed against the resistance or from its extended position.

Biceps Brachii

As biceps brachii crosses both elbow as well as shoulder joints, it has action on both the joints.

Action on Elbow

- Biceps brachii is a *powerful supinator*, particularly during rapid movement and when it acts against the resistance. This action is on *superior radioulnar joint* due to spiraling or twist of its tendon at insertion to radial tuberosity.
- Biceps brachii is also flexor of the elbow when the muscle acts *against resistance.*

Action on Shoulder

- It is a *flexor of shoulder joint* to a slight extent.
- Tension of tendon of long head of biceps brachii is more important action during abduction of shoulder by deltoid. It prevents upward displacement of head of humerus.

Brachialis

Brachialis is flexor of elbow in any of the following conditions.
- Forearm is supinated or pronated
- Movement occurs without or against resistance.

SA 3.2 Write a note on brachial artery.

BRACHIAL ARTERY (FIG. 3.2)

Brachial artery is the *artery of anterior compartment* of arm. Profunda brachii artery, one of its branches, is the artery of the posterior compartment.

Origin

The brachial artery begins **as continuation of axillary artery** at the inferolateral border of tendon of teres major in medial side of upper end of arm.

Termination

The artery terminates by dividing into two terminal branches, **radial and ulnar arteries** at the level of neck of radius *1 cm below the elbow joint.*

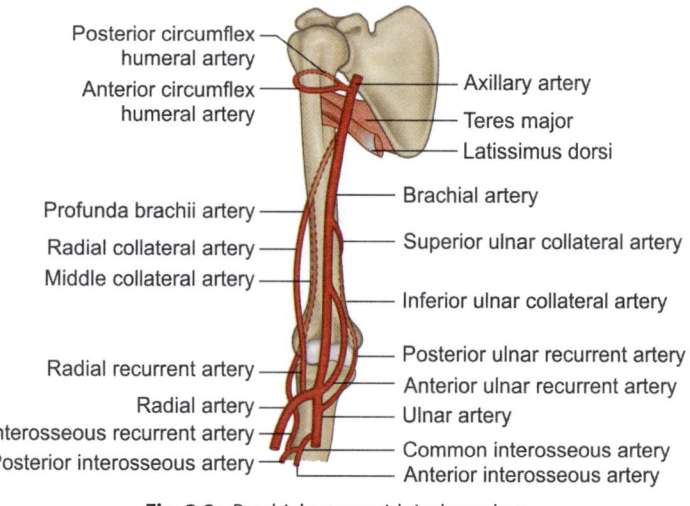

Fig. 3.2: Brachial artery with its branches.

Important Relations

- Brachial artery is superficially related only to the skin, and superficial and deep fascia.
- Median nerve runs lateral to the artery in the upper half, crosses in front of the artery in the middle of the arm to lie medially in the lower half.
- In upper half of the arm, the medial cutaneous nerve of the forearm and ulnar nerve are medial to the artery.
- In lower half, basilic vein is in relation medial to the artery.
- At the level of elbow, bicipital aponeurosis lies in front of artery to pass downwards and medially, separating the artery from the median cubital vein.

Branches

Profunda Brachii Artery

The profunda brachii artery is the large branch of brachial artery which arises from the posteromedial aspect at the level of distal border of teres major. It passes downwards and laterally along the spiral groove of humerus with the radial nerve. Here the neurovascular bundle is placed between lateral and medial heads of triceps brachii of the posterior compartment of arm. It gives muscular branches and a nutrient artery for humerus. At the end of spiral groove, the profunda brachii artery divides into two terminal branches—*radial collateral artery* and *middle collateral artery*.

Radial collateral artery pierces lateral intermuscular septum and runs down in front of lateral epicondyle of humerus. Middle collateral branch runs behind the septum and epicondyle. Both the arteries take part in anastomosis around elbow joint.

Variations

- Profunda brachii artery may take origin *from axillary artery*.
- It may have *common origin with posterior circumflex humeral artery*.

Nutrient Artery for Humerus

Nutrient artery for humerus arises at the mid level of arm enters the nutrient canal at the site of attachment of coracobrachialis. The artery is *directed downwards*.

Superior Ulnar Collateral Artery

It is the branch of brachial artery usually arising a little below the middle of arm. Occasionally it arises from profunda brachii artery. It accompanies the ulnar nerve and pierces the medial intermuscular septum along with the nerve to enter the posterior compartment of arm. After giving muscular branches, it passes behind medial epicondyle of humerus to take part in anastomosis around elbow joint. One branch form superior ulnar collateral artery may descend in front of the elbow joint.

Inferior Ulnar Collateral Artery

It is also known as **supratrochlear artery**. It arises from brachial artery 5 cm proximal to the elbow. The artery pierces the medial intermuscular septum and curves around back of lower end of humerus to anastomose with middle collateral artery. It gives off a branch which descends in front of medial epicondyle.

Middle Ulnar Collateral Artery

It may be occasionally present. If present, it arises from brachial artery, in between origin of superior and inferior ulnar collateral artery. *It descends in front of medial epicondyle.*

Muscular Branches

These branches are distributed to the biceps brachii, coracobrachialis and brachialis.

Terminal Branches

Brachial artery divides into two terminal branches, **radial and ulnar arteries** 1 cm below the level of elbow joint.

These are described in the chapter of front of forearm.

SA 3.3 Discuss the boundaries and contents of cubital fossa.

CUBITAL FOSSA

Introduction

Cubital fossa is a triangular hollow area in front of elbow.

Boundaries (Fig. 3.3)

Outlines of the triangular area are as follows.
- **Lateral side:** Medial border of brachioradialis muscle. This border is more or less straight.
- **Medial side:** It is oblique and directed downwards and laterally. Medial outline is formed by lateral border of pronator teres muscle.
- **Base:** It is horizontal and present above. Base is formed by an imaginary line formed by joining the two epicondyles of humerus.
- **Apex:** Apex is directed downwards where pronator teres meets brachioradialis.

Beside the outlines, cubital fossa has a roof and a floor, in between lie the contents.
- **Roof:** Beneath the skin and superficial fascia, roof of cubital fossa is formed by:
  - Deep fascia in front of elbow
  - Bicipital aponeurosis.

  On the deep fascia forming the roof, following structures are present (**Fig. 3.4**).
  - Lateral cutaneous nerve of the forearm—along lateral side
  - Medial cutaneous nerve of the forearm—along medial side
  - Median cubital vein—directed upwards and medially from cephalic vein to basilic vein.
- **Floor** (**Fig. 3.5**)
  - Superomedial part is formed by *brachialis*
  - Inferolateral part is formed by *supinator*.

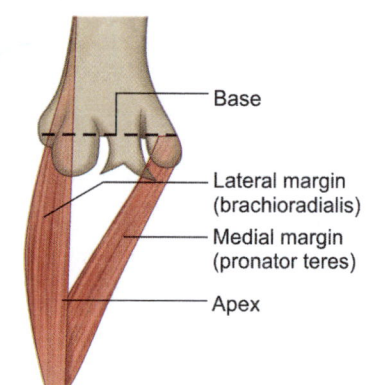

Fig. 3.3: Outline of cubital fossa (right).

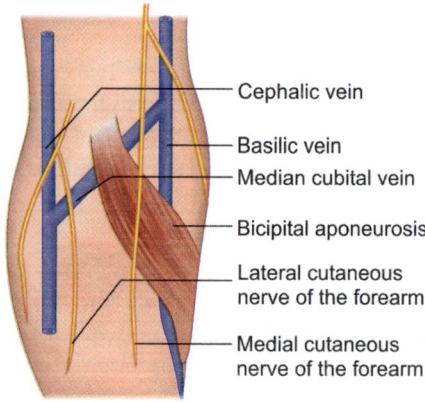

Fig. 3.4: Structures on the roof of cubital fossa (right).

Contents (Fig. 3.6)

The contents of the fossa are visualized after retraction of lateral and medial boundaries, as the fossa is a very narrow space.

From medial to lateral side the contents of cubital fossa are the following.

- **Median nerve:** The nerve is overlapped by pronator teres medially and other contents of the fossa laterally. The nerve gives some muscular branches for forearm and finally leaves the fossa to descend further passing between two heads of pronator teres.
- **Bifurcation of brachial artery:** Terminal part of brachial artery and its subdivision into radial artery and ulnar artery is usually found in cubital fossa.
  - Radial artery is always more superficial and narrower than ulnar artery.
  - Proximal parts of both radial and ulnar arteries give rise to the branches which take part in anastomosis around elbow joint. In addition, the ulnar artery gives rise to the common interosseous artery that divides into anterior and posterior interosseous arteries, which run in front of and behind the interosseous membrane of forearm respectively.
- **Tendon of biceps brachii:** Crossing the elbow joint, the tendon presents a twist in such way that, its anterior surface turns laterally to be attached to radial tuberosity. This spiraling of the tendon is the reason for the biceps to act as supinator.
- **Radial nerve:** The nerve is placed in the furrow between brachioradialis with extensor carpi radialis longus laterally and brachialis medially. *After giving branches to these three muscles, radial nerve bifurcates into superficial and deep branches in the cubital fossa.* The superficial branch runs down further and the deep branch leaves for back of the forearm passing through supinator.

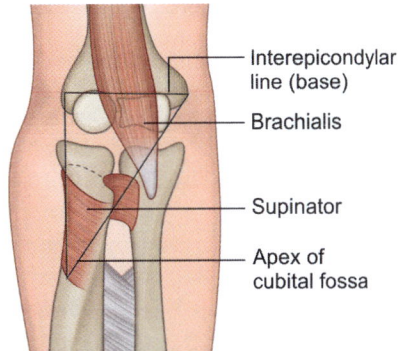

Fig. 3.5: Brachialis (superomedial) and supinator (inferolateral) forming floor of cubital fossa.

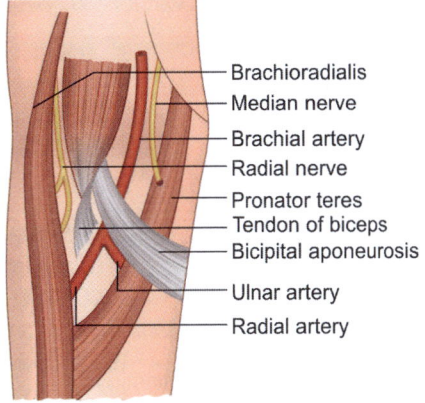

Fig. 3.6: Content of cubital fossa.

Applied Anatomy

- Median cubital vein is the common site for following clinical procedures.
  - Intravenous injection of drugs
  - Intravenous infusion of fluid or blood
  - Drawing out of blood for laboratory investigations.
- Arterial pulsation of brachial artery is heard with the help of stethoscope at cubital fossa to record blood pressure.

Chapter 4

Posterior Compartment of Arm

SA 4.1 Write a note on triceps brachii muscle.

TRICEPS BRACHII MUSCLE (FIG. 4.1)

Triceps brachii muscle takes its name from its three head of origin—long, lateral and medial.

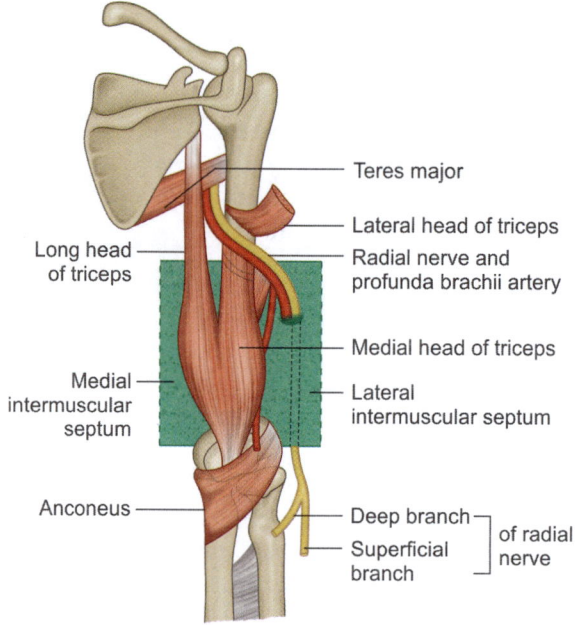

Fig. 4.1: Triceps brachii muscle.

Origin

Long head of the muscle arises by a flattened tendon from the *infraglenoid tuberosity of scapula*. The fibers fuse above with the fibers of capsular ligament of shoulder joint. The fleshy fibers of long head descend medial to lateral head and superficial to medial head of the muscle.

Lateral head take origin through a more expanded flattened tendon from:
- An oblique ridge on posterior surface of shaft of humerus above and parallel to the spiral groove.
- The lateral border of shaft of humerus above spiral groove as high as the surgical neck of the bone.
- Lateral intermuscular septum.

The fibers meet in a common tendon which overlaps the structures in the spiral groove and fuse with medial head.

Medial head is overlapped posteriorly by lateral and long heads. It arises from:
- *Entire posterior surface* of shaft of humerus *below the spiral groove*
- *Medial border* of shaft of humerus from the lower end of insertion of teres major up to 2.5 cm above trochlea
- *Medial intermuscular septum*
- *Lower part of lateral intermuscular septum.*

Insertion
The tendon of triceps brachii is found to appear near the middle of the muscle differentiated in the form of *superficial and deep laminae.*

After receiving the muscle fibers, the two layers unite above the elbow. Most of the fibers of single tendon so formed are attached to *superior surface of olecranon process. A band from the tendon* extends downwards and laterally *over anconeus muscle* **to fuse with deep fascia of forearm.**

Nerve Supply
Three heads of triceps are supplied by separate branches of *radial nerve (C_6, C_7 and C_8)* as follows:
- **Above the spiral groove:** To long and medial heads of triceps
- **In the spiral groove:** To medial and lateral heads of the muscle.

Action
- In general, triceps is *the major extensor of* the elbow joint
- Medial head is active in all forms of extension of the joint
- Lateral and long heads come into the action mostly in extension against resistance
- In addition, long head supports lower part of capsule of shoulder joint when the arm is hyperabducted.

SN 4.2 **Write a short note on anconeus muscle.**

ANCONEUS (FIG. 4.1)

Origin
Anconeus is a small triangular muscle on the back of elbow. In one side it blends with fibers of triceps and distally it fuses with the surface of capsule of elbow joint. It arises through a tendon from the *posterior aspect of lateral epicondyle of humerus.*

Insertion
Fibers of anconeus fan out downwards and medially towards ulna across the back of elbow. Spiraled fibers of the muscle are inserted on the *lateral surface of olecranon process and upper one fourth of posterior surface of ulna.* The muscle gives an *expansion to posterior aspect of capsule of elbow joint.*

Nerve Supply
Nerve to anconeus is a long slender nerve arising from radial nerve (C_6, C_7 and C_8) in the spiral groove. The nerve passes through the substance of medial head of triceps to reach anconeus.

Actions
It is not clearly known which action of anconeus is more important. But following are its actions.
- *Anconeus helps triceps* to extend the forearm on elbow joint.

- It *prevents abduction of ulna* (its widening from radius) *during pronation of forearm.*
- It increases tension of capsule of elbow joint, so that *capsular fibers are not pinched within the joint.*

SN 4.3 Write a short note on profunda brachii artery.

PROFUNDA BRACHII ARTERY (FIG. 4.2)

Introduction
Profunda brachii artery is the artery of the posterior compartment of arm and it forms a neurovascular bundle along with the radial nerve in the spiral groove.

Origin
Profunda brachii artery springs out from posteromedial aspect of brachial artery beyond the teres major muscle. It runs downwards, backwards and laterally along the spiral groove, where it lies deep to the lateral head of triceps.

Termination
At the inferolateral end of spiral groove, it divides into two terminal branches—radial collateral and middle collateral arteries.

Branches
In the spiral groove:
- Muscular branches for triceps
- Nutrient branch for humerus

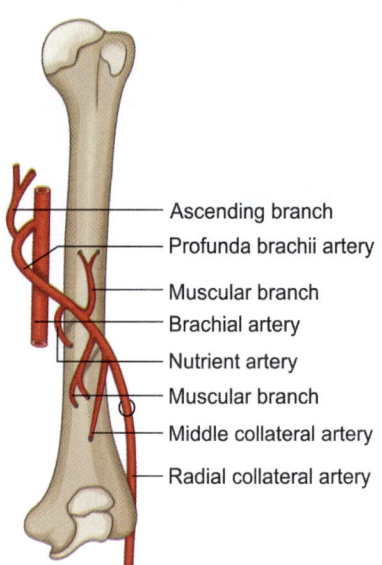

Fig. 4.2: Profunda brachii artery.

Terminal Branches
- Radial collateral artery is one of the terminal branches which pierces the lateral intermuscular septum along with radial nerve and runs downwards in front of lateral epicondyle to take part in arterial anastomosis in front of lateral side of elbow joint.
- Middle collateral artery runs downwards in the posterior compartment of arm. It takes part in anastomosis around elbow joint passing behind lateral epicondyle of humerus.

Note: The radial nerve has been described in Chapter 11: Major Nerves of the Upper Limb.

Chapter 5

Shoulder Girdle and Shoulder Joint

LA 5.1 Discuss briefly the shoulder girdle with its movements and clinical anatomy.

SHOULDER GIRDLE

Introduction

Shoulder girdle or pectoral girdle is the articulomuscular link between trunk and upper limb. It is structured by following components.
- **Skeletal framework** made up of bones and joints
- **Muscular components.**

Skeletal Framework of the Girdle

Bones of shoulder girdle are **clavicle** in front and **scapula** behind. These two bones are joined together only by a small plane variety of synovial joint known as **acromioclavicular joint**. This joint is stabilized by a *strong accessory ligament* called **coracoclavicular ligament**. Axial skeleton of the trunk is connected to medial end of the clavicle of shoulder girdle through **sternoclavicular joint** only. This joint, though not secured much, is stabilized by strong **costoclavicular ligament** below. Again the scapula of the girdle is connected to humerus of the upper limb through **glenohumeral joint** or **shoulder joint**.

Muscular Component of the Girdle

It is the clavicle of shoulder girdle only which is connected to axial skeleton through the sternoclavicular joint. But the scapula does not form any joint with any of the bones of axial skeleton. It is connected to the trunk as well as upper limb by many muscles which tie the bone in different directions. These muscles support the bone so also the shoulder girdle and helps in wide range of movements. The muscles are divided into following groups.

Muscles connecting the scapula with the ribs
- Pectoralis minor
- Serratus anterior.

Muscles connecting the scapula with the vertebral column (spines)
- Trapezius
- Levator scapulae
- Rhomboideus minor
- Rhomboideus major.

Muscles connecting the scapula with the upper end of humerus
- Deltoid

- Supraspinatus
- Infraspinatus
- Teres minor
- Teres major.

Importance of Shoulder Girdle

Through the process of evolution, attainment of erect posture made the upper limbs (forelimbs) free in bipedal animals including man. Wide range of movements of upper limb is primarily possible due to various factors. In addition, beyond certain range, further movement of shoulder joint is associated with various types of movement of scapula so also the movement of two joints of the shoulder girdle. Shoulder joint; therefore, enjoys wider range of movement for the upper limb, due to scapular movement along with movements of both the joints of shoulder girdle.

STERNOCLAVICULAR JOINT (FIGS. 5.1 AND 5.2)

Introduction

Sternoclavicular joint is a *saddle shaped synovial joint* between the clavicular notch of manubrium sterni and the medial sternal end of the clavicle.

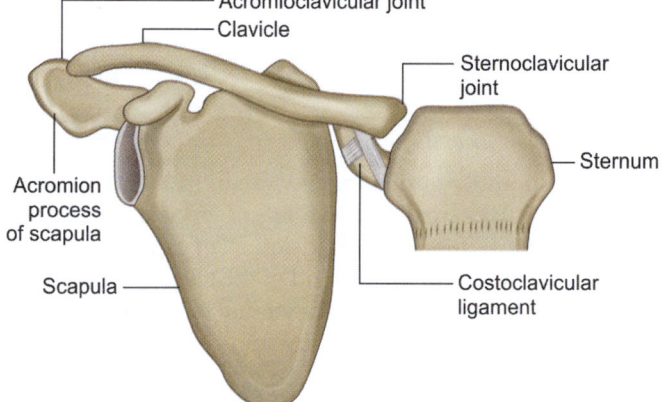

Fig. 5.1: Skeletal framework of shoulder girdle.

Bony Configuration with Articular Surface

Clavicular notch of manubrium sterni is concave from above downwards and covered by *hyaline cartilage* giving it a smoother appearance.

Sternal end of clavicle presents following characteristics:
- It is not typically convex, but **concavoconvex** which fits with concave articular surface of clavicular notch manubrium
- These two incongruent articular surfaces are adjusted with each other through interposition of a **concavoconvex articular disk**.
- Articular surface of clavicle is rough as it is **covered by fibrocartilage**, but *not hyaline cartilage* which is typically present on the articular surface of synovial joint.

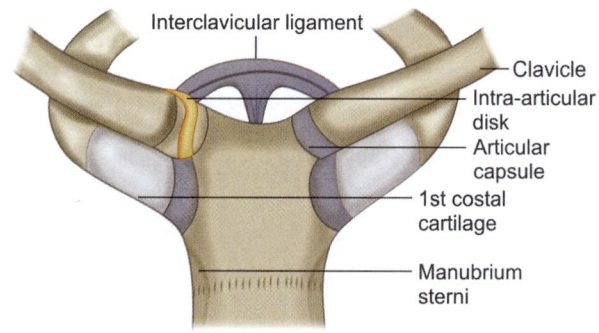

Fig. 5.2: Sternoclavicular joint.

The rough **articular surface extends** for a short distance on the **inferior surface** which comes in contact with superior surface of 1st costochondral junction.

Capsular Ligament

Capsular ligament of the sternoclavicular joint connects the margins of articular surfaces of two bones and invests the joint like a sleeve.

The fibers of capsule are thickened in front and behind to from **anterior and posterior sternoclavicular ligaments.**

Accessory Ligaments

- **Interclavicular ligament:** Function of this ligament is to bind the joints of two sides. Its transverse fibers cross the midline above suprasternal notch and connect medial ends of both the clavicle. The vertical fibers of this 'T' shaped ligament pass down to be attached to the suprasternal notch
- **Costoclavicular ligament:** This is a strong bilaminar ligament binding the sternal end of clavicle with manubrium sterni and superior surface of 1st costal cartilage with adjacent part of 1st rib. The ligament lies lateral to the joint. Fibers of the anterior layer pass downwards medially and those of posterior layer pass upward and medially. It is interesting to note that the fibers of anterior and posterior planes of costoclavicular ligament are in same direction as those of external intercostal and internal intercostal muscles of chest wall respectively.

Costoclavicular ligament is a strong accessory ligament of sternoclavicular joint which **prevents upward displacement** of the joint.

Intra-articular Disk

- It is an oval fibrocartilaginous intra-articular disk, whose peripheral margin is attached to inner surface of fibrous capsule.
- It presents concavoconvex surface to increase the congruence of articular surfaces.
- Through the capsule, the disk is attached *posterosuperiorly* to the clavicle and *anteroinferiorly* to the 1st costal cartilage.

The articular disk or the meniscus divides joint cavity into two components:
1. **Lateral = Menisco-clavicular component**: It allows **elevation** and **depression**
2. **Medial = Menisco-sternal component**: It allows **forward** and **backward movements**

Important Relations

Posterior aspect of the joint is related to *formation of brachiocephalic vein* of the respective sides. *Internal thoracic artery* also runs down behind the joint.

Arterial Supply

The joint is supplied by branch from **internal thoracic artery**.

Nerve Supply

Innervation is derived from articular branch the **medial supraclavicular nerve**.

ACROMIOCLAVICULAR JOINT (FIGS. 5.1 AND 5.3)

Introduction

Acromioclavicular joint is a small plane variety synovial joint between the facets on anterior part of medial margin of acromion process of scapula and the lateral end of clavicle.

It is the only joint connecting two bones of shoulder girdle together.

Fibrous Capsule

- Fibrous capsule is small but loose envelop attached to the margin of facets and is internally lined by synovial membrane.
- The capsule is strengthened by **acromioclavicular ligament** on its *superior aspect*.

Articular Disk or Meniscus

Unlike that of sternoclavicular joint, the fibrocartilaginous intra-articular disk of the joint is *incomplete* and attached to the inner surface of *posterosuperior aspect* of the capsule.

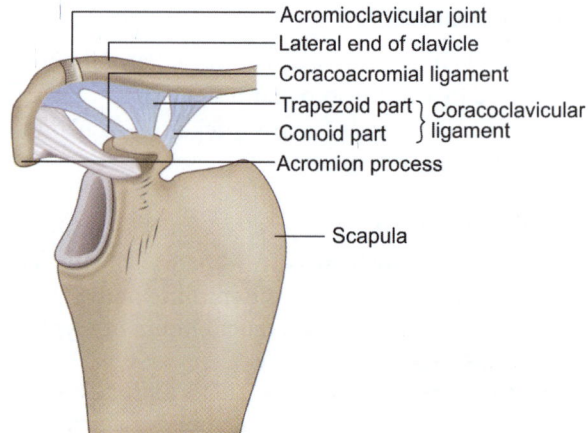

Fig. 5.3: Acromioclavicular joint.

Coracoclavicular Ligament

Coracoclavicular ligament is the accessory ligament of acromioclavicular joint.

It is a very strong ligament, acting as a secondary support of the joint. It binds the coracoid process of scapula and the lateral end of clavicle.

The ligament has conoid and trapezoid parts. **Conoid part** looks like an inverted cone. Upper basal end is attached to **conoid tubercle** on inferior surface of lateral end of clavicle. Lower tapering end is attached below to the root (knuckle) of coracoid process on the posterosuperior aspect of junction of its vertical and horizontal parts. **Trapezoid part** is rectangular extending from **trapezoid ridge** on inferior surface of lateral one-third of clavicle to an oblique line on superior surface of horizontal part of caracoid process.

Coracoclavicular ligament is important functionally to transmit the weight or force of upper limb via medial end of clavicle so the sternoclavicular joint to the trunk.

Arterial Supply

Acromial branch of thoracoacromial artery.

Nerve Supply

Suprascapular nerve.

Movements of Shoulder Girdle

Principles of Movements

- Medial component of sternoclavicular joint, i.e. menisco-sternal joint is concerned with forward and backward movements. The lateral component, menisco-clavicular joint produces elevation and depression.
- Movements of two joints of shoulder girdle, i.e. sternoclavicular and acromioclavicular joints, occur in reverse direction.
- Wide range of movement of scapula by various muscles attached to it, is associated with movements of both the joints of the girdle which are synchronized as follows:
  - **Elevation** of scapula = **Elevation** of acromioclavicular joint = **Depression** of sternoclavicular joint

- **Depression** of scapula = **Depression** of acromioclavicular joint = **Elevation** of sternoclavicular joint
- Forward movement **(protraction)** of scapula = Forward movement of acromioclavicular joint = Backward movement of sternoclavicular joint
- Backward movement **(retraction)** of scapula = Backward movement of acromioclavicular joint = Forward movement of sternoclavicular joint

- Wider range of free movement of shoulder so arm is the result of associated movement of shoulder girdle with the movement of shoulder joint in some situation. For example, upward, forward and medial movement of scapula is associated with hyperabduction of shoulder joint. It is important to note that, beyond 90° abduction of shoulder joint, for every 2° movement of this joint is associated with 1° of upward, forward and medial rotational movement of scapula.

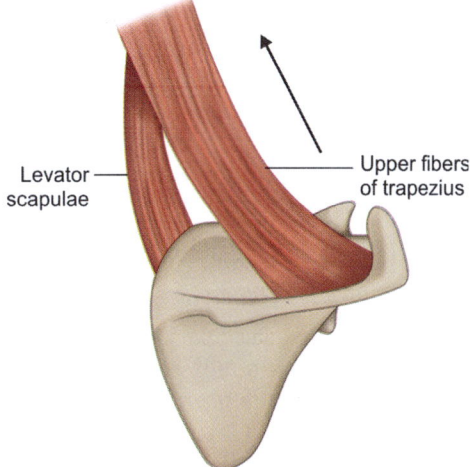

Fig. 5.4A: Elevators of scapula.

Movements of Scapula

Elevation and Depression

- **Elevation** is caused by *levator scapulae* and *upper fibers of trapezius* **(Fig. 5.4A)**. The movement is seen in *shrugging of shoulder*.
- **Depression** of scapula is caused by *pectoralis minor* and *lower fibers of serratus anterior* **(Fig. 5.4B)**. It is also assisted by **lower fibers of trapezius (Fig. 5.4C)**. The movement is manifested by *drooping of shoulder*.

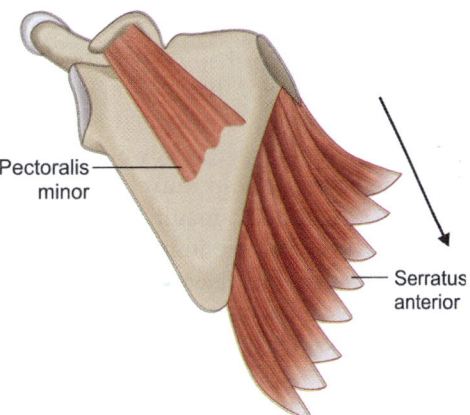

Fig. 5.4B: Depressors of scapula.

Forward Movement (Protraction) and Backward Movement (Retraction)

- **Protraction** or forward movement of scapula occurs in *pushing* or *punching* movements. It is caused by combined action of *serratus anterior* and *pectoralis minor* **(Figs. 5.5A and B)**.
- **Retraction** or backward movement occurs typically during *squaring the shoulder*. It is caused by the *middle fibers of trapezius* and the *rhomboideus* **(Fig. 5.5A)**.

Rotation of Scapula

Scapula rotates **upwards, forwards** and **medially** over the chest wall in case of **hyperabduction of**

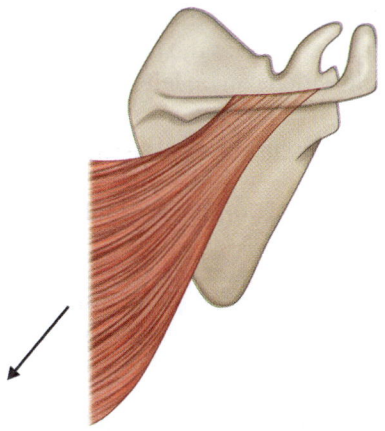

Fig. 5.4C: Lower fibers of trapezius— assists in depression.

shoulder. This movement is brought about by **upper fibers trapezius** and **lower fibers of serratus anterior**.

Clinical Anatomy

Though not very common, dislocation may occur in both sternoclavicular and acromioclavicular joints.

Sternoclavicular Joint Dislocation

Though the sternoclavicular joint is subjected to regular stress and strain, *dislocation of this joint is resisted by the strong costoclavicular ligament.* As this joint is supported inferiorly by the superior aspect of 1st costochondral junction and bound inferolaterally by strong costoclavicular ligament, upper and lower dislocations of the joint are prevented. But there is chance of anterior or posterior dislocation. **Anterior dislocation** displaces medial end of clavicle beneath the skin and it may be displaced upwards by pull of sternocleidomastoid muscle. **Posterior dislocation** usually results from direct trauma in front of the joint. This is more serious because displaced medial end of clavicle may cause pressure effect on major blood vessels related posterior to the joint.

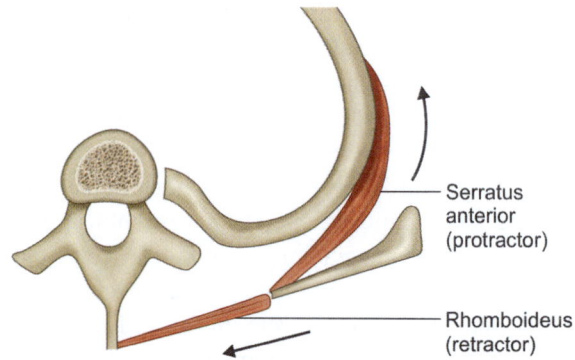

Fig. 5.5A: Protractor and retractor of scapula.

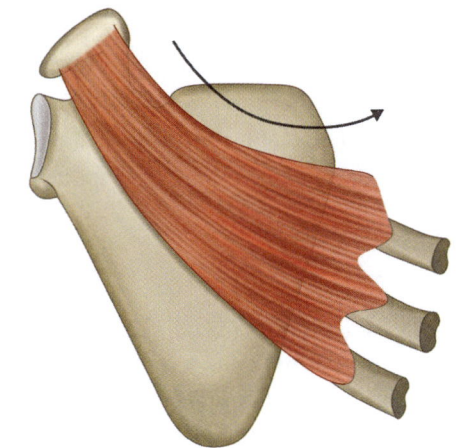

Fig. 5.5B: Pectoralis minor—assists in protraction.

Acromioclavicular Dislocation

Coracoclavicular ligament is an important support for acromioclavicular joint. But this joint also gets dislocated following a severe blow over the point of shoulder. It occurs following a severe fall. Plane of the articular surface passes downwards and medially. So force over the top of shoulder presses the acromion process downwards and medially below the lateral end of the clavicle which can be felt prominently. This condition is known as **'shoulder separation'**.

LA 5.2 **Discuss briefly the shoulder joint with a note on its movements and clinical anatomy.**

SHOULDER (GLENOHUMERAL) JOINT

Introduction

- Shoulder joint or gelnohumeral joint is the *multiaxial synovial joint* between hemispherical head of the humerus and glenoid fossa of the scapula.
- It is the joint connecting pectoral girdle with upper appendicular skeleton.

Special Characteristics of the Joint

- It is the most mobile joint possessing the freedom of wide range of mobility
- Hemispherical head of humerus is not well secured in shallow glenoid fossa of scapula

- During resting condition as well as during movement, stability of the joint is maintained mainly by the surrounding muscles and soft tissue
- It is the joint most frequently dislocated.

Articulating Surfaces (Fig. 5.6)

Convex (male) articular surface of the joint is the hemispherical head of humerus.

Concave (female) articular surface is the pear-shaped shallow glenoid fossa at lateral angle of body of scapula.

Both the surfaces are covered by hyaline articular cartilage. The cartilage is thickest at center and thinnest at periphery in case of the head of humerus. Cartilage covering the glenoid fossa of scapula is thinnest at the center and thickest at periphery. It makes articular surfaces more congruent.

In any position of the joint, only a part (about one-third) of articular surface of head of the humerus comes in contact with articular surface of the glenoid fossa of scapula. Depth of the articular surface of glenoid fossa is increased to some extent by attachment of a rim of fibrocartilage to the margin of glenoid fossa. This fibrocartilaginous rim is known as *glenoid labrum*.

Glenoid Labrum (Figs. 5.7A and B)

Glenoid labrum is the fibrocartilaginous rim attached to the margin of glenoid fossa.

Superiorly, the glenoid labrum fuses with the fibers of the tendon of long head of biceps brachii.

On cross section, the glenoid labrum is triangular with its base attached to the margin of glenoid fossa. Its apex is free. Inner surface merges with the surface of glenoid fossa of scapula.

Functions of the glenoid labrum are following:
- It *deepens the cavity* of glenoid fossa
- It *protects the bony margin* of glenoid fossa
- It assists in *lubrication of articular surface.*

Fibrous Capsule (Fig. 5.6)

Fibrous capsule is the envelop of the joint. Its attachments are as follows:
- *Medial (Proximal)*: Medial end of the capsule is attached to the neck of scapula

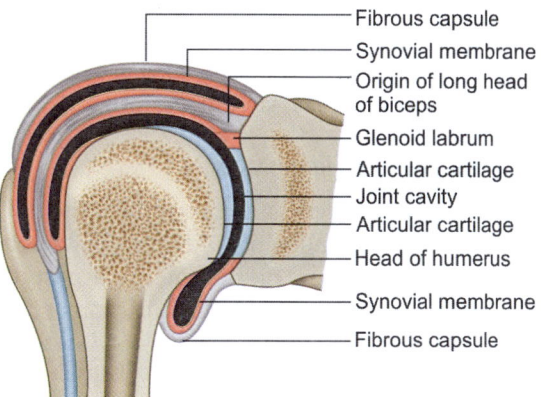

Fig. 5.6: Shoulder joint in coronal section.

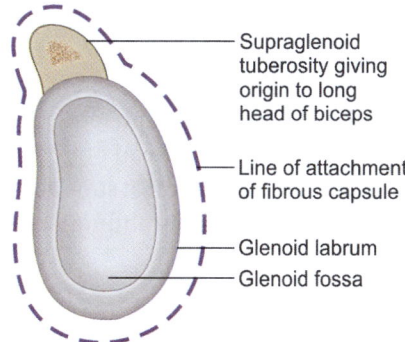

Fig. 5.7A: Glenoid labrum in relation to the margin of glenoid fossa and attachment of fibrous capsule.

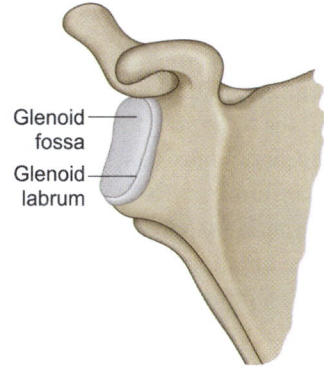

Fig. 5.7B: Glenoid labrum attached at the margin of glenoid fossa.

beyond the glenoid margin giving attachment to glenoid labrum. Superiorly the capsule extends to the lateral side of root of coracoids process to enclose the origin of long head of biceps brachii which is thus intracapsular in origin.
- *Lateral (Distal):* Laterally fibrous capsule is attached to the line of anatomical neck of the humerus which is slightly constricted margin of articular surface of head of humerus.

Inferiorly the line of attachment of capsule extends about 1.25 cm beyond the articular margin of humerus head. For this reason capsule is loose and lax inferiorly. It prevents undue stretching of capsule in abduction of shoulder joint.

Deficiency (Gap) in Fibrous Capsule
- One gap is present in the capsule at the upper end of intertubercular sulcus to allow exit of intracapsular tendon of long head of biceps brachii.
- One small aperture on the anterior aspect of capsule through which the synovial cavity of the joint communicates with the subscapular bursa.

Rotator Cuff—An Additional Support of Capsule (Fig. 5.8)

Tendons of some muscles are fused with lateral end of outer surface of capsule to give additional strength. This is known as *rotator cuff*. The tendons forming rotator cuff are as follows.
- Anteriorly: Subscapularis
- Superiorly: Supraspinatus
- Posteriorly: Infraspinatus and teres minor
- Inferiorly: Though long head of triceps takes part in formation of rotator cuff, it supports the weakest part of capsule in hyperabduction of shoulder joint.

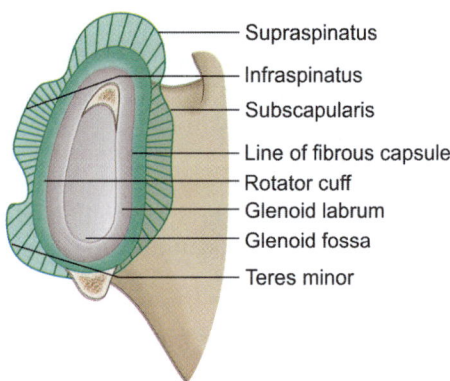

Fig. 5.8: Rotator cuff around shoulder joint.

Functions of Rotator Cuff
- It maintains a compressive force on the surface of capsule to keep proper contact between two articular surfaces
- It resists displacement of the articular surfaces.

Synovial Membrane

Synovial membrane lines the inner surface of capsule and in general it is attached to the margin of articular surface of glenoid fossa and humeral head with following special characteristics.
- In case of glenoid fossa, synovial membrane is attached along the line of peripheral margin of glenoid labrum
- On the superior aspect of glenoid fossa a gap lies between the line of attachment of synovial membrane and fibrous capsule, as origin of tendon of long head of biceps from supraglenoid tuberosity is intracapsular but extrasynovial
- Inferomedial to the head of humerus, a part of 1.25 cm of upper end of humerus is lined by synovial membrane, as this part is intracapsular
- A sheath of synovial membrane is prolonged around tendon of long head of biceps along intertubercular sulcus up to surgical neck of humerus (*see* **Fig. 5.6**).

Ligaments of the Joint

Glenohumeral Ligament (Fig. 5.9)

Special characteristic of this ligament is that, it is visible from inner surface of capsule. It strengthens anteroinferior part of fibrous capsule. Glenohumeral ligament present three bands—superior, middle and inferior.

- **Superior glenohumeral ligament** is proximally attached to supraglenoid tuberosity just in front of origin of long head of biceps. Distally it is attached to a small depression *(fovea capitis)* on superior aspect of lesser tubercle of humerus.
- **Middle glenohumeral ligament** extends from upper two-thirds of anterior margin of glenoid fossa to lesser tubercle of humerus deep to subscapularis.
- **Inferior glenohumeral ligament** is the thickest band. It supports the inferior aspect of capsule which is loose. It extends from anterior, inferior and posterior margin of glenoid labrum to the medial aspect of neck of humerus.

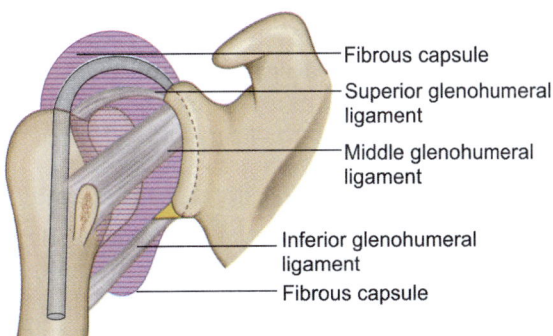

Fig. 5.9: Glenohumeral ligament.

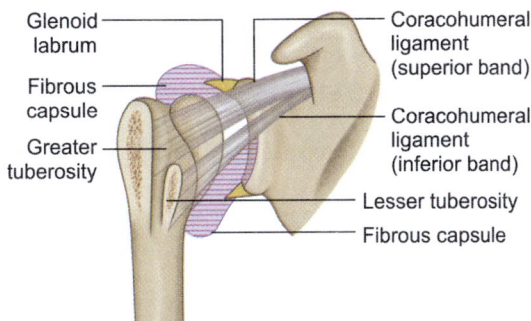

Fig. 5.10: Coracohumeral ligament of shoulder joint.

Coracohumeral Ligament (Fig. 5.10)

Root of coracohumeral ligament is attached to the dorsolateral aspect of base of coracoid process. Blending with capsule, it extends in the form of two bands to be attached to the greater and lesser tubercles of humerus.

Transverse Humeral Ligament (Fig. 5.11)

This ligament is a broad fibrous band which extends between greater and lesser tuberosities of humerus. Thus it bridges over intertubercular sulcus to convert it into a canal through which passes the long tendon of biceps brachii enclosed by a synovial sheath. The ligament acts as a retinaculum to hold the tendon in position during movement of shoulder joint.

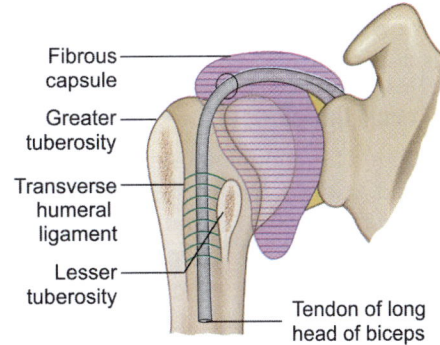

Fig. 5.11: Transverse humeral ligament of shoulder joint.

Coracoacromial Arch—An Additional Socket of the Joint (Fig. 5.12)

Coracoacromial arch is the outer protective socket for structurally less stable shoulder joint. It is formed by inferior surface of acromion, coracoid process and a flattened band-like **coracoacromial**

ligament bridging between them. This osseoligamentous structure forms a protective arch. It overlies the head of humerus and thus prevents superior displacement of humeral head from glenoid fossa.

The coracoacromial ligament forming the arch is triangular in outline and it extends from the tip of acromion to the lateral margin of horizontal part of coracoid process.

Factors Maintaining the Stability of Shoulder Joint

The articulation between relatively large hemispherical head of humerus and shallow glenoid fossa permits a wide range of mobility at the expense of stability. That is why, a variety of additional factors increase the stability of shoulder joint.
- **The glenoid labrum** increases the depth of articular surface of glenoid fossa.
- **The glenohumeral ligaments** act as static stabilizer in certain position of joint.
- **Negative pressure** within the joint also plays a role for contact of articular surfaces.
- **The coracoacromial arch** acts as a secondary socket to prevent upwards displacement of head of humerus.
- Compressive force around the joint by **rotator cuff** stabilizes the joint during active movement of the joint.
- **Long head of biceps** offers additional support superiorly.
- **Long head of triceps** offers inferior support of the joint particularly in abducted condition of shoulder joint.

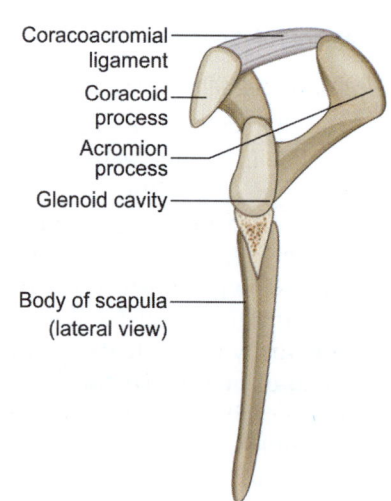

Fig. 5.12: Coracoacromial arch—a secondary socket for shoulder joint.

Important Relations
- **Anteriorly**: Subscapularis muscle, axillary vessels and brachial plexus
- **Posteriorly**: Infraspinatus and teres minor muscles
- **Superiorly**: Supraspinatus and deltoid muscles, and coracoacromial arch
- **Inferiorly**: Long head of triceps brachii muscle, axillary nerve and posterior circumflex humeral vessels.

Bursae Around the Joint

Bursae around the shoulder joint are membrane bound spaces between different aspects of fibrous capsule and tendons around it. Some important bursae are following.
- *Subscapular bursa*: This bursa is between subscapularis and capsule. It communicates with joint cavity.
- *Subacromial bursa*: It is between superior aspect of the capsule and the coracoacromial arch and deltoid overlying it.
- *Infraspinatus bursa*: It is between infraspinatus muscle tendon and posterior aspect of capsule.

Arterial Supply

Anterior and posterior circumflex humeral arteries, suprascapular artery and circumflex scapular artery.

Nerve Supply

Suprascapular nerve, axillary nerve and lateral pectoral nerve.

Movements of Shoulder Joint

Shoulder joint enjoys maximum freedom of mobility when compared with any joint of the body. This is possible at the expense of stability. Two main reasons for sacrifice of stability are laxity of articular capsule and much wider surface area of humeral head in comparison to glenoid fossa.

Multiaxial shoulder joint permits following groups of movements.
- *Flexion and extension*: Around side to side axis
- *Abduction and adduction*: Around anteroposterior axis
- *Medial and lateral rotations*: Around vertical axis
- *Circumduction*: Combination of above movements

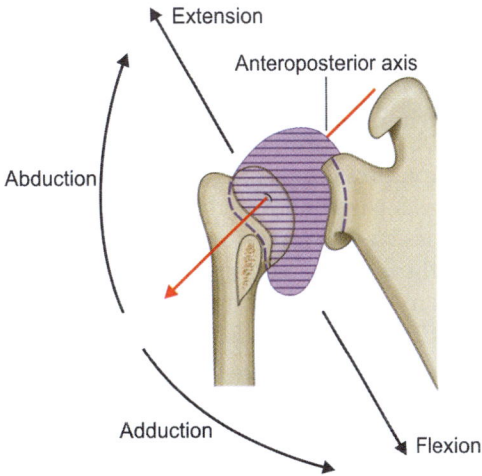

Fig. 5.13: Abduction and adduction of shoulder joint occur around anteroposterior axis.

Before the movements of the shoulder joint are studied, it is important to note that, the plane of the joint does not coincide with the side-to-side plane of the body, as **glenoid fossa is directed forwards and laterally**. So, the transverse axis of the joint coinciding with the plane of scapula is directed forwards and laterally (**Figs. 5.13 and 5.14**) forming an angle with coronal plane of body. Anteroposterior axis coinciding with the plane of the joint is directed forwards and medially (**Figs. 5.13 and 5.15**). Vertical axis passes through the head of humerus.

Following are the movements of shoulder (glenohumeral) joint:
- **Flexion and extension**: These occur at right angle to the transverse axis passing forwards and laterally and along the plane of the joint which is parallel to glenoid fossa. During flexion, the arm moves forwards and medially and during extension it moves backward and laterally (**Fig. 5.14**). Main flexor muscles are clavicular head of pectoralis major and anterior fibers of deltoid. Their actions are assisted by coracobrachialis and biceps brachii. Extensors are posterior fibers of deltoid, latissimus dorsi and teres major.
- **Abduction and adduction (Fig. 5.13)**: These movements take place round an anteroposterior axis passing forwards and medially parallel to the plane of the joint. Abduction is initiated by supraspinatus. But the chief abductor is deltoid, particularly

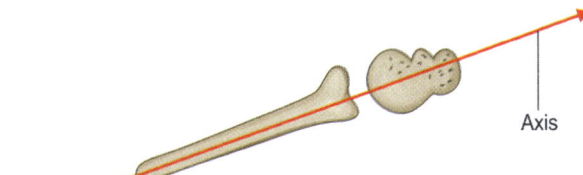

Fig. 5.14: Transverse axis for flexion—extension coincides with the plane of scapula.

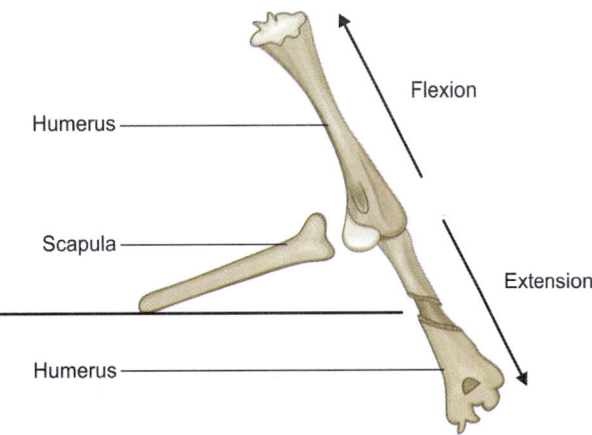

Fig. 5.15: Line of flexion—extension passing at right angle to the plane of scapula.

its middle fibers. Adduction is caused by pectoralis major, latissimus dorsi, teres major and teres minor.
- **Lateral and medial rotation**: Extensive lateral and medial rotation of shoulder joint can be demonstrated with the elbow fixed by the side of the trunk with its 90° flexed position. In this position, forearm is to be moved laterally or medially to demonstrate respective rotational movements of the shoulder joint. Rotation of the joint occurs round a vertical axis passing through the center of head of humerus. Chief lateral rotator is infraspinatus, assisted by teres minor and posterior fibers of deltoid. Medial rotation is mainly performed through the action of subscapularis. It is assisted by latissimus dorsi, teres major and anterior fibers of deltoid.
- **Circumduction:** It is the combination of above movements. This movement is classically demonstrated through the action of a cricket bowler.

Combined Movement of Shoulder Joint and Shoulder Girdle

Movement of freely mobile shoulder joint is associated with movement of shoulder girdle. This occurs at *scapulothoracic junction* leading to movement of scapula. Scapular movement is associated with similar movement (e.g. elevation or depression) of acromioclavicular joint and reverse movement of sternoclavicular joint. *Flexion and extension* movement of shoulder joint is associated with *protraction and retraction of scapula* on chest wall respectively. Again *abduction and adduction* of shoulder joint is accompanied by *elevation and depression of scapula* respectively. Out of full range of abduction of 180°, beyond 90° of abduction, every 10° of movement of shoulder joint is associated with 5° of movement of scapula.

Clinical Anatomy

Dislocation of Glenohumeral Joint

Due to maximum freedom of movement and lack of stability of the glenohumeral joint, dislocation is common as a result of direct or indirect trauma. Because of rotator cuff and coracoacromial arch, the joint is secured superiorly, anteriorly and posteriorly. So displacement of humeral head occurs inferiorly due to laxity and insecurity of capsule. Head of humerus is displaced inferoanteriorly in front of glenoid fossa deep to subscapularis muscle. Rarely it is posteriorly dislocated in the infraspinous fossa.

Rotator Cuff Injuries

In case of repetitive straining on musculotendinous rotator cuff, e.g. in swimming, fast bowling, throwing, weight lifting, its injury may result. Recurrent inflammation of the rotator cuff will lead to a painful condition. It is very common cause of shoulder pain which is due to tear of supraspinatus tendon as this is the relatively avascular area of rotator cuff.

Frozen Shoulder

This condition is also known as *adhesive capsulitis*. Usually the persons of 40 to 60 years age group are affected. The condition results after glenohumeral dislocation, supraspinatus tendinitis, rotator cuff tear and bicipital synovitis. It leads to restriction of abduction of shoulder joint up to 45°. This disability is due to adhesion of inflamed articular capsule of the joint, rotator cuff, subacromial bursa, coracoacromial arch and deltoid.

Shoulder Pain

Glenohumeral joint or shoulder joint is very sensitive to pain. The synovial membrane, capsule and ligaments are richly supplied by axillary nerve (C_5, C_6) and suprascapular nerve (C_5, C_6). Any pathological condition surrounding the joint leads to shoulder pain due to irritation of the nerves. It will result in reflex spasm of muscle around the joint which will immobilize the joint.

Referred Pain in Shoulder

Some pathological conditions, with normal shoulder joint, may cause feeling of pain in the shoulder tip. This is the pain referred to shoulder, when any area supplied by the same segmental nerve, C_5 and C_6, is diseased. The examples are:
- Diseases of spinal cord and vertebral column at C_5, C_6 level.
- Pressure of the same segmental spinal nerves by cervical rib.
- Irritation of diaphragmatic pleura, supplied by phrenic nerve (C_3, C_4, C_5). It may be due to inflammation of diaphragmatic pleura or gallbladder.

Axillary Nerve Injury

Axillary nerve may often be injured in case of dislocation of glenohumeral joint, due to its close relation with inferior aspect of capsule. Dislocated humeral head presses over the nerve at quadrangular space below the capsule. If the nerve is injured, paralysis of deltoid with impairment of sensation of the skin over the muscle results.

Chapter 6

Anterior Compartment of Forearm

LA 6.1 **Give an account of the muscles of the front of forearm.**

Individual muscle may be asked in the form of short note.

MUSCLES OF THE FRONT OF FOREARM

Introduction

Anterior compartment of forearm contains number of muscles most of which are flexor of the wrist and fingers. This compartment also contains the pronator muscles of forearm acting on radioulnar joints. The muscles are disposed in superficial and deep layers.

Muscles of front of forearm are:

Muscles of superficial layer (from lateral to medial)	Muscles of deep layer
• Pronator teres • Flexor carpi radialis • Palmaris longus • Flexor digitorum superficialis • Flexor carpi ulnaris	• Flexor pollicis longus • Flexor digitorum profundus • Pronator quadratus

Superficial Flexor Muscles

Pronator Teres (Fig. 6.1)

Pronator teres is the most lateral among the muscles of superficial plane. It is oblique in direction from medial side of elbow to the middle of lateral margin of front of forearm. The muscle forms medial boundary of the cubital fossa.

Origin

Humeral head is the larger and superficial head. It arises from:
- Lower end of medial supracondylar line just above medial epicondyle
- Common tendinous origin of flexor muscles
- Intermuscular fascial septum separating adjacent muscles
- Inner surface of deep fascia of forearm (antebrachial fascia).

Ulnar head arises from:
Medial aspect of the coronoid process of ulna beyond to the site of attachment of flexor digitorum superficialis.

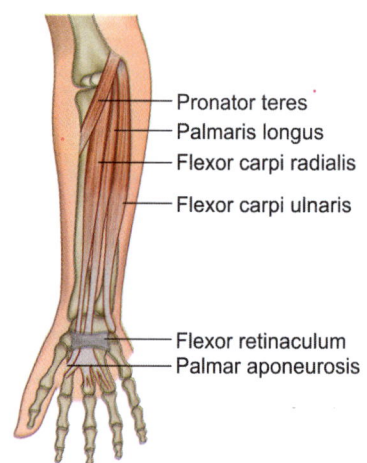

Fig. 6.1: Superficial muscles of front of forearm.

Insertion

The two heads of pronator teres muscle blend at an acute angle. The muscle extends obliquely downwards and laterally across the front of forearm. The flat tendon is inserted into middle of lateral surface of the shaft of radius at the point of maximum convexity.

Accessory slips of origin

- Supracondylar process of humerus, if present
- Medial intermuscular septum of arm
- Tendons of biceps and brachialis.

Important relations

- Between two heads of pronator teres runs down the *median nerve*
- Ulnar artery descends deep to both the heads of the muscle
- Pronator teres forms the oblique medial boundary of the cubital fossa.

Nerve supply

Pronator teres is supplied by *median nerve* (C_6 and C_7 fibers).

Actions

- Pronator teres comes into action *only during rapid and forceful pronation of forearm* along with pronator quadratus which is always active in pronation. The muscle rotates the radius medially in front of the ulna, so that palm of the hand faces backward turning dorsomedially.
- Same as all the flexor muscles arising from medial epicondyle, pronator teres is a *week flexor of the elbow joint.*

Flexor Carpi Radialis (Fig. 6.1)

Flexor carpi radialis is medial to pronator teres.

Origin

- *Medial epicondyle* of humerus through common tendinous origin of flexor muscles
- *Intermuscular fascial septum* separating adjacent muscles
- Deep fascia of forearm *(antebrachial fascia).*

Occasional sources of origin:

- Tendon of biceps
- Bicipital aponeurosis
- Coronoid process of ulna.

Insertion

In the middle of forearm, the fusiform narrow slip of muscle is continued as long tendon enclosed by synovial sheath. It *passes through a osseofibrous canal* bound dorsally by a groove on trapezium and ventrally by a slip from flexor retinaculum.

Main insertion is into the palmar surface of *base of second metacarpal bone.* A slip goes to be attached to *similar area of third metacarpal bone.*

Accessory (occasional) slip of insertion to:

- *Flexor retinaculum*—condensation of deep fascia in front of flexor tendons beyond the wrist
- *Trapezium*
- *Fourth metacarpal bone (base).*

Important relations

In lower end of front of forearm, the radial artery is placed on the ventral surface of lower end of radius between flexor carpi radialis medially and brachioradialis laterally.

Nerve supply

Median nerve (fibers of C_6 and C_7).

Actions

- *Jointly with flexor carpi ulnaris* in medial side, the muscle causes *flexion of wrist*
- *Along with radial extensors* (longus and brevis), flexor carpi radialis is an *abductor of wrist*.

Palmaris Longus (Fig. 6.1)

Origin

Palmaris longus is a thin fusiform muscle arising from:
- *Common tendon of origin* from medial epicondyle of humerus
- *Fascial septum* between adjacent muscles
- Inner surface of *deep fascia of forearm.*
  The muscle lies medial to flexor carpi radialis.

Insertion

Long thin tendon of the muscle is inserted:
- On the superficial surface of *flexor retinaculum* with interlacement of fibers
- Some fibers of the tendon of palmaris longus, passing over flexor retinaculum become broader and fuse with superficial aspect of fibers of *palmar aponeurosis*.

Nerve supply

Median nerve (*fiber of C_7 and C_8*).

Action

- The most important function of palmaris longus is to act as an anchor for the skin and fascia of the hand
- It is the weak flexor of wrist
- Morphologically the palmar aponeurosis is known to be distal part of the tendon of palmaris longus, though this aponeurosis is the defunct part of the muscle. So palmaris longus is the degenerated metacarpophalangeal joint flexor.
  Palmaris longus is absent in 10% of cases.

Flexor Digitorum Superficialis (Fig. 6.2)

Flexor digitorum superficialis (sublimis) in the largest among the muscles of the superficial plane of anterior compartment of forearm. It lies deep to pronator teres, flexor carpi radialis and palmaris longus. So, the flexor digitorum superficialis may be grouped as the muscle of the intermediate layer.

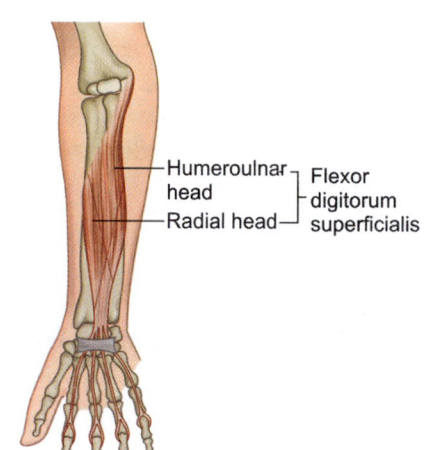

Fig. 6.2: Flexor digitorum superficialis (muscle of superficial group).

Origin

Humeroulnar head

- From medial epicondyle through common tendon of origin of flexor muscle.
- Medial aspect of coronoid process proximal to ulnar origin of pronator teres.
- Anterior band of ulnar collateral ligament of elbow joint
- Intermuscular septa separating adjacent muscles.

Radial head

From upper oblique part of anterior border (anterior oblique line) of radius in the form of a thin sheet.

Insertion

Before insertion, the muscle divides finally in four tendinous slips for medial four digits, i.e. index to little finger. But before that, beneath the flexor retinaculum, the muscle tendon will divide into superficial and deep strata. Superficial stratum is continued as two tendons for middle and ring fingers. Deep stratum forms tendons for index and little fingers.

Insertion of individual tendon slip: In the palm of hand four tendons diverge to pass towards the respective finger, superficial to respective tendon of flexor digitorum profundus. Beyond the metacarpophalangeal joint, superficialis tendon bifurcates into two slips which embress the profundus tendon from either side and is finally inserted into palmar surface of base of middle phalanx. Before getting inserted, two slips reunite. The profundus tendon passes towards the distal phalanx between two slips of superficialis tendon.

Important relations

Median nerve and ulnar artery run downwards between the proximal ends of two heads of flexor digitorum superficialis.

Nerve supply

Flexor digitorum superficialis is supplied by the median nerve through its fibers of C_8 and T_1 spinal nerve roots only.

Actions

As the tendinous slips are inserted to base of middle phalanx, prime action of flexor digitorum superficialis is to cause flexion of proximal interphalangeal joint. But it also flexes the wrist joint and metacarpophalangeal joint, over which this muscle tendon passes.

Flexor Carpi Ulnaris (Fig. 6.1)

Flexor carpi ulnaris is the most medial of the superficial muscles of the forearm.

Origin

Humeral head

From medial epicondyle via the origin of common flexor tendon.

Ulnar head

Shows extensive origin:
- Medial aspect of olecranon process of ulna
- Upper two-thirds of posterior border of ulna through a common aponeurotic origin along with extensor carpi ulnaris and flexor digitorum profundus

- Intermuscular fascial septum between it and flexor digitorum superficialis
- Occasional slips of origin from lower end of medial aspect of coronoid process of ulna. Distal half of the muscle presents a thick tendon.

Insertion
- Main insertion is in the pisiform bone
- Beyond the pisiform, the tendon is continued to be attached to the hamate and base of fifth metacarpal as pisohamate and pisometacarpal ligaments.
- Tendinous fibers may extend up to the flexor retinaculum and base of fourth metacarpal bone *occasionally*.

Important relations
The ulnar nerve passes between two heads of origin of flexor carpi ulnaris.

Nerve supply
Flexor carpi ulnaris is supplied by *the ulnar nerve* carrying fibers of C_7, C_8 and T_1 spinal nerves.

Actions
- Along with flexor carpi radialis, the muscle flexes the carpus or the wrist joint
- When the muscle jointly acts with extensor carpi ulnaris, it adducts the wrist joint.

Deep Group of Muscles

It is interesting to note that superficial flexor muscles are accompanied by one pronator (pronator teres) and deep group of muscles are accompanied by another pronator (pronator quadratus).

Deep compartment of front of forearm contains:
1. Flexor digitorum profundus } Lying in a same plane side by side
2. Flexor pollicis longus
3. Pronator quadratus: Lying deep to above two muscles.

Flexor Digitorum Profundus (Fig. 6.3)

Origin

From ulna

- Proximal (upper) three-fourths of anterior and medial surfaces of shaft of ulna
- A small depression on medial surface of coronoid process of ulna
- Upper three-fourth of posterior border of shaft of ulna through the common aponeurotic origin along with flexor carpi ulnaris and extensor carpi ulnaris.

From interosseous membrane

Medial or ulnar half of anterior surface of interosseous membrane.

Insertion

Flexor digitorum profundus divides into four slips of tendons which pass deep to the flexor retinaculum and the tendons of flexor digitorum superficialis. The part of flexor digitorum profundus for index finger is usually separate all throughout. The tendons for other

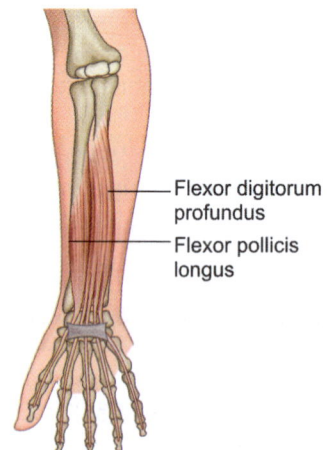

Fig. 6.3: Deep muscles of front of forearm.

fingers are joined by fibrous slips as far as the palm. At the level of proximal phalanges profundus tendons pass between the bifurcated tendon of superficialis and are finally inserted on the palmar aspect of base of distal phalanges.

Nerve supply
- Lateral half of flexor digitorum profundus giving tendon slips for index and middle fingers is supplied by the *anterior interosseous branch of median nerve*
- Medial half of the muscle for ring and little fingers is supplied by the *ulnar nerve.*
  Both the nerves carry fibers of C_8 and T_1 spinal nerve roots.

Actions
- Flexor digitorum profundus is the only muscle among all flexors which causes flexion of distal interphalangeal joint
- The muscle is also capable of flexion of all other joints over which it crosses, i.e. wrist joint, metacarpophalangeal joint and proximal interphalangeal joint.

Flexor digitorum profundus is concerned with coordinated finger flexion. It is for gentle digital flexion. The force in flexion is increased by flexor digitorum superficialis.

Flexor Pollicis Longus (Fig. 6.3)
Flexor pollicis longus is the long flexor of the thumb arising in the forearm lateral to flexor digitorum profundus.

Origin
Slightly hollowed anterior surface of radius between the radial tuberosity above, and the attachment of pronator quadratus below.

Lateral half of anterior surface of interosseous membrane.

Occasional slips of origin from:
- Lateral or medial border of coronoid process
- Medial epicondyle of humerus.

Insertion
The muscle ends in a flattened tendon which passes deep to flexor retinaculum being enclosed by independent synovial sheath. The tendon is inserted into palmar surface of base of terminal phalanx of thumb.

Variations
- A slip from flexor pollicis longus may be connected to flexor digitorum profundus or superficialis or to pronator teres. Connection with profundus is common
- Origin of the muscle from interosseous membrane may be absent
- Sometimes whole muscle may be absent.

Important relations
Anterior interosseous nerve and vessels descend between flexor pollicis longus and flexor digitorum profundus in front of interosseous membrane.

Nerve supply
Flexor pollicis longus is supplied by the anterior interosseous branch of median nerve through the fibers carried from C_7 and C_8 nerve roots.

Actions
- Flexor pollicis longus flexes both the phalanges of the thumb acting on both interphalangeal and metacarpophalangeal joints.
- It also flexes carpometacarpal joint of thumb, especially when the distal joints are fixed.

Pronator Quadratus (Fig. 6.4)
Pronator quadratus is a short flat, quadrilateral muscle which crosses over front of lower part of radius and ulna.

Origin
- From the ridge, oblique in direction, on the lower part of anterior surface of shaft of ulna
- From the anterior surface of lower end of ulna medial to the oblique ridge
- From the fibro-aponeurotic covering of the muscle.

Insertion
- *Superficial fibers* are inserted to lower one-fourth of anterior border of radius and corresponding part of anterior surface of the bone
- *Deeper fibers* are inserted to the triangular area on medial aspect of lower end of shaft of radius above its ulnar notch.
The fibers of the muscle are directed laterally and slightly downwards.

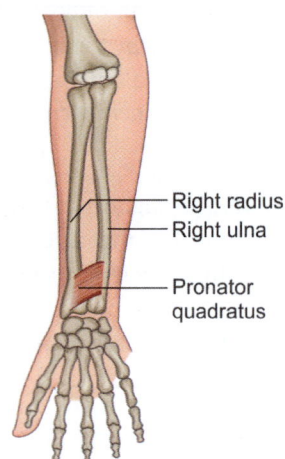

Fig. 6.4: Deep muscle of front of forearm (pronator quadratus).

Nerve supply
Pronator quadratus is supplied by anterior interosseous nerve which is a branch of median nerve. The fibers are derived from C_7 and C_8 nerves.

Actions
- Pronator quadratus is the pronator of forearm. During rapid and forceful pronation the muscle is assisted by pronator teres
- When upward thrust is transmitted through wrist, pronator quadratus prevents separation of lower ends of radius and ulna.

SA 6.2 Write a note on the anterior interosseous nerve.

ANTERIOR INTEROSSEOUS NERVE (FIG. 6.5)
Introduction
It is the deeply seated, long and slender nerve to supply the deep muscles of forearm, which are flexor pollicis longus, lateral half of flexor digitorm profundus and pronator quadratus.

Origin
It arises from the posterior aspect of median nerve in the upper end of forearm in the cubital fossa proximal to the tendinous arch of flexor digitorum superficialis.

Course and Relation
The nerve descends vertically:
- In front of interosseous membrane

- In between flexor pollicis longus and flexor digitorum profundus, but deep to these muscle
- Behind pronator quadratus muscle and in front of interosseous membrane *to end as articular branch.*

Branches
- *Muscular branches*: To the lateral and medial sides muscular branches are distributed to *flexor pollicis longus* and *lateral half of flexor digitorum profundus.*
  Distal end of the nerve passing behind the *pronator quadratus*, supplies the muscle from its deep surface.
- *Articular branches* are distributed from the terminal end of nerve to the *inferior radioulnar joint, wrist joint* and *intercarpal joints.*

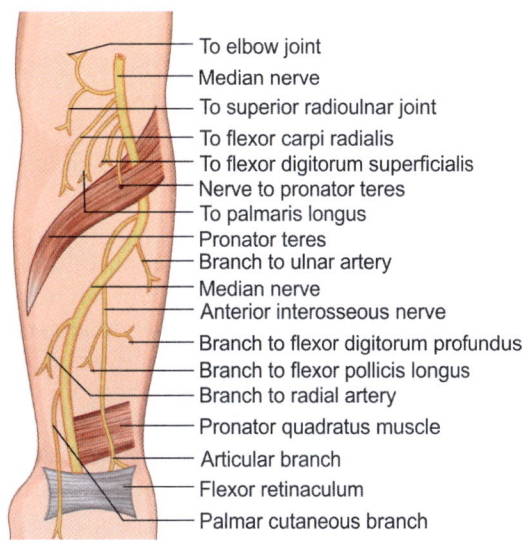

Fig. 6.5: Distribution of median nerve in the forearm.

SA 6.3 Describe the radial artery in forearm.

RADIAL ARTERY (FIG. 6.6)
Salient Points
- Radial artery in one of the two terminal branches of brachial artery 1 cm below the elbow joint.
- Radial artery appears to be more direct continuation of brachial artery.
- Radial artery is more superficial than ulnar artery being covered anteriorly only by the skin and fascia in lower part of forearm.
- In the lower end of forearm, radial artery is related to the anterior surface of shaft of radius in between tendon of flexor carpi radialis medially and prominent anterior border of lower end of radius laterally. Here pulsation of the artery is easily felt against the bony surface in clinical practice.
- The artery crosses in front of following structures successively from above downwards:
  - Tendon of biceps brachii
  - The supinator
  - Distal end of pronator teres
  - Radial head of flexor digitorum superficialis } All muscles
  - Flexor pollicis longus
  - Pronator quadratus
  - Lower end of anterior surface of radius: Bone
  - Superficial terminal division of radial nerve (superficial radial nerve) is close to its lateral side in middle third of forearm: Nerve
- Radial artery leaves the lower end of front of the forearm at the level of wrist to enter in dorsum of hand passing through the plane between abductor pollicis longus and extensor pollicis bravis superficially and radial collateral ligament of wrist joint at the deep.
- Radial artery is usually accompanied by venae comitantes.

Termination

Radial artery enters the palm at the deeper plane from the dorsum of hand passing between the two heads of 1st dorsal interosseous muscle. It forms the deep palmar arch anastomosing with the deep branch of ulnar artery.

Branches

- **Radial recurrent artery** arises just distal to elbow and it passes upwards and laterally between superficial and deep divisions of radial nerve. It ascends deep to brachioradialis and anterior to supinator and brachialis. The artery gives muscular branches to these muscles and end by anastomosing with radial collateral branches profunda brachii artery in front of elbow joint.
- **Muscular branches** are distributed to the muscles of lateral part of front of forearm.
- **Palmar carpal branch** arises from radial artery at the lower border of pronator quadratus. It passes deep to the flexor tendons and takes part in formation of palmar carpal network anastomosing with palmar carpal branch of ulnar artery.
- **Superficial palmar branch** arises from radial artery just before it leaves the forearm. This branch runs distally to the palm usually passing through the short muscles of thumb. It ends by supplying these muscles or it may join the terminal end of ulnar artery to form the superficial palmar arch.

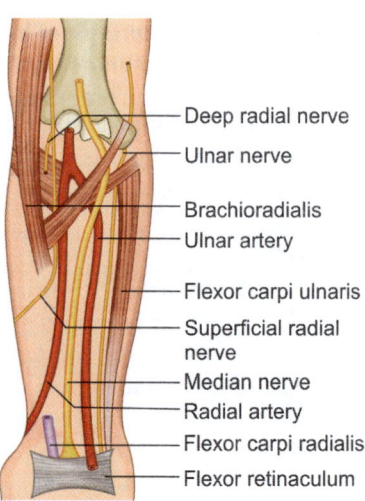

Fig. 6.6: Nerves and arteries of front of forearm.

Clinical Anatomy

The radial artery is the commonest site for clinical examination of the arterial pulse.

SA 6.4 Discuss the arterial anastomosis around the elbow joint.

ARTERIAL ANASTOMOSIS AROUND ELBOW JOINT (FIG. 6.7)

Significance

- Arterial anastomosis around elbow joint establishes an alternative channel of circulation through brachial, radial and ulnar arteries.
- Arteries of this anastomosing network are deep-seated. These arteries supply ligaments and bones of the elbow joint and superior radioulnar joint.

Source of Arteries Forming the Network

In front of lateral epicondyle of humerus
- Radial collateral branch of profunda brachii artery—from above
- Radial recurrent branch of radial artery—from below.

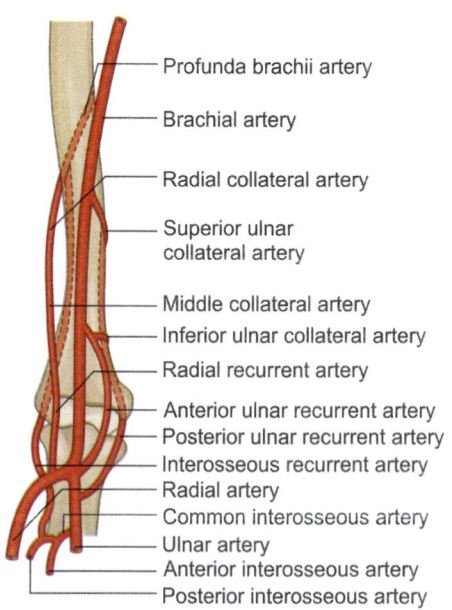

Fig. 6.7: Arterial anastomosis around elbow.

Behind lateral epicondyle of humerus:
- Middle collateral branch or posterior descending branch of profunda brachii artery from above
- Interosseous recurrent branch of posterior interosseous artery, which is a branch of common interosseous artery.

In front of medial epicondyle of humerus:
- Inferior ulnar collateral artery—a branch of brachial artery participating from above
- Anterior ulnar recurrent artery—a branch of ulnar artery joining from below.

Behind medial epicondyle of humerus:
- Superior ulnar collateral artery and posterior branch of inferior ulnar collateral artery—both are the branches of brachial artery joining from above.
- Posterior ulnar recurrent artery—a branch of ulnar artery—from below.

In addition to above communication, on the posterior aspect of elbow joint a transverse anastomosis establishes communication between arteries of lateral and medial sides.

Chapter 7

Posterior Compartment of Forearm

LA 7.1 Give a brief account of the muscles of the posterior compartment of forearm.

Individual muscle may be asked in the form of short note.

MUSCLES OF THE POSTERIOR COMPARTMENT OF FOREARM

- Among the muscles of back of forearm, anconeus muscle is not included in the list. The reasons are:
  - The muscle arises proximal to elbow joint, from lateral epicondyle of humerus.
  - It is supplied by trunk of the radial nerve, while the nerve is in the spiral groove.

  Anconeus has been discussed in the chapter of back of arm (Chapter 4).

- Muscles of posterior compartment of forearm are many. But they can be easily remembered if they are classified as per their *functional categories* which are as follows:

  Group 1:
  Muscles acting **on wrist**—extensors (abductors or adductors also) of the wrist
  - Extensor carpi radialis longus
  - Extensor carpi radialis brevis
  - Extensor carpi ulnaris.

  Group 2:
  Muscles acting **on medial four fingers**—extensors
  - Extensor digitorum
  - Extensor indicis (for index finger)
  - Extensor digiti minimi (for little finger).

  Group 3:
  Muscles acting **on thumb**—abductor and extensors
  - Abductor pollicis longus
  - Extensor pollicis brevis
  - Extensor pollicis longus.

  Besides the above groups following two other groups are also as follows:

  Group 4:
  Muscle acting **on elbow**—flexor in midprone position—brachioradialis.

  Group 5:
  Muscle acting **on radioulnar joint**—supinator—the supinator.

Anatomical Subdivision

It is in two different planes.

Superficial Plane
- Brachioradialis
- Extensor carpi radialis longus

- Extensor carpi radialis brevis
- Extensor digitorum
- Extensor digiti minimi
- Extensor carpi ulnaris.

Deep Plane

- Supinator
- Abductor pollicis longus
- Extensor pollicis brevis
- Extensor pollicis longus
- Extensor indicis.

Deep Fascia—Specialized to Bind the Posterior Compartment Muscles

Deep fascia of back of forearm is thicker than the fascia in front of forearm. It sends intermuscular septa between adjacent muscles which also give origin to the muscles.

While the tendons of back muscles cross over the back of wrist, they are bound by a thick band of fascia which acts as a retinaculum to prevent bow-stringing of the tendons of the contracting muscles.

Muscles of Superficial Group (Fig. 7.1)

Brachioradialis

Brachioradialis is the most superficially placed muscle along the lateral side of the forearm.

Origin

- From proximal two-thirds of lateral supracondylar line of humerus
- From anterior aspect of lateral intermuscular septum of arm.

Insertion

The muscle is continued as a flat tendon in the middle of forearm and is inserted on the lateral aspect of lower end of radius just above its styloid process.

Variations

- At its origin, it may be *fused with brachialis*
- Occasionally, *insertion* of the muscles is *more proximal*
- The *tendon may divide into two* or more slips
- On rare occasion, brachioradialis *may be absent*.

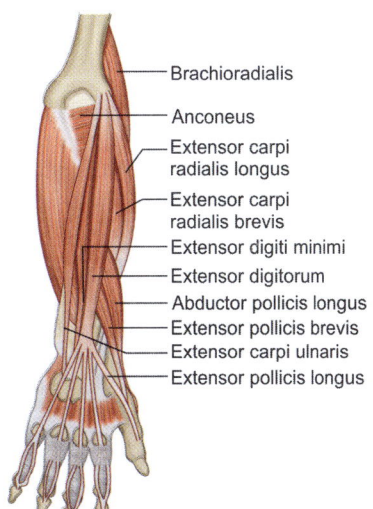

Fig. 7.1: Muscles of posterior compartment of forearm.

Important relations

- Brachioradialis forms lateral boundary of cubital fossa at the elbow
- Radial nerve in the cubital fossa lies between brachialis and brachioradialis
- Radial artery is related to the medial side of the muscle.

Nerve supply

Brachioradialis is supplied by *radial nerve* (C_5, C_6 fibers) after piercing lateral intermuscular septum of arm.

Action

It is important to note that, though brachioradialis is the muscle of extensor compartment of forearm and is supplied by the radial nerve, it is *a flexor of elbow*, especially *in midprone position* of forearm.

Extensor Carpi Radialis Longus

Origin
- Distal one-third of lateral supracondylar line of humerus
- Anterior surface of lateral intermuscular septum of arm
- Some fibers from common tendinous origin of extensors from the lateral aspect of lateral epicondyle of humerus.

Insertion
The muscle belly ends in a flat tendon at the junction of upper third and lower to thirds of forearm. It is partly covered by brachioradialis.

The tendon runs downward along the lateral surface of radius beneath the abductor pollicis longus and extensor pollicis brevis.

Passing deep to the extensor retinaculum, the tendon gets inserted on the lateral side of dorsal surface of base of second metacarpal bone. It may give slips to the base of adjacent metacarpal bone (first or third).

Nerve supply
Extensor carpi radialis longus is supplied by *radial nerve* (C_6, C_7 fibers).

Action
The muscle is extensor and abductor of wrist.

Extensor Carpi Radialis Brevis

Origin
- From lateral epicondyle of humerus along with common tendinous of origin of other extensors
- From radial (lateral) collateral ligament of elbow joint
- From the strong aponeurosis which overlies the surface of the muscle
- From adjoining intermuscular septa.

Insertion
- Radial side of dorsal aspect of base of third metacarpal bone
- Adjacent area of base of second metacarpal bone.

Nerve supply
Extensor carpi radialis brevis is supplied by *the deep branch of radial nerve* called deep radial nerve or *posterior interosseous nerve* (C_7 and C_8 fibers) before it pierces the supinator muscle.

Action
Along with extensor carpi radialis longus, this muscle acts as abductor and extensor of the wrist.

Extensor Digitorum

Extensor digitorum is the common extensor for medial four fingers. On the dorsum of hand, tendinous slips for the fingers will be inserted to the phalanges of respective fingers as stated below:

Origin
- From lateral epicondyle of humerus through origin of common extensor tendon
- From adjacent intermuscular septa
- From deep fascia of forearm.

Important points
- Proximal to the wrist, extensor digitorum divides into four tendinous slips.
- Four tendons pass under extensor retinaculum in a common synovial sheath with tendon of extensor indicis.
- The tendons diverge on dorsum of hand to proceed for respective fingers.
- Tendinous slips for index finger and little finger are joined from their medial side by tendon of extensor indicis and extensor digiti minimi respectively.
- On the dorsum of hand, the tendons, while diverging are connected by aponeurotic sheet called *intertendinous connections*.

Insertion
On the dorsum of fingers, tendon divides into a central and two collateral slips at the level of metacarpophalangeal joint. The three slips are connected by a triangular aponeurotic band, base of which is directed proximally. This triangular aponeurosis is known as *dorsal digital expansion* or *extensor expansion*. Through this expansion, the intermediate tendinous slip is inserted into the dorsal aspect of base of middle phalanx. Two collaterals fuse to be inserted into the dorsum of base of distal phalanx. Further details of the extensor expansion is discussed in the chapter of hand (Chapter 9).

Nerve supply
Extensor digitorum is supplied by the deep branch of radial nerve called deep radial nerve or posterior interosseous nerve (fibers of C_7 and C_8 nerves).

Actions
- Extensor digitorum can extend any or all of the joints it crosses over, i.e. wrist, metacarpophanlageal, and proximal and distal interphalangeal joints. Extension of interphalangeal joints occurs through dorsal digital expansion.
- Intertendinous connections probably helps in extension of any finger independently.

Extensor Digiti Minimi
Extensor digiti minimi is a thin muscle and its tendon blends with the medial side of tendon of extensor digitorum for little finger.

Origin
- From lateral epicondyle of humerus through common tendinous origin of extensors. Its origin is in the form of thin tendinous slip.
- From adjacent fascial intermuscular septa
- From deep fascia of back of the forearm.

Insertion
The tendon of extensor digiti minimi, sometimes divided into two slips, is joined on its lateral side by tendon of extensor digitorum. Through dorsal digital expansion (extensor expansion), all the tendons are inserted into the base of the middle and distal phalanges of little fingers.

Nerve Supply

Extensor digiti minimi is supplied by the posterior interosseous nerve (C_7, C_8 fibers).

Actions

- Extensor digiti minimi causes extension of any of the joints of little finger even independently.
- It can extend the wrist joint also to some extent.

Extensor Carpi Ulnaris

Origin

- Lateral epicondyle of humerus through common tendinous origin of extensor muscles.
- Sharp posterior border of ulna through common aponeurotic origin of flexor carpi ulnaris and flexor digitorum profundus
- Deep fascia of back of forearm covering the muscle.

Insertion

The tendon of extensor carpi ulnaris passes through a groove in between head and styloid process of ulna, deep to the extensor retinaculum in a separate compartment. Finally, it is inserted into a tubercle on medial aspect of base of fifth metacarpal bone.

Nerve supply

Extensor carpi ulnaris is supplied by the posterior interosseous nerve (C_7, C_8 fibers).

Actions

- Combined with extensor carpi radialis longus and brevis, extensor carpi ulnaris causes extension of wrist. Extension along with fixation of wrist by extensor carpi ulnaris is important for gripping an object in hand and to tighten the fist.
- Acting with flexor carpi ulnaris, extensor carpi ulnaris leads to adduction of hand.

Muscles of Deeper Layer of Back of Forearm

Muscles of deeper layer of back of forearm are the following:
- Abductor pollicis longus ⎫
- Extensor pollicis brevis ⎬ Acting on thumb
- Extensor pollicis longus ⎭
- Extensor indicis—acting on index finger
- The supinator—acting on radioulnar joints

Fundamental Points on Attachments (Fig. 7.2)

- The first four muscles take origin from back of shaft of radius and/or ulna
- Abductor pollicis longus takes origin from both the bones
- Extensor pollicis brevis arises from radius only
- Extensor pollicis longus and extensor indicis take origin from ulna only
- The supinator muscle arises from ulna and is inserted into radius encircling the posterolateral aspect of the bones.

Abductor Pollicis Longus

Origin

- From the radial or lateral side of upper part of **posterior surface of shaft of ulna** *below the attachment of anconeus*

- From the ulnar side of middle third of **posterior surface of shaft of radius** *below the attachment of the supinator*
- Posterior surface of interosseous membrane between origin of the muscle from the radius and ulna.

Insertion

The muscle descends downwards and laterally and becomes superficial in distal part of forearm. It becomes tendinous just proximal to the wrist. The tendon passes over the lateral aspect of lower end of radius accompanied by tendon of extensor pollicis brevis.

The muscle is usually inserted as follows:

It subdivides into two slips. One of the slips is inserted on the *lateral aspect of base of first metacarpal bone*. Another gets attached to the *trapezium*.

Nerve supply

Abductor pollicis longus is supplied by the posterior interosseous nerve (C_7, C_8) which is the deep branch of radial nerve.

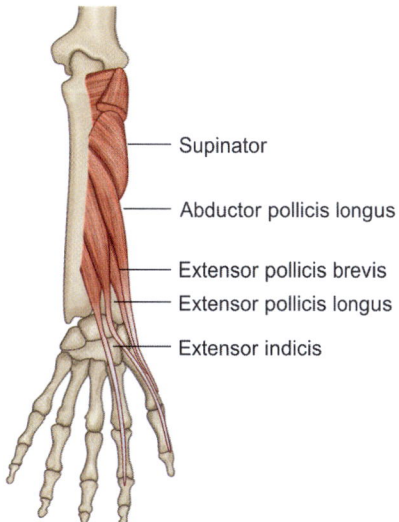

Fig. 7.2: Deep muscles of posterior compartment of forearm.

Actions

- Abductor pollicis longus *is the abductor of the wrist joint.*
- Acting together with abductor pollicis brevis, it causes *abduction of the thumb.*
- Acting with extensors of the thumb, the muscle causes *extension of carpometacarpal joint.*
- Tendinous slip attached to the trapezium *stabilizes the trapezium.* So the first metacarpal bone can move on it.

Extensor Pollicis Brevis

In the back of forearm, extensor pollicis brevis is the companion of abductor pollicis longus.

Origin

- **Posterior surface of radius** distal to origin of abductor pollicis longus
- Adjacent area of *interosseous membrane.*

Insertion

- The tendon is attached on the dorsal surface of *base of proximal phalanx of thumb.*
- *Additional insertion* is sometimes found on the dorsal aspect of *base of distal phalanx of thumb.*

Nerve supply

Extensor pollicis brevis is supplied by the posterior interosseous nerve (C_7, C_8).

Actions

Extensor pollicis brevis extends the proximal phalanx of thumb and the first metacarpal also.

Extensor Pollicis Longus

It is not only longer, but also larger than extensor pollicis brevis.

Origin
- Radial (lateral) part of **posterior surface of shaft of ulna** below the origin of abductor pollicis longus
- Adjoining part of *interosseous membrane*.

Insertion
- The tendon of extensor pollicis longus passes through a separate tunnel beneath the extensor retinaculum
- The tendon *bends round the dorsal tubercle or Lister's tubercle* of radius to change its direction downwards and laterally towards the thumb from dorsal aspect of the wrist
- It is inserted to the dorsal surface of base of distal phalanx of thumb.

Nerve supply
Extensor pollicis longus is supplied by the posterior interosseous nerve (C_7, C_8).

Actions
- Extensor pollicis longus *is extensor of the distal phalanx of thumb*
- In combination with extensor pollicis brevis and abductor pollicis longus, it *extends proximal phalanx and metacarpal of thumb*
- During prolonged action, due to obliquity of the tendon, extensor pollicis longus *adducts the thumb*.

Extensor Indicis

Extensor indicis is the additional extensor muscle for index finger, which strengthens the index finger slip of extensor digitorum. This thin long muscle lies medial to extensor pollicis longus.

Origin
- Radial (lateral) part of **posterior surface of shaft of ulna** below the origin of extensor pollicis longus
- Adjoining part of interosseous membrane.

Insertion
- The tendon of extensor indicis descends through the common tunnel under extensor retinaculum along with the tendon of extensor digitorum.
- At the level of head of second metacarpal bone, it blends with the ulnar side of tendon of extensor digitorum for index finger.
- Insertion of slips of extensor digitorum for the medial four digits has been described in connection with the same muscle.

Nerve supply
Extensor indicis is supplied by the posterior interosseous nerve (C_7, C_8).

Actions
- Extensor indicis helps in *extension of index finger independently*, even in any position of wrist
- Additionally, the muscle may cause *extension of wrist*.

Supinator

The muscles, described so far, act on finger and wrist. But supinator, being the muscle of posterior or extensor compartment of forearm, *acts on the radioulnar joints*.

Origin

- Lateral epicondyle of humerus
- Radial collateral ligament of elbow joint
- Annular ligament of superior radioulnar joint
- Supinator crest of upper end of ulna
- Posterior part of hollow area in front of supinator crest
- Aponeurosis covering the muscle.

Insertion

Musculotendinous fibers of supinator wraps around posterolateral aspect of upper end of shaft of radius and is inserted into a 'V' shaped area on upper part of lateral surface of shaft of the same bone between its anterior and posterior oblique lines.

Nerve supply

Supinator muscle is supplied by the deep radial nerve or the posterior interosseous nerve (C_6 and C_7) before the nerve passes through the muscle to enter the posterior compartment of forearm from the front.

In addition, the nerve gives a branch while traversing through the muscle.

Actions

- Supinator causes supination of radioulnar joints by rotating the radius outwards (laterally), so that the palm of the hand faces forwards. It acts alone in slow unopposed supination.
- In case of fast and forceful supination, the supinator muscle comes into action along with the biceps brachii which is a powerful supinator.

SA 7.2 Discuss briefly the posterior interosseous nerve.

POSTERIOR INTEROSSEOUS NERVE

The nerve of posterior compartment of forearm (Fig. 7.3).

Origin

The nerve of the posterior compartment of forearm is usually named as the posterior interosseous nerve, which is the deep terminal branch of radial nerve. Radial nerve, after giving 3 muscular branches in the cubital fossa, to brachioradialis, extensor carpi radialis longus and brachialis, divides into superficial and deep terminal branches, called superficial radial and deep radial nerves.

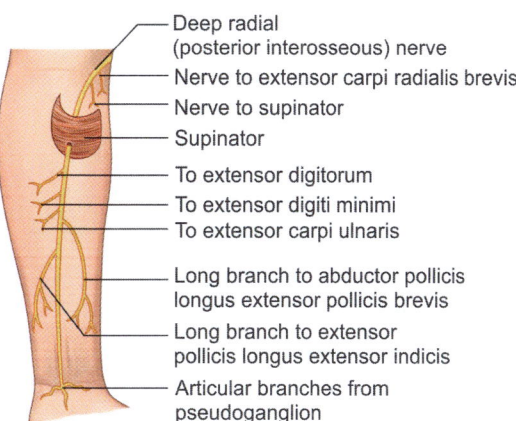

Fig. 7.3: Distribution of deep radial (posterior interosseous) nerve.

Entry in Back of Forearm

Posterior interosseous nerve, arising in the furrow between brachioradialis and brachialis, curves round the lateral aspect of upper end of shaft of radius and enters back of forearm running between two planes of supinator muscle.

Course and Relations
- Emerging from supinator at the posterior compartment of forearm, posterior interosseous nerve initially lies between the superficial and deep planes of muscles.
- At the lower border of extensor pollicis brevis, it runs further deeper underneath extensor pollicis longus along the surface of interosseous membrane.
- While running on the interosseous membrane after giving muscular branches, posterior interosseous nerve is reduced to a fine thread to end on the back of wrist, where it passes deep to extensor retinaculum in the compartment of extensor digitorum and extensor indicis.
- On the dorsum of wrist, the nerve is expanded and flattened, called 'pseudoganglion'.
- From the pseudoganglion filamentous nerve fibers are distributed to the wrist joint, distal radioulnar joint, intercarpal joints and intermetacarpal joints.

Branches
- **Proximal to the supinator**
  Before passing through the supinator, while the posterior interosseous nerve is in front of forearm, it gives branches to:
  - Extensor carpi radialis brevis
  - Supinator.
- **Within the supinator:** It gives additional branch to supinator
- **Distal to the supinator**
  - Three short branches to the following three muscles:
    ◊ Extensor digitorum
    ◊ Extensor digiti minimi
    ◊ Extensor carpi ulnaris
  - Two long branches—lateral and medial
      Lateral long branch to— 1. Abductor pollicis longus
                              2. Extensor pollicis brevis
      Medial long branch to— 1. Extensor pollicis longus
                             2. Extensor indicis.
- **Terminal branches**—from 'pseudoganglion'
  All these are *articular branches* to:
  - Wrist joint
  - Distal radioulnar joint
  - Intercarpal joints
  - Intermetacarpal joints.

Clinical Anatomy
Posterior Interosseous Nerve Palsy
Causes
Posterior interosseous nerve may be compressed or entrapped in its course through supinator due to trauma or inflammation. It may be injured during surgical operation for exposure of head of the radius.
Effect
- Inability to extend the fingers at metacarpophalangeal joints
- Difficulty in extension and abduction of thumb.
- Weakness and radial deviation of wrist extension due to loss of function of extensor carpi ulnaris. Nerve supply of extensor carpi radialis longus and brevis is not affected.

Chapter 8

Elbow Joint and Radioulnar Joints

LA 8.1 Describe the elbow joint. Add a note on its movements and clinical anatomy.

ELBOW JOINT

Introduction

The elbow joint is a complex synovial joint between lower end of humerus and upper ends of radius and ulna. The joint is more complex because of following reasons:
- It includes two articulations as follows:
  - *Humeroulnar joint*: Articulation between the trochlea (pulley) of the humerus and the trochlear notch of the ulnat
  - *Humeroradial* joint: Articulation between the capitulum of humerus and the head of radius.
- Joint cavity of elbow joint communicates with the cavity of superior radioulnar joint.

Articular Surfaces

Articular surfaces are:
- Trochlea (pulley) and capitulum of humerus
- Trochlear notch of ulna
- Round and concave superior surface of head of radius.

All the articular surfaces are covered by hyaline articular cartilage.

The trochlea of humerus shows special design through more downward projection of its medial edge. Due to this reason, transverse axis of the joint passing side to side shows slight downward and medial inclination.

Trochlear notch of ulna is also not ideally designed for full congruence (full contact). Olecranon and coronoid parts of trochlear notch are separated by a narrow nonarticular strip.

Capitulum of the humerus and head of the radius are reciprocally curved.

Elbow joint is most congruent, therefore, it is the most stable joint of the body. The joint is most fully congruent when the forearm is positioned midway between pronation and supination position and is flexed at right angle.

Elbow joint is a **modified hinge joint** because the forward and backward swinging movement of the joint around the slightly oblique transverse axis is associated with conjunct rotation.

Fibrous Capsule

Fibrous capsule of elbow joint is lax and loose anteriorly and posteriorly. It is reinforced in both lateral and medial side by respective collateral ligaments.

Attachment of the capsule is somewhat complicated and is as follows:

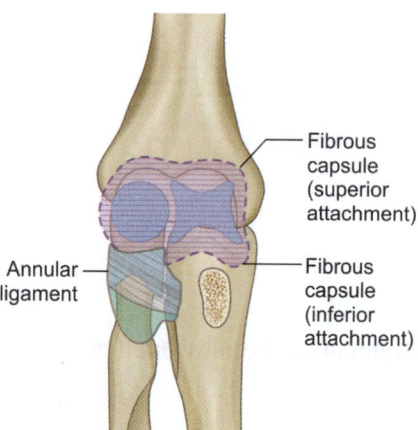

Fig. 8.1A: Fibrous capsule of elbow joint (anterior aspect).

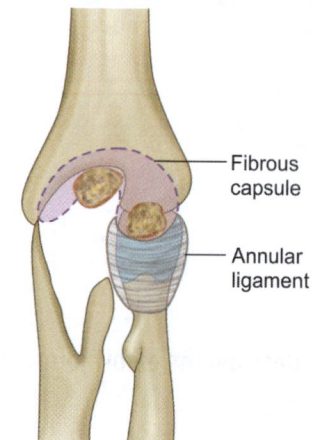

Fig. 8.1B: Fibrous capsule of elbow joint (posterior aspect).

Proximal Attachment
- *In front,* the fibrous capsule is attached on to the front of epicondyles on either side. In the middle, the line of attachment is extended over the superior aspect of radial and coronoid fossae beyond the superior margins of capitulum and trochlea **(Fig. 8.1A)**.
- *Behind,* the line of attachment of capsule extends from the back of epicondyles to the superior margin of olecranon fossa **(Fig. 8.1B)**.

Distal Attachment (Figs. 8.1A and B)
- *On the ulnar side,* the capsule is attached to the margins of olecranon and coronoid components of trochlear notch.
- *On the lateral side,* the capsule is attached to the superior margin of annular ligament of superior radioulnar joint which encircle the anterior, lateral and posterior aspects of circumference of head of the radius.

Some tendinous fibers of *brachialis* blends with anterior aspect of capsule. Its posterior aspect is overlapped by the tendon of *triceps brachii*.

Synovial membrane is attached to the margin of articular surfaces of the bones and it lines the intracapsular areas of humerus, namely the radial, coronoid and olecranon fossae but it does not cover the articular surfaces. Synovial membrane of elbow joint is continuous inferiorly with the synovial membrane of superior radioulnar joint.

Ligaments

The elbow joint is supported medially and laterally by the ulnar and radial collateral ligaments respectively.

Ulnar Collateral Ligament (Fig. 8.2)
- Ulnar collateral ligament is triangular in appearance with thick anterior, posterior and inferior bands connected by intermediate thin part.
- **Anterior band** is strongest and thick cord like. Its apex is attached to the front of medial epicondyle of humerus. Its distal basal end is attached to the tubercle on medial margin of coronoid process of ulna.

- **Posterior band** is broader and weaker. It extends from back of medial epicondyle to the medial margin of olecranon.
- **Inferior band** is oblique and is often weak, between olecranon and coronoid.
- The gap in between the three bands is filled up by a *thin intermediate part*.
- Ulnar collateral ligament is related to *flexor carpi ulnaris and ulnar nerve*.
- The ligament *gives origin to some fibers of flexor digitorum superficialis* between medial epicondyle and coronoid process.

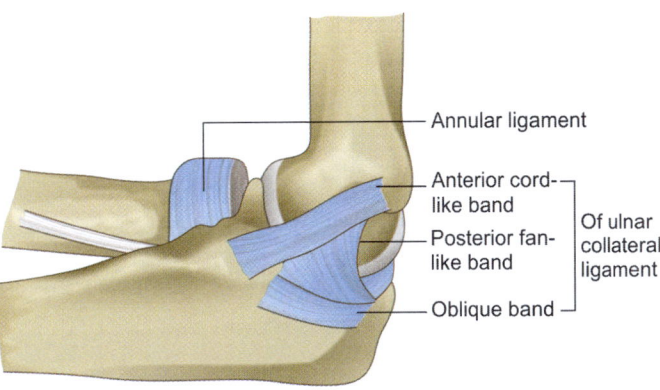

Fig. 8.2: Ulnar collateral ligament of elbow joint.

Radial Collateral Ligament (Fig. 8.3)

Radial collateral ligament is fan shaped on the lateral aspect of the joint. Its proximal apical end is attached to the inferior aspect of lateral epicondyle of humerus. Distal end widens to blend on the surface of annular ligament of superior radioulnar joint. Some of the fibers of the ligament are continued up to proximal end of the supinator crest of ulna. Supinator and extensor carpi radialis brevis partly originate from this ligament.

Relation of the Joint

- **Anteriorly:** Tendon of brachialis, Tendon of biceps brachii, brachial artery and median nerve.
- **Posteriorly:** Triceps brachii and anconeus
- **Laterally:** Common tendon of origin of extensor muscles, extensor carpi radialis brevis and supinator
- **Medially:** Common tendon of origin of flexor muscles, flexor carpi ulnaris and ulnar nerve.

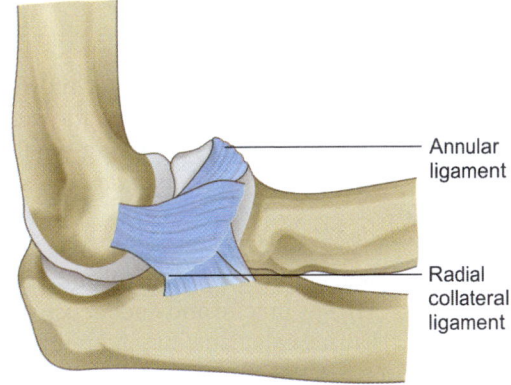

Fig. 8.3: Radial collateral ligament of elbow joint.

Arterial Supply

The elbow joint is supplied by arterial anastomosis around the joint which is contributed by following arteries:
- **In front of lateral epicondyle:**
  - Radial collateral artery
  - Radial recurrent artery.
- **Behind lateral epicondyle:**
  - Middle collateral artery
  - Interosseous recurrent artery.
- **In front of medial epicondyle:**
  - Inferior ulnar collateral artery
  - Anterior ulnar recurrent artery.

- **Behind medial epicondyle:**
    - Superior ulnar collateral artery
    - Posterior ulnar recurrent artery.

Nerve Supply
- **Chief source:**
    - Musculocutaneous nerve
    - Radial nerve.
- **Additional source:**
    - Median nerve
    - Ulnar nerve.
        Nerve to brachialis and *nerve to anconeus* give articular branches to the joint.

Factors Maintaining the Stability
- Full congruence of the articular surfaces
- Ulnar and radial collateral ligaments
- Muscles attached *close to the joint*, e.g. origin of common tendons of extensors laterally and flexors medially, brachialis and biceps in front and triceps behind.

Movements
As the elbow joint is uniaxial hinge joint, movements are *flexion and extension around the transverse axis*. The ulna moves on trochlea and the radial head moves on capitulum together. Flexion and extension of the joint is not a pure swing, but these are associated with *conjunct rotation*. The radius becomes slightly *pronated during extension* and *supinated during flexion*.

Muscles Producing Movements
Flexion: Brachialis, biceps brachii and, brachioradialis (in midprone position)
Extension: Triceps brachii and anconeus.
During extension, brachioradialis may come into function.

Clinical Anatomy
- **Posterior dislocation of elbow** may occur due to fracture of olecranon process of ulna. Anterior dislocation is prevented by the strong tendons of brachialis and biceps in front of the joint. In case of posterior dislocation of elbow, the normal triangular outline formed by tip of olecranon and two epicondyles is lost.
- **Effusion of elbow** due to trauma or infection causes swelling over the back of the elbow as the capsule of the joint is thin and loose posteriorly. Moreover the joint capsule is subcutaneous posteriorly.
- **Tennis elbow** is also known *as lateral epicondylitis*. It is characterized by pain over the lateral epicondyle of humerus during abrupt pronation of forearm. Causes of tennis elbow may be any of the following:
    - Tear of the fibers of common extensors arising from lateral epicondyle
    - Tear of fibers of extensor carpi radialis brevis only.
    - Sprain of radial collateral ligament of elbow joint.
    - Inflammation of the bursa beneath extensor carpi radialis brevis.
- **Student's elbow** results from the inflammation of the subcutaneous bursa over the posterior surface of olecranon. Patient presents a soft painful swelling over the back of olecranon.
- **Compression of nerves around the elbow** is found very often as these nerves, while crossing the elbow, are either related to the surface of bone (ulnar nerve) or the fibromuscular arch (median

nerve or deep branch of radial nerve). Clinical presentations are pain, loss of function of the muscles supplied by the nerve and even wasting (atrophy) of the muscles.

SA 8.2 Write a brief note on the superior radioulnar joint.

PROXIMAL (SUPERIOR) RADIOULNAR JOINT (SEE FIG. 8.1)

Introduction

Proximal or superior radioulnar joint is a *pivot type of synovial joint* between the upper ends of radius and ulna.

Articulating Surfaces (Fig. 8.4)

- **Pivot:** It is the smooth circumferential surface of head of radius.
- **Ring:** It is an osseofibrous ring having two parts.
  - *Osseous (bony) part (1/5th)* is formed by a depressed articular surface at lateral aspect of upper end of ulna called *radial notch* which fits with medial aspect of head of radius.
  - *Fibrous part (4/5th)* is formed by annular ligament which encircle posterior, lateral and anterior aspect of head of radius.

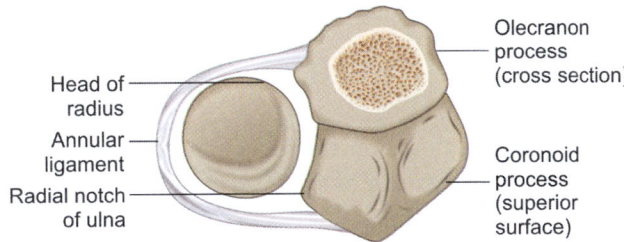

Fig. 8.4: Annular ligament and articular surfaces of proximal (superior) radioulnar joint.

All the above-mentioned articulating surfaces are covered by thin layer of hyaline cartilage.

Axis of the joint passes vertically through the center of head of radius. Head of radius (pivot) rotates around this axis within the ring.

Fibrous Capsule of the Joint

It is the fibrous capsule of the elbow joint which is continued down to enclose superior radioulnar joint. It is attached below to the annular ligament (*see* **Fig. 8.1**).

Synovial membrane of the joint lines not only the fibrous capsule but also the annular ligament and it is continuous with the synovial membrane of the elbow joint.

Ligaments of the Joint

Annular ligament (*see* **Figs. 8.2 to 8.4**) is a strong circular fibrous band forming the 4/5th of the osseofibrous ring of the joint. It encircles the head of radius and is attached to the anterior and posterior margins of the radial notch of ulna which form the 1/5th of the ring. Upper margin of annular ligament fuses with the capsular ligament of elbow joint. The circumference of the ligament fitting as a tight collar round the radial head helps in secured rotation of the head of the bone. Lower part of annular ligament is narrow and it encircles loosely the neck of radius.

Synovial membrane is continuous below the annular ligament over the neck of radius as the *sacciform recess*.

Quadrate ligament is a small thin quadrangular fibrous band, disposed horizontally from lower margin of radial notch of ulna to medial aspect of neck of the radius.

Relations of the Joint

Anterolaterally: *Supinator muscle* and terminal end of *radial nerve* dividing into superficial and deep divisions.

Posteriorly: *Anconeus muscle*.

Arterial Supply

- Arterial supply of the joint is derived from the lateral side of anastomosis around elbow. The main arteries are following:
  - *In front*: Anastomosis between radial collateral and radial recurrent arteries.
  - *Behind*: Anastomosis between middle collateral and interosseous recurrent arteries.

Nerve Supply

Articular branches of musculocutaneous, radial and median nerves supply the proximal radioulnar joint.

Movements

Supination and pronation, the rotatory movements of the joint, are described below. *(For detailed movements and clinical anatomy—vide answer of Question No. 8.4)*

SN 8.3 Write a short note on the antebrachial interosseous membrane.

INTEROSSEOUS MEMBRANE (FIG. 8.5)

Introduction

Interosseous membrane of the forearm is known as *antebrachial interosseous membrane* which acts as an elongated and flattened ligament of *radioulnar syndesmosis*.

Attachments

Lateral

From interosseous border or medial (ulnar) border of shaft of radius. This attachment extends upwards up to the level of 2.5 cm below the radial tuberosity. Distally, this attachment extends up to lower end of radius along the posterior margin of medial triangular surface of lower end of the bone.

Medial

To the radial (lateral) or interosseous border of shaft of ulna. Below, the attachment extends up to the lower end of the ulna.

Direction of Fibers

The fibers are directed downwards and medially from radius to ulna. Above the free upper margin of the membrane, a gap exist between the two bones.

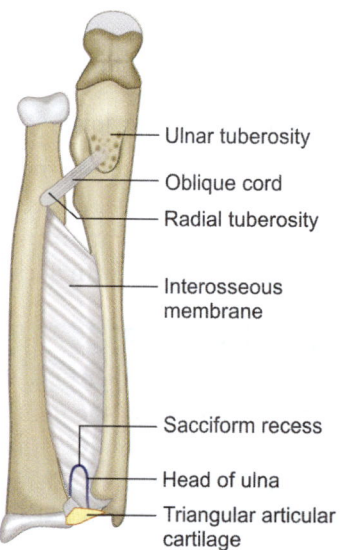

Fig. 8.5: Distal (inferior) radioulnar joint and interosseous membrane.

Surfaces
- Anterior or flexor surface
- Posterior or extensor surface.

Relations and Attachments of the Surfaces
Anterior Surface
- It gives origin to flexor pollicis longus, flexor digitorum profundus and pronator quadratus.
- Anterior surface is related to anterior interosseous artery and nerve.

Posterior Surface
- From the posterior surface of interosseous membrane muscles originating are—abductor pollicis longus, extensor pollicis brevis, extensor pollicis longus and extensor indicis.
- It is related to posterior interosseous nerve and artery.
- Lower part of the posterior surface is in relation with the terminal part of anterior interosseous artery which *pierces the membrane* to go backwards.

Functions of Interosseous Membrane
- The membrane binds the shafts of radius and ulna.
- Oblique direction of fibers of the membrane transmits the force downwards and medially from radius to ulna when the limb is supported through the hand.
- It provides the surface for attachment of muscles.

Oblique Cord
It is a cord like fibrous band which extends from the medial aspect of ulnar tuberosity to the lower end of radial tuberosity. The band is directed downwards and laterally, i.e. opposite to the direction of fibers of interosseous membrane.

Structures passing through the gap between oblique cord and upper margin of interosseous membrane is *posterior interosseous artery* arising from common interosseous artery.

Morphologically the oblique cord represents the degenerated part of *flexor pollicis longus.*

SA 8.4 Write a brief note on the pronation and supination movements of the forearm.

PRONATION AND SUPINATION
Pronation and supination are the rotational movements of forearm occurring at the *radioulnar joint complex*. This rotational movement occurs between the head of ulna and ulnar notch of radius below and between the head of radius and radial notch of ulna above.

In pronation, the radius along with the hand turns *anteromedially and obliquely across the ulna*, so that the proximal end of the radius remains lateral, but the *distal end becomes medial to ulna*. During this movement, *the fibers of interosseous membrane becomes spiralled*.

In supination, the radius goes back to the position lateral and parallel to the ulna and the fibers of the interosseous membrane becomes *unspiralled*.

The axis of pronation and supination is an oblique line which passes proximally through the radial head and distally through the site of ulnar attachment of the triangular articular disk on a small depression between the head and styloid process of ulna. Truly, this is the line of axis of movement of radius relative to ulna. The radial head rotates within the osseofibrous ring spinning on the capitulum of the humerus and its lower end and the triangular articular disk swing round the ulnar head.

Movement of the hand is associated with the pronation and supination of forearm. The palm of the hand turns backwards in pronation and forwards in supination. When the elbow is extended, the hand can be turned through 140° to 150°. This can be increased up to 360° by humeral rotation and scapular movement. *Power is greater in pronation* and it becomes evident when the nuts, bolts and screws are tightened by right handed persons.

Clinical Anatomy

Subluxation (incomplete dislocation) or **'pulled elbow'** is a common complication among the preschool children. It occurs when a child is suddenly lifted up by pulling the upper limb in pronated position of forearm. It displaces the radial head due to tear in lower loose part of anular ligament of superior radioulnar joint. Sublaxation may finally pull the radial head upwards out of the annular ligament due to muscular contraction.

Chapter 9

Hand

SN 9.1 Write a short note on flexor retinaculum of hand.

FLEXOR RETINACULUM OF HAND

Introduction

Flexor retinaculum is a strong fibrous band which *crosses in front of the carpal bones* in the proximal end of the hand *distal to the wrist joint*.

Its proximal margin corresponds to the level of *distal dominant skin crease* in front of wrist.

- **Measurement**: 2–3 cm both transversely as well as longitudinally.
- **Attachments:** Main attachment of flexor retinaculum is at the following four prominence of carpal bones.
  Laterally:
  1. Tubercle of scaphoid
  2. Crest of trapezium.
  Medially:
  1. Pisiform
  2. Hook of hamate bone.

Proximally the flexor retinaculum blends with the deep fascia of the forearm and *distally*. It is continuous with the palmar aponeurosis.

Formation of Carpal Tunnel (Figs. 9.1A and B)

Palmar aspect of articulated carpal bones presents a forward concavity which is bridged ventrally by the band of flexor retinaculum. The retinaculum, along with the concavity of the carpal bones forms a osseofibrous tunnel called *carpal tunnel*. The space within the carpal tunnel is overcrowded by the flexor tendons with their synovial sheath and some of the nerves and vessels for the palm.

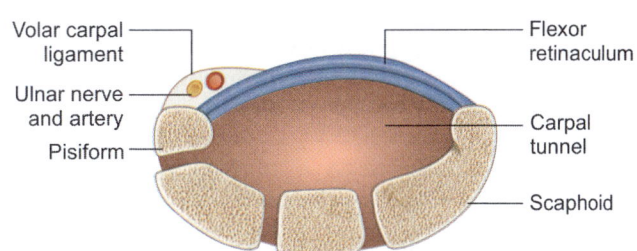

Fig. 9.1A: Carpal tunnel with medial accessory slip of flexor retinaculum.

Accessory Slips of Retinaculum (Figs. 9.1A and B)

Both the lateral and the medial sides of flexor retinaculum send accessory slip as follows:

- **Medial slip** is *superficial*. This slip is called **volar carpal ligament**. It sweeps over the ulnar artery and ulnar nerve and is attached to the pisiform bone along with the main band. The

space between the superficial slip and medial end of main band of the retinaculum is called *canal of Guyon* inside which the ulnar nerve may be compressed occasionally.
- **Lateral slip** *is deep*. It is attached to the medial ridge of the groove on palmar aspect of trapezium. An osseofibrous tunnel thus formed transmits the tendon of flexor carpi radialis.

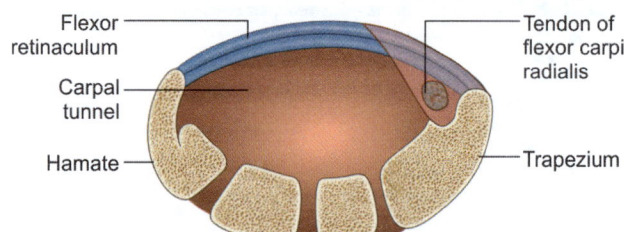

Fig. 9.1B: Carpal tunnel with lateral accessory slip of flexor retinaculum.

Structures Attached to the Retinaculum

- Tendon of *palmaris longus* is attached to the proximal border and adjacent part of palmar surface of the flexor retinaculum.
- Proximal apical end of triangular *palmar aponeurosis* is attached to the distal border.
- Muscles of thenar and hypothenar eminences originate partly from the lateral and medial side of the retinaculum respectively.

Relations

Superficial Relations (Medial to Lateral)

- Ulnar nerve end ulnar artery
- Palmar cutaneous branch of the ulnar nerve
- Tendon of palmaris longus
- Palmar cutaneous branch of the median nerve
- Superficial palmar branch of the radial artery

Deep Relations

- Median nerve
- Tendon of flexor pollicis longus
- Four tendinous bands of flexor digitorum superficialis
- Four tendinous slips of flexor digitorum profundus.

Functions

- Flexor retinaculum of hand acts as a *natural wrist band* to protect the structures crossing the wrist deep to it.
- As it is called retinaculum, it guards the flexor tendons passing deep to it to *prevent their bow-stringing* displacement during contractions.

Clinical Anatomy

Carpal tunnel syndrome is a clinical condition due to compression of median nerve within the rigid osseofibrous tunnel tightly packed by flexor tendons with their synovial sheath. The condition is characterized by burning sensation of skin of lateral side of palm supplied by the median nerve.

SA 9.2 Write a brief note on palmar aponeurosis.

PALMAR APONEUROSIS (FIG. 9.2)

Introduction

Palmar aponeurosis is the condensed and thickened deep fascia over the central hollow of the palm. It provides additional protection for the blood vessels and nerves of the palm lying beneath it. Laterally and medially palmar aponeurosis merges with the deep fascia over thenar and hypothenar muscles.

Shape and Extent

It is triangular in outline with its apex directed towards the flexor retinaculum and base towards the distal end of the palm.

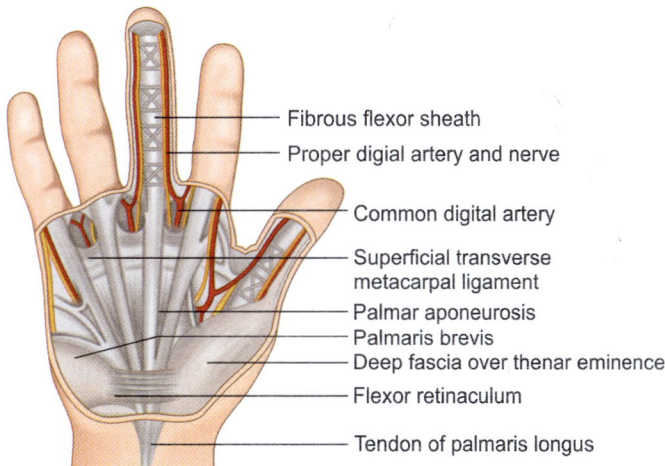

Fig. 9.2: Palmar aponeurosis.

Planes of Fibers

Palmar aponeurosis is composed of the following two planes of fibers:
1. **Superficial longitudinal fibers**
   - Proximal end of longitudinal fibers is continuous with the fibers of tendon of palmaris longus crossing over and fusing with the fibers of flexor retinaculum.
   - Distally the longitudinal fibers divides into four bands for medial four fingers. Each of the bands is continuous distally with the fibers of fibrous flexor sheath of respective fingers.
2. **Deep transverse fibers** interconnect the distal end of longitudinal slips of the palmar aponeurosis. Here these fibers form *superficial transverse metacarpal ligament* at the level of heads of the metacarpal bones.

   Deeper fibers of transverse lamina pass to connect heads of metacarpal bones as *deep transverse metacarpal ligament*.

Apex of the palmar aponeurosis blends with the superficial surface of flexor retinaculum. Proximal to the retinaculum the fibers of the palmar aponeurosis are also continuous with the thin tendon of palmaris longus. This interrelation establishes the view that morphologically palmar aponeurosis represents the spread out distal part of tendon of palmaris longus continued beyond the superficial surface of flexor retinaculum.

Base of the palmar aponeurosis extends distally up to the level of distal palmar crease where it splits into four slips to extend up to the base of medial four fingers. Each of the slips divides into two collaterals which fuse with the proximal end of fibrous flexor sheath of the corresponding digit.

Margins of the palmar aponeurosis are lateral and medial, which fuse with the thinner deep fascia over thenar and hypothenar eminence respectively. Medial margin gives *origin to palmaris brevis muscle*.

Palmar fascial septa are medial, lateral and intermediate. *Medial palmar septum* connects the medial margin of palmar aponeurosis with the palmar surface of shaft of fifth metacarpal bone.

Lateral palmar septum passes from lateral margin of the aponeurosis to the palmar surface of shaft of first metacarpal bone. Intermediate palmar septum connects the deep surface of palmar aponeurosis with the palmar surface of shaft of third metacarpal bone.

Functions
- Thick and condensed fibrous sheet of palmar aponeurosis protects underlying blood vessels, nerves and tendons.
- Due to its fixation with the skin, the palmar aponeurosis improves the firmness of the grip of the hand.

Clinical Anatomy
Progressive increase of fibrous tissue in the medial part of palmar aponeurosis causes shortening (*contracture*) of this part. The condition is known as **Dupuytren's contracture.** It causes *flexion deformity* (bending) of little and ring fingers. Surgical incision through the shortened part of the aponeurosis (*fasciotomy*) may be required to normalize the bent fingers.

SA 9.3 Discuss briefly the fibrous flexor sheath of fingers.

FIBROUS FLEXOR SHEATH OF FINGERS (FIG. 9.3)

Introduction
Fibrous flexor sheaths are deep fascial encasing on the palmar aspect of flexor tendon in each finger. Along with the palmar aspect of the phalanges and interphalangeal joint, the sheath forms an osseofibrous tunnel for smooth passage of digital slip of flexor tendons along with their respective synovial sheath.

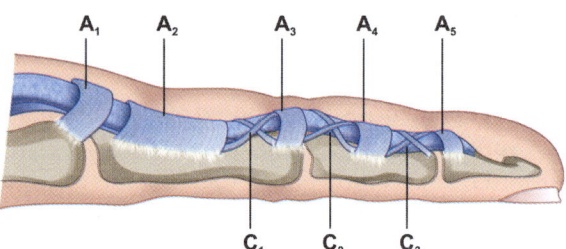

Fig. 9.3: Components of fibrous flexor sheath of fingers.

Functions
- As already stated, the fibrous flexor sheath takes part in formation of smooth osseofibrous tunnel for passage of digital slip of flexor tendons.
- During flexion of the fingers, fibrous flexor sheath holds the digital tendon in proper position.

Extent
From the head of metacarpal bone to the base of terminal phalanx.

Attachments
- Head of metacarpal bone
- Sides of proximal and middle phalanges
- Palmar ligaments of interphalangeal joints
- Base of terminal phalanx.

Parts (Fig. 9.3)
Basically, the fibrous flexor sheath is composed of following two types of fibers:
1. **Annular fibers (A fibers):** These are attached to the sides of the bones (metacarpal heads and phalanges).

2. **Cruciform fibers (C fibers):** These are attached to the sides of palmar ligaments of interphalangeal joints.

   These two kinds of fibers are further subdivided as follows **(Fig. 9.3):**
   - *A1 fibers*: Attached to the sides of heads of metacarpal and base of proximal phalanx.
   - *A2 fibers*: Attached to the sides of shaft of proximal phalanx
   - *A3 fibers:* Attached to the sides of head of proximal phalanx
   - *A4 fibers*: Attached to the sides of shaft of middle phalanx
   - *A5 fibers*: Attached to the sides of base of distal phalanx.
   - *C1 fibers*: Attached to the *proximal end* of *proximal interphalangeal joint*
   - *C2 fibers*: Attached to the *distal end* of *proximal interphalangeal joint*
   - *C3 fibers*: Attached to *the proximal end of distal interphalangeal joint.*

Clinical Anatomy

Trigger Finger

Normally, flexor tendons move smoothly within the osseofibrous tunnel formed by fibrous flexor sheath on the palmar aspect of phalanges. Thickening of fibrous flexor sheath or localized thickening of flexor tendon interferes with the free movement of the tendon within the tunnel. When forceful or passive flexion and subsequent extension of the finger is attempted, it is leads to a sudden audible 'click' or 'snap'. This condition is named as *'trigger finger'* or *'snapping finger'*.

SA 9.4 Classify intrinsic muscles of the hand. Write a brief note on thenar and hypothenar muscles.

INTRINSIC MUSCLES OF THE HAND

Intrinsic muscles of the hand are so called because each of these small muscles are *confined within the palm of hand.* They are 20 in number (4 × 5). Each of the 5 groups comprises 4 muscles. The groups are as follows:

A. **Thenar muscles (4 = 3 + 1):** *All are the muscles of thumb (pollex).* They are as follows:
   a. *3 superficial*
      i. One short abductor of thumb
      ii. One short flexor of thumb
      iii. One for opposition of the thumb (for approximation of tip of thumb to the tips of other fingers)
   b. *1 deep* = Adductor of thumb.
B. **Hypothenar muscles (4 = 1 + 3)**
   a. *1 superficial* = Palmaris brevis
   b. *3 deep* = For little finger
      i. One short abductor
      ii. One short flexor
      iii. One for opposition, as in thumb.
C. **4 lumbrical muscles** are short slender muscles ending in thin tendon. They are related to four slips of tendon of flexor digitorum profundus.
D. **4 palmar interossei** = Present in intermetacarpal space
E. **4 dorsal interossei** = Present in intermetacarpal space.

Thenar Muscles

Name of the muscles	Origin	Insertion	Actions
Abductor pollicis brevis	• Tubercle of scaphoid • Crest of trapezium • Flexor retinaculum	Lateral side of base of proximal phalanx of thumb	Abduction of the thumb
Flexor pollicis brevis	**Superficial head** • Crest of trapezium • Flexor retinaculum **Deep head** • Trapezoid • Capitate	United tendon is inserted to the lateral side of base of proximal phalanx of thumb	Flexor of the thumb
Opponens pollicis	• Crest of trapezium • Flexor retinaculum	Lateral half of palmar surface of 1st metacarpal bone	Opposition of thumb for making its tip to be in contact with tips of other fingers
Adductor pollicis (It is deep seated)	**Oblique head** • Capitate • Bases of 2nd and 3rd metacarpal bone **Transvers head** Palmar surface of shaft of 3rd metacarpal bone	Common tendon of two heads is inserted into medial side of base of proximal phalanx of thumb	Adduction of thumb used for gripping

Nerve Supply

By median nerve. Flexor pollicis brevis may receive an additional supply from the deep branch of ulnar nerve.

Hypothenar Muscles

Name of the muscles	Origin	Insertion	Actions
Palmaris brevis (*subcutaneous muscle*)	• Flexor retinaculum • Apical part of palmar aponeurosis (medial side)	Deep surface of skin of medial margin of hypothenar eminence	Improves the grip of hand
Abductor digiti minimi	• Pisiform bone • Pisohamate ligament • Tendon of flexor carpi ulnaris	Medial side of base of proximal phalanx of little finger	Abduction of little finger moving it away from ring finger
Flexor digiti minimi	• Hook of hamate • Flexor retinaculum	Medial side of base of proximal phalanx of little finger	Flexion of little finger at metacarpophalangeal joint
Opponens digiti minimi	• Hook of hamate • Flexor retinaculum	Medial side of shaft of palmar surface of 5th metacarpal bone	Deepening of hollow of palm by opposition of tip of little finger to the tip of thumb

Nerve Supply

Palmaris brevis is supplied by the superficial branch of ulnar nerve. The deep branch of the nerve supplies the other three muscles.

SA 9.5 Write a note on the synovial sheath of flexor tendons. Add a note on its clinical anatomy.

SYNOVIAL SHEATH OF FLEXOR TENDONS (FIGS. 9.4A AND B)

While the long flexor tendons of the digits cross over the wrist, palm and fingers, they invaginate the elongated thin-walled fibroserous membranous sacs which form the synovial sheath of the flexor tendons. Due to invagination by the tendon, a synovial sheath forms one *visceral layer* and one *parietal layer* which are continuous with each other through a *mesotendon*. Through the line of mesotendon, blood vessels reach to the tendon.

In between two layers of the synovial sheath, a very thin amount of lubricating fluid prevents the friction of the tendons which are always subjected to the stress and strain.

Flexor synovial sheaths are classified as follows:
1. Synovial sheath for tendon of flexor pollicis longus named as *Radial bursa*.
2. Common synovial sheath for tendons of flexor digitorum superficialis and flexor digitorum profundus known as *ulnar bursa*.
3. *Digital synovial sheaths of the fingers.*

Radial Bursa (Fig. 9.4A)

It is the synovial sheath which covers the tendon of flexor pollicis longus while it passes from the level a little above the flexor retinaculum up to its site of insertion.

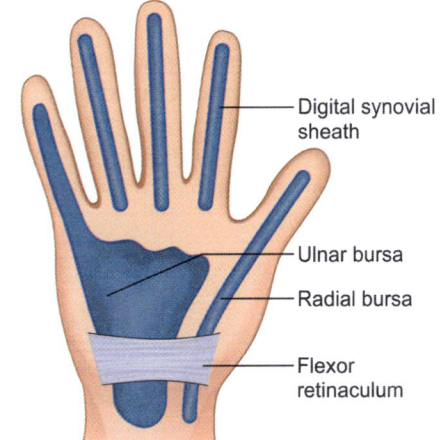

Fig. 9.4A: Synovial sheath of flexor tendons.

Extent

It extends *proximally* 2.5 cm above the flexor retinaculum and *distally* up to the base of terminal phalanx of thumb.

Ulnar Bursa (Fig. 9.4A)

It is the synovial sheath common for all the tendon slips of flexor digitorum superficialis and flexor digitorum profundus. The sheath is invaginated from its lateral side by the tendons.

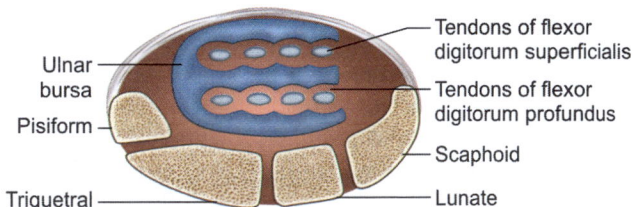

Fig. 9.4B: Synovial sheath related to flexor tendons seen on cross section.

Extent

The ulnar bursa extends *proximally* 2.5 cm above the flexor retinaculum.

Distally, the extent of the ulnar bursa shows following two characteristics:
1. For the both superficial and profundus tendons of little finger the ulnar bursa extends up to the site of insertion of the tendon of profundus at the *base of terminal phalanx of little finger.*
2. Sheath around the tendon slips for index, middle and ring finger extends *up to the midlevel of the palm* where it *ends in a blind sac.*
   Occasionally radial and ulnar bursa may communicate beneath the flexor retinaculum.

Digital Synovial Sheath (Fig. 9.4A)

These are the synovial sheaths which enclose the flexor tendons in the fingers extending *from the level of head of metacarpal bone* to the *base of distal phalanx*.

Digital synovial sheaths are disposed *within the fibrous flexor sheaths*. These are of following three types:
1. Digital synovial sheath *for the thumb is continuation of the radial bursa.*
2. Digital synovial sheath *for the little finger is the extension of the ulnar bursa.*
3. The similar digital sheaths for index, middle and ring fingers are *independent*. Each of them extends from the head of metacarpal bone to the base of terminal phalanx of respective finger.

Vincula of the Tendons (Fig. 9.5)

As the flexor tendons glide within the fibrous flexor sheath, they require special arrangement for blood supply. These blood vessels reach the distal parts of the tendons through the *thin synovial folds with networks of delicate connective tissue fibers* which are called **vincula tendinum**. They are of following two types:
1. **Vincula brevia** are smaller and triangular in appearance. They are *two in number in each finger,* one for the superficial flexor tendon and one for deep flexor tendon. They extend from the deep surface of tendon at the site of insertion to the palmar aspect of interphalangeal joint close to the site of insertion.
2. **Vincula longa** are thiner and more elongated. Two from the superficials and one from the profundus tendon are attached to the palmar aspect of proximal parts of proximal and middle phalanges respectively.

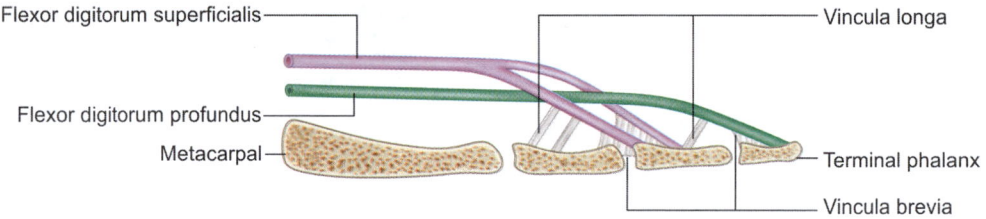

Fig. 9.5: Insertion of digital slips of common flexor tendon.

Clinical Anatomy

Tenosynovitis is the clinical condition characterized by inflammation of the synovial sheath of the flexor tendons which are deeply seated in the palm. It is a very painful condition. Prick in the tip of little finger may give rise to inflammation of the ulnar bursa resulting in a painful swelling on the hollow of the palm. Inflammation of the radial bursa due to pricking injury to the tip of the thumb causes painful swelling over the thenar eminence.

SN 9.6 Write a short note on the lumbrical muscles.

LUMBRICAL MUSCLES (FIG. 9.6)

General Points
- Lumbrical muscles are four thin elongated muscle ending in thin tendon.
- These muscles are four in number. They are numbered as 1st, 2nd, 3rd and 4th from lateral to medial.

- Their origins are adhered to the four slips of tendon of flexor digitorum profundus.
- 'Lumbrical' is a latin ward which means earthworm. The muscles are so called because they look like elongated worms.

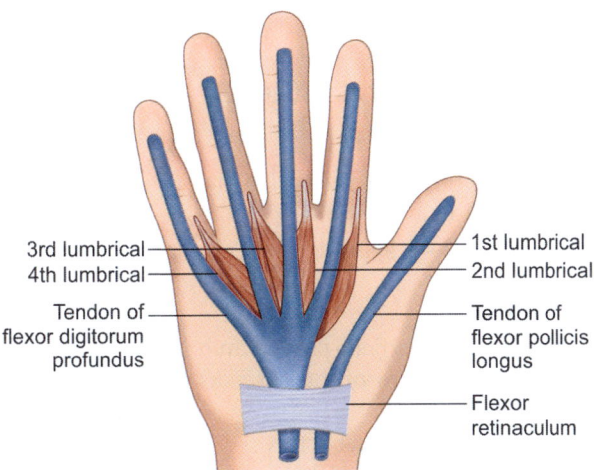

Fig. 9.6: Lumbrical muscles.

Origin

1st and 2nd lumbricals are *unipennate in origin* and *3rd and 4th lumbricals are bipennate in origin*. All originate from the tendons of flexor digitorum profundus.

1st lumbrical arises from radial (lateral) side of the *tendon for index finger*.

2nd lumbrical arises form radial (lateral) side of the *tendon for middle finger*.

3rd lumbrical arises from adjoining sides of the *tendons for middle and ring fingers*.

4th lumbrical arises from the adjoining sides of *tendons for ring and little fingers*.

Insertion

Each of the tendons passes across the lateral side of corresponding metacarpophalangeal joint and is *inserted into the radial (lateral) side* of the dorsal digital expansion on the dorsal aspect of corresponding fingers.

Nerve Supply

First and second lumbricals receive nerve supply from **the median nerve**. *Third and fourth lumbricals* are innervated by **the deep branch of ulnar nerve**.

Actions

Lumbrical muscles result in flexion of metacarpophalangeal joint and extension of both interphalangeal joints of respective finger through their attachment in dorsal digital expansion.

Clinical Anatomy

A narrow fascial canal around the slender tendon of each lumbrical muscle extends up to the site of insertion. These are called **lumbrical canals**. 1st lumbrical canal extends from lateral palmar fascial space (thenar space) to the radial side of base of index finger. 2nd, 3rd and 4th lumbrical canals connect the medial palmar fascial space (midpalmar space) with the web spaces between the bases of medial four finger. So infection from web spaces can spread through the lumbrical canals to the deep seated palmar spaces.

SN 9.7 Write a short note on the superficial palmar arch.

SUPERFICIAL PALMAR ARCH (FIG. 9.7)

Introduction
It is *the superficial arterial arch* of the palm formed almost entirely by the ulnar artery in the palm.

Formation
Formation of superficial palmar arch occurs in one third of the cases as one of the following:
- Entirely by the ulnar artery
- Superficial palmar branch of radial artery joining the ulnar artery
- Arteria radialis indicis, arteria princeps pollicis or median artery uniting with the ulnar artery.

Situation
Superficial palmar arch shows distal convexity and is situated at the level of distal border of fully extended thumb.

Relations
The arterial arch lies **deep to** *palmaris brevis muscle and palmar aponeurosis.* It passes from medial to lateral **superficial to** *flexor digiti minimi, branches of median nerve, flexor tendons and lumbricals.*

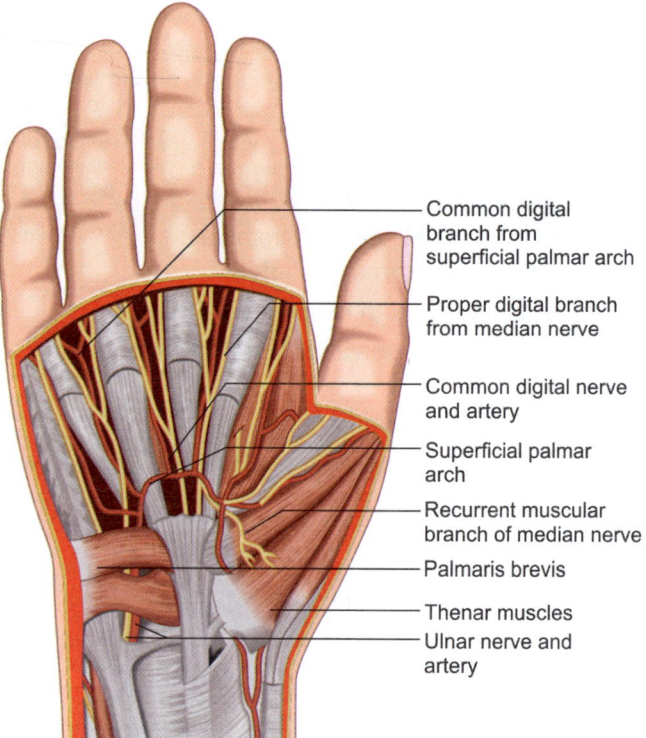

Fig. 9.7: Superficial arteries and nerves of the palm.

Branches
- **Common palmar digital arteries** are three in number which originate from the corvex side of the superficial palmar arch:
  - They run distally superficial to the 2nd, 3rd and 4th lumbrical muscles.
  - Reaching the level of respective interdigital cleft between the medial four fingers, they are *joined by the corresponding palmar metacarpal arteries* which arise from deep palmar arch.
  - Finally, each of the three common palmar digital arteries bifurcates **into two proper palmar digital arteries** which run along the contiguous sides of the adjacent fingers.
- **Proper palmar digital artery for the medial side of little finger** takes origin directly from the medial end of superficial palmar arch.
- **Proper palmar digital arteries for the radial side of index finger and both the sides of thumb** are called **arteria radialis indicis** and **arteria princeps pollicis** respectively. These arteries usually arise from the terminal part of radial artery while the later enters the palm from the dorsum of hand. These two proper digital arteries may **occasionally arise from the lateral end of superficial palmar arch**.

Distribution of Proper Palmar Digital Artery

Each proper palmar digital artery runs distally along the side of finger dorsal to the proper digital nerve. Each of these arteries gives **two dorsal branches** *which anastomose with dorsal digital artery* and supply the dorsum of finger opposite the middle and terminal phalanges including the nail bed. Apart from the soft tissue of palmar aspect of fingers, the palmar digital artery also supplies metacarpophalangeal and interphalangeal joints.

Two proper palmar digital arteries of each finger from both sides of finger anastomose with each other at the level of interphalangeal joints and in the subcutaneous tissue of finger tips. Terminal branches of digital arteries form a number of vascular arcades which provide a rich vascular supply to the distal part of the fingers.

SA 9.8 Write a brief note on the interossei muscles of hand.

INTEROSSEI MUSCLES OF HAND

- Interossei of the hand are the deepest sets of muscles. They are so called because they occupy the intervals between adjacent metacarpal bones.
- Interossei muscles are divided into 4 palmar and 4 dorsal sets out of 20 (5 sets × 4) intrinsic muscles of hand.

Palmar Interossei (Fig. 9.8)

- They are four in number and are numbered serially from lateral to medial side.
- The palmar interossei are unipennate in origin.
- They arise from the palmar surface of shaft of metacarpals rather than lying in the intervals between the two.

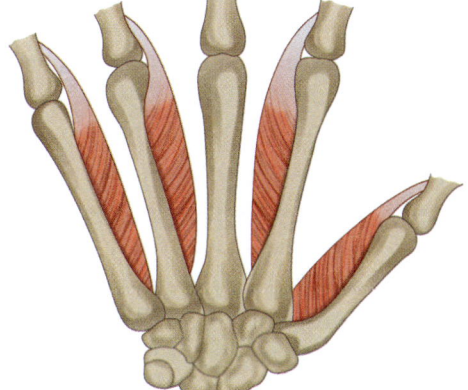

Fig. 9.8: Palmar interossei (right side—palmar view).

Third metacarpal out of the five, **does not give origin to any palmar interosseous**.

Considering the axis passing through the long axis of 3rd metacarpal, all the palmar interossei take origin from *adductor side* of palmar surface of 1st, 2nd, 4th and 5th metacarpal bones. *First palmar interosseous is occasionally less developed.*

Insertion of the tendon of each interosseous is **on the adductor side of dorsal digital expansion** (extensor expansion) of respective finger.

Dorsal Interossei (Fig. 9.9)

All the four dorsal interossei are bipennate muscles. Each of them arise from adjacent sides of two metacarpals extending proximally up to their bases, the tendons of their *insertion converge towards the hand axis* passing through the third metacarpal bone. So each of the tendons *is inserted into the abductor side* of base of proximal phalanx as well as dorsal digital expansion of corresponding finger. So proximal

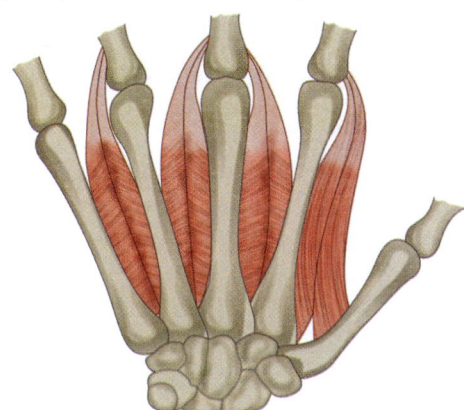

Fig. 9.9: Dorsal interossei (right side—palmar view).

phalanx of **middle fingers gives insertion to the two dorsal interossei,** the second on the radial side and the third on the ulnar side (**Fig. 9.9**).

Nerve Supply of the Interossei

All the palmar as well as dorsal interossei are supplied by **deep branch of ulnar nerve** carrying fibers from C_8 **and** T_1 segments of spinal cord.

In addition, **the first dorsal interossei is occasionally supplied** by an additional branch from **recurrent muscular branch of median nerve** in the palm.

Actions of Interossei

Before the actions of the interossei are to be understood, a fundamental point of abduction and abduction of finger is to be clarified. The types of movements are considered in relation to the axis passing through the center of middle finger. From the **Figures 9.8 and 9.9**, it is clear that four *palmar interossei are inserted away from the axis with none of these attached to the middle finger.* It means that their insertions are divergent from the axis. Again, the dorsal interossei are convergent towards the axis with two of them inserted to the middle finger, one from either side.

Therefore palmar interossei adduct the medial two (ring and little) and lateral two (thumb and index finger) fingers towards the axis of middle finger. Again the dorsal interssei abduct these fingers away from the same axis.

Action through extensor expansion: Along with the lumbrical inserted on the radial side of corresponding finger, the interossei on the radial or ulnar side (both sides in the middle finger), through the extensor expansion or dorsal digital expansion, leads to flexion of metacarpophalangeal joints and extension of interphalangeal joints. The movement pattern is very useful for *precision grip* (writing and buttoning a cloth) and *pinch grip*.

Clinical Anatomy

Paralysis of the interossei due to lesion of C_8, T_1 fibers for central cause (Klumpke paralysis) or peripheral injury of median and ulnar nerves results in 'claw-hand'. The deformity is manifested by extension of metacarpophalangeal joint and flexion of interphalangeal joints.

LA 9.9 Discuss briefly the distributions of the median nerve and ulnar nerve in the palm of the hand.

MEDIAN NERVE IN THE PALM (*SEE* FIG. 9.7)

Entry in Palm

To enter the palm of hand, the median nerve passes deep to the flexor retinaculum *in the carpal tunnel* where it may be compressed on rare occasion. Distal to the retinaculum the nerve becomes *thickened* and *flattened*. It divides to end into five to six branches. The *nature and level of division are variable.*

Palmar Cutaneous Branch

It takes origin 3 cm proximal to the flexor retinaculum. It divides into lateral and medial branches. *The lateral division* supplies the skin over thenar eminence and communicates with the distal end of the lateral cutaneous nerve of the forearm. *The medial division* supplies skin over central part of palm and joins with the palmar cutaneous branch of ulnar nerve.

Motor (Recurrent) Branch

It is a short thick branch which arises from the lateral aspect of median nerve just below the flexor retinaculum with a *slight recurrent course*. It gives branches to *flexor pollicis brevis, abductor pollicis brevis* and *opponens pollicis*. Occasionally, it is found to give a branch to the *first dorsal interosseous*.

The motor (recurrent) branch of median nerve often may arise in the carpal tunnel and then pierces the flexor retinaculum.

Palmar Digital Branches

After giving the recurrent muscular branch, the median nerve divides into lateral and medial palmar branches. The usual distributions of these two divisions are as follows:
1. **Lateral palmar division** usually gives rise to into **three proper digital branches** which supply both sides of the thumb and the radial side of index finger. The branch to the radial (lateral) side of index finger sends a **nerve to the first lumbrical**.
2. **Medial palmar division** divides into **two common digital nerves** which run distally in between the slips of flexor tendons. The lateral branch bifurcates into two proper digital nerves for *adjacent sides of index and middle fingers*. Proper digital nerves from medial division supply *adjacent sides of middle and ring fingers*.

So, ultimately it is seen that palmar surface of lateral three fingers and a half receives innervation from digital branches of median nerve.

Proper palmar **digital nerve for radial (lateral) side of middle finger** gives out **branch to second lumbrical**.

Beyond the base of terminal phalanx, each digital nerve gives off a **dorsal branch** which runs dorsally to supply the corresponding half of the **nail bed** of the respective fingers.

Other Branches

Besides the muscular (recurrent) branch and digital branches, the median nerve gives out **vasomotor branches** to the radial and ulnar arteries and their branches. Digital nerves of the median nerve give also **articular branches** to the small joints of the hand.

ULNAR NERVE IN THE PALM

Beyond the level of wrist to enter the palm of hand the ulnar nerve runs through the **Guyon's canal**, lateral to the pisiform and medial to the ulnar artery. It passes superficial to the main band of flexor retinaculum but under to its superficial slip (volar carpal ligament). At the base of hypothenar eminence, it divides into *superficial and deep terminal branches*.

Dorsal branch of ulnar nerve, which is not the nerve of the palm, arises from the ulnar nerve *5 cm above the wrist* and passes dorsally under cover of flexor carpi ulnaris and pierces the deep fascia for cutaneous distribution on the medial side of dorsum of the hand with medial one and a half fingers. Its distribution is discussed in the chapter of dorsum of hand.

Superficial Terminal Branch of Ulnar Nerve

Superficial palmar division of ulnar nerve initially supplies following two branches:
1. **Motor branch**: To *palmaris brevis*
2. **Sensory branch**: To the skin over the hypothenar eminence.

Finally, the superficial division divides **into two palmar digital nerves** which are as follows:
1. **Medial:** *Proper palmar digital branch* for the medial side of little finger
2. **Lateral**: *Common palmar digital branch* which divides into *two proper digital nerves* for adjacent sides of little and ring finger.

At the level of base of terminal phalanx, each of the proper digital branches sends a **dorsal branch** which supplies the nail bed on the dorsum of the fingers.

Common digital branch of superficial division of ulnar nerve sends a **communicating branch** to the most medial common digital branch of median nerve.

Deep Terminal Branch of Ulnar Nerve (Fig. 9.10)

Deep terminal branch of ulnar nerve *accompanies the deep branch of ulnar artery* and it passes between abductor digiti minimi and flexor digiti minimi. Then it perforates the opponens digiti minimi to pass from medial side to lateral side of palm deep to the long flexor tendons. The nerve lies here within the curve of deep palmar arch formed by terminal part of the radial artery joining with deep branch of ulnar artery.

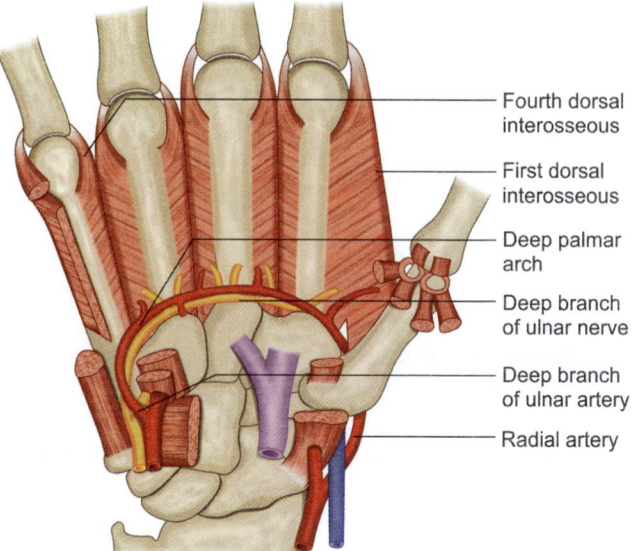

Fig. 9.10: Deep branch of ulnar nerve and deep palmar arch.

Branches of deep terminal branch of ulnar nerve are following from its medial end to lateral end.
- **Muscular branches at its origin**: These are for *abductor digiti minimi, flexor digiti minimi* and *opponens digiti minimi*.
- **Muscular branches at the center of palm**: Passing along the planes between long flexor tendons and the interossei:
    - To all the *palmar* and *dorsal interossei*
    - To the *3rd and 4th lumbricals*. In addition, *occasionally 3rd lumbrical* may be also supplied by the median nerve.
- **Terminal muscular branches**: Deep branch of ulnar nerve terminates by supplying:
    - *Adductor pollicis*
    - *First palmar interossei*
    - *Flexor pollicis brevis*
- **Articular branches are for:**
    - Wrist joint
    - Intercarpal, carpometacarpal and intermetacarpal joints.
- **Vascular branches** are to supply ulnar artery and its branches.

Clinical Anatomy

Ulnar tunnel syndrome is a clinical condition in which case the ulnar nerve is entrapped or compressed in the *Guyon's canal* between the main band of flexor retinaculum and its superficial part (volar carpal ligament). **Causes** of this syndrome may be trauma, ganglion (swelling of synovial sheath of tendons) or compression by nearby accessory muscles.

Clinical manifestations are:
- *Pain in the hand*
- *Paresthesia* (altered sensation) of the palmar aspect of little finger and medial half of ring finger.

- *Weakness and wasting* of intrinsic muscles of the hand supplied by the ulnar nerve.
- *Ulnar claw hand* in extreme cases.

LA 9.10 **Give and account of the facial spaces of the hand. Add a note on their clinical anatomy.**

Short notes: Digital pulp space; midpalmar space; space of parona; lumbrical canals.

FASCIAL SPACES OF HAND
Introduction
Beneath the skin and superficial fascia, the deep fascia of palm of hand with its central thickened part called palmar aponeurosis overlies multiple groups of intrinsic muscles of hand, long extrinsic flexor tendons, blood vessels and nerves. Again these structures lying in different planes are either covered by fascia (e.g. interossei) or embedded in a fascial plane (e.g. flexor tendons with lumbricals). So fasciae of multiple planes enclose some spaces with limited room and unyielding outlines.

Besides, the pulp of fingers, the lower end of forearm and the dorsum of hand covered by loose skin present some spaces.

Anatomical knowledge of these fascial spaces are important to be acquired because, very often a minor injury to the hand gives rise to infection of these spaces which requires proper management clinically.

Classification of Spaces
- **Fingers:** Digital pulp space
- **Palm:**
  - Midpalmar space
  - Thenar space
  - Adductor space
  - Web space
- **Lower end of forearm:** Forearm space of Parona
- **Dorsum of hand:**
  - Dorsal subcutaneous space
  - Dorsal subaponeurotic space.

Digital Pulp Space (Fig. 9.11)
Introduction
Digital palp space is the subcutaneous space on the pulp of finger between the skin and periosteum covering the palmar surface of distal phalanx. This space is closed proximally, as the deep fascia of the finger, represented by fibrous flexor sheath is attached to the palmar surface of base of distal phalanx.

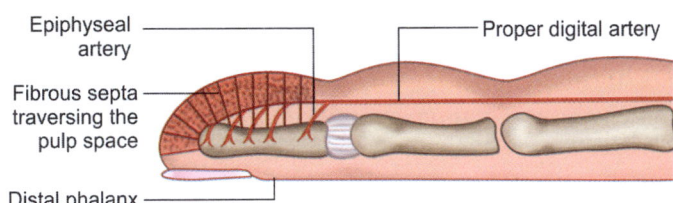

Fig. 9.11: Digital pulp space.

Contents
- *Subcutaneous fatty tissue* fills up the whole of pulp space. Fibrous tissue septae extend from periosteum of distal phalanx to the deep surface of skin. It divides the subcutaneous fat into small loculi.
- Proper digital vessels and nerves.

Branches of digital arteries passing through the pulp space

Distal part of the proper digital artery, while passing through the pulp space, gives branches to the soft tissue of the digital pulp as well as the distal four fifth of the terminal phalanx. These branches traverse through the fibrous septal compartment. But the *epiphyseal branch* to supply the proximal one fifth of the distal phalanx arises from the digital artery before it enters the pulp space.

Clinical anatomy

As the tips of the fingers are very frequently subjected to contact and pressure in daily life, pulp space are very often infected to due to trauma. Infection of pulp space give rise to formation of abscess. This condition is known as **whitlow**. Because of the fibrous tissue septae passing through the pulp space, there is no provision for expansion of the tissue affected by whitlow. It gives rise to a throbbing pain. In addition, the arteries supplying the distal four fifth of the distal phalanx are compressed by the inflammatory pressure. It results in **avascular necrosis** *of the distal four fifth of the phalanx*. But the proximal one fifth of the phalanx is saved as its artery originates more proximally and does not traverse through the pulp space.

Drainage of abscess: The complication of avascular necrosis of the distal phalanx can be prevented by surgical drainage of the abscess in proper time. *Incision* for drainage of pulp space should be *ideally made at the side of the finger dorsal to the posterior limit of flexor creases*. The incision will therefore pass through the plane between the phalanx dorsally and digital nerves and vessels ventrally.

Midpalmar Space (Fig. 9.12)

Midpalmar space is located beneath the medial half of palmar aponeurosis.

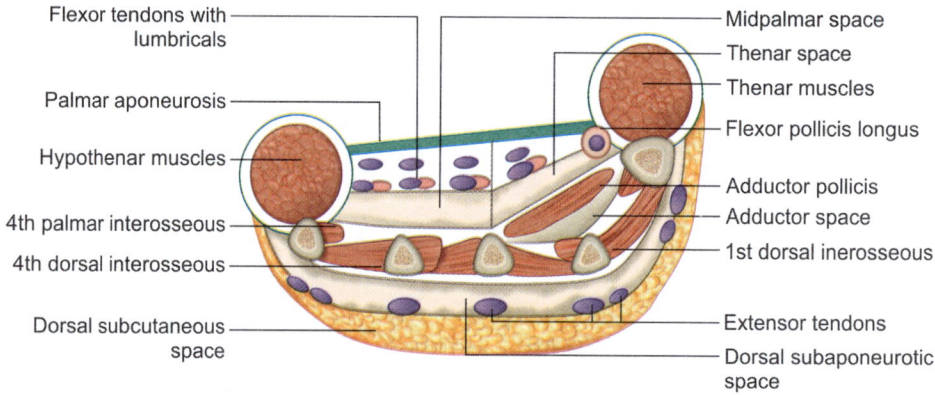

Fig. 9.12: Fascial spaces of hand.

Boundaries

Ventral
- Loose and thin fascial layer of the plane of flexor tendons (superficialis as well as profundus) for little, ring and middle finger with corresponding medial three lumbricals forms the *direct ventral boundary* of the midpalmar space.
- This boundary is further *reinforced* by medial half of the palmar aponeurosis and superficial palmar arch.

Dorsal
Fascia covering the medial two pairs of interossei with the adjacent metacarpal bones.

Medial

Medial palmar septum from the medial margin of palmar aponeurosis to the long axis of palmar surface of shaft of 5th metacarpal bone. This septum passes lateral to the hypothenar eminence.

Lateral

Intermediate palmar septum extending from deep surface of the thin fascia of flexor tendons opposite the line of the tendons for middle finger to the palmar surface of the shaft of third metacarpal bone.

Extent (Fig. 9.13)

Proximal

Midpalmar space extends proximally up to the distal margin of flexor retinaculum. Occasionally this space is continuous with the space in the forearm beneath the flexor tendons.

Distal

The space extends up to the level of the *distal palmar crease*. Beyond this level, the midpalmar space extends distally as three narrow *lumbrical canals* formed by the fascial sheath of the medial three lumbrical tendons. The lumbrical canals *extends up to the lateral side of the base of the medial three fingers* (Fig. 9.13).

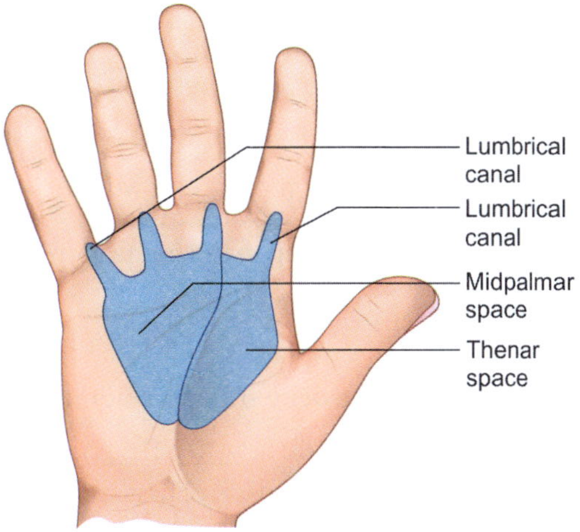

Clinical anatomy

See below.

Fig. 9.13: Lumbrical canals extending from palmar spaces.

Thenar Space (Fig. 9.12)

Thenar space is situated beneath the lateral half of the palmar aponeurosis deep to lateral part of the central hollow of the palm. *Thenar space is medial to the thenar eminence* from which it is separated by a fascial septum. The space is triangular in cross section.

Boundaries

Ventral

- Long flexor tendons (superficialis as well as profundus) and first lumbrical muscle embedded in a thin layer of fascia.
- Further superficially—superficial palmar arch, division of the median nerve and lateral half of palmar aponeurosis.

Dorsal

Fascia covering the ventral surface of adductor pollicis muscle.

Medial

Intermediate palmar septum which extends from palmar surface of shaft of third metacarpal bone to the thin fascia binding the slips of flexor tendons.

Lateral
- Lateral palmar septum demarcating the muscles of thenar eminence and extending up to lateral margin of palmar aponeurosis.
- Tendon of flexor pollicis longus covered by synovial sheath (radial bursa).

Extent (Fig. 9.13)

Proximal

Up to the distal border of flexor retinaculum

Distal

Up to the level of *proximal transverse palmar crease*. Thenar space is prolonged further distally through the narrow *lumbrical canal* around the tendon of *first lumbrical muscle* to the lateral side of the base of index finger.

Clinical anatomy

See below.

Adductor Space (Fig. 9.12)

This is a thin space deep to the plane of the adductor pollicis muscle.

Boundaries

Ventral

Fascia covering the deep surface of adductor pollicis muscle.

Dorsal

Fascia covering the interossei of first and second intermetacarpal space with palmar surface of shaft of second metacarpal bone.

Medial

Shaft of third metacarpal bone.

Lateral

Shaft of first metacarpal bone.

Web Spaces

Web spaces are four subcutaneous spaces deep to the folds of skin connecting the bases of fingers.

Extent

Web space extends *distally* up to its free skin margin.

Proximally, it extends up to the level of metacarpophalangeal joint.

Contents

- Subcutaneous fat
- Superficial transverse metacarpal ligament
- Tendons of lumbricals and interossei
- Bifurcations of common digital vessels and nerves into their proper digital branches.

Forearm Space of Parona (Fig. 9.14)

This is an intermuscular space in the lower end of forearm deep to the plane of long flexor tendons.

Boundaries

Ventral

- Tendons of flexor digitorum profundus and flexor digitorum superficialis enclosed by synovial sheath (*ulnar bursa*)
- Tendon of flexor pollicis longus enclosed by its synovial sheath (*radial bursa*).

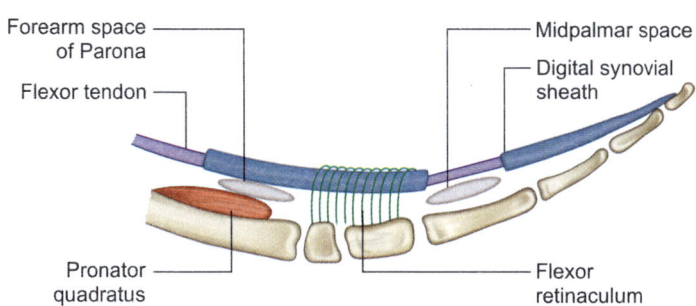

Fig. 9.14: Forearm space of Parona.

Dorsal

- Pronator quadratus muscle with its covering fascia.
- Lower end of interosseous membrane.

Extent

Proximal

Forearm space of Parona is continuous above for a short distance deep to tendons of long flexor and in front of interosseous membrane. Infection may spread above into this plane.

Distal

Beyond the level of flexor retinaculum, space of Parona reaches the level of proximal end of midpalmar and thenar spaces demarcated by fascial lining. But in case of abscess formation of in palmar spaces, it may spread proximally into Parona's space.

At the sides

Parona's space extends to the subcutaneous plane both at the lateral and medial borders of forearm. Superficial extention of the space gives an advantage of drainage of the abscess along the borders of lower end of forearm.

Clinical anatomy

See below.

Dorsal Spaces of Hand (see Fig. 9.12)

Skin of the dorsum of hand is thin and very loose. Beneath the loose subcutaneous tissue plane, slips of extensor digitorum for the medial four fingers are connected by intertendinous aponeurotic band. Deep to this, dorsum of hand presents the fascial covering of dorsal interossei muscles and the dorsal surface of shaft of metacarpal bones.

So, the dorsum of hand presents two spaces as follows:
1. **Dorsal subcutaneous space** is between the skin with subcutaneous tissue plane and the flattened sheet like intertendinous aponeurotic band connecting extensor tendon slips.
2. **Dorsal subaponeurotic space** is bounded between aponeurotic band superficially and fascia over the dorsal interossei at the deeper plane.

Clinical Anatomy of Spaces of Hand

Digital Pulp Space

Infections of digital pulp space occur very often as the finger tips are always subjected to all the times exposure, contact and pressure or prick. Infection is characterized by throbbing pain, as the inflammatory tissue traversed by fibrous septa gets limited space for expansion and is richly supplied by sensory nerves.

Inflammation and subsequent abscess formation in the digital pulp space may lead to avascular neurosis of distal four fifth of the distal phalanx as this area's blood vessels are traversed and so entangled by the fibrous tissue septa of the space.

Thenar and Midpalmar Space

These palmar spaces lie beneath the central hollow of the palm of hand. Palmar hollow, being the important area related to all kinds of grip, is very often subjected to the injury from a minor prick to a cut wound. This may lead to palmar space infection.

Lumbrical canals extend from the distal end of the palmar space to the web spaces of the finger base. Subcutaneous **web spaces** are often prone to be infected. This infection may extend from the web space to the palmar spaces through the lumbrical canal.

Space of Parona

Deep to flexor retinaculum, forearm space of Parona may extend up to the proximal end of midpalmar space, usually separated by a fascial barrier. Midpalmar space abscess may break this fascial barrier and spread into the forearm space of Parona. Pus from the Parona's space points to the surface on either the lateral or the medial border of lower end of forearm. Abscess is drained approaching the one of these two borders of forearm.

Dorsal Spaces of Hand

Infection of the spaces of the dorsum of hand may occur due to trauma on the knuckles, otherwise their infection is uncommon. But these spaces, particularly the loose subcutaneous space are very often swollen due to infection in the other fascial spaces.

SA 9.11 **Write a brief note on the cutaneous nerves of dorsum of hand.**

CUTANEOUS NERVES OF DORSUM OF HAND (FIG. 9.15)

Cutaneous innervation of the dorsum of hand is shared by:
- Superficial branch of the radial nerve
- Dorsal branch of ulnar nerve

Superficial branch of the radial nerve, named as superficial radial nerve, arises as one of the two terminal branches of the radial nerve along with its deep branch just below the bend of the elbow. It passes through the forearm *to supply the skin of dorsum of the hand only.* About 7 cm proximal to the wrist the superficial branch, winds around the radius deep to brachioradialis. It perforates the deep fascia above the wrist and runs down over the extensor retinaculum. The nerve then crosses over the *anatomical snuff box* bounded laterally by abductor pollicis longus and extensor pollicis brevis and medially by extensor pollicis longus. Appearing of the dorsum of hand, the superficial radial nerve supplies the

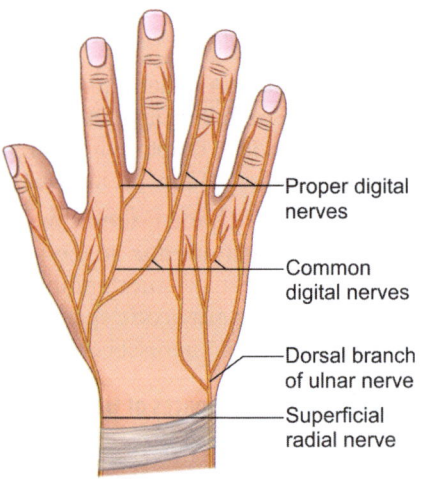

Fig. 9.15: Cutaneous nerves of dorsum of hand.

skin of lateral two thirds of dorsum of hand and divides into digital branches to supply the skin of dorsum of thumb, and index and middle fingers and also the lateral half of ring finger. Nail beds with the dorsum of these fingers opposite the distal phalanx are supplied by dorsal twigs of palmar digital branches of median nerve.

Dorsal branch of ulnar nerve is also a purely sensory nerve which supplies the skin of medial one third of dorsum of hand and medial 1½ fingers. It arises from the ulnar nerve 5 cm proximal to the front of wrist at the medial side of front of forearm. It curves around the ulna deep to flexor carpi ulnaris tendon and descends superficial to the extensor retinaculum. Appearing at the dorsum of hand, the dorsal branch of ulnar nerve gives rise to cutaneous branches to the skin of medial one third of dorsum of hand and finally divides into digital branches for the skin of dorsum of little finger and medial half of ring finger. Skin over the distal phalanx with nail beds of these fingers is supplied by the dorsal branches of proper palmar digital division of superficial terminal branch of ulnar nerve.

Variations of Cutaneous Innervation of Dorsum of Hand

- Each of the two nerves of the dorsum of hand may take pant 50% of cutaneous innervation. In such cases, 2½ fingers will be supplied by both the superficial branch of radial nerve and the dorsal branch of ulnar nerve.
- In some cases, in addition to the usual pattern, lateral half of the dorsum of ring finger may be additionally supplied by a branch of the ulnar nerve.

SN 9.12 **Write a short note on the extensor retinaculum of hand.**

EXTENSOR RETINACULUM OF HAND (FIG. 9.16)

Introduction
Extensor retinaculum of hand is a thick band of deep fascia crossing over the tendons at the back of wrist.

Measurement
It is 2 cm broad from above downwards.

Direction of Fibers
Fibers of the retinaculum are slightly oblique and directed *downwards and medially*.

Attachments
Laterally: Lower end of anterior border of the radius.

Medially: The fibers curve round the medial border of the wrist, pass ventrally and are attached to the *triquetral* and *pisiform* bones.

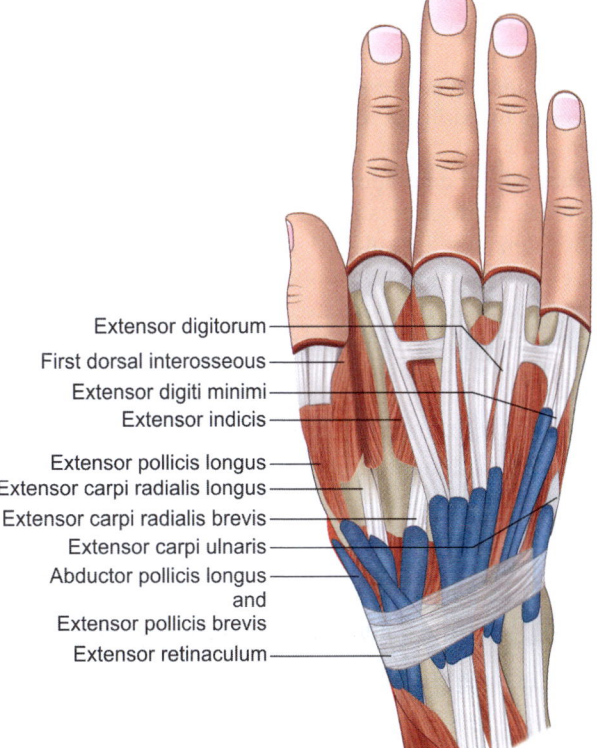

Fig. 9.16: Extensor retinaculum and tendons of dorsum of hand with synovial sheath.

Compartments Beneath the Retinaculum (Fig. 9.17)

The space beneath the extensor retinaculum is divided into six compartments by the fibrous septae which pass from deep surface of the retinaculum to the dorsal aspect of lower ends of radius and ulna. Structures passing through these six osseo-fascial compartments are divided in following groups from lateral to medial.

Tendons of Ist to IVth compartments are in relation to lateral and posterior aspect of lower end of radius. The tendon of Vth compartment passes along the plane of interval between lower end of radius and ulna. The tendon of VIth compartment runs through the groove bounded by head and styloid process of ulna.

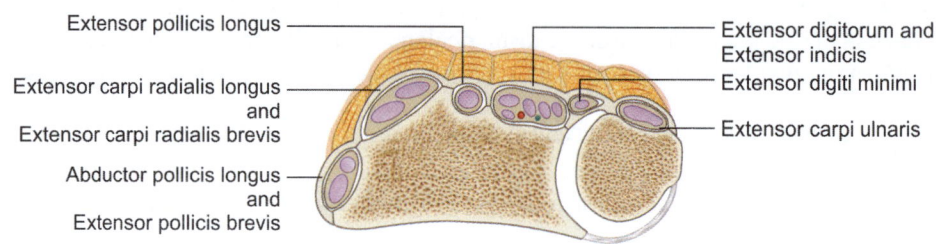

Fig. 9.17: Tendon compartments beneath extensor retinaculum.

Synovial Tendon Sheaths Related to Extensor Retinaculum (see Fig. 9.16)

Tendons passing through each of the six osseofibrous tunnels deep to the extensor retinaculum are covered by their respective synovial sheath. Tendons of abductor pollicis longus and extensor pollicis brevis passing through the tunnel I may have independent synovial sheath. Proximal ends of the tendon sheaths are just a little above the extensor retinaculum. Distally, they reach up to the bases of metacarpal bones. Tendons sheaths of extensor digitorum, extensor indicis and extensor digiti minimi may be continued more distally up to the midmetacarpal level.

Compartments (From lateral to medial)	Structures
I	Abductor pollicis longus Extensor pollicis brevis
II	Extensor carpi radialis longus Extensor carpi radialis brevis
III	Extensor pollicis longus
IV	Extensor digitorum Extensor indicis Deep branch of radial nerve (posterior interosseous nerve) Anterior interosseous artery
V	Extensor digiti minimi
VI	Extensor carpi ulnaris

Functions of Extensor Retinaculum

Extensor retinaculum crossing over the back of wrist keep the tendons, passing deep to it, in position. It prevents the bowstringing of the tendons during contraction of their fleshy parts.

Synovial sheaths facilitate smooth movement of the tendons under the retinaculum.

SN 9.13 Write a short note on dorsal digital expansion.

DORSAL DIGITAL EXPANSION (EXTENSOR EXPANSION) (FIG. 9.18)

Introduction

It is also known as *extensor tendon apparatus*. It is a composite tendinous band formed on the extensor surface of digits. The tendon apparatus is formed by tendons of following muscles in each of the medial four digits.

- Extensor digitorum
- Dorsal interosseous
- Palmar interosseous
- Lumbrical
- Tendon of extensor indicis in index finger
- Tendon of extensor digiti minimi in little finger.

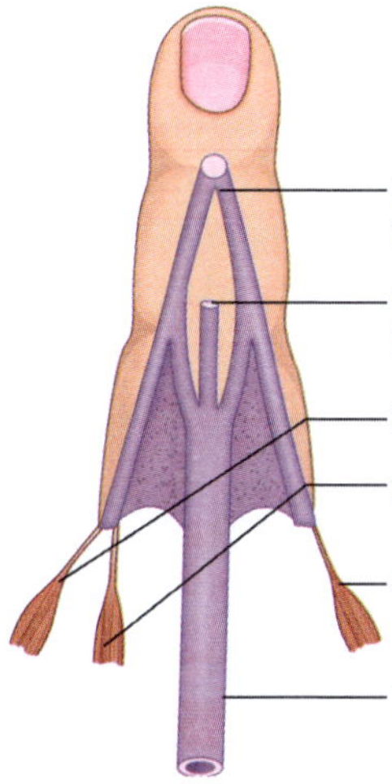

Formation

Initially, the divided four tendons of extensor digitorum are interconnected on the dorsum of hand by *obliquely directed* fibers of *intertendinous junctions*. This tendinous interconnection is functionally important because it will help in extension of a finger, even when the individual tendon of this finger is cut or lacerated at a proximal point.

Fig. 9.18: Dorsal digital expansion (extensor expansion) of right middle finger.

On the dorsal aspect of metacarpophalangeal joint each of the tendon of extensor digitorum is expanded into a triangular band with the apex directed distally. It is named **extensor expansion or dorsal digital expansion**. It forms a triangular *movable hood* over the dorsal aspect of proximal phalanx. The hood moves proximally and distally during extension and flexion of the finger respectively. It is separated from the metacarpophalangeal joint by *a small bursa*.

The margins of the expansion are thickened *on the radial (lateral) side* by the tendon of *lumbrical and interosseous muscles* and *on the ulnar (medial) side* by the tendon of *interosseous only*. But the tendons of interossei unite at the level of proximal end and the tendon of lumbrical fuses at the level of distal end of the middle phalanx.

Division of Slips

Proximal to the proximal interphalangeal joint, the extensor expansion divides into *a central slip* and *two lateral bands*. There occurs interchange of fibers among them through criss-cross disposition of fibers.

Attachments

- The *central slip* gets attached to the dorsal aspect of base of *middle phalanx*.
- The *lateral bands* are prolonged distally and finally *fuse together* to be attached to the dorsal aspect of *distal phalanx*.

Functions

- Fundamentally, the extensor expansion acts for extension of fingers at the metacarpophalangeal joint as well as interphalangeal joint.
- In addition, due to the attachments of interossei and lumbricals, the extensor expansion causes flexion of metacarpophalangeal joint and extension of both the interphalangeal joints. This mechanism can be simply understood through the fact that, *the interossei and lumbrical cross the palmar aspect of metacarpophalangeal joint and dorsal aspects of interphalangeal joints*.

This action is essential for some kinds of precise finger movements, e.g. during writing or buttoning a cloth.

Clinical Anatomy

Mallet Finger (Baseball Finger)

If the distal phalanx is flexed forcibly in full extended position of the finger, it may cause avulsion or tear of the insertion of the extensor tendon. It results in deformity manifested by extension of proximal interphalangeal joint and flexion of distal interphalangeal joint.

SN 9.14 Write a short note on anatomical snuff box.

ANATOMICAL SNUFF BOX (FIG. 9.19)

Definition

Anatomical snuff box is a triangular depression with its apex directed distally on the lateral side of dorsum of hand.

This triangular depression becomes more prominent during full extension of the thumb.

Boundaries

- **Lateral**: Tendons of *abductor pollicis longus* and *extensor pollicis brevis*
- **Medial**: Tendon of *extensor pollicis longus*
- **Apex:** Convergence of lateral and medial tendons
- **Base**: Level of lateral side of lower end of radius
- **Roof**: Subcutaneous fascia crossed by the formation of *cephalic vein* and the terminal divisions of superficial branch of *radial nerve*
- **Floor:** Dorsal surface of *scaphoid and trapezium*.

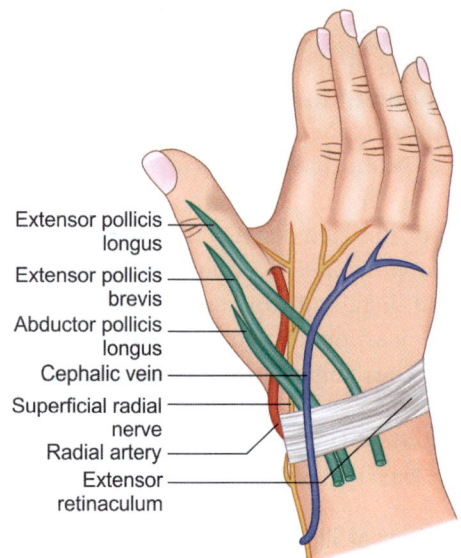

Fig. 9.19: Anatomical snuff box.

Contents

Radial artery, before it enters the palm of the hand between two heads of first dorsal interosseous muscle.

Clinical Anatomy

- Pulsation of the radial artery can be felt at the site of anatomical snuff box.
- In case of fracture of scaphoid bone, patient complains of pain at this site.
- Cephalic vein is often chosen at this site of intravenous fluid transfusion.

Chapter 10

Joints of the Wrist and Hand

LA 10.1 Describe the radiocarpal (wrist) joint.

RADIOCARPAL (WRIST) JOINT

Introduction
Radiocarpal or wrist joint is the articulation between the inferior surface of lower end of radius and carpal bones of the proximal row.

Out of the two bones of the forearm, as only the radius takes part in formation of wrist joint, keeping the ulna free, radius can move the hand with it during pronation and supination.

Type of the Joint
Radiocarpal joint is considered to be the ellipsoid variety of synovial joint as both the articular surfaces of the joint are elliptical in outline.

Articulating Surfaces (Fig. 10.1)
Proximal articular surface is formed by:
- *Inferior surface of lower end of radius* which is covered by hyaline cartilage. The surface is divided by a smooth anteroposterior ridge into lateral triangular and medial quadrangular areas.
- *Inferior surface of triangular articular disk* of the inferior radioulnar joint.

Basal aspect of the triangular disk is attached to inferior margin of ulnar notch of radius and apex is attached to a small depression between the head and styloid process of ulna.

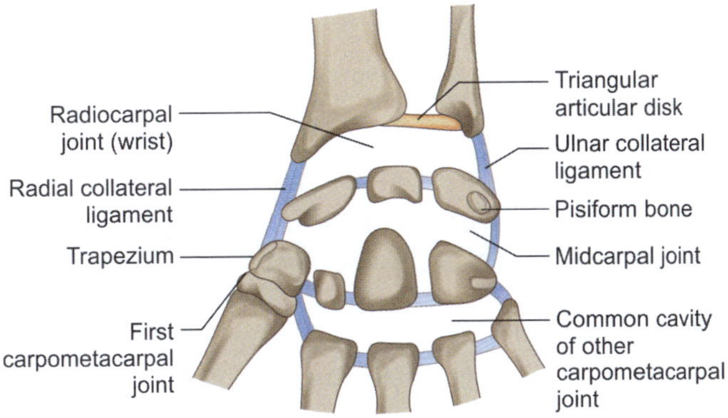

Fig. 10.1: The joints of wrist and hand.

Distal articular surface is formed by the proximal convex articular surfaces of:
- Scaphoid
- Lunate
- Triquetral.

These are the three lateral bones of proximal row. The pisiform, the medial most bone does not have the chance to articulate, because it lies ventral to the triquetral.

In neutral position of the wrist, scaphoid and lunate form the articulation. Triquetral comes in contract in full adduction of the wrist.

Ligaments

Capsular Ligament (Fibrous Capsule)

Attachments of fibrous capsule of the wrist joint are as follows.

Proximal

- Anterior and posterior margins of inferior surface of lower end of radius
- Anterior and posterior margins of triangular articular disk of inferior radioulnar joint
- Margin of head of ulna.

Distal

Margins of proximal (superior) articular surface of the scaphoid, lunate and triquetral bones.

Synovial membrane lines the inner surface of the capsule. It is usually separate from distal radioulnar joint and also intercarpal joints. A small protrusion of synovial lining extend upwards in front of the triangular articular disk close to the ulnar styloid process. It is called **prestyloid recess** or **processus sacciformis**.

Radial collateral ligament (Fig. 10.1): It extends from lateral aspect of tip of styloid process of radius to the nonarticular lateral surface of the *scaphoid* and *trapezium*. Radial artery crosses obliquely over this ligament from ventral to the dorsal aspect.

Ulnar collateral ligament (Fig. 10.1): It is attached to the tip of styloid process of ulna proximally and to the nonarticular medial surface of the *triquetral* and *pisiform bones* distally.

Palmar radiocarpal ligament: It extends from the anterior ridge-like margin of lower end of radius to the palmar surface of *scaphoid, lunate* and *triquetral bones*. The fibers are formed by thickening of anterior fibers of capsule and may extend even up to the bone of the distal row. This ligament is strong enough to carry the hand with radius during supination and pronation of forearm.

Palmar ulnocarpal ligament: It extends from the base of styloid process of ulna and adjoining part of anterior margin of triangular articular disk to the palmar aspect of *lunate* and *triquetral bones*. Thickened medial part of anterior aspect of the fibrous capsule forms this ligament.

Dorsal radiocarpal ligament: Fibers of this ligament extend from posterior margin of lower end of radius to the dorsal surface of *scaphoid, lunate* and *triquetral bones*.

Important Relations

Anterior

- Flexor carpi radialis tendon with its synovial sheath
- Tendon of flexor pollicis longus enclosed by radial bursa
- Tendons of flexor digitorum superficialis and profundus covered by ulnar bursa
- Median nerve
- Ulnar vessels and ulnar nerve.

Posterior

- **Extensor tendons of the wrist:** Tendons of extensor carpi radialis longus and brevis, extensor carpi ulnaris.

- **Extensors of the digit:** Extensor digitorum, extensor pollicis longus, extensor indicis and extensor digiti minimi.
- Terminal part of *anterior interosseous nerve and the anterior interosseous artery.*

Lateral
- Radial artery
- Tendons of abductor pollicis longus and extensor pollicis brevis.

Medial
Dorsal branch of ulnar nerve, while crossing obliquely from the anterior aspect of forearm to dorsum of hand.

Arterial Supply
Arteries supplying the wrist joint are derived from *palmar and dorsal carpal arches.*

Nerve Supply
- *Anterior interosseous branch* of median nerve
- *Posterior interosseous branch* of radial nerve *(deep radial nerve)*
- *Dorsal and deep branches* of ulnar nerve.

Movements of Wrist Joint
Joint line passes through the tips of radial and ulnar styloid processes.

Movements of the wrist joint are:
- Flexion and extension (forward and backward bending of wrist)
- Abduction and adduction (radial deviation and ulnar deviation)
- Circumduction (combination of above movements).

Range of flexion of hand on forearm is more than that of extension. During these movements, wrist movements are associated with the corresponding *movements in the midcarpal joint* between proximal and distal rows of carpal bones.

Adduction of the hand is greater than the abduction. Adduction occurs from the neutral position mostly in the midcarpal joints.

In circumduction, succession of movements are flexion, adduction, extension and abduction.

Muscles Producing Movements

Flexion
- Flexor carpi radialis and flexor carpi ulnaris, acting jointly
- Flexors of the fingers and thumb
- Palmaris longus.

Extension
- Extensor carpi radialis longus and brevis and, extensor carpi ulnaris
- Extensors of the fingers and thumb

Abduction
- Abductor pollicis longus

- Flexor carpi radialis acting jointly
- Extensor carpi radialis longus and brevis.
  Abduction movement is limited within the range of 15° due to projection of radial styloid process.

Adduction

Simultaneous contraction of extensor and flexor carpi ulnaris.

Clinical Anatomy

Wrist Fracture

Various types of fracture dislocations around the wrist are common due to fall with various positions of open hand. Some important clinical conditions are following.
- *Colle's fracture*: Fracture of lower end of radius in adults. It is a complete transverse fracture within distal 2 cm of radius. This fracture results from *forced dorsiflexion of wrist*.
- *Smith's fracture of radius*: It is less common in incidence. It occurs in young men due to fall on the dorsum of hand in flexed position of wrist.
- *Fracture of scaphoid*: It usually results from fall on the outstretched hand with the wrist extended and abducted.
- *Fracture separation of distal epiphysis of radius* is common in children due to frequent falls in which forces are transmitted from hand to radius.

Wrist Injuries

Various tendons, nerves and vessels lying superficial to the wrist joint all around are very often subjected to the injury.

Ganglion

It is a common Greek terminology which means a swelling or knot. It is a cystic swelling usually lying on the dorsal aspect of wrist. It occurs due to *swelling* of tendon synovial sheath followed by subsequent *mucoid degeneration*. The small cystic swelling is *filled up with mucinous fluid*.

Rheumatoid Arthritis

Wrist joint is often swollen in **rheumatoid arthritis** which is a *collagenous disease* leading to more deposition of collagen fibers in the vicinity of the joint.

Immobilization of Wrist

In case of fracture dislocation in and around wrist, to allow proper union, the wrist joint is immobilized in its optimum position of **30° dorsiflexion**.

LA 10.2 Describe the first carpometacarpal joint.

FIRST CARPOMETACARPAL JOINT (FIG. 10.2)

Introduction

First carpometacarpal joint is the independent joint because it has a separate joint cavity. Movements of the human hand are very specialized for the following two important reasons.
- Long axis of the 1st metacarpal bone is ventrally rotated for 90^0 from the plane of the other metacarpals which facilitates opposition movement.
- First carpometacarpal joint is independent from adjacent joints. It allows wide range of mobility of the thumb.

Type
It is a saddle variety of synovial joint as the articular surfaces are concavoconvex.

Articular Surfaces
- Distal surface of the trapezium
- Proximal surface of the base of first metacarpal bone.

Concavoconvex nature of both the articular surfaces is the reason for wide range of mobility of the joint.

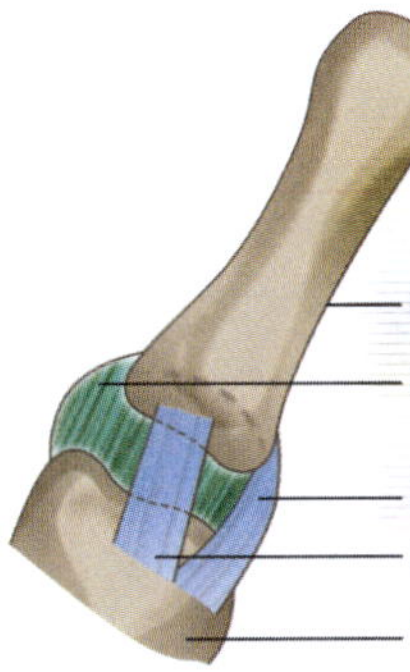

Ligaments (Fig. 10.2)
Fibrous capsule is a *thick but loose* fibrous envelope which encloses the joint cavity. The capsule is attached to the margins of both the articular surfaces and is lined by **synovial membrane**.

Lateral ligament is a wide and thick fibrous band which connects the lateral aspects of the trapezium and the base of first metacarpal. It strengthens the lateral aspect of the joint capsule.

Both the palmar and dorsal ligaments are directed *downwards and medially. They extend* from the respective surfaces of the trapezium to the ulnar sides of the corresponding surfaces of the base of first metacarpal bone.

Fig. 10.2: First carpometacarpal joint (right side).

Relations
Anterior
The joint is covered by muscles of the thenar eminence ending in tendons.

Posterior
- Tendon of extensor pollicis brevis
- Tendon of extensor pollicis longus.

Lateral
Abductor pollicis longus.

Medial
- First dorsal interosseous muscle
- Radial artery—crossing the dorsomedial aspect of the joint to pass between two heads of 1st dorsal interosseous.

Arterial Supply
Articular branch from the radial artery.

Nerve Supply
A twig from the first digital branch of median nerve.

Movements (Fig. 10.3)
Movements of first metacarpophalangeal joint is reflected on the movements of the thumb.
- **Flexion and extension**: The thumb moves across the plane of the palm.

- **Abduction and adduction**: The thumb moves at right angle to the plane of the palm.
- **Opposition**: The thumb crosses the palm and touches the other fingers.
- **Rotation**: Medial rotation is associated with *flexion*. *Lateral rotation* is associated with *extension*.

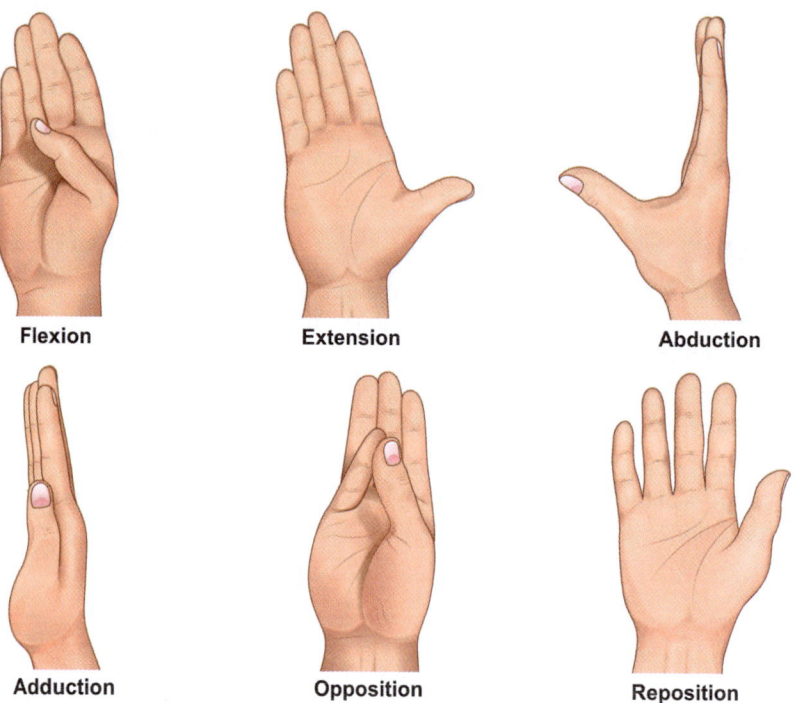

Fig. 10.3: Movements of first carpometacarpal joint.

Muscles Producing Movements

Flexion: Flexor pollicis brevis
Extension: Extensor pollicis brevis
  and
  Extensor pollicis longus
Abduction: Abductor pollicis brevis
  and
  Abductor pollicis longus
Adduction: Adductor pollicis
Opposition: Opponens pollicis.

Clinical Anatomy

Concavoconvex articular surfaces and 90° rotation of plane of 1st metacarpal in relation to the plane of other metacarpals are the two basic reasons for wide range of movement of 1st carpometacarpal joint. This free movements of the joint may be restricted in *traumatic and rheumatoid arthritis*.

Chapter 11

Major Nerves of the Upper Limb

SA 11.1 Describe the axillary nerve. Add a note on its clinical anatomy.

AXILLARY NERVE (FIG. 11.1)

Introduction
Axillary nerve is so called because it arises in the axilla and most of its course is confined in and around the axilla.

Origin
Axillary nerve arises from the posterior cord of brachial plexus (C_5, C_6) in the posterior wall of axilla, in front of subscapularis muscles, behind the third part of axillary artery and lateral to the radial nerve.

Course
Axillary nerve has a circumflex course for which it is often called *circumflex nerve*. Basically, its course can be better understood in relation to the surgical neck of humerus as follows:
- First the axillary nerve goes backwards along the medial side of surgical neck of humerus
- Then it passes laterally along the posterior aspect of the bone
- Finally the nerves turns forwards along the lateral aspect of the surgical neck.

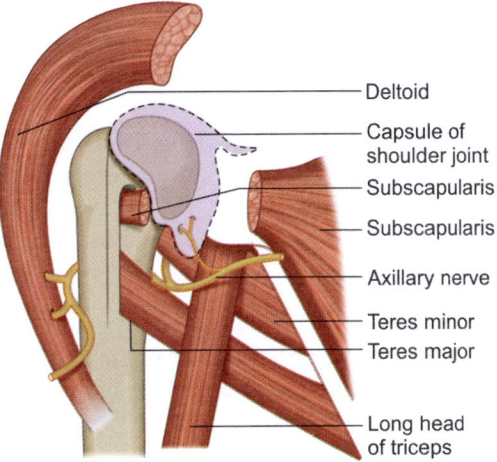

Fig. 11.1: Course of axillary nerve.

Relations
- From the level of origin, the **first part of axillary nerve** passes backwards *through the quadrangular space* which is bounded as follows **(Fig. 11.1):**
  - *Above* (from before backwards): Subscapularis muscle, capsule of shoulder joint and teres minor muscle.
  - *Below*: Teres major muscle.
  - *Medially:* Long head of triceps brachii muscle.
  - *Laterally*: Surgical neck of humerus.

  While the trunk of the nerve passes through the quadrangular space, it divides into *anterior and posterior divisions.* Here the nerve is accompanied by posterior circumflex humeral vessels.

- **In the second part**, the anterior division of the nerve curves round the back of humerus along with the posterior circumflex humerus vessels.
- **In the third part of the course**, *anterior division* of the nerve winds forwards along the lateral aspect of the surgical neck of humerus undercover of the deltoid muscle till it reaches its anterior border. After supplying the muscle it is continued as cutaneous branch.

In the quadrangular space, the posterior division passes backwards and medially below the level of glenoidal margin. It sends branch to the *teres minor muscle* and is continued as *upper lateral cutaneous nerve of the arm*. The nerve to the teres minor supplies branch to the *posterior part of the deltoid*. The branch to the posterior part of the deltoid occasionally arise directly from the posterior division or as a common mixed root with the upper lateral cutaneous nerve of the arm. There is often a swelling or *pseudoganglion* on the *nerve to the teres minor*.

Branches (Figs. 11.2 and 2.11)

Trunk

Articular branch to the *shoulder joint*.

Anterior Division

- Motor branch—to the *deltoid muscle*
- Cutaneous branch—continuation of the anterior division to supply skin over the anteroinferior part of deltoid.

Posterior Division

1. Nerve to the teres minor } Motor braches
2. Nerve to the posterior part of the deltoid
3. Upper lateral cutaneous nerve of the arm: Sensory branch

Clinical Anatomy

Most common causes of axillary nerve lesion are the following:
- Trauma, e.g. constant pressure on the nerve by a badly adjusted crutch.
- Fracture dislocation of the shoulder joint
- Fracture of surgical neck of humerus which is closely related to the nerve.

Clinical manifestations are the following:
- **Motor loss**: Paralysis of deltoid causes impairment of abduction of shoulder joint.

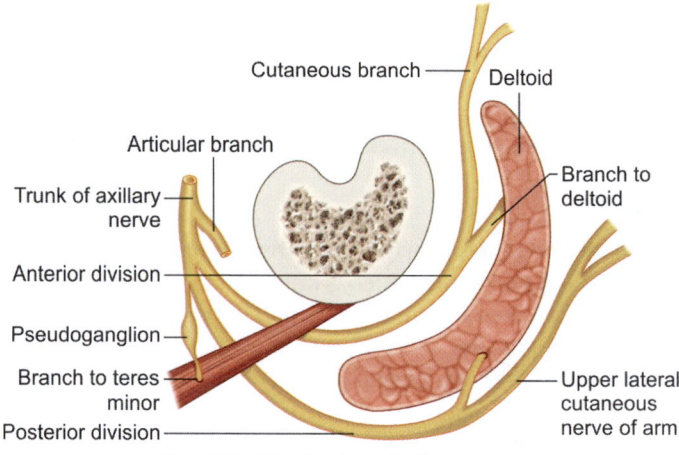

Fig. 11.2: Distribution of axillary nerve.

Progressive wasting of deltoid will be evident by prominence of greater tuberosity. Paralysis of

teres minor will not produce any effect, as infraspinatus will compensate its loss of function as lateral rotator of shoulder.
- **Sensory loss**: Loss of sensation over a patchy area on the outer aspect of arm.

SA 11.2 Describe the musculocutaneous nerve.

MUSCULOCUTANEOUS NERVE (FIG. 11.3)

Introduction
Musculocutaneous nerve is so called because it is a mixed nerve having specific motor and sensory (cutaneous) components.

Motor component of the musculocutaneous nerve is to supply the *muscles of anterior (flexor) compartment of the arm*.

Sensory component is for *cutaneous innervation of lateral half of front of forearm*.

Origin
Musculocutaneous nerve originates from the lateral cord of brachial plexus (C_5, C_6, C_7) at the level of distal border of pectoralis minor.

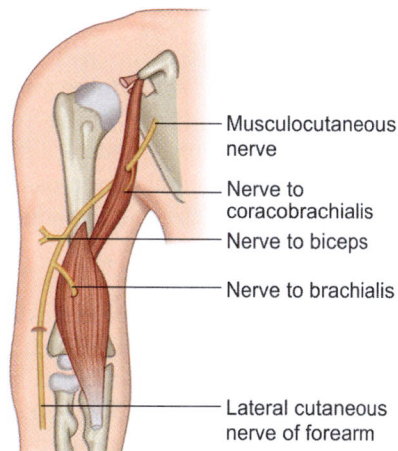

Fig. 11.3: Musculocutaneous nerve.

Course and Relations
The nerve passes through the coracobrachialis muscle and is directed downwards and laterally to pass between biceps brachii and brachialis muscles. In the next part of its course it appears lateral to the biceps brachii underneath of deep fascia. The nerve perforates the deep fascia just beyond the elbow and is continued as *lateral cutaneous nerve of the forearm*.

Branches

Motor
- Before piercing coracobrachialis: To coracobrachialis
- Within coracobrachialis: To coracobrachialis
- After coracobrachialis: To biceps brachii and brachialis.

Sensory
- **Cutaneous:** Lateral cutaneous nerve of the forearm: To the lateral half of skin of the front of forearm.
- **Articular:** To the elbow joint from the *nerve to brachialis*.

Clinical Anatomy
Individual or isolated lesion of musculocutaneous nerve is rare, as protected undercover of the biceps. It may occur in fracture of shaft of humerus. Main disability is the remarkable weakness in elbow flexion, because the biceps brachii and much of the brachialis are paralyzed. Loss of supination due to paralysis of the biceps, the chief supinator, will be compensated by action of the supinator. Sensory loss is the impairment of cutaneous sensation on lateral half of front of forearm.

LA 11.3 Describe the median nerve with its clinical anatomy.

MEDIAN NERVE

Introduction
Median nerve is so called because, throughout almost whole of its course, in the arm as well as forearm it is median in position.

Origin
It is formed by union of fibers of lateral and medial cords of brachial plexus.
- *Fibers of lateral cord*: Come *from ventral division* of C_5, C_6, C_7 nerve roots (lateral root).
- *Fibers of medial cord*: Come from ventral division of C_8 and T_1 nerve roots (medial root).
- Fibers from medial cord cross the front of third part of axillary artery and join the lateral cord.

Principle of Distribution
Though the median nerve arises in the axilla, it is *almost not for distribution of any branch in axilla and arm. Along with the ulnar nerve*, the median nerve supplies *muscles of anterior compartment of forearm and palm of hand*. It has major contribution to supply the muscles of forearm whereas most of the muscles of palm of the hand are supplied by the ulnar nerve.

Course and Important Relations

In the Axilla
Median nerve is formed through the union of lateral and medial roots. Medial root runs in front of axillary artery to join the lateral root. The nerve reaches the arm lateral to the brachial artery at the lower border of teres major muscle.

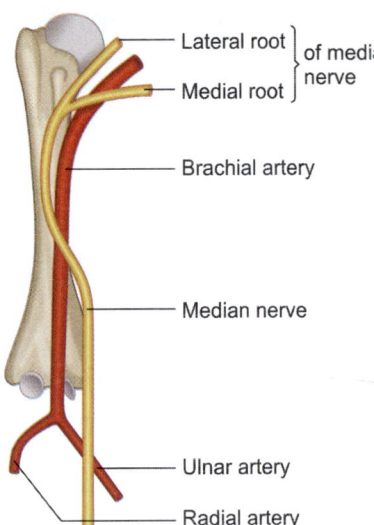

Fig. 11.4: Median nerve.

In the Arm (Fig. 11.4)
Descending vertically, the median nerve crosses the front of brachial artery from lateral to medial side at the middle of arm at the level of insertion of coracobrachialis.

The nerve crosses the elbow joint in front of brachialis and deep to the bicipital aponeurosis.

In the Forearm
In the upper end of forearm the median nerve presents important course and relation **in the cubital fossa.**

In the cubital fossa, as one of its contents, the median nerve presents important relationship with the tendon of biceps and the terminal end of brachial artery. *From lateral to medial*, the relationship is tendon, artery and nerve **(TAN)** (Fig. 11.5).

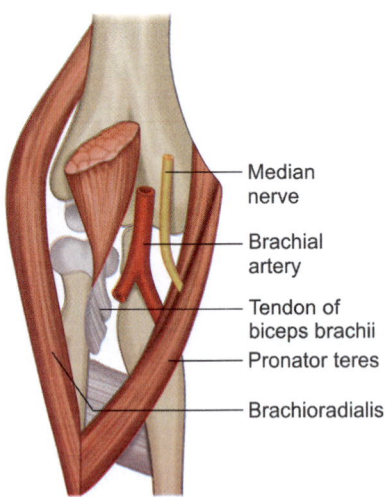

Fig. 11.5: Median nerve in cubital fossa.

In the cubital fossa, median nerve gives *muscular branches* to supply all the *superficial flexors of forearm*. It goes out of the cubital fossa passing between two heads of pronator teres.

Beyond cubital fossa, median nerve passes through the plane between fleshy bellies of flexor digitorum superficialis and flexor digitorum profundus running deep to the tendinous arch of the former muscle. While leaving cubital fossa, the median nerve gives out a branch from its back called *anterior interosseous nerve*.

About 5 cm above the level of the wrist, the median nerve appears on the lateral aspect of the tendon of flexor digitorum superficialis undercover of palmaris longus. It enters palm of the hand passing deep to flexor retinaculum.

Anterior interosseous nerve, along with the anterior interosseous artery, descends in front of interosseous membrane in between and deep to flexor pollicis longus and flexor digitorum profundus. It gives muscular branches to flexor pollicis longus and lateral half (for index and middle fingers) of flexor digitorum profundus. Finally the nerve passes deep to pronator quadratus to supply the muscle from its deep surface. Anterior interosseous nerve ends by giving articular branches of distal radioulnar, radiocarpal (wrist) and intercarpal joints.

In the Palm of Hand

Before the median nerve crosses the wrist, it gives palmar cutaneous branch. In the palm of hand, the median nerve gives muscular branch having recurrent direction for muscles of thenar eminence. Finally, it divides into digital branches for palmar aspect of lateral 3 ½ fingers with their nail beds and dorsal aspect of distal phalanges. First and second lumbricals are also supplied by the digital branches of the median nerve.

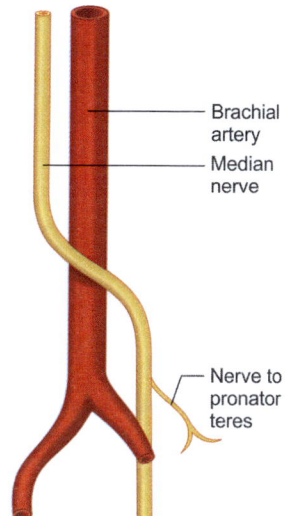

Fig. 11.6: Median nerve in the arm.

Branches

In the Arm (Fig. 11.6)
- **Muscular:** Pronator teres
- **Vascular:** Brachial artery.

In the Forearm (Fig. 11.7)
- Muscular (flexor)
  - Flexor carpi radialis
  - Palmaris longus
  - Flexor digitorum superficialis
- Anterior interosseous nerve (mixed nerve)
- Articular: Elbow joint
- Cutaneous: Palmar cutaneous nerve for lateral half of skin of the palm.

Anterior Interosseous Nerve (Fig. 11.8)
- **Muscular:**
  - Flexor pollicis longus

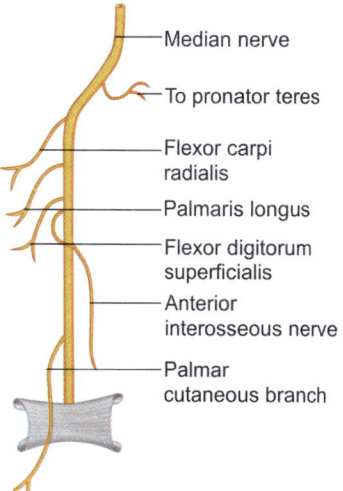

Fig. 11.7: Distribution of median nerve.

- Flexor digitorum profundus (lateral half)
- Pronator quardatus (from deep surface)
- **Articular:**
  - Distal radioulnar joint
  - Radiocarpal (wrist) joint
  - Intercarpal joints.

In the Palm of Hand (Fig. 11.9)

- **Recurrent (muscular) branch:** Abductor pollicis brevis, flexor pollicis brevis and opponens pollicis.
- **Digital (cutaneous) branches:** Common digital branches dividing into proper digital branches for palmar aspect of lateral 3 ½ fingers, each of which gives dorsal branches for corresponding areas of nail beds with skin over the distal phalanx.
- **Lumbrical branches:** 1st and 2nd lumbricals are supplied by proper digital branches for radial side of index and middle finger respectively.

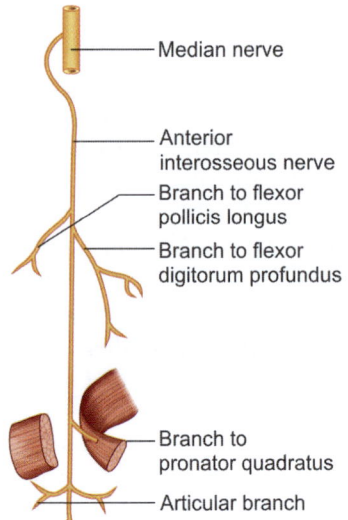

Fig. 11.8: Distribution of anterior interosseous nerve.

Clinical Anatomy

Median nerve is usually injured at the following two sites.
1. At the elbow
2. At the wrist.

Lesion at the Elbow

Motor loss

Paralysis of *pronators of forearm* and *long flexor muscles* of wrist and fingers *except flexor carpi ulnaris* and *medial half of flexor digitorum profundus* gives rise to following effect.

- Forearm is kept in supine position.
- Weakness of flexion of wrist.
- Wrist is in adducted position due to strength of flexor carpi ulnaris and medial half of flexor digitorum profundus associated with paralysis of flexor carpi radialis.
- Inability to flex interphalangeal joints of the index and middle fingers due to loss of function of lateral half of flexor digitorum profundus. Weak flexion of metacarpophalangeal joint is possible by the action of interossei.
- During an attempt to make a fist, though ring and little finger flex, index and to a lesser extent middle finger remain straight.
- Loss of flexion of terminal phalanx of thumb due to paralysis of flexor pollicis longus.
- *Flattening of hand* due to *wasting of thenar muscles* and *abduction and lateral rotation of thumb*. The deformity gives rise to *'ape-like'* hand.

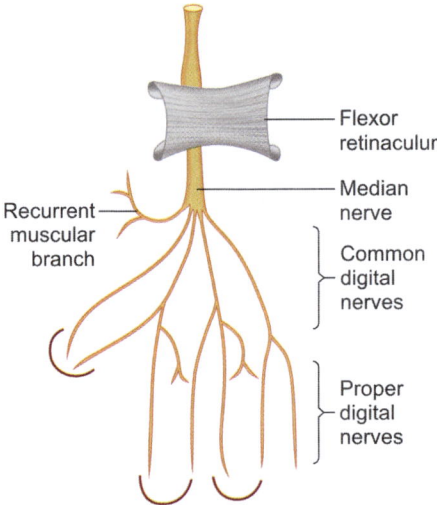

Fig. 11.9: Median nerve in the palm.

Sensory loss

Loss of sensation of the following areas of hand:
- Lateral 2/3 of palm of hand or a little less
- Palmar aspect of lateral 3 ½ fingers
- Dorsal surface of distal phalanx of the same fingers.

Lesion at the Wrist

Motor loss

Functions of forearm muscles are normal as their supply remains intact. Paralysis of thenar muscles leads to the *'ape-like'* deformity of the hand with following features:
- Wasting of thenar muscles with *'flattening'* of hand
- Thumb is *abducted* and *rotated laterally*.

In median nerve injury most serious motor defect is loss of opposition of thumb to the other fingers. This will affect 'pincer-like' skilled action of the hand.

Sensory loss

Loss of sensation of skin of palmar aspect of lateral 3 ½ finger with their dorsum opposite the distal phalanx will be evident.

Sensation of lateral half or 2/3 of palm of the hand will be preserved if the injury of the median nerve occurs distal to the origin of its palmar cutaneous branch above the wrist.

CARPAL TUNNEL SYNDROME

Carpal tunnel is the osseofibrous tunnel bounded by the concavity of palmar aspect of carpal bones and the deep surface of flexor retinaculum. Carpal tunnel syndrome occurs due to compression of the median nerve while passing through the tunnel which is tightly packed with flexor tendons with synovial sheath, nerves and vessels.

Effects of the syndrome are the following:
- Sensation of *'pins and needles'* or burning sensation over the skin of palmar aspect of lateral 3 ½ fingers.
- *Weakness of the thenar muscles.*

Causes of compression over the median nerve is either *synovial sheath inflammation* or *osteoarthritis of carpal bones*.

LA 11.4 Describe the ulnar nerve with its clinical anatomy.

ULNAR NERVE

Introduction

The ulnar nerve is so called because its course with most of its distribution are along the ulnar (medial) side of the upper limb.

Origin

Ulnar nerve originates in the axilla from the medial cord of brachial plexus carrying fibers of C_8 and T_1 nerve roots. A contribution from C_7 nerve is received from the median nerve. These fibers join at any level from the level of axilla to forearm.

Principle of Distribution

Ulnar nerve gives no branches in the axilla and arm. Along with the median nerve, motor fibers of ulnar nerve are distributed for flexor muscles of forearm and intrinsic muscles of palm of hand. It takes the minor share (only 1 ½ muscles) in forearm and major share (15 out of 20 muscles) in palm of the hand.

Course and Important Relations

In the Axilla and the Arm (Fig. 11.10)

In the axilla, the ulnar nerve is situated between axillary artery laterally and axillary vein medially. Here it is posterior to medial cutaneous of the forearm.

In the arm, the ulnar nerve runs medial to the brachial artery. *At the middle of arm*, opposite the level of insertion of coracobrachialis, the nerve *pierces the medial intermuscular septum of arm* and runs vertically downwards in the lower half of posterior compartment of arm. At the level of elbow, the ulnar nerve passes over the groove on the posterior surface of medial epicondyle. Here the nerve is superficial and passes through an osseofibrous tunnel whose boundary is as follows:
- Bony outline:
  - Lateral: Olecranon process of ulna
  - Medial: Medial epicondyle
- Fibrous outline:
  - Floor: Medial collateral ligament of elbow joint
  - Roof: A fibrous band (subcutaneous).

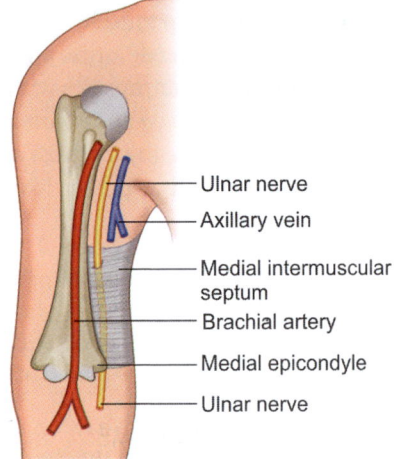

Fig. 11.10: Ulnar nerve in the arm.

In the Forearm (Fig. 11.11)

The ulnar nerve appears in the forearm *passing between the two heads of flexor carpi ulnaris*. Beyond the upper third of forearm, the nerve runs downwards in relation to the following structures.
- Lateral to flexor carpi ulnaris
- Medial to ulnar artery
- In front of flexor digitorum profundus.

After giving the muscular and the dorsal cutaneous (sensory) branches, the ulnar nerve reaches the front of wrist.

In Front of Wrist

In front of wrist, the ulnar nerve becomes superficial appearing in between the tendon of flexor carpi ulnaris and the ulnar artery. At the level of carpal tunnel, the nerve passes superficial to the flexor retinaculum but deep to its superficial slip called volar carpal ligament. Here the nerve passes between the pisiform bone medially and the hook of hamate laterally.

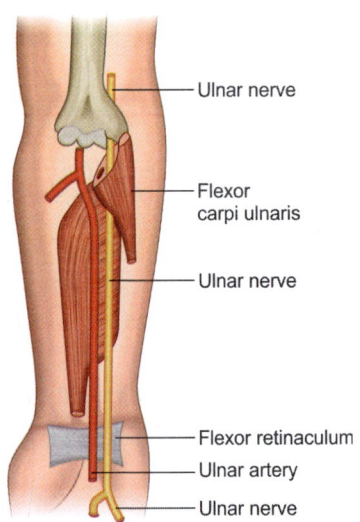

Fig. 11.11: Ulnar nerve in the forearm.

In the Palm of Hand

While crossing the flexor retinaculum or just distal to it, the ulnar nerve divides into superficial and terminal deep branches which reach the base of hypothenar eminence.

Superficial terminal branch supplies motor branch to palmaris brevis and sensory branch to skin of medial side of palm. It divides into two palmar digital nerves. One supplies the medial side of little finger. Other gives a twig to the median nerve and bifurcates into two proper digital branches for adjoining side of little and ring finger. Dorsal branches from the proper digital nerves supply nail bed and skin over distal phalanx of medial 1 ½ fingers.

Deep terminals branch, accompanied by deep branch of ulnar artery passes between abductor digiti minimi and flexor digiti minimi and then perforates opponens digiti minimi. The nerve passes from medial to lateral side of palm proximal to the concavity of deep palmar arch. It lies in the plane between flexor tendons and interossei. From proximal to the distal ends, the nerve gives branches to following muscles.

- Three hypothenar muscles
- 3rd and 4th lumbricals
- All the palmar and dorsal interossei
- Adductor pollicis
- Flexor pollicis brevis.
  It also gives articular branch to the wrist joint.

Dorsal branch of ulnar nerve originates in the forearm 5 cm above the wrist. It passes dorsally beneath the flexor carpi ulnaris. Piercing the deep fascia of forearm, it runs down along the medial side of back of the wrist. In the dorsum of hand, it bifurcates into two branches to supply medial side of little finger and adjacent sides of little and ring fingers. If the third branch is found to be present, it supplies adjacent side of ring and middle fingers. These dorsal digital branches reach up to the base of distal phalanx. In case of ring finger, it may supply even only up to the base to middle phalanx.

Branches

The ulnar nerve gives **no branches in axilla and arm**.

In the Forearm

- **Articular branch:** Gives to the elbow joint
- **Muscular branches:** To supply flexor carpi ulnaris and medial half of flexor digitorum profundus
- **Cutaneous branches:** Two in number
  i. Palmar cutaneous branch
  ii. Dorsal cutaneous branch
- **Superficial terminal branch:** It supplies palmaris brevis muscle of hypothenar region and skin of palmar surface of medial 1 ½ fingers
- **Deep terminal branch:** As muscular fibers to three hypothenar muscles, 3rd and 4th lumbricals, all interossei, adductor pollicis and usually flexor pollicis brevis
- Articular branch to radiocarpal joint.

Clinical Anatomy

Injury at Wrist

The ulnar nerve is **most commonly injured at the wrist**. This will give rise to following effects.

Motor loss

If injury occurs at the level of wrist, innervation of muscles in the forearm will not be affected. So, the flexor carpi ulnaris and the medial half of flexor digitorum profundus supplied by the ulnar nerve will function normally. Disability will be due to paralysis of 15 out of 20 intrinsic muscles of hand. All muscles of the hand except three thenar muscles and 1st and 2nd lumbricals will be paralyzed. So, following deformity will be observed.

- Due to paralysis of the both palmar and dorsal introssei, both **adduction as well as abduction of fingers will not be possible**. The patient will not be able to grip a piece of paper in between two fingers tightly.
- **Positive Froment's sign**: When the patient is asked to grip a piece of paper tightly between the thumb and the index finger, due to paralysis of adductor pollicis, he/she tries to do this through contraction of flexor pollicis longus tightly, which results in flexion of distal phalanx of thumb.
- **Ulnar claw hand:** Due to paralysis of all the interossei and 3rd and 4th lumbricals, there will be impairment of flexion of metacarpophalangeal joints and extension of interphalangeal joints. Due to unopposed action of extensor digitorum, metacarpophalangeal joints will be in extended position and interphalangeal joints will be in flexed position due to unopposed action of long flexor tendons. This deformity is known as *'Claw hand'*. As the 1st and 2nd lumbricals, supplied by the median nerve, are functioning, clawing of the index and middle finger will be partial. Full deformity of little and ring fingers and partial deformity of index and middle fingers lead to a condition called ulnar claw hand.
- *Paralysis of hypothenar muscles* leading to **'disuse atrophy'** will cause **flattening of medial side of the palm of hand**.
- Dorsum of hand will show **'hollowing'** of the spaces between metacarpal bones *due to wasting of the dorsal interossei muscles.*

Sensory loss

- Loss of sensation over the skin of palmar aspect of medial one and a half fingers will be evident due to lesion of superficial branch of ulnar nerve.
- If palmar cutaneous branch is affected, there will be loss of sensation over the skin of ulnar one-third of palm of the hand.

Lesion at Elbow

If the ulnar nerve is injured **at the level of elbow** *in addition to the abovementioned motor and sensory loss,* following effects are also observed.

Motor loss

Flexor carpi ulnaris and medial half of flexor digitorum profundus, giving tendons to ring and little fingers, are paralyzed. Following effects will be observed.

- When the patient is asked to make a tightly clenched first, tightening of tendon of flexor carpi ulnaris will be absent.
- Due to paralysis of flexor carpi ulnaris, flexion of wrist will be associated with abduction of wrist due to action flexor carpi radialis only.
- Due to paralysis of medial half of flexor digitorum profundus, remarkable flexion of terminal phalanges of ring and little finger will not be possible.
- Due to wasting of above two muscles, there will be flattening of medial border of front of forearm.

Sensory loss

In addition to the sensory loss on medial side of palm and medial one and a half fingers, *lesion of dorsal cutaneous branch* will give rise to following effects.
- Loss of cutaneous sensation over medial one third of dorsum of hand.
- Loss of cutaneous sensation on the dorsum of medial one and a half fingers.

LA 11.5 Describe the radial nerve with its clinical anatomy.

RADIAL NERVE

Introduction

Radial nerve is the thickest of the nerves arising from brachial plexus passing through the upper limb. It is so called, because in the most of its course, it passes along the radial (lateral) side of upper limb.

Radial nerve is the only nerve in the upper limb which are distributed to axilla, arm, forearm and hand.

Origin

Radial nerve originates from the posterior cord of brachial plexus and it contains the fibers arising from all the nerve roots (C_5 to C_8 and T_1) forming brachial plexus. However, *fibers of T_1 nerve are occasionally absent*.

Radial nerve, being the thickest and longest among the nerves of posterior cord, is *considered as continuation of the posterior cord*.

Principles of Distribution

- Radial nerve supplies all the muscles of posterior (extensor) compartments of arm and forearm.
- It gives cutaneous branches to the back of arm as well as forearm and to the major areas of dorsum of hand and fingers.
- It gives articular branches to all the joints it crosses.

Course, Important Relations and Distribution

In the Axilla

In the axilla, the radial nerve lies:
- In front of the muscles of posterior wall
- Behind the axillary artery (3rd part)
- Medial to the axillary nerve.

While the radial nerve passes through the axilla, it gives following branches:
- **Muscular branches**: To the long and medial head of triceps brachii
- **Sensory branches**: Posterior cutaneous nerve of the arm which supplies skin of the back of arm.

Entry from axilla to arm (Fig. 11.12)

Radial nerve *leaves the axilla at the lower border of teres major*.

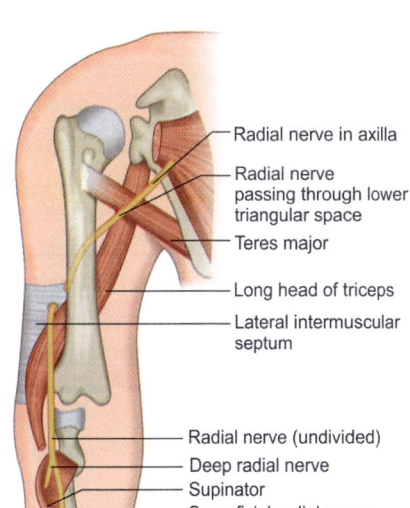

Fig. 11.12: Radial nerve in the arm.

It enters the back of arm passing through the **lower triangular space** which is bounded as follows:
- **Base:** Lower border of teres major
- **Medial side:** Long head of triceps
- **Lateral side:** Shaft of humerus.

In the Back of Arm (in the Spiral Groove) (Fig. 11.13)

In the posterior compartment of arm, the radial nerve is directly related to the spiral (radial) groove of shaft of the humerus. Here, the nerve is in direct contact with the bone undercover of lateral head of triceps arising from the oblique ridge of humerus above and parallel to the spinal groove.

Radial nerve *in the spiral groove* is the part of the nerve which passes through the *posterior compartment of the arm.* Here the radial nerve gives following branches.

Muscular branches to:
- Lateral head of triceps
- Medial head of triceps
- Anconeus: It is a long thin nerve passing through the fibers of medial head of triceps.

Sensory branches are the following:
- Lower lateral cutaneous nerve of the arm: It supplies the skin of lower part of posterolateral aspect of the arm.
- Posterior cutaneous nerve of the forearm: It gives branches to the skin of back of the forearm up to the level of wrist.

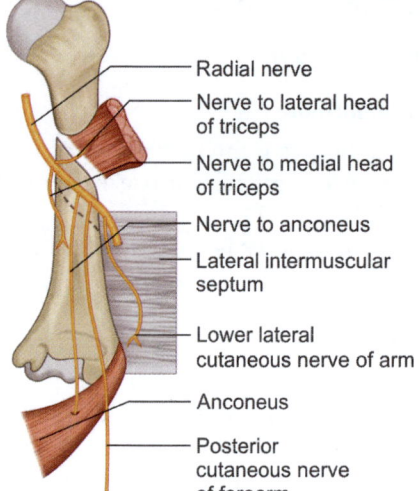

Fig. 11.13: Radial nerve in spiral groove.

After spiral groove:
The trunk of the radial nerve **after spiral groove** is the part in the lower third of **front of arm after piercing the lateral intermuscular septum** of arm.

The nerve lies here is the intermuscular furrow which is bounded as follows:
- **Medially:** Brachialis
- **Laterally:** Brachioradialis and extensor carpi radialis longus.

Here the radial nerve presents following characteristics:
- It gives branches to these three muscles
- It lies here in the lateral part of cubital fossa
- While it is on supinator muscle, the radial nerve divides into:
  - **Superficial terminal branch** (also called **superficial radial nerve**)—is a *purely sensory nerve* and *distributed to dorsum of hand.*
  - **Deep terminal branch** (also called **posterior interosseous nerve**)—almost *motor branch for muscles of back of forearm* with some articular filaments.

Deep Branch of Radial Nerve (in the Back of Forearm) (Fig. 11.14)

Deep branch of radial nerve is also called **posterior interosseous nerve** as it runs vertically on the posterior aspect of interosseous membrane.

The nerve enters the back of forearm winding round the lateral aspect of radius through the supinator muscle.

It lies initially in the plane between the superficial and deep group of extensor muscles. Beyond the extensor pollicis longus tendon, it is continued on the dorsal surface of interosseous membrane *in the form of a fine thread*. On the dorsal surface of carpus, the posterior interosseous nerve presents a thickening called '*pseudoganglion*' from which filaments are distributed to the carpal joints.

Branches of posterior interosseous nerve are grouped as follows.
- **Proximal to supinator:**
  - Supinator
  - Extensor carpi radialis brevis
- **In the supinator**: Additional branch to supinator
- **Distal to supinator**

Three short branches:
- Extensor digitorum
- Extensor digiti minimi
- Extensor carpi ulnaris

Two long branches:
- **Lateral**: To abductor pollicis longus and extensor pollicis brevis
- **Medial**: To extensor pollicis longus and extensor indicis.

Terminal branches (*articular*):
- Inferior radioulnar joint
- Wrist joint
- Intercarpal joints.

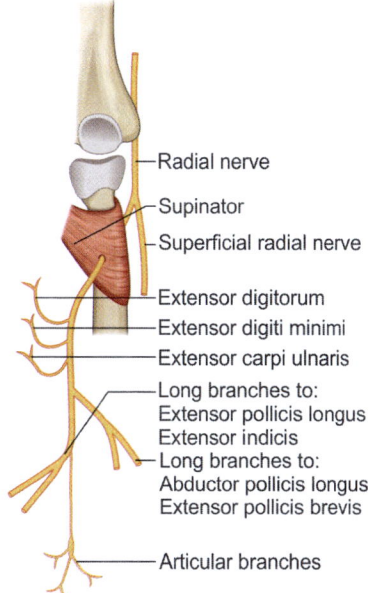

Fig. 11.14: Deep radial (posterior interosseous) nerve.

Superficial Terminal Branch (for the Dorsum of Hand)

This nerve is also called **superficial radial nerve**. Though it arises in the cubital fossa as one of the two terminal divisions of radial nerve, it is *for sensory innervation in the dorsum of hand*.

Superficial radial nerve descends along the lateral side of front of forearm lateral to the radial artery deep to brachioradialis. It winds around the lateral side of radius deep to brachioradialis 7 cm above the wrist. It pierces deep fascia on the lower part of back of forearm and enters the dorsum of hand crossing over the anatomical snuff box. On the dorsum of hand, it **divides into digital nerves** to supply the skin of dorsal aspect of lateral 3 ½ fingers up to the level of base of terminal phalanx.

Clinical Anatomy

Injuries to the radial nerve is common in the axilla and in the spiral groove.

Injuries in the Axilla

The most common causes of injuries to the radial nerve are the following.
- Pressure of the upper end of a badly fitting crutch in armpit
- Pressure on the axilla when a drunken person falls asleep with one arm over the back of the chair
- Pressure on the nerve by fracture dislocation of upper end of humerus.

Effect of the nerve injury in the axilla will be due to loss of functions of all the branches of radial nerve including those arising in the axilla.

Motor loss

All extensors of the elbow (triceps and anconeus), wrist and fingers are paralyzed. So disabilities will be following:
- Patient is unable to extend the elbow joint, the wrist joint and the fingers. Elbow will remain in flexed position.
- Wrist will remain in flexed position. The deformity is known as **wrist drop**. Due to this position of the wrist, a tight grip to hold an object by full flexion of the fingers is not possible. Wrist drop occurs due to unopposed action of the flexor muscles.
- Though supinator and brachioradialis are paralyzed, so supination of forearm is not possible when the elbow is in extended position. In flexed position of elbow, supination of forearm can be performed by biceps brachii.

Sensory loss

- Skin over the back and lower lateral part of the arm.
- A narrow strip of skin over the back of forearm.
- Lateral part of dorsum of hand and the dorsal aspect of lateral three and a half fingers except the area over the distal phalanges.

Injury at the Spiral Groove

Causes

- Fracture of the shaft of humerus and subsequent union of the bone trapping the nerve
- Pressure over the nerve by the edge of the operation table
- Prolonged application of tourniquet in the arm.

Effect

Motor loss

The patient will be unable to extend the wrist and fingers with the presentation of **wrist drop** deformity.

Extension of the elbow will not be affected if the nerve supply of triceps and anconeus is preserved.

Sensory loss

- Loss of cutaneous sensation over the skin of the larger lateral area of dorsum of hand and the dorsal aspect of lateral three and a half fingers due to loss of function of superficial branch of the radial nerve.
- As the injury site is the spiral groove, loss of sensation over the skin of back of arm as well as forearm will be observed if the posterior cutaneous nerves of the arm and the forearm are involved.

Chapter 12

Explanatory Notes (Clinical/Embryological/Morphological)

12.1 The clavicle is the specialized long bone.

The clavicle is a long bone as it has a length with medial (sternal) and lateral (acromial) ends with the shaft in between.

It is considered as a specialized long bone because the bone has the following special character by which it differs from all other long bones of the body.
- The clavicle is the long bone having *no medullary cavity*.
- It develops through the *membranous type of ossification*.
- *Two primary centers* of ossification appear at the shaft.
- *One secondary center* appears for the medial (sternal) end of the clavicle only. The lateral (acromial) end grows as an extension of the diaphysis (shaft).
- It is the long bone (except the metatarsals) which is *horizontally placed* in the body.

Apart from the above-mentioned special character, the clavicle presents also following two features when compared to all the bones of the body.
1. It is the first bone to ossify. Two primary centers appear at 5th to 6th week of intrauterine life.
2. It is the bone which may be pierced through and through by a cutaneous nerve (middle supraclavicular nerve).

12.2 Fracture of the clavicle commonly occurs at the junction of medial two-thirds and lateral one-third.

Fracture of the clavicle occurs very commonly due to indirect violence as a result of blows or impact on the shoulder or fall on outstretched hand. Fracture occurs at the junction of medial two-thirds (presenting anterior convexity) and lateral one-third (anterior concavity). This is the weakest *point of the bone* due to following reasons.
- Two curvatures of this bone meet at this point.
- This point is weakest because the medial two-thirds are cylindrical and the lateral one-third is flattened.
- The junctional point of the two curvatures is the site where two primary centers of ossification appear side by side. From this point of cleavage between the two centers, ossification process extends towards both the ends.
- At the junction of two curvatures, the surface of the bone does not give attachment to any muscle, so this site is less secured.
- The junction between medial and lateral curvatures is pierced by following structures:
  - Nutrient artery
  - Middle supraclavicular nerve (occasionally).

12.3 Breast abscess is always drained through a radial incision, and never through the circular incision.

A localized breast abscess develops due to infection and inflammation of the breast tissue by microorganism. Glandular parenchyma of the breast tissue is made up of 15–20 lobules. Adjacent lobules are separated by the fibrous septa demarcating the compartments. These septa act as the first line of barrier against the spread of infection from one lobule to the adjacent one. Each of the glandular lobules drains through one lactiferous duct from the periphery of the breast centrally to the nipple through centripetal direction. It means that the lactiferous ducts are radially arranged. So, for drainage of the breast abscess through radial incision has following advantages when compared to the circular or elliptical incision.

- The lactiferous duct, radially directed, so parallel to the radial incision will have little chance of injury.
- Unlike the circular or elliptical incision, the radial incision will not cause spread of infection from the affected compartment to the adjacent healthy one.

12.4 An elderly lady presenting a nodular swelling in the axilla must be given proper clinical attention.

A blunt conical prolongation of the breast tissue extends upwards, backwards and laterally from the superolateral quadrant of the organ to the axilla. It is called the *axillary tail of Spence*. Though the whole breast lies in the plane of superficial fascia of the pectoral region, the axillary tail is more deeply placed beneath the axillary fascia passing through the fascial opening called the *foramen of Langer*.

Occasionally, the carcinoma of the breast may start growing from the axillary tail of the gland, in which case, initially the whole of the breast may be found normal and healthy. For this reason, when an elderly lady complains of a nodular swelling in the axilla, probability of the carcinoma of the breast arising from the axillary tail is to be ruled out through proper clinical examination and investigations.

12.5 A patient suffering from carcinoma of breast may present the following signs—(a) peau d'orange appearance of the breast skin, (b) dimple or puckering of the skin, (c) retraction of the nipple and (d) fixation of the breast over the deeper structures.

Peau d'orange is a Latin term which means the orange peel. The orange peel looks glossy and swollen with number of small pits. In case of carcinoma of breast, the skin of the breast show glossy and swollen appearance like the orange peel, if the subcutaneous lymph vessels get obstructed due to infiltration by the cancer cells. The pitted appearance of the skin is due to infiltration and also retraction of the connective tissue septa attached to the deep surface of the skin.

Dimple or puckering of the skin overlying the breast is due to retraction of fibers of the suspensory ligament of Cooper as a result of infiltration by the cancer cells.

Retraction of the nipple is due to infiltration of the lactiferous duct by the cancer cells and subsequent fibrosis.

Fixation or adhesion of the breast to the underlying pectoral fascia and pectoral muscles is due to direct spread of the cancerous growth of breast to the deeper structures.

12.6 Krukenberg's tumor of the ovary is one of the example of metastasis (secondary spread) of carcinoma of the breast.

Because of the widespread lymphatic drainage of the breast, metastasis of the breast through lymphatic channels occurs in various sites all around the organ. Lymph vessels from the lower medial quadrant of the breast follow through a peculiar route. They pass along the pectoral region and anterior abdominal wall. Piercing the linea alba, the vessels drain into the subdiaphragmatic and subperitoneal lymph nodes. First the cancer cells spread along this route. The disseminated cancer cells thus reach the peritoneum from where finally the cancer cells may drop down through peritoneum (transperitoneal route) to cause ovarian metastasis which is called *Krukenberg's tumor*.

12.7 Upper lesion of the brachial plexus causes Erb-Duchenne paralysis.

The upper lesion of brachial plexus affects the upper trunk of the plexus which is formed by the union of the C_5 and C_6 nerve roots. It results from the sudden forceful increase of the angle between the side of the neck and the top of the shoulder. It occurs if the neck with the head is displaced to the opposite side and/or the shoulder is abnormally depressed to the same side. This kind of injury will cause excessive traction or even tearing of the C_5 and C6 roots. So, the function of the suprascapular (C_5, C_6), axillary (C_5, C_6) and musculocutaneous (C_5, C_6, C_7) will be affected. The effect of the lesion will be as follows:

Motor Loss
- Lesion of the suprascapular nerve will cause paralysis of:
  - Supraspinatus: Loss of abduction of shoulder
  - Infraspinatus: Loss of lateral rotation of shoulder
- Lesion of the axillary nerve will cause paralysis of:
  - Deltoid: Loss of abduction of shoulder
  - Teres minor: Loss of lateral rotation of shoulder
- Lesion of the musculocutaneous nerve will cause paralysis of:
  - Biceps brachii: Loss of supination of forearm and flexion of elbow
  - Brachialis: Loss of flexion of elbow
  - Corachobrachialis: Loss of flexion of shoulder.

Deformity in Erb-Duchenne paralysis will be as follows:
- The limb will hang by the side of the body with medial rotation due to unopposed action of pectoralis major. The elbow will be extended and the forearm will be pronated because of the loss of action of biceps and brachialis.
- The position of the upper limb in this condition is like that of a porter or waiter hinting for a tip. That is why the lesion is also called '*porter or waiter tips paralysis*'.

Sensory Loss
Loss of cutaneous sensation along the lateral sides of the arm (C_5) and forearm (C_6).

12.8 Lower lesion of the brachial plexus causes Klumpke paralysis.

The lower lesion of brachial plexus affects the lower trunk of the plexus which is formed by the union of C_8 and T_1 nerve roots. It results from the sudden increase of the angle between the medial side of the arm and the lateral chest wall. It may occur due to hyperabduction of the shoulder when a person attempts to save himself/herself by clutching an object with the help of hand while falling from a height. Sudden forceful overstretching of the arm will cause tearing of C_8 and T_1 roots forming the lower trunk of brachial plexus. This lesion called Klumpke paralysis, will give rise to the following motor and sensory dysfunction.

Motor Loss

Motor fibers of C_8 and T_1 roots are distributed through the lower trunk and finally through the median and ulnar nerve to all the small muscles of the hand. Among the small muscles, the lumbricals and the interossei are concerned with flexion of the metocarpophalangeal joints and extension of the interphalangeal joints. In Klumpke paralysis, not only these functions are lost, the hand will be deformed showing hyperextension of the metacarpophalangeal joint and hyperflexion of the interphalangeal joints. These two kinds of the deformities are due to the unopposed action of the extensor and flexor tendons of the fingers respectively. The deformed condition is known as *full claw hand*.

In addition, the hand will show flattening of the thenar and hypothenar eminences due to wasting of the respective group of the muscles.

Sensory Loss

The Klumpke paralysis is also associated with the loss of the cutaneous sensation over the medial two fingers, medial side of the hand and forearm (C_8) and the medial side of the arm (T_1).

12.9 Lesion of the long thoracic nerve results in winging of the scapula.

Long thoracic nerve arises in the supraclavicular part of the brachial plexus by union of the fibers from the roots of 5th, 6th and 7th cervical nerves. The nerve then runs along the upper part of anterolateral chest wall to supply the only muscle, serratus anterior.

The nerve may be injured due to the following causes.
- A blow to or pressure on the root of the neck of the lower end of the posterior triangle
- A major surgical operation like radical mastectomy to treat carcinoma of the breast.

The serratus anterior has the following roles in our daily life.
- The tone of the muscle keeps the scapular costal surface with its vertebral border and inferior angle in close contact with the chest wall
- The muscle helps in protraction (forward gliding) of the scapula along the chest wall when a pressure of the hand is applied to push an object forwards
- It rotates the scapula upwards, forwards and laterally when the arm is abducted beyond 90° to raise the hand above the head.

So, paralysis of serratus anterior muscle due to lesion of the long thoracic nerve will give rise to following disabilities.
- Inability to raise the hand above the head through upward and forward rotation of scapula
- Lack of power to push a fixed or heavy object forwards.

While the above-mentioned movements are attempted, the vertebral border and inferior angle of the scapula will no longer remain closely applied to the chest wall and will be protruded called *winging of scapula*.

12.10 Injury to the axillary nerve gives rise to a typical abduction disability of the shoulder.

Axillary nerve is often injured due to the any of the following reasons.
- Pressure by a badly adjusted crutch which presses the nerve upwards in the axilla
- Following anteroinferior dislocation of the shoulder joint the dislocated humeral head may press the nerve downwards
- Fracture of surgical neck of humerus may cause entrapment of the nerve.

Disability for the nerve injury is due to paralysis of the deltoid muscle which is the powerful abductor of the shoulder. The patient will be able to abduct the shoulder up to 15° due to action of supraspinatus muscle. But further abduction from 15° to 90° will be impaired due to paralysis of deltoid.

Teres minor, one of the lateral rotators of shoulder and supplied by the axillary nerve, will also be paralyzed. But it will not produce any impact in lateral rotation which is mainly done by the infraspinatus muscle.

Cutaneous sensation will be lost over the lower half of deltoid.

Remote effect of axillary nerve lesion will be *prominence of the greater tuberosity* of humerus as a result of *disuse atrophy of deltoid*.

12.11 Effect of the radial nerve injury—(a) at the axilla and (b) at the spiral groove.

RADIAL NERVE INJURY AT THE AXILLA

It occurs usually due to prolonged use of a badly adjusted crutch which presses over the nerve in the axilla. It is the example of more central lesion of the radial nerve before its branches are given out. This lesion is typically called **crutch paralysis** having the following effects.

Motor Effects

- Loss of extension of the elbow due to paralysis of the *triceps brachii*. The elbow will remain in flexed position due to the unopposed action of the flexor muscle.
- Flexor deformity of the wrist, called wrist drop due to loss of extension of wrist as a result of paralysis of all extensors supplied by the deep branch of radial nerve and due to the unopposed action of the flexor muscles of the wrist.
- Supination of the forearm in extended position of the elbow will not be possible due to paralysis of the *supinator* muscle. However, supination can be carried out in semiflexed position by the biceps.

Sensory Loss

- Loss of sensation (anesthesia) over the lower part of the back of the arm
- Loss of sensation over the narrow strip of skin over the back of forearm
- Loss of sensation over the skin of lateral two-thirds area of the dorsum of hand and dorsum of lateral 3 ½ fingers up to the proximal and middle phalanx.

RADIAL NERVE INJURY AT THE SPIRAL GROOVE

This lesion may occur in the following cases:
- In case of fracture of the shaft of humerus at the spiral groove
- Where a drunken person falls asleep overnight with his arm pressed against the backrest or arm of the chair. It is called 'Saturday night paralysis'. As it is the more peripheral lesion of the nerve, the effect of the lesion will be a little different as follows:

Motor Loss

- Triceps brachii will not be functionless as the two heads of the muscles out of the three, long and medial, receive their supply from the radial nerve proximal to the spiral groove. So extension function of the elbow will not be impaired.
- Other effects, e.g. the wrist drop and loss of supination in extended position of the elbow will be same as the previous lesion.

Sensory Loss

Loss of sensation over the lateral two-thirds of the dorsum of hand and the dorsum of the lateral three and a half fingers up to the proximal and middle phalanges.

12.12 Discuss the difference between full claw hand and ulnar claw hand.

Claw hand is the deformity of hand which shows following presentations.
- Hyperextension of the metacarpophalangeal joints
- Hyperflexion of the proximal and distal interphalangeal joints
- Hyperextension of the wrist joint.

The deformity is called full claw hand when it affects all the five fingers of the hand. In case of ulnar claw hand, the only medial two fingers, the ring and little, are affected. The finger deformities are due to loss of function of the lumbricals and interossei which causes flexion of metacarpophalangeal joints and extension of the both proximal as well as distal interphalangeal joints.

FULL CLAW HAND

This clinical condition is the effect of the central lesion of brachial plexus. It is due to injury of the lower trunk of brachial plexus which is formed by union of C_8 and T_1 nerves. The injury to the lower trunk occurs due to sudden, forceful hyperabduction of the shoulder. C_8 and T_1 fibers of lower trunk shared by the median and ulnar nerve are distributed to the small muscles of hand including the lumbricals and interossei. As these nerve fibers are commonly lesioned at the lower trunk level in the axilla, the full claw hand affecting all the fingers results. Again it may be found in case of injury to both the median and ulnar nerves at the level of elbow. The deformity of the full claw hand will show following features.

- Hyperextension of the metacarpophalangeal joint: Caused by unopposed action of extensor tendons of the fingers.
- Flexion of both the proximal as well as distal interphalangeal joint: Caused by unopposed action of superficial and deep flexor tendons of the fingers.

  } Due to loss of function of lumbricals and interossei

- Hyperextension of the wrist: Caused by unopposed action of extensors of the wrist, e.g. extensor carpi radialis (longus and brevis) and ulnaris.

  } Due to loss of function of flexor carpi radialis and ulnaris

ULNAR CLAW HAND (MAIN-EN-GRIFFE)

The ulnar claw hand is the more peripheral lesion of selective fibers of C_8 and T_1 nerves passing through the ulnar nerve. This is due to lesion of the ulnar nerve which occurs commonly due to fracture dislocation of the elbow. In this case, typical claw hand deformity will be obvious in ring and little fingers due to loss of both lumbricals and interossei of these two fingers. As the 1st and 2nd lumbrical muscles, which are for the index and middle fingers, are supplied by the median nerve, the claw hand deformity is not manifested in lateral two fingers.

Associated Deformities in Ulnar Claw Hand

- Because of the paralysis of the palmar and dorsal interossei, power of abduction and adduction of the fingers is abolished. That is why, when asked for, the patient will fail to grip a piece of paper tightly between two adjacent fingers.
- **Positive Froment's sign**: Patient fails to adduct the thumb due to paralysis of adductor pollicis. It asked, the patient attempts to grip a piece of paper between the thumb and index finger, he does it by tight contraction of flexor pollicis longus along with flexion of the terminal phalanx.
- Flattening of the hypothenar eminence and loss of the convexity of the medial border of the hand due to paralysis and disuse atrophy of the hypothenar muscles.

- Appearance of hollowing between the metacarpal bones on the dorsum of hand due to wasting of the dorsal interossei muscle.

12.13 Hand shows 'ape-like' deformity in case of the median nerve injury.

'Ape-like' hand is formed if the median nerve is injured far more distally at the level of the wrist. It gives rise to the following deformities or disabilities.
- The thenar eminence is flattened as the thenar muscles are finally wasted following their paralysis.
- The thumb is adducted and laterally rotated. Adduction deformity is due to paralysis of abductor pollicis brevis and so unopposed action of adductor policis supplied by ulnar nerve. Lateral rotation is due to paralysis of opponens pollicis and flexor pollicis brevis.
- Opposition movement of the thumb towards the tips of other fingers become impossible due to paralysis of opponens pollicis.
- As the first and second lumbricals are paralyzed. If a patient is asked to make a fist slowly, the movement of the index and middle finger lags behind the movements of the ring and little finger.

12.14 Carpal tunnel syndrome gives rise to the sensation of 'pins and needles' along the lateral aspect of palm of the hand.

Carpal tunnel is an osseofibrous tunnel on the front of the wrist. It is bounded posteriorly by the concave anterior surface of the carpal bones and anteriorly by the fibrous band of the flexor retinaculum. The tunnel is tightly packed by their synovial sheaths and the median nerve.

Carpal tunnel syndrome is a clinical condition causing compression of the median nerve within the tunnel. The causes may be the following.
- Tenosynovitis: Inflammation of the synovial sheath of flexor tendons.
- Osteoarthritic changes or fracture dislocation of the carpal bones.
- Fluid accumulation in the tunnel due to some diseases like hypothyroidism.

Clinically the syndrome is manifested by:
- Burning pain, classically termed as 'pins and needles' along the distribution of the median nerve to the lateral three and a half fingers.
It is to be noted that no paresthesia occurs over the thenar eminence because this area is supplied by the palmar cutaneous branch of the median nerve, which passes superficial to the flexor retinaculum.
- Weakness of the thenar muscles.
The condition is dramatically relieved if the tunnel is decompressed by making a longitudinal incision through the flexor retinaculum.

12.15 Various factors maintain the stability of the multiaxial shoulder joint having wide range of mobility.

The articulation between relatively large hemispherical head of humerus and shallow glenoid fossa of the shoulder joint permits a wide range of mobility at the expense of stability. That is why, following factors come into action to increase the stability of the joint.
- The glenoid labrum: It is a fibrocartilaginous rim attached to the margin of glenoid fossa. It increases the depth of the fossa. Thus it increases the congruence of the articular surface.
- The glenohumeral ligaments act as static stabilizer in certain positions of the joint.
- Negative pressure within the joint plays a role for contact of the articular surfaces.
- Coracoacromial arch act as s secondary socket to prevent upward displacement of the head of humerus.

- Rotator cuff: Tendons of some muscles are fused with the outer surface of the capsule of shoulder joint to give additional strength. This is called rotator cuff. The tendons forming the cuff are as follows:

Anteriorly:	Subscapularis
Superiorly:	Supraspinatus
Posteriorly:	Infraspinatus
Posteroinferiorly:	Teres minor

  The rotator cuff maintains the compressive force on the surface of the capsule to keep proper contact between two articular surfaces.
  It resists the displacement of the articular surfaces.
- Long head of triceps offers inferior support of the joint particularly in abducted condition of the shoulder joint.
- Long head of biceps offers additional support superiorly.

12.16 The shoulder joint is commonly dislocated inferiorly.

Due to maximum freedom of movement and the lack of stability of the shoulder joint, dislocation is common as a result of direct or indirect trauma. The stability of the shoulder joint depends to a great extent on the surrounding muscles, specially the short muscles which form the *rotator cuff*. Through the rotator cuff the joint capsule is strengthened superiorly by supraspinatus, anteriorly by subscapularis and posteriorly by infraspinatus and teres minor. In addition, superior displacement is further prevented by the secondary socket formed by the *coracoacromial arch*.

Inferior dislocation of the humeral head from the glenoid fossa is therefore common due to the following two fundamental reasons.
1. The rotator cuff is deficient inferiorly.
2. To allow hyperabduction of the shoulder, the capsule is very loose inferiorly.

Following inferior dislocation, the head of the humerus is displaced inferoanteriorly in front of the glenoid fossa deep to the subscapularis muscle.

12.17 Tennis elbow.

Considering the pathology, this clinical condition is known as *lateral epicondylitis*. It is characterized by the inflammation of the tissue surrounding the lateral epicondyle of humerus.

This condition is called *tennis elbow* because this type of injury results very commonly among the tennis players during sudden forceful extension of the elbow in pronated condition of the forearm. This type of movement occurs during backhand strokes in the lawn tennis. Of course the same kind of injury may be found in cricketers. The patient complains of pain over the lateral epicondyle of the humerus. The pain occurs on extension of the wrist and elbow in pronated condition of the forearm.

The lesions in the 'tennis elbow' may be the following:
- Sprain or the tear of the common extensor origin
- Tearing of the independent fibers of extensor carpi radialis brevis muscle
- Sprain of the radial collateral ligament of the elbow joint
- Inflammation of the bursa beneath the extensor carpi radialis brevis muscle.

12.18 Younger children often suffer from 'pulled elbow'.

The head of the radius is kept well secured within the osseofibrous ring of the superior radioulnar joint. The major part of the circumference of the ring is formed by the tough fibers of the annular ligament. In case of adults the annular ligament is funnel shaped. Its upper cylindrical part encircles the head of the radius and the lower conical part fits as a tight coller around the neck of the bone. But in case of young children, whole of the ligament is vertically cylindrical. So, when a child is lifted off the ground suddenly by pulling up his/her arm in pronated condition of the forearm, the head of the radius slips partially downwards out of the annular ligament. It results in partial dislocation (subluxation) of the head of the radius. The radius head is displaced distally, partially out of the torn annular ligament. The proximal part of the ligament may be trapped between the head of the radius and the capitulum of the humerus. Clinically this condition is known as *'pulled elbow'* characterized by the pain due to pinched annular ligament.

12.19 Fracture of the bones around the elbow results in Volkmann's ischemic contracture.

Volkmann's ischemic contracture is the deformity characterized by contracture (shortening) due to fibrosis of the muscles of the flexor and/or extensor group of the forearm. It results a complication of the fracture of lower end of humerus or, upper end of radius or ulna. The disorder is the effect of spasm of a localized segment of the brachial artery either due to fracture itself or due to overtight plaster cast. The muscles of the forearm undergo ischemic necrosis because of the reduced arterial blood flow to them due to arterial spasm. The flexor muscles are mainly affected because they are longer than the extensors.

The deformity is one of the following types:
- The long flexor muscles of the wrist and fingers are *more contracted* than extensor muscles.
  Defect: The wrist joint is flexed and the fingers are extended.
- The long extensor muscles of the fingers, which are inserted through the extensor expansion to the proximal phalanx, are greatly contracted.
  Defect: The wrist and metacarpophalangeal joints are extended and the interphalangeal joints of the finger are flexed.
- Both the flexor as well as the extensor muscles of the forearm are contracted.
  Defect:
  – Wrist joint—flexed
  – Metacarpophalangeal joints—extended
  – Interphalangeal joints—flexed.

12.20 Dupuytren's contracture results in flexion deformity of the ring and little finger.

Dupuytren's contracture is the clinical condition characterized by progressive fibrosis of the ulnar side of the palmar aponeurosis. It leads to contracture of the digital slips of the palmar aponeurosis for the ring finger and the little finger. The deformity usually starts at the root of the ring finger and bends the finger into the palm flexing the metacarpophalangeal joint. Later, the little finger is affected in the same manner. When the condition becomes long standing, as the fibrous flexor sheaths of the corresponding fingers are pulled, the proximal interphalangeal joints are also flexed. But the distal interphalangeal joints are not involved. These remain extended and come in contact with the palm.

The deformity is corrected through the following procedures.
- When *collagenase enzyme* is injected into the contracted band of the fibrous tissue, it gives rise to remarkable improvement of the contracture.
- *Surgical resection* of the fibrous bands is followed by *physiotherapy*.

12.21 Trigger finger.

It is a clinical condition characterized by a palpable or audible *'snapping'* of a finger when asked to flex or extend it. It occurs if there is narrowing of the space deep to fibrous flexor sheath or thickening of the flexor tendon in front of the metacarpophalangeal joint.

Normally the long flexor tendons enclosed by the synovial sheath move freely and smoothly inside the space of fibrous flexor sheath of the fingers. Trigger finger is so called because in this condition the long flexor tendons find less space to play smoothly within the fibrous flexor sheath leading to perception of 'palpable or audible snapping' like the trigger of a gun when the finger is flexed or extended.

12.22 Knowledge of anatomical snuff box is important for the clinicians.

Anatomical snuff box is a narrow triangular depression located just proximal to the dorsolateral aspect of the base of the thumb. It is more clearly visible on extension of the thumb. This small fossa is bounded laterally by the tendons of abductor pollicis longus and extensor pollicis brevis and medially by the tendon of extensor pollicis longus. The floor is formed by the scaphoid bone. The contents are the formation of cephalic vein, a segment of the radial artery and terminal branching of the superficial radial nerve. Because of the crowding of these structures, special attention is to be given for this fossa by the clinicians for the following reasons.
- Deep tenderness is felt at the floor of the fossa for the fracture of scaphoid.
- The cephalic vein is commonly selected for venepuncture at the roof of the anatomical snuff box.
- The pulsation of the radial artery can be felt here against the scaphoid bone at the floor.
- Terminal branches of superficial radial nerve, if pressed here, may give rise to paresthesia (altered sensation) on the lateral aspect of the dorsum of hand.

12.23 Digital pulp space infection may be very serious causing avascular necrosis of the distal 4/5th of the terminal phalanx sparing its proximal 1/5th.

The pulp space of the fingers is a closed fascial compartment filled up with locules of fat on the palmar aspect of the distal phalanx. These spaces, specially of the thumb and index finger, are very often infected by the micro-organisms following a simple pricking injury. A pair of proper digital artery traverses this space along the two margins of the fingers. Before the artery enters the space a branch is given off to supply the proximal 1/5th epiphysis of the distal phalanx freely. The remaining distal 4/5th receive branches which are entangled by the fibrous septa traversing the space. Because of the unyielding nature of the pulp space, as it is traversed by the fibrous septa, the digital artery supplying the distal 4/5th of the distal phalanx is compressed by the inflammatory tissue. If the infection is left out or neglected, the compressed artery will lead to jeopardization of the blood supply to the distal 4/5th of the terminal phalanx. Ultimately, it may be serious to cause avascular necrosis of this part of terminal phalanx sparing its proximal 1/5th (epiphysis) supplied by the branch of the digital artery which arises proximal to the pulp space.

12.24 A pricking injury at the tip of thumb or little finger may give rise to the painful swelling in the palm of the hand.

This complication results from the spread of infection from digital synovial sheath of the thumb and little finger. The condition, known as *tenosynovitis* results from a small penetrating wound, made by point of a needle or thorn. On rare occasion, the sheath may becomes infected by extension of the pulp space infection.

The digital synovial sheath of the index, middle and ring finger extend proximally up to the level of the head of the metacarpal at the base of the corresponding finger. The digital sheath for the thumb is continued from the *radial bursa* which is the synovial sheath of the tendon of flexor pollicis longus. The ulnar bursa is the synovial sheath of the tendons of flexor digitorum superficialis and profundus. It extends in the palm of the hand at the midmetacarpal level from where it is continued further distally in the little finger as digital synovial sheath for the same finger.

So, when infection starts due to pricking injury at the tips of the thumb and little finger, it spreads through the radial and ulnar bursa respectively to the palm of the hand. Infection results in distension of the sheath with pus. The finger and the palm are swollen due to accumulation of pus. The distended finger is held in semiflexed position. Passive extension of the finger is extremely painful as the distended sheath is stretched.

12.25 Infection of palmar spaces (thenar and midpalmar spaces) may give rise to the swelling in the web spaces, dorsum of hand and margins of lower end of forearm.

Hand infection is very common in the group of people who are in habit of manual labor through grip functions. Pricking injury may lead to infection in thenar and midpalmar spaces of the palm. Though these spaces are deep to the palmar aponeurosis and flexor tendons, but superficial infection may spread to the deep through the thin fascial lining of the spaces. Again the infection can spread from one space to the another through the thin barrier of intermediate septum attached to palmar aspect of the shaft of the third metacarpal bone. Pus or infected fluid, accumulated initially in the palmar spaces fails to bulge out towards the palmar surface due to the thick skin and tough palmar aponeurosis. But infected fluid and edema spread through the following lines of less resistance.

- Infection spreads through lumbrical canals from the thenar and midpalmar spaces to the web spaces between the bases of adjacent fingers.
- As the lymph vessels pass through the intermetacarpal spaces from palm to dorsum, edematous fluid fills up the dorsal subaponeurotic space.
- Though the thenar and midpalmar spaces are closed proximally by the fascial lining, gradually increasing inflammatory fluid breaks the fascial barrier and extends proximally to the forearm space of Parona between the strong bunch of flexor tendons superficially and the pronator quadratus in the deep. Finally inflammatory swelling may be found to bulge out at the lateral as well as medial margins of the lower end of the forearm.

Chapter 13

SECTION 2: LOWER LIMB

Front of Thigh

SN 13.1 Write a short note on inguinal lymph nodes.

INGUINAL LYMPH NODES

Inguinal lymph nodes which are present in the plane of subcutaneous fatty tissue are known as **superficial inguinal lymph nodes**. These lymph nodes are important because they receive lymph vessels from lower limb, perineum with external genitalia and infraumbilical part of the body wall.

Superficial Inguinal Lymph Nodes (Fig. 13.1)

These are about 10 in number and arranged in following two groups:
1. **Proximal**: Below and parallel to the inguinal ligament. These are also known as **horizontal group** divided into **lateral** and **medial sets**.
2. **Distal** or **vertical**: These are parallel to the terminal part of great saphenous vein.

Area of Drainage (Afferents)

Upper lateral group receives lymph vessels from:
- The posterior part of the body wall and the flank below the level of umbilicus
- The gluteal region and the upper and lateral side of the thigh.

Upper medial group receives lymph vessels from:
- Anterior wall of abdomen below the level of umbilicus
- Soft tissue of perineum
- External genitalia except glans penis or clitoridis. It includes the vagina below the hymen in females
- Lower anal canal
- Superolateral angle of uterus—the lymph vessels reach along the route of round ligament of uterus.

Lower vertical group receives lymph vessels from:
- Area of skin and fascia of lower limb which is drained by great saphenous vein.

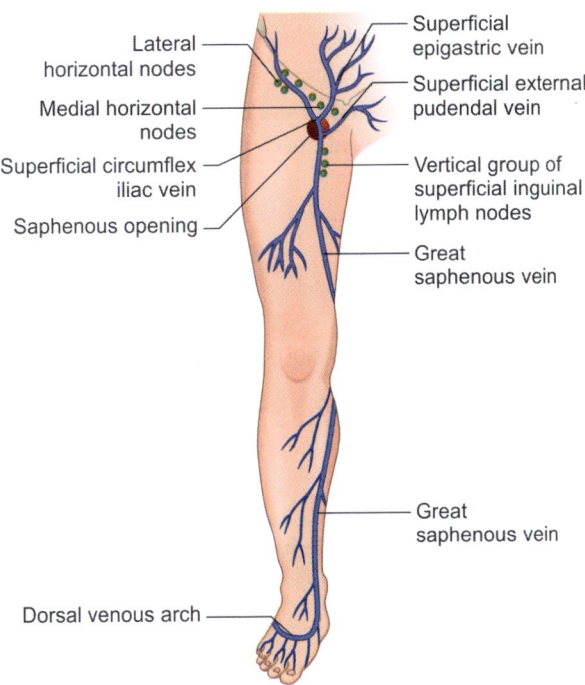

Fig. 13.1: Great saphenous vein and superficial inguinal lymph nodes.

- A few lymph vessels from the route of short shaphenous vein may drain in this group of lymph nodes crossing the knee joint.

Efferents
- Efferent vessels from all the groups of superficial lymph nodes pass through the cribiform fascia and drain into the **deep inguinal lymph nodes**.
- A few lymph vessels cross over the inguinal ligament and drain into the **external iliac lymph nodes.**

Deep Inguinal Lymph Nodes

These are three to four in number and lie underneath the fascia lata. These nodes are on the medial side of the femoral vein. One or two may be deeply situated inside the femoral canal.

Afferents
- Lymph vessels from the deeper tissue of the lower limb. These vessels run along the course of the femoral vein and its tributaries.
- Efferent lymph vessels arising from the superficial inguinal lymph nodes.

Efferents

All the efferent vessels ascends through the femoral canal. Deep lymph node situated inside the femoral canal is known as Cloquet's lymph node. Finally the efferents pierce the femoral septum and drain into the external iliac group of lymph nodes.

Clinical Anatomy

- Inguinal lymph nodes receive lymph from some remote areas of lower limb. So the lymph has to travel a large distance. This is clinically significant. For example, inguinal lymph nodes may be inflamed and enlarged in case of an infection at the great toe.
- Inguinal lymph nodes not only receive the lymph from the whole lower limb, but also from the external genitalia, perineum, lower part of anal canal and even pelvic organs like uterus. So in case of pathological condition (inflammation or malignancy), the medial group of superficial inguinal lymph nodes is affected.

SN 13.2 Write a short note on saphenous opening.

SAPHENOUS OPENING (FIG. 13.2)

Introduction

Saphenous opening is an oval aperture on the fascia lata in the upper medial part of front of thigh below the inguinal ligament.

Situation

About 4 cm below and lateral to the pubic tubercle.

Size and Shape

It is oval in outline with 2.5 cm vertical and 2 cm horizontal measurements.

Formation

Saphenous opening is formed due to a vertical cut or slit of anterior aspect of upper end of sleeve of fascia lata into a lateral and medial part and overlapping of the medial slip by the lateral slip.

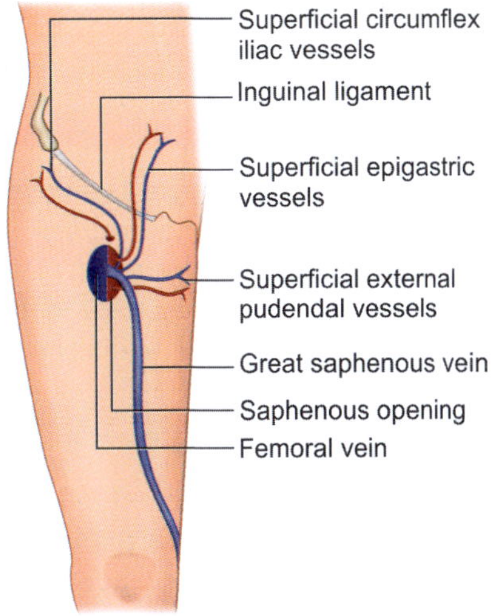

Margin

- The lateral slip presents a free crescentic margin which is called **falciform margin**. This margin forms the superior, lateral and inferior boundary of the opening.
- Medial margin of the opening is rounded and formed by the medial slip of cut sleeve of fascia lata which covers the pectineus but runs behind the femoral vessels to be attached to the pectineal line of pubis.

Fig. 13.2: Saphenous opening.

Structures at the Opening

The saphenous opening is bridged by a layer of superficial fascia. This fascial covering of the saphenous opening is sieve-like for which it is called **cribriform fascia** which is pierced by the following structures:
- Superficial external pudendal artery
- Superficial epigastric artery
- Lymph vessels from superficial inguinal lymph nodes to the deep lymph node in the femoral canal.

Cribriform fascia is not pierced by:
- *Superficial circumflex iliac artery which pierces fascia lata lateral to the saphenous opening.*
- *Corresponding superficial veins which open superficial to the cribriform fascia in the great saphenous vein.*

Clinical Anatomy

Saphenous opening is the deficiency in the deep fascia of front of thigh through which the **femoral hernia** bulges out superficially.

SN 13.3 **Write a short note on iliotibial tract.**

ILIOTIBIAL TRACT (FIG. 13.3)

Introduction

Iliotibial tract is the condensation of fascia lata on the lateral aspect of thigh.

Extent and Attachment

- **Inferiorly**, the iliotibial tract is attached to a smooth circular facet-like area on the *anterolateral aspect of lateral condyle of the tibia*.
- **Superiorly**, the fascial band subdivides into two laminae to enclose the insertion of **tensor fascia latae** and three-fourths of the muscle fibers of **gluteus maximus**. *Superficial lamina* is attached to the anterior 5 cm of the outer lip of ventral segment of iliac crest from the anterior superior iliac spine to the tubercle of iliac crest. *Deep lamina* passes upwards and medially to fuse with the capsule of the hip joint.

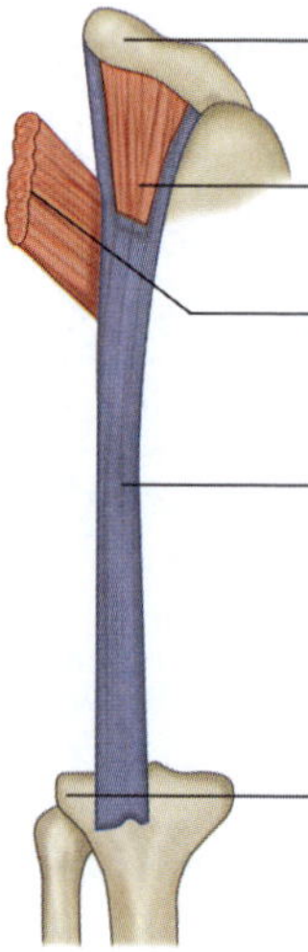

Functions

- Iliotibial tract, attached below at the lateral condyle of the tibia, receives insertion of tensor fascia latae and gluteus maximus. Thereby, it acts as the tendons of these two muscles. In erect posture, these two muscles, acting from below through the iliotibial tract fix the pelvis, when they work simultaneously on both the sides.
- In hyperextended position, when the foot is on the ground, quadriceps femoris is supposed to be tonically contracted. But on prolonged standing, the iliotibial tract maintains the hyperextended position of the knee keeping the quadriceps in relaxed condition and the patella freely mobile.

Fig. 13.3: Iliotibial tract.

SA 13.4 Write a brief note on boundaries and contents of the femoral triangle.

FEMORAL TRIANGLE

Introduction

When the fascia lata is dissected and reflected from the front of the thigh, the muscles deep to it are exposed. Among this muscles, most superficial, long, ribbon-like muscle is identified to cross the thigh obliquely downwards and medially. It is *sartorius*. Medial to the sartorius, in the upper third of the front of thigh a triangular hollow area is detected. It is the femoral triangle with its base directed proximally towards the groin line.

In living body, the hollow of femoral triangle is better identified in flexed position of the hip.

Boundaries (Figs. 13.4 and 13.5)

Outlines of the triangle are base, lateral and medial margins with the apex. The triangle has a gutter like *floor*.

Outlines

- **Base** is formed by the inguinal ligament.
- **Lateral margin** is formed by the medial border of sartorius.
- **Medial margin** is formed by the **medial border** of adductor longus as this muscle takes part in the formation of floor of the triangle.

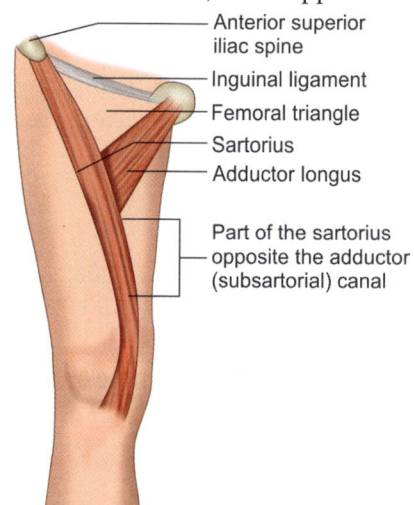

Fig. 13.4: Outline of femoral triangle and location of adductor canal.

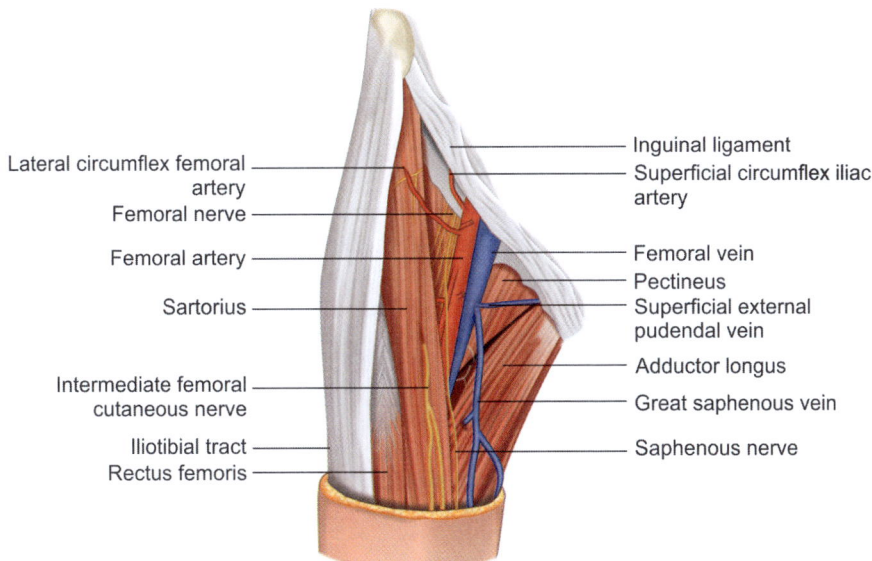

Fig. 13.5: Boundaries and content of femoral triangle.

- **Apex of the triangle** is formed at the site where the sartorius muscle overlaps the adductor longus.
- **Roof** of the femoral triangle is formed by the deep fascia of thigh or *fascia lata* which presents *the saphenous opening* bridged by *the cribriform fascia*.

  Structures lying on the roof are the following:
  - Terminal part of *the great saphenous vein* with its distal sets of tributaries.
  - *Superficial subcutaneous branches of the femoral artery.*
  - *Superficial inguinal lymph nodes* with terminal parts of its afferent lymph vessels.
  - Terminal part of *the ilioinguinal nerve* and *the femoral branch of genitofemoral nerve.*
- **Floor** of the triangle is formed by the following muscles from *lateral to medial side*.
  - Iliacus
  - Psoas major
  - Pectineus
  - Adductor longus.

Contents

Most important content of the femoral triangle is the large **neurovascular bundle** made up of the *femoral nerve* and *femoral vessels*. From lateral to medial they are:

- **Femoral nerve**: This is to be identified and its branches are to be exposed in the first step of dissection. The femoral nerve is found in the groove between iliacus and psoas major muscles of the floor. The nerve lies lateral to the proximal part of femoral vessels enclosed by a fascial sheath called femoral sheath. The femoral nerve is found to divide into **anterior and posterior divisions** each of which again divides into branches.
- **Femoral artery** is on the lateral side of the femoral vein and is situated on the medial side of the femoral nerve. The artery extends from the midinguinal point (of the base) to the apex of the triangle. In the femoral triangle, the femoral artery gives rise to the following branches:

Section 2: Lower Limb

- Superficial circumflex iliac artery ⎫
- Superficial epigastric artery   ⎬ Superficial branches
- Superficial external pudendal artery ⎭
- Deep external pudendal artery ⎫
- Profunda femoris artery   ⎬ Deep branches
- Muscular arteries   ⎭

- **Femoral vein** is medial to the femoral artery at the upper end of the triangle, but as it approaches the apex, the vein is posteromedial to the artery. In the femoral triangle, the femoral vein receives the great saphenous vein and the veins corresponding to the deep branches of femoral artery. In the femoral triangle, proximal end of the femoral vessels are enclosed by the fascial femoral sheath.
- **Other contents** of the femoral triangle are listed below:
  - Deep inguinal lymph nodes
  - Femoral branch of genitofemoral nerve
  - Nerve to pectineus
  - Lateral cutaneous nerve of the thigh.

Clinical/Applied Importance of Femoral Triangle

- Hollow of the femoral triangle is the site for the protrusion of the bulge of **femoral hernia** passing successively through the femoral ring, femoral canal and saphenous opening. The bulge is located inferolateral to the pubic tubercle.
- Iliopsoas muscle inserted at the floor of the femoral triangle is covered by terminal end of iliopsoas sheath. Accumulation of casseous (necrotic) material from tuberculosis of lumbar vertebrae (**caries spine**) may trickle down deep to iliopsoas sheath up to the femoral triangle presenting a lump (swelling or bulge).
- Femoral artery in the femoral triangle lies against the head of femur separated by the iliopsoas tendon. **Arterial pulse** is clinically felt at this site of femoral artery.
- Femoral artery at the femoral triangle is chosen for injection of formalin solution for preservation of cadavers. The procedure is known as **embalming**.

SA 13.5 Give a brief account on the femoral sheath. Add a note on its clinical anatomy.

FEMORAL SHEATH (FIG. 13.6)

Introduction

The femoral vessels, behind the inguinal ligament, take along a funnel-shaped prolongation of fascia, contributed from fascia transversalis in front and iliopsaos fascia behind. This fascial prolongation for about 4 cm length below the inguinal ligament is fused with the adventitia of the artery and the vein to form the femoral sheath.

Shape and Size

- Femoral sheath is funnel shaped with its border end upwards behind inguinal ligament and narrower end fusing with the adventitial coat of femoral vessels.
- Length is 4 cm.

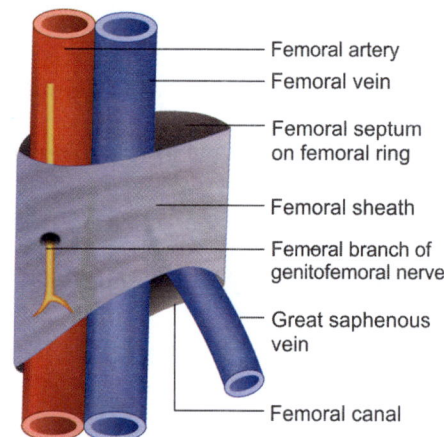

Fig. 13.6: Femoral sheath.

Walls of the Sheath

- **Anterior wall** is formed by the extension of fascia transversalis.
- **Posterior wall** is formed by the extension of iliopsoas fascia.

On both the sides, the anterior and posterior fascial layers fuse with each other. The femoral nerve lies outside the sheath on the lateral aspect. Medial wall of the sheath is shorter and passes downwards and laterally.

Compartments

Femoral sheath is subdivided into following three compartments by the anteroposteriorly running vertical septa.
1. **Lateral compartment** lodges the *femoral artery* and the *femoral branch of genitofemoral nerve*. The nerve comes out of the sheath by piercing the anterior wall of the sheath.
2. **Intermediate compartment** is occupied by the *femoral vein*.
3. **Medial compartment** is the shortest. It is called the femoral canal.

Femoral Canal

Femoral canal is the shortest and narrowest *medial compartment* of the femoral sheath. It is conical in shape with the base directed upwards and apex downwards. At the apex the wall of the canal is fused with the adventitial coat of femoral vein.

Length of the canal is 2.5 cm and the base at the upper end also measures 2.5 cm.

Femoral ring is the broader upper aperture of the femoral canal. The ring is bounded as follows:
- **Anteriorly**: *Inguinal ligament*
- **Posteriorly**: *Pectineal fascia* covering pectineus muscle
- **Laterally**: *Fascial septum* separating femoral vein
- **Medially:** Concave free margin of *lacunar ligament*.

Femoral septum is a condensation of extraperitoneal fatty tissue bridging over the femoral ring. It is pierced by efferent lymph vessels from the lymph node in the femoral canal to the external iliac group of lymph nodes.

Superior surface of the femoral septum is covered by a layer of *partietal peritoneum*. The upward concavity on the peritoneum is known as **femoral fossa**.

Contents of the Femoral Canal

- A single lymph node called **Cloquet's lymph node** or **Rosenmuller's lymph node.**
- Lymph vessels
- A small quantity of loose areolar tissue.

Function of Femoral Canal

Space inside the femoral canal acts as a 'dead space' which accommodates distended femoral vein during increased venous return which occurs during physical exercise or prolonged walking.

Clinical Anatomy of Femoral Canal (Femoral Sheath or Femoral Ring)

Femoral canal so also the femoral ring is a deficiency at the bottom of abdominal as well as peritoneal cavity through which abdominal contents may be protruded causing **femoral hernia**.

A femoral hernia is more common in females because the femoral ring as well as the femoral canal are wider due to following reasons:
- Lacunar ligament is smaller
- Other outlines of the femoral ring are larger due to wider pelvis
- Femoral vein is narrower.

Direction of bulge of femoral hernia is specific. First it bulges downwards through the femoral ring. Then to follow the line of least resistance, it protrudes forwards through saphenous opening and finally upwards and laterally towards anterior superior iliac spine below and parallel to the groin line following the line of least resistance.

Clinical differentiation between femoral hernia and inguinal hernia

Pubic tubercle is the guide to differentiate the femoral hernia from inguinal hernia clinically. *Femoral hernia protrudes inferolateral* to the pubic tubercle. Protrusion of inguinal hernia occurs superomedial to the pubic tubercle. **Obstruction** followed by **strangulation** of femoral hernia is common complication due to the narrow neck at the femoral ring. The strangulation is relieved by widening the femoral ring through resection of the base of lacunar ligament.

Precaution during ligament resection

The pubic branch of obturator artery anastomoses with the pubic branch of inferior epigastric artery. This anastomosis may be sometimes very prominent which itself may take the place of obturator artery. It is called *abnormal obturator artery*. Usually this artery lies in relation to the femoral vein at the lateral wall of femoral ring. *Sometimes, the artery may lie in relation to the base of lacunar ligament at the medial margin of the femoral ring.* So before resection of the base of lacunar ligament to reduce the obstructed and/or strangulated hernia, a surgeon must take care of the artery.

SN 13.6   Write a short note on the sartorius muscle.

SARTORIUS (FIG. 13.7)

Sartorius is the longest muscle of the body.

Origin

It arises from the anterior superior iliac spine and the upper part of the notch below it. The fibers of sartorius are all parallel to each other and run for whole length of the muscle.

The muscle crosses the thigh obliquely. In the upper third it forms lateral boundary of the femoral triangle. In the middle third of the thigh it passes over the fascio-aponeurotic roof of subsartorial canal or adductor canal. In lower third, it descends more vertically to cross the anteromedial aspect of knee joint.

Insertion

At the lower end, sartorius becomes aponeurotic and flattened to be inserted into upper part of

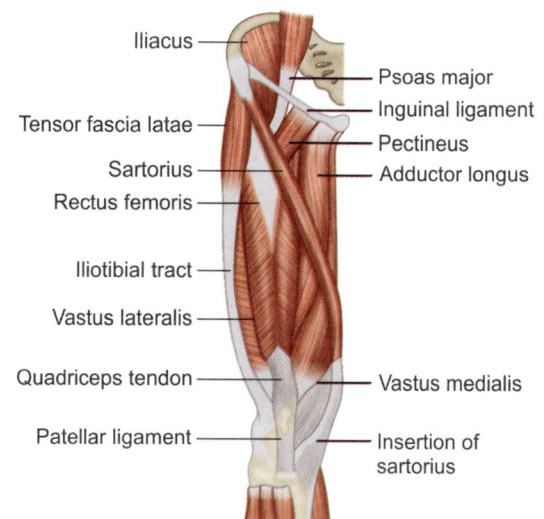

Fig. 13.7: Muscles of front of thigh.

medial surface of shaft of tibia, in front of insertions of gracilis and semitendinosus. The upper end of the aponeurosis of sartorius arches backwards over the insertions of tendons of gracilis and semitendinosus.

Nerve Supply

From anterior division of femoral nerve (L_2, L_3, L_4).

Actions

Sartorius causes flexion, lateral rotation and abduction of hip joint and flexion of the knee joint. During contraction of sartorius when this composite movement of the hip and knee joint occurs, it gives the lower limb a position when a tailor is working. That is why sartorius is called *tailor's muscle*.

SN 13.7 Write a short note on the pectineus muscle.

PECTINEUS (FIG. 13.7)

Pectineus is a flat quadrilateral muscle which forms the floor of femoral triangle between psoas major laterally and adductor longus medially.

Origin

- Pectineal line and the narrow area adjacent to it (pecten pubis)
- Pectineal surface of superior ramus of pubis
- Deep surface of the fascia covering the muscle itself.

Insertion

The muscle slopes downwards and backwards to be inserted into the *spiral line* extending from the lesser trochanter to the upper end of linea aspera of femur.

Pectineal Fascia

This is the fascia covering the pectineus muscle which is formed by *infolding of the fascia lata*. It passes behind the femoral vein and femoral canal to reach beneath the falciform margin of the saphenous opening.

Nerve Supply

Pectineus is the example of hybrid or composite muscle which is composed of a ventral flexor part and a dorsal adductor part.
- The ventral flexor part is supplied by the trunk (or anterior division) of femoral nerve (L_2, L_3)
- The dorsal adductor part is supplied by the anterior division of obturator nerve (L_2, L_3).

Actions

Ventral part of pectineus is flexor and its dorsal part is adductor of the hip joint.

SA 13.8 Write a brief note on the quadriceps femoris muscle.

QUADRICEPS FEMORIS

Quadriceps femoris is the chief extensor muscle of the knee joint and is made up of four components—*rectus femoris* and three vastus muscles named *vastus lateralis, vastus intermedius* and *vastus medialis*.

All the four parts of the muscle converge towards each other to form *quadriceps tendon* which contains the patella, the largest sessamoid bone. It continues downwards beyond patella as patellar ligament (*ligamentum patellae*) which is attached to upper part of the tuberosity of tibia.

Rectus Femoris (Figs. 13.7 and 13.8)

It is only part of the quadriceps femoris which takes its origin *proximal to the hip joint* from the ilium of hip bone. It arises by two heads as follows.
1. **Straight head** arises from the *upper half of anterior inferior iliac spine* above the site of attachment of iliofemoral ligament of the hip joint.
2. **Reflected head** arises from the broad shallow sulcus on the lower part of dorsal surface of ilium *above the acetabulum*. Two heads unite to form a fusiform muscle containing superficial and deep plane of fibers. *Superficial fibers* are *bipennate* and *deep fibers* are *parallel*. At a lower level it *forms the anterior lamina of the quadriceps tendon*. The posterior surface of the muscle forms a shining aponeurosis which glides on the anterior surface of vastus intermedius. Anterior surface of the muscle presents a similar aponeurosis in its upper part.

Vastus Lateralis (Figs. 13.7 and 13.8)

Vastus lateralis has an *extensive linear origin* from:
- Upper half of intertrochanteric line
- Anterior and inferior margins of lateral surface of greater trochanter
- Lateral lip of the gluteal tuberosity
- Upper half of the lateral lip of linea aspera
- Lateral intermuscular septum.

At the lower end of thigh, the muscle is incorporated in the quadriceps tendon. Anterior margin of the muscle is separated from the vastus intermedius by a shallow vertical groove. Along this vertical groove the *nerve to the vastus lateralis* and the *descending branch of lateral circumflex femoral artery* run downwards.

Vastus Intermedius (Figs. 13.7 and 13.8)

It arises from upper two-thirds of anterior and lateral surfaces of shaft of femur. The muscle wraps over the femoral shaft and its anterior surface is covered by an aponeurosis which merges below in the quadriceps tendon.

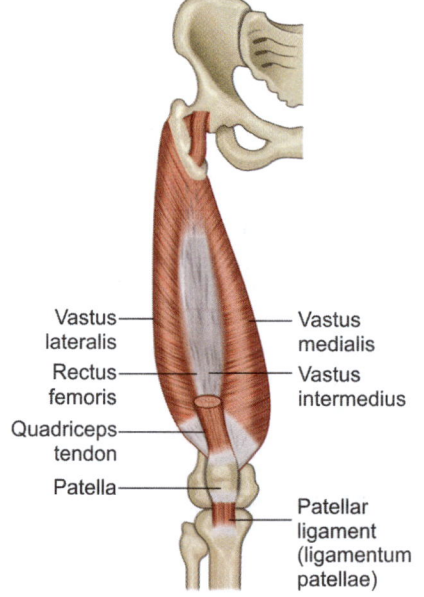

Fig. 13.8: Components of quadriceps femoris.

Vastus Medialis (Figs. 13.7 and 13.8)

This muscle arises from:
- Lower half of intertrochanteric line
- Spiral line
- Medial lip of linea aspera
- Upper part of the medial supracondylar line
- *Lower part of the tendon of adductor magnus.*

The muscle descends along the medial aspect of the femoral shaft. Most of its fibers merge with the vastus intemedius and is continuous below with the quadriceps tendon. **The lowest fibers** of vastus medialis show the specialized insertion. These fibers are more or less **horizontal** and are **inserted directly into the medial border of patella**. These fibers have an important role **to maintain the stability of the patella**.

Tendon of quadriceps femoris is inserted into the base (upper margin) and the sides of the patella. A *thin sheet* from the tendon passes over the front of the patella into the patellar ligament.

Patellar ligament (ligamentum patellae) connects the apex and adjacent lower rough part of posterior surface of patella with the upper part of the tuberosity of the tibia. It represents the continuation of the quadriceps tendon beyond the patella.

Patellar retinacula are the outward expansion from the quadriceps tendon and the patellar ligament which connect the *margins of the patella* with *the condyles of the tibia and the collateral ligaments* of the knee joint. In addition, the lateral patellar retinaculum is further strengthened by the iliotibial tract.

Nerve Supply

Each of the four components of quadriceps femoris is supplied by a branch from the posterior division of femoral nerve (L_3, L_4).

Actions

Quadriceps femoris is the main extensor of the knee joint. Rectus femoris, in addition, assists the iliopsoas to flex the hip joint.

Factors Maintaining Stability of Patella

The patella, developed as a sessamoid bone in the quadriceps tendon, is mobile from side to side against the patellar surface of femoral condyles. Though the patellar ligament is vertical in direction, the pull of quadriceps tendon is *oblique*, parallel to the line of shaft of femur. So, when the muscle contracts, it tends to pull the patella obliquely upwards and laterally, leading to a chance for lateral dislocation of patella from the patellar surface of femoral condyles. This is prevented by following three factors.
1. **Ligamentous factor:** It is the vertical direction of the pull by the patellar ligament and the tension of the medial patellar retinaculum.
2. **Bony factor:** It is the more forward projection of patellar articular surface on the lateral condyle of femur.

   But unless the muscular factor comes into action, these two factors are not capable to prevent the lateral displacement of patella.

3. **Muscular factor**: The lowest fibers of vastus medialis which are inserted into the medial border of patella, are horizontal in direction at their insertion end. This plays the most important role to correct the lateral dislocation.

ARTICULARIS GENU

It is also known as **the articular muscle of the knee.** This muscle is a *derivative of the vastus intermedius* and it consist of *variable number of slips of origin.*

Origin

Articularis genu arises by multiple slips from the lower part of anterior surface of shaft of femur below the lower limit of origin of the vastus intermedius.

Insertion

The muscle is inserted into the summit of the *suprapatellar bursa* which is a superior outpouching of the synovial membrane of the knee joint.

Nerve Supply

Articularis genu is supplied by the *nerve to the vastus intermedius* which arises from the posterior division of femoral nerve. The same nerve also gives an *articular branch to the knee joint.*

Actions

Articularis genu pulls the suprapatellar bursa with the synovial membrane upwards during extension of the knee joint. This prevents compression of the synovial fold between hard surfaces of the femur and the patella.

SA 13.9 Discuss briefly the boundaries and contents of the adductor canal. Add a note on its clinical anatomy.

ADDUCTOR CANAL

Introduction

Adductor canal is also called **subsartorial canal** or **Hunter's canal**. Adductor canal is an intermuscular cleft situated on the medial aspect of middle third of front of thigh. It is beneath the sartorius muscle for which it is called subsartorial canal.

Extent

Above: Apex of femoral triangle where the sartorius muscle crosses over the adductor longus.

Below: The osseoaponeurotic opening bounded by shaft of femur and the deficiency (gap) in the line of insertion of the adductor magnus muscle.

Cross Section (Fig. 13.9)

Adductor canal is triangular in outline in cross section of thigh having *anteromedial, posterior* and *lateral walls.*

Boundaries (Fig. 13.9)

Lateral wall is formed by *the vastus medialis*.

Posterior wall is formed by the *adductor magnus*. Upper part of the boundary is additionally formed by the *adductor longus*.

Anterior wall is also represented as the **roof**. It is *aponeurotic in nature*. It is formed by a *strong fibrous membrane* joining the muscles of the lateral and posterior wall. Sartorius is placed over this fibrous roof. Beneath the sartorius lies a plexus of sensory nerves called subsartorial plexus. **Subsartorial plexus** is formed by union of following sensory nerves.

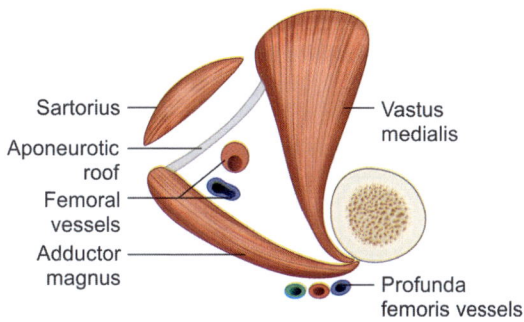

Fig. 13.9: Boundaries and contents of adductor canal through cross section of middle third of right thigh.

- A branch from the medial cutaneous nerve of thigh
- A branch from the saphenous nerve
- A branch from the anterior division of obturator nerve.
  The nerve plexus supplies the fascia lata and the skin of medial side of the thigh above the knee.

Contents (Fig. 13.10)

- **Femoral artery**: It extends throughout the whole length of the canal, from the apex of femoral triangle up to the opening in the adductor magnus. At the beginning of the canal, the femoral artery crosses in front of the femoral vein. So in the canal, the artery lies on the *anteromedial aspect of the vein*.
  In the lower part of the canal, the femoral artery gives rise to its *last branch*, the **descending genicular artery** which divides into superficial and deep branches. The superficial branch runs with the saphenous nerve. The deep branch takes part in anastomosis around the knee joint.

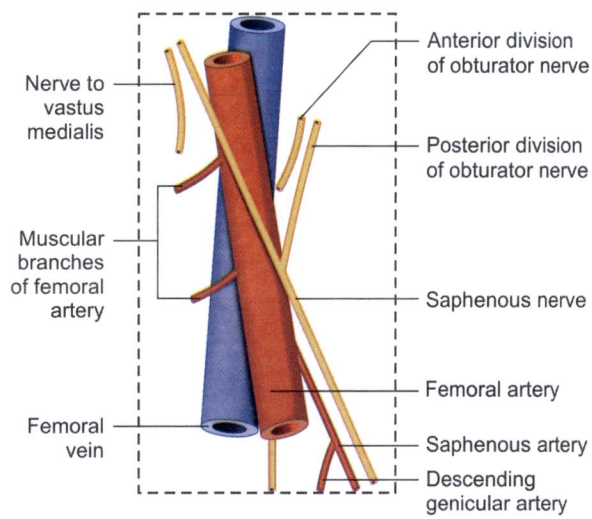

Fig. 13.10: Contents of adductor canal.

- **Femoral vein**: The femoral vein is overlapped in front by the artery in the upper part of the canal. The artery lies medial to the vein in the lower part of the canal.
- **Saphenous nerve**: This only sensory branch from the posterior division of femoral nerve, crosses the femoral artery from lateral to medial side. *It goes out of the canal by piercing the aponeurotic roof.*
- **Posterior division of the obturator nerve**, after supplying the adductor muscles, runs in front of adductor magnus as the sensory component. It passes down along with the femoral vessels to leave the canal through the adductor magnus hiatus. It ends by supplying the back of the knee joint.

- **Nerve to vastus medialis** is the branch from posterior division of femoral nerve. It lies lateral to the femoral artery and enters into the muscle in the upper part of the canal.

Clinical Anatomy

Exposure of femoral artery is needed in cases of various kinds of vascular surgery of lower limb.
If the ligature of the femoral artery is to be done for any indication, collateral circulation will be established more richly through the following anastomosis.
- The descending branch of lateral circumflex femoral and the descending genicular arteries.
- Perforating branch of profunda femoris artery and muscular branch of popliteal artery.

History of Clinical Anatomy

Due to complication of aneurysm of popliteal artery of John Hunter, a famous British anatomist, femoral artery was ligated at the adductor canal. It is the reason for which the adductor canal is named Hunter's canal.

SA 13.10 Write a brief note on the femoral artery.

Short notes: Profunda femoris artery.

FEMORAL ARTERY (FIG. 13.11)

Introduction

Femoral artery is the main artery supplying the lower limb.

Origin

Femoral artery starts as the continuation of the external iliac artery behind the inguinal ligament at *midinguinal point*, which is the midpoint between the anterior superior iliac spine and the *pubic symphysis*.

Termination

At the junction of middle third and lower third of thigh, the femoral artery passes through the hiatus of adductor magnus to be continued as popliteal artery on the back of knee.

Course and Important Relations

Throughout its course the femoral artery is accompanied by the femoral vein. Its course and relations are divided as follows.

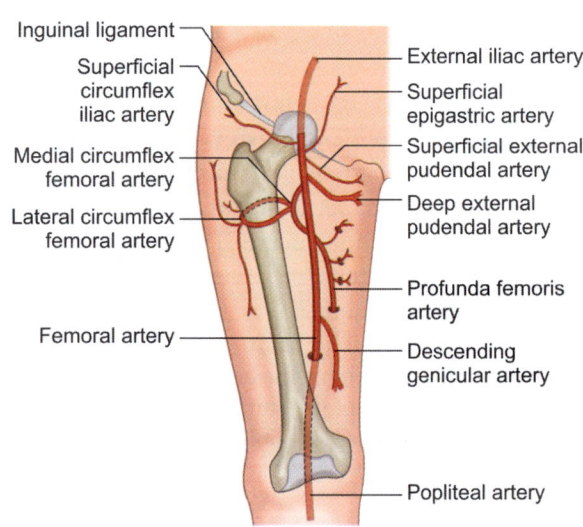

Fig. 13.11: Femoral artery with its branches.

In the Femoral Triangle

- Along with the vein, proximal 4 cm of the femoral artery is enclosed by the *femoral sheath*. The artery lies in the lateral compartment of femoral sheath along with the *femoral branch of genitofemoral nerve*. The artery lies on the psoas major and is medial to the *femoral nerve*.
- While descending over the floor of femoral triangle, the artery crosses successively psoas major, pectineus and adductor longus.
- At the apex of femoral triangle, slight medial inclination of the femoral artery, brings it in front of the femoral vein.

In the Adductor Canal

Due to narrow space inside the adductor canal the structures of the neurovascular bundle are very closely related as stated below.
- From the front of the femoral vein, the femoral artery inclines just medial to the vein. The saphenous nerve crosses the artery from lateral to medial side.

Branches

In the Femoral Triangle

- **Superficial circumflex iliac artery** appears in the superficial plane by *piercing the fascia lata just lateral to the saphenous opening* and passes upwards and laterally below and parallel to the lateral half of inguinal ligament. It takes part in arterial anastomosis near anterior superior iliac spine.
- **Superficial epigastric artery** comes out through the saphenous opening and passes upwards and medially towards the umbilicus crossing the inguinal ligament.
- **Superficial external pudendal artery** becomes superficial piercing through the saphenous opening and passes medially to supply the region of external genitalia.
- **Deep external pudendal artery** runs deep to the spermatic cord or round ligament of uterus to supply the scrotum or labium majus.

Profunda Femoris Artery

Introduction

Profunda femoris artery is the largest branch of femoral artery. It is mainly for distribution in the medial or adductor compartment but gives also the branches to the other two (flexor and extensor) compartments of thigh.

Origin

Profunda femoris artery arises from the lateral side of the femoral artery 4 cm below the inguinal ligament.

Termination

Terminal end of the artery, running down in the adductor (medial) compartment, pierces the adductor magnus to go backwards in the back of thigh to anastomose with the upper muscular branch of popliteal artery.

Course

Arising from the lateral side of the femoral artery, the profunda femoris artery lies in the femoral triangle. It leaves the femoral triangle between adductor longus and pectineus and runs behind the former muscle.

The artery descends then behind adductor longus and in front of adductor bravis above and adductor magnus below. It leaves the medial compartment perforating the adductor magnus and reaches the back of knee.

Branches

- **Medial circumflex femoral artery** leaves the femoral triangle to reach the back of thigh passing between pectineus and psoas major. It curves round the medial side of upper end of shaft of femur to take part in the cruciate anastomosis.
- **Lateral circumflex femoral artery** runs also horizontally towards the lateral side initially passing between two divisions of the femoral nerve and then deep to the sartorius and rectus femoris. It gives rise to ascending, horizontal and descending branches.
    - *The ascending branch* runs upwards and laterally undercover of the tensor fascia latae. It supplies the hip joint and finally ends by anastomosing with superior gluteal artery.
    - *The horizontal branch* participates in cruciate anastomosis below the greater trochanter on the back of thigh.
    - *The descending branch* runs down along the line of anterior border of vastus lateralis accompanied by the nerve to the vastus lateralis
- **Perforating arteries** are three in number which originate from the profunda femoris artery in a vertical row. They perforate adductor magnus to go backwards for the formation of *chain anastomosis* in the back of thigh.
- **Muscular arteries** originate from the femoral artery to supply the muscles of anterior compartment of thigh. Muscular branches also arise from the profunda femoris artery which are mainly for the muscles of adductor compartment.

Clinical Anatomy

- Close relation of the femoral artery against the tough iliopsoas tendon and the head of femur gives an **advantage for compression of the artery** to arrest the bleeding distal to it.
- **Pulsation of femoral artery** can be felt at the above-mentioned site, as and when required for various clinical indications.
- **Cannulation**: Femoral artery is the second to the radial artery as the choice for the placement of arterial line through cannulation.
- **Aneurysm of femoral artery**: Expansile swelling along the line of femoral artery which fluctuates with the arterial pulse helps in diagnosis of aneurysm of femoral artery.

LA 13.11 **Discuss briefly the femoral nerve.**

FEMORAL NERVE (FIG. 13.12)

Introduction

Femoral nerve is the nerve of anterior compartment of thigh which contains mainly the extensor muscles of the knee.

Origin

Femoral nerve originates from the lumbar plexus. It is formed by union of posterior divisions of anterior rami of L_2, L_3 and L_4 nerves.

Course and Important Relations

- Femoral nerve originates in the posterior abdominal wall within the substance of the psoas major muscle. It runs downwards and laterally to appear lateral to the psoas major muscle.
- In the false pelvis, the nerve lies in the groove between iliacus and psoas major muscles to reach the level of inguinal ligament.
- Along the iliopsoas groove the nerve enters the femoral triangle in the front of thigh passing behind the inguinal ligament.
- Just a little below the inguinal ligament, lying lateral to the femoral sheath, the femoral nerve divides primarily into *anterior* and *posterior divisions* which give rise to many branches.

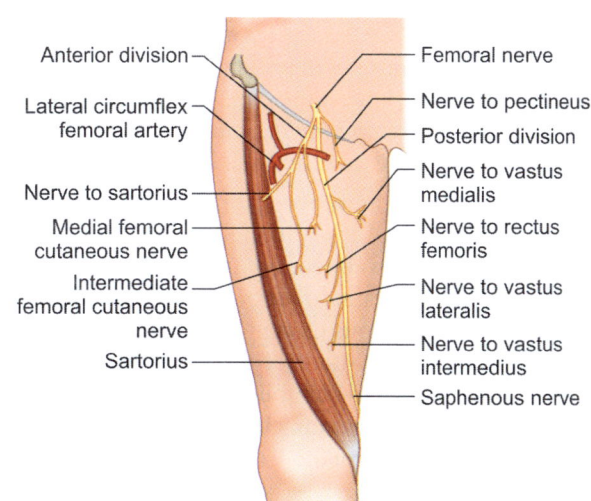

Fig. 13.12: Distributions of femoral nerve.

Branches

From the Trunk

- *To iliacus*: This branch arises when the femoral nerve lies in the iliopsoas groove between iliacus and psoas in the false pelvis.
- *To pectineus*: Nerve to pectineus arises from the trunk of femoral nerve just after it reaches the femoral triangle passing behind the inguinal ligament. It supplies the muscle passing behind the femoral sheath.

From Anterior Division

Branches are *mainly cutaneous* and *one muscular* to the sartorius
- *Medial cutaneous nerve of thigh* perforates the fascia lata at the middle of thigh and supplies the skin on the medial side of thigh.
- *Intermediate cutaneous nerve of the thigh* proceeds vertically downwards and pierces the fascia lata at a higher level. It may also pierce the sartorius muscle. It supplies the skin of front of thigh as low down the knee.
  Both the cutaneous branches give twigs to form the *patellar plexus*
- *Nerve to sartorius* is the only muscular branch that arises from anterior division. But, after supplying the sartorius, it may be continued as intermediate cutaneous nerve of thigh.

From Posterior Division

Branches are mainly muscular and one cutaneous, which is the saphenous nerve.
- *Nerve to rectus femoris* is *usually double*. The upper nerve gives articular branch to *the hip joint*.
- *Nerve to vastus medialis* is the largest and most prominent muscular branch. It is placed lateral to the femoral vessels in the adductor canal. Here it gives *vascular branch* to the femoral artery. Supplying the muscle, it continues downwards to give *articular branch* for the knee joint.

- *Nerve to vastus lateralis* runs along the anterior border of the muscle along with the descending branch of lateral circumflex femoral artery. Supplying the muscle, the nerve continues as *articular branch* for the knee joint.
- *Nerve to vastus intermedius* enters the muscle through its anterior surface. It gives branches also to the *articularis genu* and the *knee joint*.

Saphenous nerve is the only sensory branch from the posterior division of femoral nerve. It descends lateral to the femoral artery in the femoral triangle and enters the adductor canal where it crosses in front of the artery to appear on its medial side. At the lower end of the canal, the saphenous nerve pierces the fibroaponeurotic roof and gives out the *infrapatellar branch for the patellar plexus*. It becomes subcutaneous piercing the fascia lata in between the tendons of sartorius and gracilis. It descends along the medial border of the tibia accompanied by the great saphenous vein and divides into two branches. One supplies the skin at the ankle and another continues beyond the ankle to supply the skin of the medial border of dorsum of foot *as far as the first metatarsophalangeal joint*. At the level of middle of thigh the saphenous nerve gives *a branch to the subsartorial plexus*.

Chapter 14

Medial Side of the Thigh

LA 14.1 Discuss briefly the muscles of medial compartment of thigh.

Individual muscle may be asked in the form of short notes

MUSCLES OF MEDIAL COMPARTMENT OF THIGH

Gracilis (Figs. 14.1A and 14.2)

Gracilis is the most superficial muscle of the medial side of the thigh.

Origin

Gracilis takes origin in the form of flattened sheet from the whole of the edge of femoral surface of the inferior ramus of pubis and adjoining part of the ramus of ischium.

Insertion

The muscle tappers down in a triangular fashion finally and it is replaced by a cylindrical tendon which is inserted into the upper end of the medial surface of the shaft of the tibia just posterior to the insertion of sartorius.

Blood Supply

Arterial supply of the gracilis is important for the purpose of reconstructive surgery. It receives segmental blood supply from the medial circumflex femoral, profunda femoris and femoral arteries from above downwards.

Nerve Supply

Anterior division of obturator nerve.

Actions

- Gracilis is a week adductor of the thigh
- It is also flexor and medial rotator of thigh.

Clinical Anatomy

A gracilis muscular flap related to pedicle of profunda femoris artery is used in *perineal reconstructive surgery*.

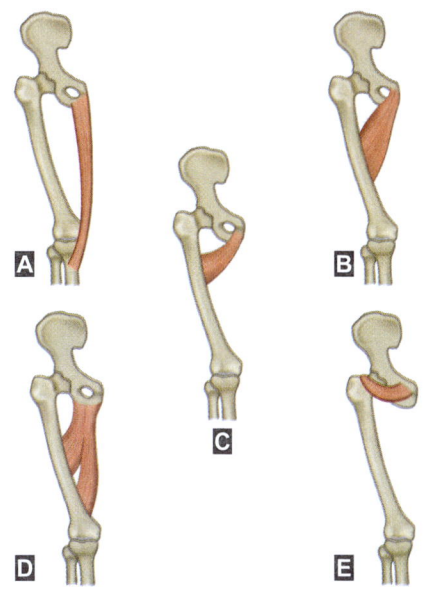

Figs. 14.1A to E: Muscles of medial compartment of thigh: (A) Gracilis; (B) Adductor longus; (C) Adductor brevis; (D) Adductor magnus; (E) Obturator externus.

Adductor Longus (Figs. 14.1B and 14.2)

Adductor longus is most superficial of the three adductors. It arises through a round tendon form the circular area on the anterior surface of the body of pubis, in the angle between pubic crest and pubic symphysis. The tendon is sometimes ossified, called **'rider's bone'**. The tendon becomes fleshly and it becomes flattened to be inserted finally through a *flat tendon* in the middle third of linea aspera of the femur.

Nerve Supply

Anterior division of obturator nerve.

Action

Along with other adductors, it is a powerful adductor of thigh.

Adductor Brevis (Figs. 14.1C and 14.3)

Adductor brevis, obviously shorter than the adductor longus, lies deep to adductor longus and pectineus. It arises from the body and inferior ramus of the pubis. It widens to become triangular in outline and is inserted into the upper part of the linea aspera just behind the insertion of pectineus and adductor longus. Anterior and posterior divisions of obturator nerve run downwards to lie over the anterior and posterior surfaces of adductor brevis respectively.

Nerve Supply

Both anterior as well as posterior divisions of obturator nerve.

Action

Adductor of thigh.

Adductor Magnus (Figs. 14.1D and 14.3)

Adductor magnus is a composite muscle formed by fusion of *hamstring* and *adductor* muscle masses.

Hamstring part of the adductor magnus is morphologically the muscle of flexor compartment of the thigh. As this has been incorporated with the adductor part of the muscle to give rise to the big muscle mass, the posterior intermuscular septum between the flexor and

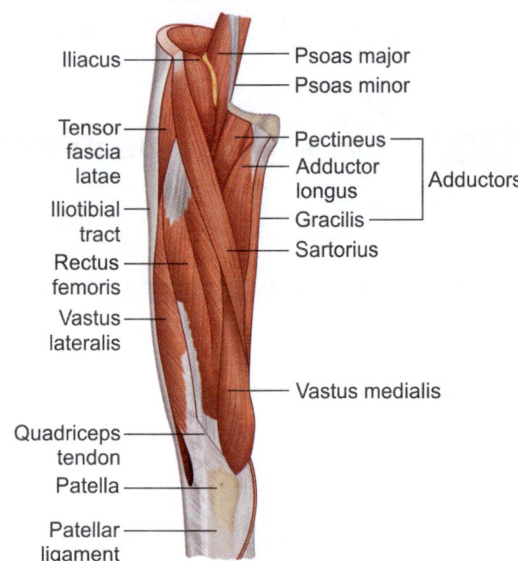

Fig. 14.2: Muscles of adductor region with front of thigh (superficial plane).

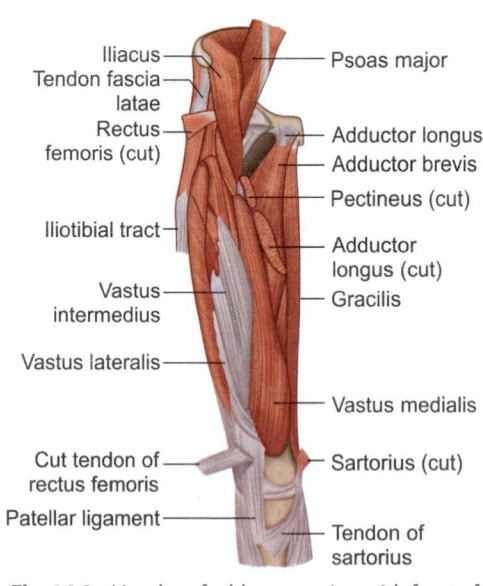

Fig. 14.3: Muscles of adductor region with front of thigh (deeper plane).

adductor compartments are poorly defined. The hamstring part arises from the lateral part of lower triangular area of ischeal tuberosity. These fibers pass vertically downwards to become tendinous. This tendon is inserted into the *adductor tubercle* of the femur *with an expansion to the medial supracondylar line.*

The hamstring part of the muscle is supposed to be inserted beyond the knee joint, as this part is functionally supposed to be the flexor of the knee. But, as this has been incorporated with the adductor part, distal part of the muscle, beyond adductor tubercle, is considered to be degenerated to form *the medial* (tibial) *collateral ligament of the knne joint.*

Adductor part of the muscle takes origin from the ischiopubic ramus, extending along the whole length of ischial ramus and adjacent part of inferior ramus of pubis. These fibers have extensive insertion extending upwards along the medial supracondylar line and the linea aspera up to the medial lip of gluteal tuberosity. The upper border of the muscle is horizontal and it is related edge to edge with the quadratus femoris. Medial circumflex femoral artery passes between the two muscles backwards to take part in the cruciate anastomosis. Near the junction of the mdial supracondylar line and the linea aspera, there is a gap in the muscular insertion, through which femoral vessels pass from the front of thigh to the popliteal fossa to be continued as popliteal vessels. Along the line of attachment of the muscle to the linea aspera, there are four small openings. Profunda femoris artery passes backwards through the lowest one and the other three transmit its perforating branches. Ascending and descending branches of all these arteries anastomose on the back of adductor magnus to form the chain anastomosis.

Nerve Supply

Adductor magnus is a *composite* or *hybrid muscle* having double nerve supply. Hamstring part is supplied by *the tibial component of the sciatic* nerve and adductor part is supplied by *the posterior division of obturator nerve.*

Actions

- Adductor magnus is a *powerful adductor* of the hip joint. But the extreme and forcible adduction is not always required.
- Action of adductors comes into a complex muscular action *in gait* and to some extent *during control of posture.*
- Adductor magnus, along with the adductor longus is *medial rotator* of thigh.
- Adductor magnus *assists in extension* of thigh at the hip joint.

Obturator Externus (Fig. 14.1E)

Origin

Obturator externus arises from the outer surface of *the obturator membrane* and the outer surface of the margin of *the obturator foramen.* Both the obturator membrane as well as origin of the muscle fibers are deficient at the site of obturator sulcus of the hip bone to convert the sulcus into a canal called *obturator canal.* Through this canal obturator nerve, artery and vein come out from the pelvis. If the nerve divides early into two divisions, they are separated by highest fibers of the obturator externus.

Direction of the Muscle Fibers

The muscle first passes laterally and backwards beneath the neck of the femur where it narrows into a tendon. Then the tendon winds in a spiral fashion around the back of the neck of femur.

Insertion

The tendinous end of the muscle is inserted into the *trochanteric fossa*, or a depression on the medial aspect of greater trochanter of femur.

Nerve Supply

Posterior division of obturator nerve.

Actions

- Along with the other short muscles around the hip, obturator externus *stabilizes* and *supports* the proximal part of the limb.
- As the line of pull of the muscle passes across the back of the hip joint, obturator externus is a *lateral rotator* of the hip joint.

LA 14.2 Discuss briefly the obturator nerve.

OBTURATOR NERVE (FIG. 14.4)

Introduction

Obturator nerve is the nerve for distribution in the medial or adductor compartment of the thigh.

Origin

The obturator nerve arises from the lumbar plexus in the posterior abdominal wall. It is formed by union of *ventral branches* of anterior primary rami of L_2, L_3 and L_4 nerves.

Entry to the Thigh

Obturator nerve lies initially in the posterior abdominal wall medial to the psoas major. Then it runs along the lateral wall of true pelvis. Finally it leaves the pelvis passing through the obturator canal to reach the medial compartment of thigh along with the obturator vessels.

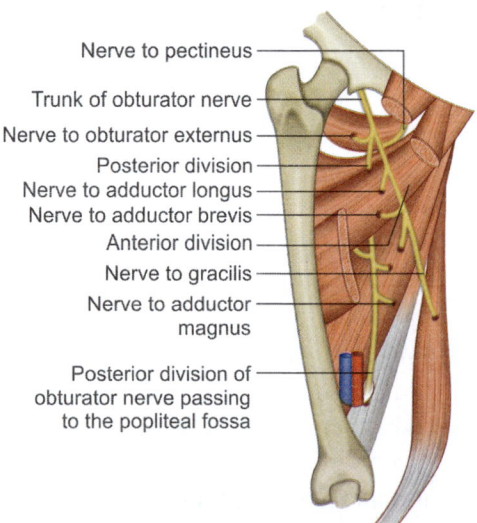

Fig. 14.4: Distribution of obturator nerve.

Bifurcation of the Nerve

While passing through the obturator canal, obturator nerve bifurcates into *anterior* and *posterior divisions*. While coming out through the obturator canal, two divisions are separated by upper fibers of obturator externus muscle.

Course and Distribution

- **Anterior division** appears in the thigh passing in front of obturator externus. Then it runs down in front of adductor brevis and behind pectineus and adductor longus. The branches from the anterior division are as mentioned below:
    - **Muscular branches**: To supply dorsal (adductor) part of pectineus, adductor longus, adductor brevis and gracilis.
    - **Articular branch**: To supply the hip joint
    - **Cutaneous branch**: To the skin of medial side of thigh through subsartorial plexus
    - **Vascular branch**: To the femoral artery
- **Posterior division** enters the thigh passing through the upper fibers of obturator externus. In the adductor canal, the posterior division passes over the posterior surface of adductor brevis and in front of adductor magnus up to the hiatus magnus of the latter muscle. Through this opening the nerve enters the popliteal fossa along with the femoral vessels.
  In the popliteal fossa, the terminal end of posterior division the obturator nerve enters inside the knee joint piercing the oblique popliteal ligament and the fibrous capsule of the joint. The branches from the posterior division are the following:
- **Muscular branches**: To obturator externus, adductor part of adductor magnus, occasionally to adductor brevis.
- **Articular branch**: To the knee joint
- **Vascular branch**: To popliteal artery.

Accessory Obturator Nerve

- It is present in 30% of individuals
- It arises in the lumbar plexus by union of fibers of anterior divisions of L_3 and L_4 nerves
- It enters the thigh *crossing over the superior ramus of the pubis* and deep to pectineus
- Branches of accessory obturator nerve are:
    - To pectineus
    - To hip joint
    - A communicating branch to the obturator nerve.

Clinical Anatomy

- Patient with cerebral palsy may show *marked spasticity of adductor group of muscles*. For relief of the severe spasm, sectioning of tendon of adductor longus and anterior division of obturator nerve is done. In severe cases, posterior division of the nerve is also sectioned.
- In painful diseases of the knee joint, *referred pain* in the hip joint is also felt due to common innervation of both the joints by the obturator nerve.

SA 14.3 Discuss briefly the profunda femoris artery.

PROFUNDA FEMORIS ARTERY (FIG. 14.5)

Introduction

Profunda femoris artery is the largest branch of the femoral artery. It is considered to be the artery of the medial or adductor compartment of the thigh. But it gives branches to all the three compartments.

Origin

Profunda femoris artery arises from the lateral side of the femoral artery 3–4 cm below the inguinal ligament.

Course

Arising in the femoral triangle, the profunda femoris artery forms a spiral turn round the femoral artery to pass between pectineus and adductor longus. Then the artery passes in front of adductor brevis above and adductor magnus below. Finally the profunda femoris artery perforates through the adductor magnus muscle to participate in anastomosis in the back of thigh.

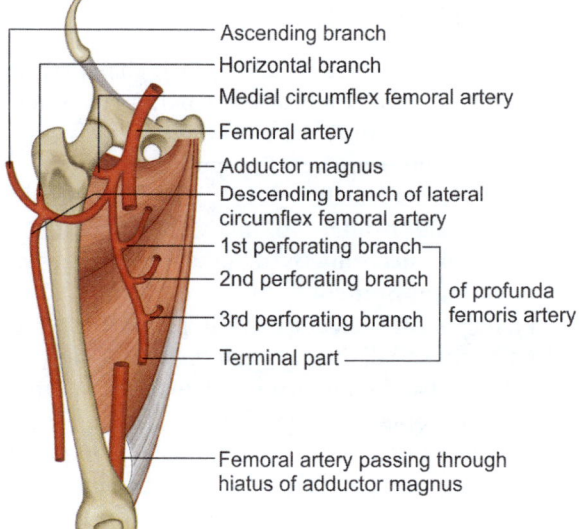

Fig. 14.5: Profunda femoris artery.

Branches

Lateral circumflex femoral artery arises from the lateral side of the profunda artery. Occasionally it arises from the femoral artery. First it passes between anterior and posterior divisions of femoral nerve. It leaves the femoral triangle passing beneath sartorius and passes laterally deep to rectus femoris. Here it divides into three branches.

Ascending branch passes upwards on the vastus lateralis under cover of sartorius and tensor fasciae latae. It gives a branch to take part in *trochanteric anastomosis*. Finally it reaches the anterior superior iliac spine to anastomose with:
- Superficial circumflex iliac artery
- Deep circumflex iliac artery
- Iliac branch of iliolumbar artery
- Superior branch of superior gluteal artery.

Transverse branch winds around the femur to take part in the cruciate anastomosis.

Descending branch runs along the anterior border of vastus lateralis accompanying the nerve for the same muscle. After giving muscular branches, it ends by dividing into terminal branches for the anastomosis around the knee joint.

Medial circumflex femoral artery originates from the medial side of the profunda femoris artery. It may also arise directly from the femoral artery. It passes backwards between pectineus and psoas major. Then it passes backwards first between obturator externus and adductor brevis and then between quadratus femoris and adductor magnus. Reaching the gluteal region, it gives an *ascending branch* for trochanteric anastomosis and a *horizontal branch* to take part in cruciate anastomosis.

Perforating arteries are four in number including the terminal end of the profunda artery itself which is considered as fourth one. All the four are called 'perforating' because they penetrate the adductor magnus to go to the back of thigh. All of them divide into ascending and descending branches. Their adjacent branches anastomose with each other to form a 'chain anastomosis'. This, in turn, anastomose with the cruciate anastomosis above and upper muscular branch of popliteal artery below.

Chapter 15

Gluteal Region, Back of Thigh and Popliteal Fossa

SN 15.1 Write short notes on sacrotuberous and sacrospinous ligaments.

SACROTUBEROUS LIGAMENT (FIG. 15.1)

It is attached medially by its broad base to the lateral margin of lower part of sacrum and upper part of coccyx. Superiorly, its attachment over the posterior sacroiliac ligament extends up to the posterior superior iliac spine. Its fibers pass obliquely downwards and laterally to be converted into a slender thick band which widens again to be attached to the medial margin of ischial tuberosity. Finally, it spreads along the ischial ramus as *falciform process*.

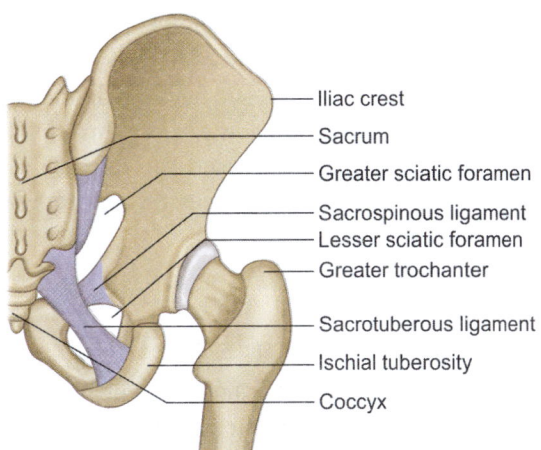

Fig. 15.1: Skeletal background of gluteal region.

Muscles Attached
- Lowest fibers of gluteus maximus.
- Some fibers of the ligament are continued in the tendon of long head of biceps femoris.

Structures Piercing
- Perforating cutaneous nerve of thigh
- Coccygeal branch of inferior gluteal artery.

SACROSPINOUS LIGAMENT

It is thin and triangular ligament. It extends from the lateral margin of sacrococcygeal junction, lying in front of sacrotuberous ligament, to the ischial spine. On its anterior aspect lies the coccygeus muscles, with which it is coextensive. Sacrospinous ligament is considered as degenerated part of coccygeus muscle.

SA 15.2 Write a brief note on gluteus medius and gluteus minimus muscles.

GLUTEUS MEDIUS AND GLUTEUS MINIMUS

Origin and Insertion

Gluteus medius takes origin from the dorsal or gluteal surface of ilium *between posterior and anterior gluteal lines*. Its posterior one-third is covered by gluteus maximus and anterior two-thirds are undercover of thick deep fascia.

The muscle is narrowed into a flat tendon which is inserted to the lateral surface of the greater trochanter. A bursa is lodged between the muscle and the trochanter.

Gluteus minimus originates under over the gluteus medius from the area of dorsal or gluteal surface of ilium *between anterior and inferior gluteal lines.*

The muscle fibers converge to form a tendon which is inserted into the anterior surface of greater trochanter. A bursa is interposed between the tendon and the front of trochanter.

Nerve Supply

Both the gluteus medius and minimus are supplied by *superior gluteal nerve* (L_4, L_5, S_1).

Actions

- These two muscles *abduct the hip joint.*
- Their anterior fibers causes *medial rotation of thigh.*
- Most important function of the muscles *along with tensor fasciae latae is to keep the pelvis steady* while walking and running. During these kinds of movements, when the foot of one side is off the ground, the pelvis will have a tendency to sag or drop downwards on that side. This will be prevented by contraction of these three muscles of opposite side acting from lower end. So, if these muscles are paralyzed, the gait will be markedly affected. During movement, pelvis will be tilted down on the normal unsupported side repeatedly. This disability is known as **positive Trendelenburg sign.**

Clinical Anatomy

Paralysis of Gluteus Medius and Minimus

Though poliomyelitis has been eradicated now-a-days, unfortunate incidence of the disease involving the lower lumbar and the sacral segments of spinal cord causes paralysis of gluteus medius and minimus supplied by the superior gluteal nerve (L_4, L_5, S_1). This causes side-to-side tilling of the pelvis during walking showing a typical **waddling gait** or **lurching gait.** When this sign is observed clinically, it is called **positive Trendelenburg sign.**

SN 15.3 **Write a short note on tensor fasciae latae muscle.**

TENSOR FASCIAE LATAE

Origin

- It takes origin from anterior 5 cm of outer lip of ventral segment of iliac crest from the anterior superior iliac spine to the tubercle of iliac crest.
- It is thin at its origin and thicker towards its insertion end.

Insertion

Tensor fasciae latae is inserted in between two laminae of the iliotibial tract, which spits up at its upper end to receive the muscle fibers.

Nerve Supply

The muscle is supplied by the superior gluteal nerve (L_4, L_5, S_1) which supplies also the gluteus medius and minimus.

Actions
- Tensor fasciae latae pulls upon the iliotibial tract and thus *assists gluteus maximus in extending the knee joint*.
- Acting along with gluteal medius and minimus, it helps to stabilize the pelvis on the unsupported side during walking or running.

Clinical Anatomy
Lesion of superior gluteal nerve causes paralysis of tensor fasciae latae with gluteus medius and minimus leading to positive Trendelenburg sign.

LA 15.4 Give a brief account of the structures undercover of gluteus maximus muscle.

Individual structure may be asked in the form of short note.

STRUCTURES UNDER GLUTEUS MAXIMUS (FIG. 15.2)

Structures under cover of gluteus maximus are divided into two groups:
1. Some muscles which are confined in the gluteal region which are *gluteus medius, gluteus minimus* and *quadratus femoris*.
2. Muscles, blood vessels and nerves which *come out through greater and lesser sciatic foramina*.

Structures Passing through Greater Sciatic Foramen (Fig. 15.2)

- *Piriformis* is the muscle which takes origin inside the pelvis but it comes out through greater sciatic foramen dividing it into upper and lower compartments.
- Structures coming out through upper compartment: *Superior gluteal vessels and nerve.*
- Structures coming out through lower compartment:
  - Inferior gluteal vessels and nerve
  - Sciatic nerve
  - Posterior cutaneous nerve of the thigh
  - Nerve to quadratus femoris
  - Nerve to obturator internus
  - Internal pudendal vessels
  - Pudendal nerve.

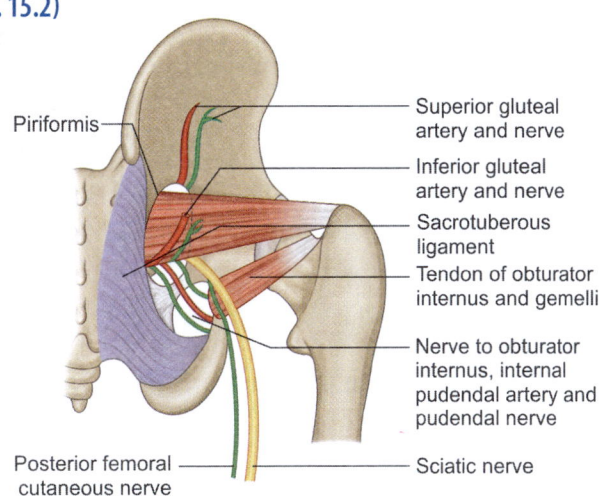

Fig. 15.2: Structures passing through greater and lesser sciatic foramina.

Structures Passing through Lesser Sciatic Foramen (Fig. 15.2)

- **Structure coming out**: *Tendon of obturator internus*
- **Structures going in**: *Nerve to obturator internus, internal pudendal artery accompanied by the vein* and *pudendal nerve*. Coming out through the greater sciatic foramen, these three structures reenter the pelvis through the lesser sciatic foramen.

Piriformis (Fig. 15.3)

Piriformis deserves its importance as the 'key muscle' of the gluteal region for its relationship with other structures. It takes origin from the *pelvic surface of the middle three pieces of sacrum*. It passes laterally to come out through the greater sciatic foramen which is almost completely filled up by the muscle. Some of the muscle fibers take origin from the upper margin of greater sciatic notch. The muscle ends into a tendon which is inserted into the medial aspect of *upper border of the greater trochanter*. Piriformis muscle is supplied by the fibers from ventral rami of S_1 and S_2 nerves. Piriformis acts as the *lateral rotator* of hip joint.

Obturator Internus and Gemelli (Fig. 15.3)

Obturator internus arises from *the internal surface of lateral wall of true pelvis* and its tendon makes *a right angle bend* around the lesser sciatic notch to appear in the gluteal region. The tendon is separated from the bony margin of lesser sciatic notch by a bursa. When the obturator internus comes out through lesser sciatic foramen, it is reinforced above and below by the fibers arising from the margins of lesser sciatic notch. These are gemellus superior and gemellus inferior. They fuse with the tendon of obturator internus which is inserted into the *medial surface of greater trochanter* just above trochanteric fossa. Obturator internus is supplied by its own independent nerve, called *nerve to obturator internus* (L_5, S_1, S_2).

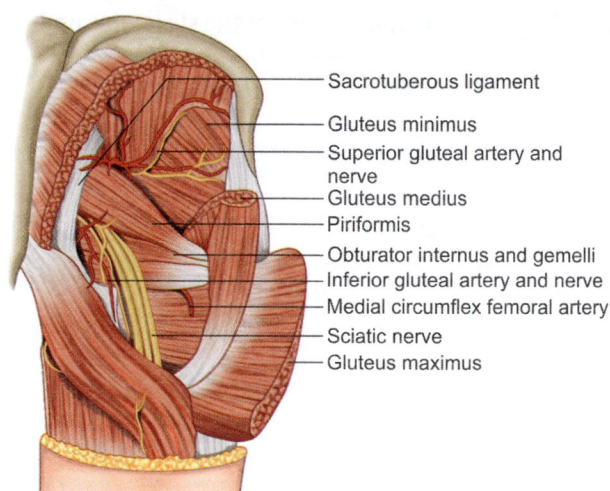

Fig. 15.3: Structures undercover of gluteus maximus.

Gemellus superior arises from the ischial spine which is above the lesser sciatic foramen and is supplied by nerve to obturator internus (L_5, S_1, S_2).

Gemellus inferior arises from the anterior margin of lesser sciatic foramen close to the ischial tuberosity and is supplied by the *nerve to quadratus femoris* (L_4, L_5, S_1).

Action

Obturator internus along with the gemelli is *lateral rotator* of the hip joint.

Quadratus Femoris

This is so called because of its rectangular outline with horizontal upper and lower margins. Quadratus femoris takes origin from the *lateral border of ischial tuberosity* and is inserted into the *quadrate tubercle of the femur*. The muscle is separated from the back of neck of femur by the tendon of obturator externus. Quadratus femoris is supplied by its own nerve called *nerve to quadratus femoris* (L_4, L_5, S_1).

Actions

- Acting along with piriformis, obturator internus and gemelli, quadratus femoris *stabilizes the hip joint.*

- Acting as prime mover, all these short muscles are *lateral rotator of extended thigh* and *abductor of flexed thigh*.

Nerves of the Gluteal Region

All the nerves arise from the sacral plexus in the pelvis.

Superior gluteal nerve, the nerve of sacral plexus, takes origin from the *dorsal branches* of ventral rami of L_4, L_5, S_1 nerves. It comes out of the pelvis through the greater sciatic foramen above piriformis and soon goes undercover of gluteus medius. It proceeds then upwards, forwards and laterally between *gluteus medius* and *gluteus minimus*. It gives branches to both the muscles and appears in between anterior borders of two muscles to supply *tensor fasciae latae*. It gives one articular branch to supply the *hip joint*.

Inferior gluteal nerve arises from the *dorsal branches* of ventral rami of L_5, S_1, S_2 nerves. It emerges from the pelvis below the piriformis along with inferior gluteal vessels. It ends by giving branches to the **gluteus maximus** from its deep surface.

Sciatic nerve appears in the gluteal region emerging from the pelvis through the lower compartment of greater sciatic foramen below the piriformis. It is the thickest nerve of the body made up of tibial and common fibular (common peroneal) components. Tibial component is formed by union of *ventral divisions* of ventral rami of L_4, L_5, S_1, S_2, S_3 nerves and common fibular component is formed by union of *dorsal division* of ventral rami of L_4, L_5, S_1, S_2 nerves. It is most lateral in position among all the structures coming out through greater sciatic foramen. It runs downward and slightly laterally with slight convexity outwards under the gluteus maximus muscle lying between greater trochanter and ischial tuberosity. Beyond the lower border of gluteus maximus, the sciatic nerve appears in the back of thigh.

Posterior cutaneous nerve of the thigh (S_1, S_2, S_3) is also known as posterior femoral cutaneous nerve. It emerges from the pelvis below the level of piriformis. It runs downwards on the sciatic nerve undercover of gluteus maximus. The nerve descends along the midline of back of thigh and back of the leg as low down as the middle of calf. It supplies the fascia lata and the overlying skin by number of branches. Gluteal branch curls around the lower border of gluteus maximus to supply the skin of lower part of buttock. *Perineal branch* of the nerve supplies scrotum or labium majus.

Patient with the diseases of pelvic viscera may experience *referred pain* along the area of distribution of posterior femoral cutaneous nerve because autonomic fibers for the pelvic viscera arise from the same sacral segments (S_2, S_3) of spinal cords. In these cases, pain along the back of thigh may be wrongly thought to be due to sciatic neuralgia.

Nerve to quadratus femoris (L_4, L_5, S_1) descends over the ischium deep to or in front of sciatic nerve. While it passes over the back of the hip joint, it gives an *articular branch* to the joint. Then it passes beneath the obturator internus with the gemelli to end on the deep surface of quadratus femoris to give *muscular branch*. It also gives a *branch to gemellus inferior*.

Nerve to obturator internus (L_5, S_1, S_2) appears for a while after it comes out of pelvis through the lower compartment of greater sciatic foramen. It crosses over the ischial spine and enters through the lesser sciatic foramen to sink into obturator internus muscle in the lateral wall of ischiorectal fossa. It gives *a branch to gemellus superior*.

Pudendal nerve (S_2, S_3, S_4) makes a brief appearance in the gluteal region. The nerve emerges below the piriformis and soon turns forwards *over the sacrospinous ligament* medial to the ischial spine. It leaves the gluteal region entering through the lesser sciatic foramen to enter the pudendal canal.

Perforating cutaneous nerve (S_2, S_3) is so called because, arising from sacral plexus, it becomes superficial after perforating through the lower part of sacrotuberous ligament and then curves around the lower border of gluteus maximus to supply the skin of inferomedial quadrant of gluteal region.

Arteries of the Gluteal Region

Superior gluteal artery is the branch arising from the posterior division of internal iliac artery in the pelvis. It appears in the gluteal region passing through the greater sciatic foramen above the piriformis. It divides into superficial and deep branches. *Superficial branch* pierces through the gluteus maximus to supply it and the overlying skin. *Deep branch* divides into superior and inferior divisions. *Superior division* takes part in anastomosis at the anterior superior iliac spine. *Inferior division* first gives branches to gluteus medius and gluteus minimus and finally takes part in trochanteric anastomosis.

Inferior gluteal artery is the branch from the anterior division of internal iliac artery and it appears in the gluteal region between piriformis and gemellus superior. The artery breaks up into multiple branches which are following:
- *Muscular branches* to gluteus maximus, piriformis and obturator internus with gemelli.
- *Anastomotic arteries* for trochanteric and cruciate anastomosis.
- *Artery for sciatic nerve:* It is called arteria nervi commitans ischiadici. It is a long but very thin artery which ultimately enters within the thick sciatic nerve. Morphologically, it represents the original **axis artery of the lower limb**.

Internal pudendal artery is also the branch arising from anterior division of internal iliac artery. It follows the similar *course like the pudendal nerve* lying lateral to it. It crosses over the bony structure of ischial spine against which it can be compressed to arrest the bleeding in the perineum. It is accompanied by the veins on its either side.

LA 15.5 Give a brief account on the Hamstring muscles.

Individual muscle may be asked as a short note

HAMSTRING MUSCLES

Hamstring muscles are so called as their distal tendinous ends cross over the lower part of thigh which is known as **ham**.

Characteristics of Hamstring Muscles
- All the hamstring muscles take origin from the ischial tuberosity
- They are inserted beyond the knee joint in the upper end of tibia or fibula
- They are innervated by the tibial component of sciatic nerve
- As they cross the back of both hip and knee joint, they are primarily extensor of hip and flexor of the knee joint.

Hamstring muscles are:
- Semimembranosus
- Semitendinosus
- Biceps femoris (long head)
   Short head of biceps femoris takes origin from the femur.
- Ischial part (hamstring part) of adductor magnus.
   Hamstring part of adductor magnus is inserted proximal to the knee joint (in adductor tubercle). Part of the tendon beyond this point is converted into tibial (medial) collateral ligament of knee joint.

Semimembranosus (Figs. 15.4A and B)

This muscle passes along the medial side of the back of thigh and it extends from the ischial tuberosity to the medial condyle of tibia. It takes origin from *upper lateral part* of ischial tuberosity.

The origin of the muscle is in the form of *a long flat tendon*. It becomes fleshly at about the middle of thigh. At the insertion end, it is again a *rounded tendon* and its main insertion is into the *horizontal concavity* on the back of medial condyle of tibia.

Expansions of Semimembranosus

From the insertion end of the muscle, three expansions diverge in different directions.
1. One passes forwards underneath to the tibial collateral ligament of the knee joint to be attached *to the medial surface of medial condyle* of tibia, being interposed by a bursa.
2. The second expansion passes *upwards and laterally* to be attached to the superior margins of the intercondylar area and also back of lateral condyle of femur. This is known as the **oblique popliteal ligament.**
3. The third tendinous expension passes downwards and laterally to form the **fascia covering popliteus** which is attached to the soleal line of tibia.

Semitendinosus (Figs. 15.4A and B)

Semitendinosus arises from the upper medial area of ischial tuberosity is common with the origin of long head of biceps femoris. At its origin side it presents fleshly belly which gradually diminishes in size from above downwards and is converted into a cord-like tendon. The tendon passes behind medial condyle of femur and then curves forwards to be inserted into the upper part of medial surface of shaft of tibia, posteroinferior to the insertions of sartorius and gracilis.

Biceps Femoris (Figs. 15.4A and B)

This muscle has two heads of origin. The **long head** takes origin, in common with semitendinosus, form the *upper medial part of ischial tuberosity*. It passes downwards and laterally crossing over the sciatic nerve, and joins with the **short head** of the muscle which has an extensive origin from the *whole length of linea aspera* and *upper part of lateral supracondylar line of femur*. Distally, the

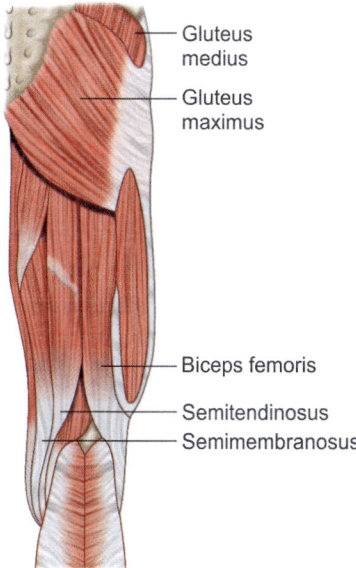

Fig. 15.4A: Superficial muscles of back of right thigh with gluteal region.

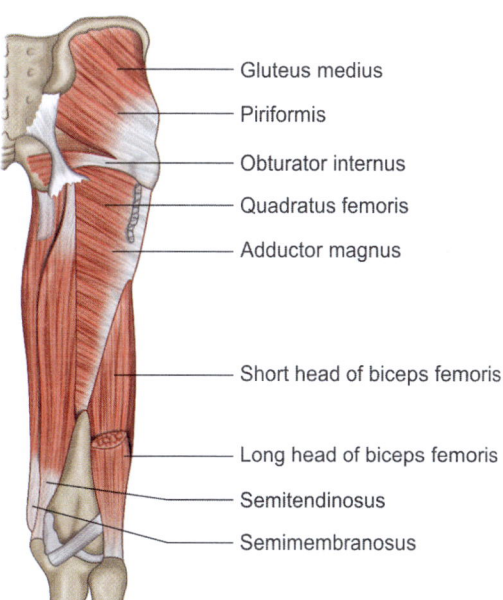

Fig. 15.4B: Deep muscles of back of right thigh with gluteal region.

single tendon of the muscle is split to enclose the fibular collateral ligament of the knee joint and is inserted into the head of the fibula.

Nerve Supply of the Hamstrings

All the three above-mentioned true hamstring muscles, namely semimembranosus, semitendinosus and biceps femoris (only long head) along with the ischial part of adductor magnus are supplied by the **tibial component of the sciatic nerve. The short head of biceps femoris** receives its nerve supply from the **common fibular (peroneal) component of the sciatic nerve.**

Actions

- Acting from above, the hamstring muscles are flexor of the knee joint
- Acting from below, they are extensor of the hip joint
- In semiflexed position, the biceps femoris is lateral rotator and, the semimembranosus and semitendinosus are medial rotator of the leg.

SA 15.6 Discuss briefly different arterial anastomoses in the back of thigh.

ARTERIES OF BACK OF THIGH

The main source of the arterial supply of back of thigh is **profunda femoris artery** with its **lateral** and **medial circumflex femoral branches** which may arise independently from the femoral artery. In addition descending branches of **superior** and **inferior gluteal arteries** and **ascending branch of popliteal artery**, from above and below respectively, contribute in arterial supply of back of thigh including gluteal region. These arteries form anastomosis which are named as follows:
- Trochanteric anastomosis
- Cruciate anastomosis
- Vertical chain anastomosis.

Trochanteric Anastomosis (Fig. 15.5)

This anastomosis lies near the trochanteric fossa. It forms the main source of blood supply of the head of femur. The anastomosis is formed by:
1. Descending branch of superior gluteal artery
2. Descending branch of inferior gluteal artery.
3. Ascending branch of medial circumflex femoral artery.
4. Ascending branch of lateral circumflex femoral artery.

Branches form this anastomosis pass accompanying the retinacular fibers of hip joint capsule along the neck of femur to supply the head of femur.

Cruciate Anastomosis (Fig. 15.5)

This anastomosis is situated at the back of middle of lesser trochanter of femur. This is formed by:
1. Descending branch of inferior gluteal artery
2. Ascending branch of first perforating artery, which is the branch of profunda femoris artery.

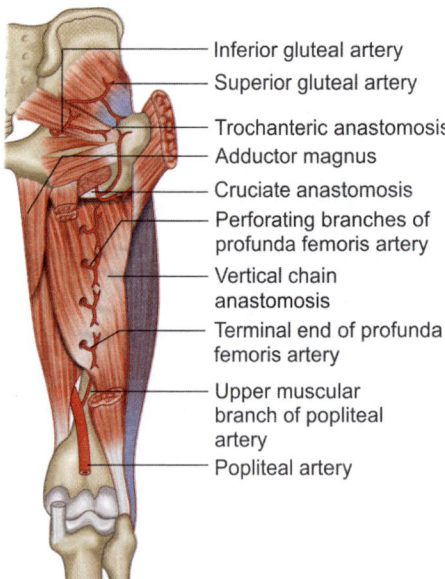

Fig. 15.5: Arterial anastomosis in back of thigh.

3. Horizontal branch of medial circumflex artery
4. Horizontal branch of lateral circumflex femoral artery

Through the descending branch of inferior gluteal artery, the descending limb of the cross, cruciate anastomosis makes the communication with the trochanteric anastomosis. Again, through the ascending branch of the first perforating artery, the ascending limb of the cross, it establishes communication with the vertical chain anastomosis below.

Vertical Chain Anastomosis (Fig. 15.5)

This is the main source of arterial supply of hamstring muscles. This arterial chain represents the artery of the back of thigh due to rudimentary form of the axis artery of the lower limb which accompanies the sciatic nerve.

Situation
The vertical chain of anastomosis lies on the posterior surface of adductor magnus muscle close to its line of insertion.

Formation
The anastomosis is formed by union of adjacent descending and ascending branches of following arteries all of which perforate the adductor magnus to pass from its front to back.
- **Three perforating branches of profunda femoris artery**, which divide into ascending and descending branches to anastomose with each other. Ascending branch of first perforating artery ascend upwards to form the lower limb of the cruciate anastomosis.
- **Terminal end of the profunda femoris artery**, which is considered as the **fourth perforating artery**, pierces adductor magnus and divides similarly into ascending and descending branches. Its ascending branch communicates with the descending branch of the third perforating artery.
- **The popliteal artery**, as the continuation of the femoral artery is considered as **the fifth perforating artery** which reaches the popliteal fossa passing through the *hiatus magnus* of adductor magnus muscle. **Upper muscular branch of the popliteal artery** ascends to anastomose with the descending branch of the terminal end of profunda femoris artery.

Clinical Anatomy
Vertical chain anastomosis on the back of thigh constitutes a collateral channel of blood supply to the lower limb as an alternative pathway parallel to the external iliac and femoral arteries. When there is necessity to ligate the femoral artery above the origin of profunda femoris artery, it establishes the collateral circulation for the lower limb.

SA 15.7 Give an account of boundaries and contents of the popliteal fossa. Add a note on clinical anatomy.

INTRODUCTION
Popliteal fossa is a diamond-shaped space behind the knee joint. This hollow of the fossa becomes more prominent during flexed position of the knee. The fossa is important because, the vessels and nerves passing over the fossa are related to the back of the knee joint.

BOUNDARIES OF POPLITEAL FOSSA

Outlines (Fig. 15.6)
- **Superomedially:** Semitendinosus and semimembranosus
- **Superolaterally:** Biceps femoris
- **Inferomedially:** Medial head of gastrocnemius
- **Inferolaterally:** Lateral head of gastrocnemius with plantaris

At the upper limit of the fossa, semitendinosus and semimembranosus diverge from biceps femoris at an acute angle which is called *apex of the popliteal fossa*.

Lower limit of the fossa is overlapped by convergence of two heads of gastrocnemius.

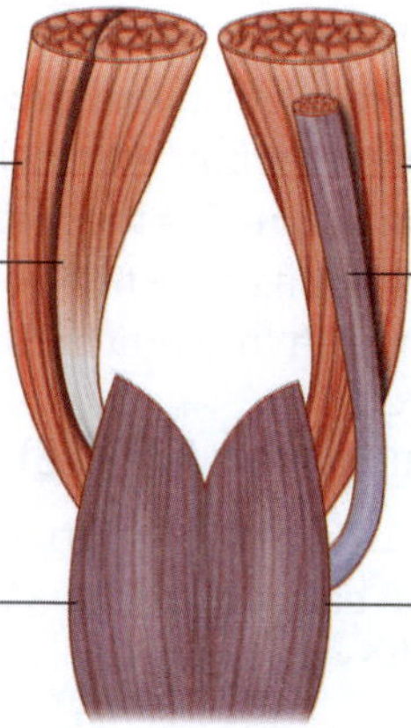

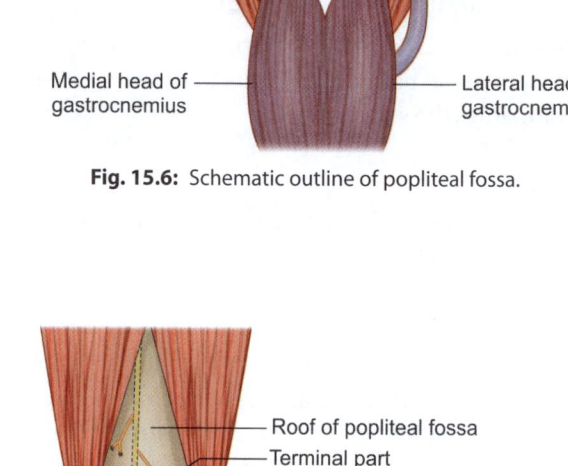

Fig. 15.6: Schematic outline of popliteal fossa.

Roof (Fig. 15.7)
Roof of popliteal fossa is formed by extension of fascia lata which is reinforced here by the transverse fibers. The fascia of the roof is known as **popliteal fascia**. Superficial fascia over the roof contains the following:
- Short saphenous vein
- Terminal part of posterior femoral cutaneous nerve
- Terminal part of medial cutaneous nerve of thigh
- Sural communicating nerve
- Lateral cutaneous nerve of the calf.

All these structures pierce the fascial roof except the medial cutaneous nerve of the thigh.

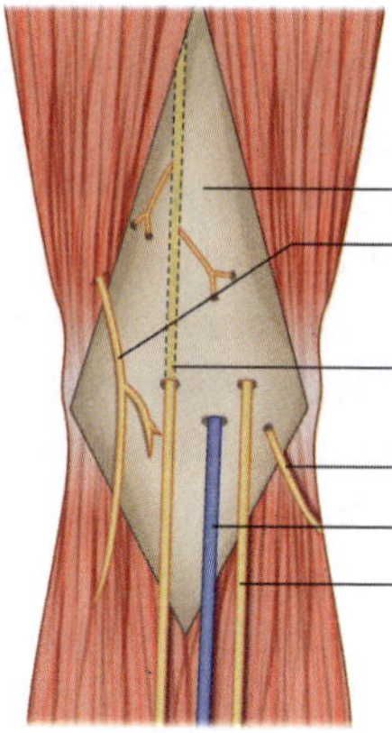

Fig. 15.7: Roof of popliteal fossa and related structures.

Floor (Fig. 15.8)
It is formed by the following structures from above downwards.
- *Popliteal surface of femur* covered by *popliteal pad of fat*
- *Capsule of knee joint* reinforced by *oblique popliteal ligament*
- *Popliteus muscle* covered by its *fascia*.

Contents
- Popliteal artery
- Popliteal vein
- Tibial nerve
- Common fibular (common peroneal) nerve

All these structures traverse through the whole length of the fossa

- Popliteal lymph nodes lying in relation to the popliteal vein.

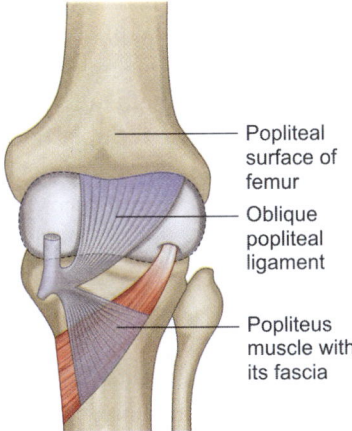

Fig. 15.8: Floor of popliteal fossa.

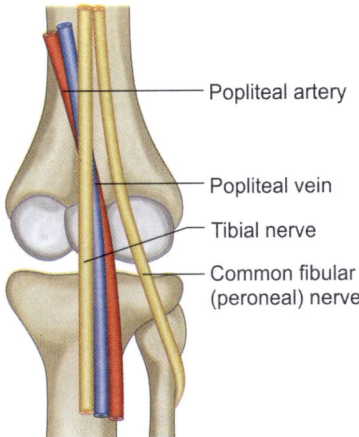

Fig. 15.9: Contents of popliteal fossa.

Interrelations of the Structures of Neurovascular Bundle (Fig. 15.9)
- Popliteal artery is crossed by popliteal vein from *lateral to medial side*
- Again, popliteal vein itself is crossed by the tibial nerve *from lateral to medial side*
- Common fibular (peroneal) nerve, lying most laterally at the apex of the popliteal fossa descends downwards and laterally *towards the lateral angle of the fossa.*

MUSCLES OF THE POPLITEAL FOSSA

Among the muscles related to popliteal fossa, the hamstring muscles have been discussed in the section of back of thigh. Gastrocnemius and plantaris is discussed in Back of the Leg and Sole of the Foot (Chapter 17). Popliteus muscle is discussed below after the section of nerves and vessels of popliteal fossa.

NEUROVASCULAR STRUCTURES OF POPLITEAL FOSSA

Tibial Nerve (Figs. 15.10 and 15.11)

The tibial nerve, the larger division of sciatic nerve, runs vertically downwards along the midline of popliteal fossa and disappears by passing deeply between the two heads of gastrocnemius. If the two heads of the muscle are separated, the nerve is found to pass along with the popliteal vessels deep to the fibrous origin of the soleus muscle, called soleal arch. Distal to the soleal arch the tibial nerve appears in the back of leg or the calf.

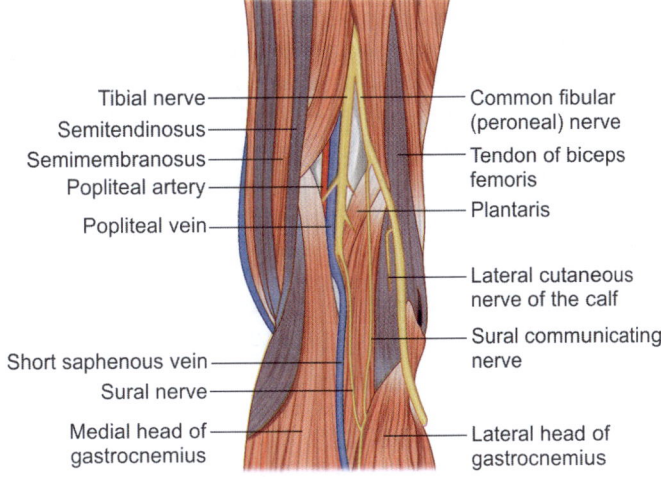

Fig. 15.10: Boundaries and content of right popliteal fossa.

In the popliteal fossa, the tibial nerve gives off following group of branches:
- **Muscular branches:** All the muscles of popliteal fossa are supplied by the tibial nerve, namely, *both the heads of gastrocnemius, plantaris, soleus* and *popliteus*. The branch to the popliteus hooks round the lower border of the muscle and supply the muscle through the deep surface.
- **Cutaneous branch: Sural nerve** is the only cutaneous branch arising from the tibial nerve. It runs vertically downwards along the narrow interval between two heads of gastrocnemius. It pierces the deep fascia of leg in the middle of calf. In the plane of superficial fascia, it communicates with the sural communicating nerve distal to the bellies of gastrocnemius. Here it is related to the short saphenous vein. The nerve is lateral to the vein.
- **Articular branches:** These are **genicular nerves**, which are three in number. **Superior** and **inferior medial genicular nerves** lying medially accompany the corresponding genicular arteries and supply the medial (tibial) collateral ligament and medial side of the capsule of the knee joint. **Middle genicular nerve** perforates the oblique popliteal ligament along with the middle genicular artery to supply cruciate ligaments of knee joint inside the capsule.

Common Fibular Nerve (Fig. 15.11)

Common fibular (common peroneal) nerve is the narrower division of sciatic nerve. It passes downwards and laterally medial to the biceps femoris and disappears in the substance of fibularis (peroneus) longus to lie in relation to the neck of fibula. The nerve can be rolled against the neck of fibula in living individual. Here the nerve is vulnerable to injury in case of fracture of neck of fibula.

Before the common fibular nerve divides into superficial and deep terminal branches, it does not give any muscular branch. The trunk of common fibular nerve gives following sensory branches.
- **Sural communicating branch** pierces the roof of popliteal fossa and runs downwards in the superficial fasica and joins with the sural nerve in the lower half of the calf.

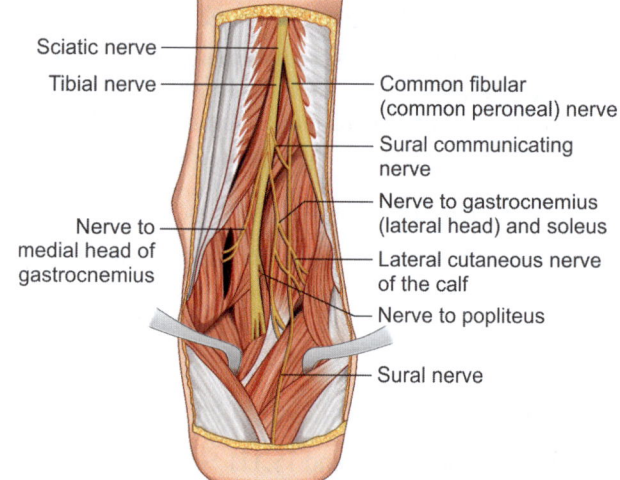

Fig. 15.11: Nerves of the popliteal fossa.

- **Lateral cutaneous nerve of the calf** pierces the deep fascia of the roof of popliteal fossa on the lateral head of gastrocnemius. It supplies the skin of upper part of anterolateral aspect of leg.
- **Superior and inferior lateral genicular nerves** are the lateral group of articular branches. They accompany the corresponding arteries and supply the fibular (lateral) collateral ligaments and the lateral part of capsular ligament of the knee joint.
- **Recurrent genicular nerve** arises from the parent trunk within the substance of fibularis (peroneus) longus. It presents a recurrent course to supply the *superior tibiofibular joint* along with the *knee joint*.

Popliteal Artery (Fig. 15.12)

Popliteal artery begins at the hiatus (opening) of adductor magnus at the upper end of popliteal fossa as continuation of the femoral artery. It ends at the lower border of popliteus opposite the level of fibrous soleal arch by dividing into anterior and posterior tibial arteries. Throughout the whole length of the popliteal fossa, the popliteal artery and the vein, and the tibial nerve are closely related to each other. At the middle of popliteal fossa the artery is crossed from lateral to medial side by the popliteal vein, which again, is crossed by the tibial nerve form lateral to medial side. So, at the middle of the fossa, tibial nerve, popliteal vein and popliteal artery are interrelated successively from superficial to deep plane. The popliteal artery runs from above downwards on popliteal surface of femur covered by popliteal pad of fat, oblique popliteal ligament and fascia covering the popliteus. Rarely the popliteal artery may divide above the level of the popliteus. In that case, the anterior tibial artery descends in front of popliteus.

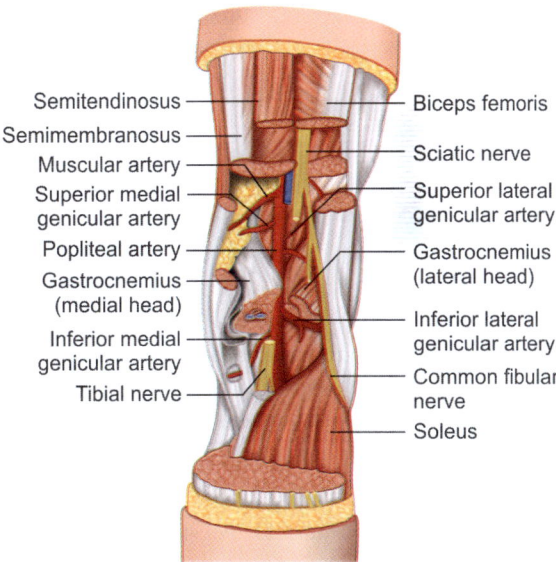

Fig. 15.12: Popliteal artery with branches.

Branches of Popliteal Artery

- **Cutaneous:** These branches become superficial piercing the roof of popliteal fossa. They supply the skin and fascia overlying popliteal fossa.
- **Muscular:** These are multiple and subdivided into upper and lower muscular groups. **Upper muscular branches** supply hamstring muscles with adductor magnus, one of these branches anastomoses with descending branch of terminal end of profunda femoris artery which is considered as the fourth perforating artery. **Lower muscular branches** supply gastrocnemius and soleus.
- **Genicular (Fig. 15.13):** These are articular branches for the knee joint and are *five in number*. These branches are a pair of *superior genicular (lateral and medial)*, a pair of *inferior genicular (lateral and medial)* and *one middle genicular arteries*.
  - **Medial superior genicular artery** lies deep to semitendinosus, semimembranosus and tendon of adductor magnus. **Lateral superior genicular artery** lies deep to the tendon of biceps femoris. Both the superior genicular arteries encircle the lower end of femur from behind forwards proximal to the attachment of two heads of gastrocnemius muscle.
  - **Middle genicular artery** pierces the oblique popliteal ligament to supply intra-articular structures including the cruciate ligaments. It is accompanied by the terminal part of the *posterior division of obturator nerve* and a *genicular branch of tibial nerve*.
  - **Medial inferior genicular artery** passes deep to medial head of gastrocnemius and tibial (medial) collateral ligament of knee joint. **Lateral inferior genicular artery** passes deep to lateral head of gastrocnemius and fibular (lateral) collateral ligament of knee joint. This artery crosses over the tendon of popliteus. Inferior genicular arteries encircle the upper end of tibia.

Clinical Anatomy

- **Popliteal pulsation:** Pulsation of the popliteal artery is felt against the back of the knee. For clinical diagnosis of the disease like **coarctation of aorta**, examination of popliteal pulse is important. Because in this condition popliteal pulse is found to be feeble in comparison to the upper limb arterial pulse.

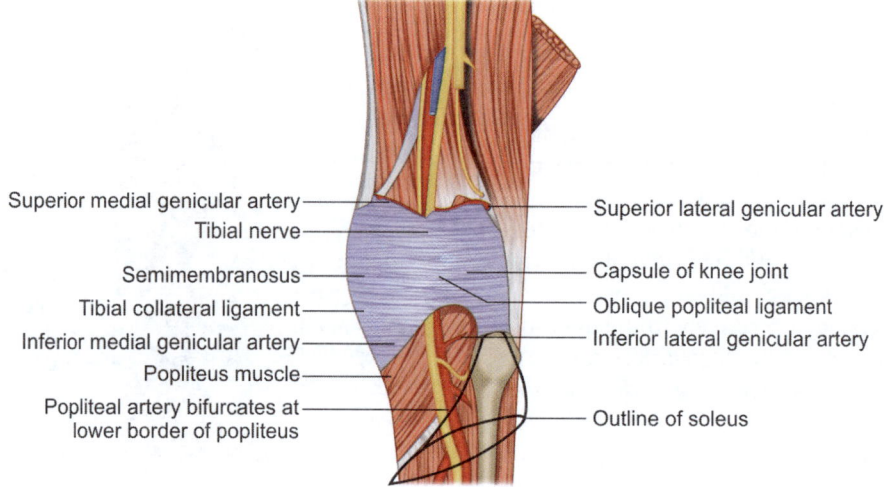

Fig. 15.13: Popliteus muscle with deeper structures of popliteal fossa.

- **Popliteal aneurysm**: Arterial aneurysm is a clinical condition characterized by localized 'ballooning' of arterial wall. This is due to congenital thinning or absence of tunica media of arterial wall. Aneurysm of popliteal artery is more common incidence.
- **Popliteal thrombosis**: Popliteal artery may be fixed to the capsule of knee joint by a fibrous band. This may cause continuous stretching of the artery leading to primary thrombosis in the popliteal artery.
- **Baker's cyst**: This is a clinical condition presenting a cystic swelling on the back of knee joint. It results from inflammation of the pouch of synovial membrane of the knee joint protruding out through the capsule of knee joint.

SA 15.8 Write a note on arterial anastomosis around the knee joint (genicular anastomosis).

GENICULAR ANASTOMOSIS (FIG. 15.14)

Genicular anastomosis is a communication network of the four genicular branches of popliteal artery with branches of femoral, profunda femoris, and anterior and posterior tibial arteries.

Fundamental Points on Branching and Communication

- Both the superior and inferior pairs of genicular arteries (branches of popliteal artery) divide into ascending and descending branches.
- *On both sides*, **descending branch of superior genicular artery** anastomoses with **ascending branch of inferior genicular artery of the corresponding side**.

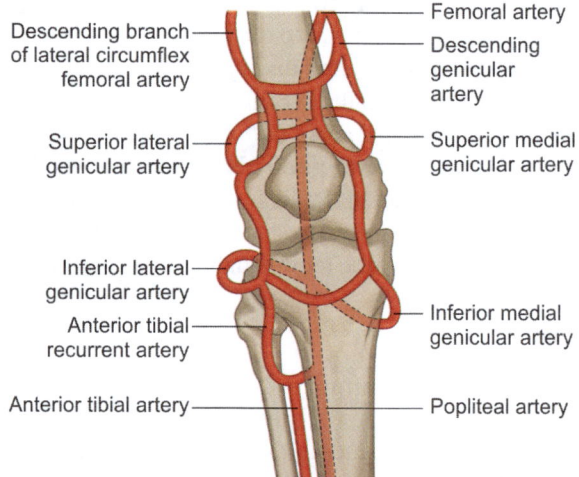

Fig. 15.14: Genicular anastomosis around the knee.

- **Ascending branches of superior genicular arteries** anastomose with the descending arteries coming from above as follows:
  - Ascending branch of lateral superior genicular artery joins with the **descending branch of lateral circumflex femoral artery coming from above.**
  - Ascending branch of medial superior genicular artery anastomoses with the **descending genicular branch of femoral artery.**
- **Descending branch of lateral inferior genicular artery** communicates with:
  - Anterior and posterior recurrent branches of **anterior tibial artery**
  - Circumflex fibular branch of **posterior tibial artery.**

SN 15.9 Write a short note on the popliteus muscle.

POPLITEUS (FIG. 15.13)

Introduction
Popliteus is a flat triangular muscle which forms the most distal part of the floor of popliteal fossa. It is covered by a fascia named fascia covering popliteus.

Origin
Popliteus *takes origin within the capsule* of the knee joint by a strong tendon which is 2.5 cm long. The tendon arises from *a depression* on the anterior part of the *groove* on the lateral surface of lateral condyle of femur. The posterior part of the groove is to accommodate the tendon during extreme flexion of knee joint.

Additional Slips
While the tendon of popliteus comes out of the joint through the capsule, it is joined on the medial side by collagenous fibers from:
- Fibrous capsule
- Arcuate popliteal ligament
- Outer margin of the lateral meniscus.
  Additional head of popliteus may arise from the sesamoid bone in lateral head of gastrocnemius.

Insertion
Inferior end of the tendon expands into fleshy fibers which forms a triangular muscle. It is inserted into the *medial two-thirds* of the triangular area above the soleal line on the posterior surface of the tibia.

Fascia Covering Popliteus
From the main insertion of semimembranosus on the back of medial condyle of tibia, an expansion extends downwards and laterally to form a fascial sheet over the popliteus muscle and is attached to the soleal line beyond the muscle fibers of the popliteus muscle.

Important Relations
While coming out through the joint capsule the tendon of popliteus is related to *a groove* on the posterior aspect of lateral meniscus and emerges below the arcuate popliteal ligament.
  The fleshy part of the muscle is overlapped by popliteal vessels, gastrocnemius, plantaris and tibial nerve.

Nerve Supply

Popliteus is supplied by a branch of tibial nerve which winds round the lower border of the muscle to enter the deep (anterior) surface.

The nerve also supplies:
- *Superior tibiofibular joint*
- *Interosseous membrane of the leg.*

Actions

- Most important action of popliteus takes place in fully extended knee. During this position, when the limb is on the ground, the femur rotates medially through the twist of the capsule and collateral ligaments which causes 'locking' of the knee joint to make it secured. On prolonged standing, the quadriceps tendon is relaxed for rest. From this position of the joint, popliteus acts from below **to unlock the joint** by rotating the femoral condyles laterally on tibial condyles. This will permit initiation of flexion of the joint.

  Attachment of fibers on lateral meniscus gives an advantage of retraction of posterior horn of the meniscus backward to prevent its crushing between the femoral and tibial condyles during full extension of the knee joint.
- In supine and seated position, the popliteus rotates the mobile tibia medially at the commencement of flexion.

Popliteus Minor

On very rare occasions, this muscle is present. It extends from posterior surface of lateral condyle of tibia to the oblique popliteal ligament.

Chapter 16

Anterolateral Compartment of Leg and Dorsum of Foot

LA 16.1 Give an account of the muscles of anterior compartment of leg.

Individual muscle may be asked in the form of short notes

MUSCLES OF ANTERIOR COMPARTMENT OF LEG

Tibialis Anterior (Fig. 16.1)

Origin
- Upper two-thirds of lateral surface of shaft of tibia extending above up to the lateral condyle.
- Adjacent part of the interosseous membrane.
- Deep surface of the deep fascia of leg (fascia cruris).

Insertion
The muscle fibers end into a strong tendon which descends over lower one-third of leg. It descends *through* medial parts of **superior extensor retinaculum** and **superior band of inferior extensor retinaculum**. It then runs *deep to* **inferior band of inferior extensor retinaculum** and inclines medially to be inserted into:
- Inferomedial aspect of medial cuneiform
- The adjoining part of the inferomedial aspect of the base of first metatarsal bone.

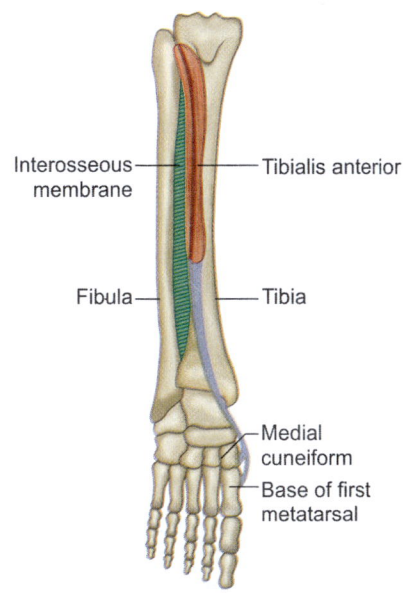

Fig. 16.1: Tibialis anterior muscle.

Occasional Slips of Insertion
- Extensor retinaculum
- **Talus**
- Head of first metatarsal bone
- Base of proximal phalanx of great toe.

Nerve Supply
Deep fibular (peroneal) nerve (L_4, L_5), which is the nerve of anterior compartment of leg.

Actions
- Tibialis anterior is *main dorsiflexor* and *powerful invertor* (to raise medial border of foot) when the foot is raised off the ground during walking.
- It *maintains the medial longitudinal arch* of foot.
- When the leg is *on the ground*, the muscle helps to *balance the leg* and *talus* over the tarsal bones.

Extensor Hallucis Longus (Figs. 16.2 and 16.4)

The muscle is interposed in between as well as overlapped by tibialis anterior and extensor digitorum longus.

Origin
- *Medial half (tibial) of middle two-fourths* of the medial surface of the shaft of fibula.
- Adjoining part of interosseous membrane.

Insertion
The muscle fibers forms a tendon which passes *deep to* the superior extensor retinaculum and traversing *through* the inferior extensor retinaculum.

The tendon then crosses superficial to anterior tibial vessels and is inserted on the dorsal surface of base of distal phalanx of great toe (hallux).

Variations
- At the level of metatarsophalangeal joint of great toe, a collateral slip from each side of the tendon covers the dorsal aspect of the joint.
- A slip of the tendon is often found to be inserted on the base of proximal phalanx of hallux.
- Extensor hallucis longus may occasionally blend with extensor digitorum longus.
- A slip of the tendon may be attached to the second toe.

Nerve Supply
Deep fibular (peroneal) nerve (L_5).

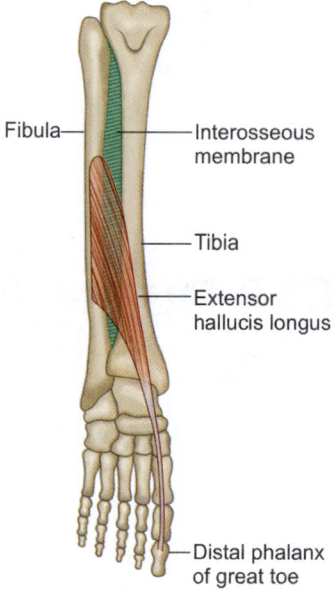

Fig. 16.2: Extensor hallucis longus muscle.

Actions
- Extensor hallucis longus, as it is called, causes extension of phalanges of hallux.
- It also dorsiflexes the foot.
- In extended position of great toe, it may be used for inversion (raising the medial border) of foot.

Extensor Digitorum Longus (Figs. 16.3 and 16.4)

Origin
The muscle presents following extensive sources of origin.
- Inferior surface of lateral condyle of the tibia
- Upper three fourths of medial surface of shaft of fibula (*whole of the surface in upper one-fourth and lateral half of the surface of middle two-fourths*).
- Adjacent part of anterior surface of interosseous membrane
- Undersurface of the deep fascia of the leg

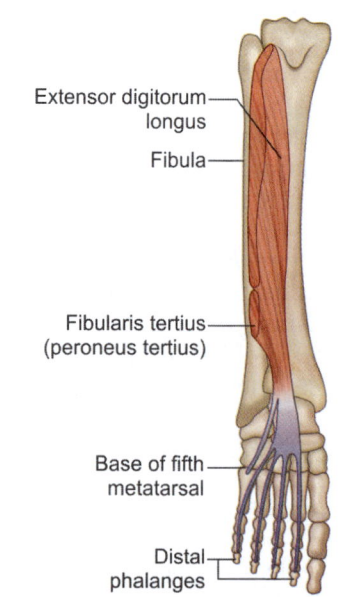

Fig. 16.3: Extensor digitorum longus and fibularis (peroneus) tertius muscle.

- Anterior intermuscular septum
- Intermuscular fascia between it and tibialis anterior.

Insertion

For insertion, extensor digitorum longus presents following characteristics:
- **Formation of tendon**: The muscle ends in a tendon in lower end of front of leg.
- **Division into four slips**: After the main tendon passes through the extensor retinacula, it divides into four slips for the lateral four toes.
- **Contribution from the other sources**:
  - On the dorsum of foot, opposite to the metatarsophalangeal joint, tendon slips for second, third and fourth toes, are joined by the respective slip of tendon of extensor digitorum brevis from the lateral side.
  - Like the extensor tendon of hand, *dorsal digital expansions* are formed on the dorsum of proximal phalanges. They receive attachment of tendon of respective lumbricals and interossei.
- **Division into central and collateral slips:** At the level of proximal interphalangeal joint, the dorsal digital expansion or expansion divides into a central and two collateral slips.
- **Attachment:** The central slip is attached to the dorsal aspect of base of middle phalanx. Two collateral slips proceed distally and reunite to be attached to the dorsum of the base of distal phalanx.

Nerve Supply

Extensor digitorum longus is supplied by deep fibular (peroneal) nerve (L_5, S_1).

Actions

- Extensor digitorum longus acts for extension of lateral four toes.
- Acting in combination with the other muscles of front of leg, it causes dorsiflexion of foot.
- Acting together with extensor hallucis longus only, it makes the plantar aponeurosis tense, thus it increases the height of medial longitudinal arch of foot through bow stringing mechanism.

Fibularis Tertius (Peroneus Tertius) (Figs. 16.3 and 16.4)

It is a specialized muscle of human body. Very often, peroneus tertius or fibularis tertius appears to be the part of extensor digitorum longus and is described as 'fifth tendon' of the muscle.

Origin

- Distal one-fourth of medial surface of shaft of fibula
- Adjacent part of interosseous membrane
- Anterior intermuscular septum of leg.

The tendon of the muscle passes *deep to* the superior extensor retinaculum and finally *through* the loop of interior extensor retinaculum.

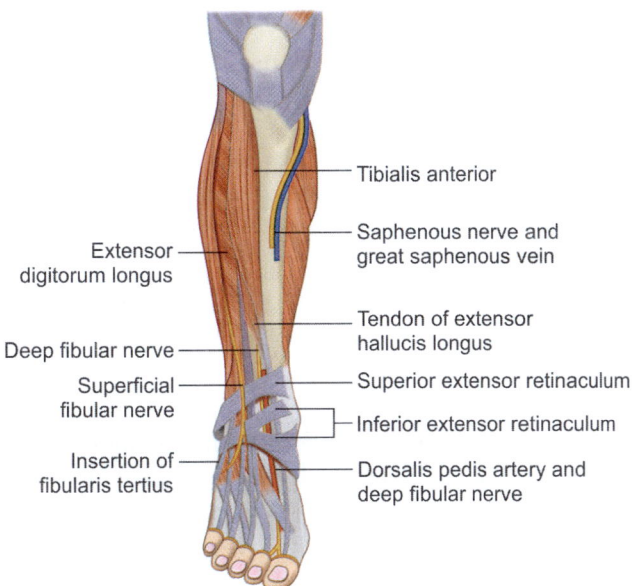

Fig. 16.4: Structures of front of leg and dorsum of foot.

Insertion
- *Medial part of dorsal aspect* of the base of the fifth metatarsal bone.
- *A thin expansion* of the tendon is continued forwards along the *medial border of the shaft* of the fifth metatarsal bone.

Nerve Supply
Deep peroneal nerve (*deep fubular nerve*) carrying fibers of L_5 and S_1 roots.

Actions
- Acting with extensor digitorum longus and tibialis anterior, peroneus tertius (fibularis tertius) causes *dorsiflexion of foot*.
- Acting with peroneus longus (fibularis longus) and peroneus brevis (fibularis brevis), it helps in *eversion of foot*.

During the swing phase of the gait, the abovementioned two conjoint actions *level the foot* and helps to clear the toes off the ground. This action improves the efficiency and increases the economy of bipedal locomotion.

The nerve and the artery of the anterior compartment of leg (the deep peroneal nerve or deep fibular nerve and the anterior tibial artery) are described after the section of 'dorsum of foot'.

SA 16.2 Discuss briefly the cutaneous nerve supply of dorsum of foot.

CUTANEOUS NERVE SUPPLY OF DORSUM OF FOOT (FIG. 16.5)

Maximum area of skin of dorsum of foot is supplied by the *superficial peroneal (fibular) nerve*. It is assisted by other nerves as mentioned below.

- **Superficial peroneal nerve (superficial fibular nerve)** perforates the deep fascia in the lower third of the leg and bifurcates into lateral and medial divisions which supply the skin of the dorsum of foot. The medial division further subdivides to supply the skin of *medial side of great toe* and that of the *second digital cleft*. The lateral division of the nerve also bifurcates to supply the skin of *third and fourth digital clefts*.
- **Saphenous nerve** supplies the skin along the medial margin of dorsum of foot up to the extent of ball (base) of the great toe.
- **Sural nerve** supplies the skin of the lateral side of dorsum as well as the lateral side of the little toe.
- **Deep peroneal (deep fibular) nerve** supplies the skin of the first interdigital cleft between great toe and second toe.
- **Medial and lateral plantar nerves,** through their respective dorsal, branches, supply the nail beds. Medial plantar nerve supplies medial three and a half toes, whereas the lateral plantar nerve supplies lateral one and a half toes.

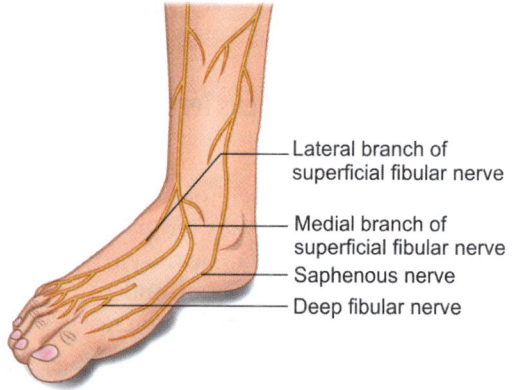

Fig. 16.5: Cutaneous nerves of dorsum of foot.

SA 16.3 Write a brief note on the extensor retinacula of the foot.

EXTENSOR RETINACULA OF THE FOOT

Superior Extensor Retinaculum (Fig. 16.6)

Introduction
Superior extensor retinaculum is a condensed band of deep fascia of lower end of front of leg which straps over the tendons of anterior compartment of leg.

Attachment
Laterally: Distal end of anterior border of fibula

Medially: Anterior border of tibia above the medial malleolus.

Location
Immediately proximal to the talocrural (ankle) joint.

Above, its proximal border is continuous with *fascia cruris*. Its distal border is connected to the inferior extensor retinaculum by *dense connective tissue*.

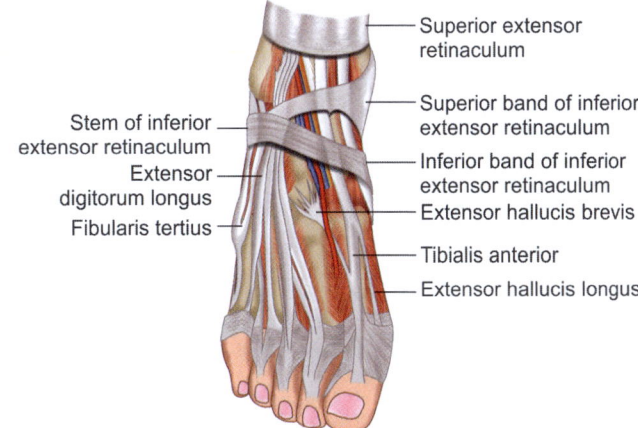

Fig. 16.6: Extensor retinacula of foot.

Superficial Relations
From medial to lateral:
- Saphenous nerve
- Great saphenous vein
- Medial and lateral divisions of superficial fibular (peroneal) nerve.

Deep Relations
From medial to lateral:
- Tendon of tibialis anterior
- Tendon of extensor hallucis longus
- Anterior tibial vessels
- Deep fibular nerve (deep peroneal nerve)
- Tendon of extensor digitorum longus
- Tendon of fibularis tertius (peroneus tertius).

Beneath the superior extensor retinaculum, only the tendon of tibialis anterior is enclosed by its synovial sheath.

Function
Extensor retinacula keep the tendons of anterior crural muscles in position during their contraction by preventing their bowstringing.

Inferior Extensor Retinaculum (Fig. 16.6)

Introduction

Inferior extensor retinaculum is a 'Y' shaped thickened band of deep fascia lying anterior to the talocrural (ankle) joint.

Stem of the 'Y' is lateral and two limbs are medial in position.

Attachment and Relations

Lateral stem is attached to the superior surface of calcaneus in front of sulcus calcanei.
- From lateral side of the ankle the stem of the retinaculum passes medially forming a *strong loop* around the tendons of fibularis (peroneus) tertius and extensor digitorum longus.
- From the deep surface of the loop, a slip passes back laterally to be attached to the sulcus calcanei. From the medial side of the loop two limbs of Y shaped band diverge from each other.

Proximal or upper limb of the retinaculum is divided into *two layers*. **The deep layer of the proximal limb** passes beneath the tendons of the extensor hallucis longus and the tibialis anterior, but superficial to the anterior tibial vessels and deep fibular (peroneal) nerve to be attached to the *medial malleolus of tibia*. **The superficial layer** loops around the tendon of extensor hallucis longus to fuse with the deep layer.

Distal or lower limb extends downwards and medially and *joins with the plantar aponeurosis*. This limb passes superficial to the tendons of extensor hallucis longus, and tibialis anterior, dorsalis pedis artery (continuation of anterior tibial artery) and deep fibular (deep peroneal) nerve.

Function

Like the superior extensor retinaculum above the ankle, the inferior extensor retinaculum binds the tendons of anterior compartment of leg in front of the ankle. During contraction of these muscles, the inferior extensor retinaculum prevents bowstringing of their tendons in front of ankle joint.

SN 16.4 Write a short note on extensor digitorum brevis muscle.

EXTENSOR DIGITORUM BREVIS

Extensor digitorum brevis is a thin muscle lying on the dorsum of foot. It is a thin muscle which arises from the distal part of the superolateral surface of the calcaneus, the talocalcaneal ligament and the deep surface of the inferior extensor retinaculum. The muscle inclines distally and medially over the dorsum of foot and ends in four tendinous slips.

The medial part of the muscle usually presents a distinct slip. It ends in a tendon that crosses the dorsalis pedis artery superficially and is inserted into the dorsal aspect of the base of proximal phalanx of the hallux. This is independently called **extensor hallucis brevis**. The other three tendon slips are attached to the lateral sides of the tendons of extensor digitorum longus for the second, third and fourth toes.

Variations

- Extensor digitorum brevis **may have accessory slips of origin from the talus and navicular.**
- It may have an **extra tendinous slip for the fifth digit.**
- One or more tendinous **slip of the muscle may be absent**.
- It may be **connected to the any of the adjacent dorsal interosseous muscles**.

Nerve Supply

Lateral terminal branch of the deep fibular (deep peroneal) nerve.

Actions

- Extensor digitorum brevis helps in extending the phalanges of the middle three toes via the respective tendons of extensor digitorum longus.
- In the hallux, it helps in extension of metatarsophalangeal joint.

Clinical Anatomy

- The tendon of extensor hallucis brevis can be used as a local graft.
- Extensor hallucis brevis muscle and tendon can serve as guide for location of the dorsalis pedis artery and the deep fibular (deep peroneal) nerve.

LA 16.5 Discuss briefly the deep fibular (peroneal) nerve.

DEEP FIBULAR (DEEP PERONEAL) NERVE

Introduction

Deep peroneal nerve is also called deep fibular nerve. It is the nerve for innervation of the muscles of anterior compartment of the leg. In addition, its terminal part carries mixed fibers for motor supply to the extensor digitorum brevis and sensory supply to small area of skin of dorsum of foot.

Origin

Deep fibular (deep peroneal) nerve begins at the bifurcation of the common fibular (common peroneal) nerve between the neck of fibula and the proximal part of fibularis (peroneus) longus muscle.

Course and Important Relations (see Fig. 16.7)

At the site of its origin, the nerve is situated in the upper end of lateral compartment of leg. Piercing the anterior crural intramuscular septum, the deep fibular nerve passes obliquely beneath the extensor digitorum longus to reach anterior to the interosseous membrane. At the junction of upper and middle thirds of the leg the nerve comes adjacent to the lateral aspect of the anterior tibial artery. It then runs vertically downwards adjacent to the artery up to ankle, where it bifurcates into lateral and medial terminal branches.

While the deep fibular nerve descends, it is initially lateral to the anterior tibial artery, then anterior and ultimately lateral to it.

Branches

In the Leg

Muscular: To tibialis anterior, extensor hallucis longus, extensor digitorum longus and fibularis (peroneus) tertius.

Sensory (articular): To ankle joint.

In the Dorsum of Foot (Terminal Branches)

Lateral terminal branch passes under the extensor digitorum brevis in front of ankle and gets swollen to form a **pseudoganglion**. It supplies *muscular branch* to extensor digitorum brevis. From the pseudoganglion, *three articular branches* go to supply tarsal and metatarsophalangeal joints of middle three digits.

Medial terminal branch runs distally over the dorsum of foot on the lateral side of the dorsalis pedis artery and gives an *articular branch* to supply first metatarsophalangeal joint. Finally the nerve subdivides into *two dorsal digital branches* for adjacent sites of great toe and second toe.

Variation

The deep fibular nerve may divide into three terminal branches.

LA 16.6 Discuss briefly the anterior tibial artery.

ANTERIOR TIBIAL ARTERY (FIG. 16.7)

Introduction

Anterior tibial artery is the smaller terminal branch of the popliteal artery.

Origin

It arises in the popliteal fossa at the lower border of popliteus where the popliteal artery bifurcates into anterior and posterior tibial arteries.

Course and Important Relations

- **Short course in the posterior compartment:** It passes between two heads of origin of tibialis posterior.
- **Entry in the anterior compartment:** Anterior tibial artery enters the anterior compartment of leg coming forwards through the oval gap at the upper end of interosseous membrane.

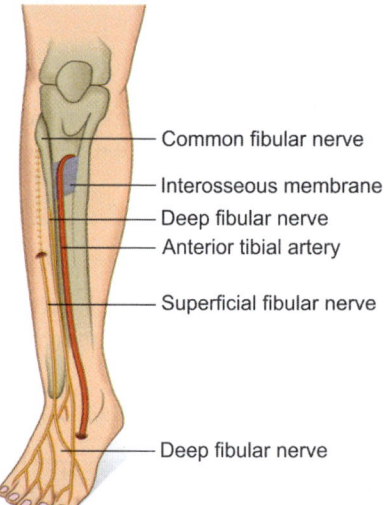

Fig. 16.7: Anterior tibial artery and deep fibular nerve.

Course in Anterior Compartment

Entering the anterior compartment of leg, in upper two-thirds, it runs in front of the interosseous membrane. First it lies between tibialis anterior and extensor digitorum longus, then between tibialis anterior and extensor hallucis longus. In lower third of front of leg, anterior tibial artery crosses over the tibia up to the midmalleolar point. The deep fibular (deep peroneal) nerve, lying lateral to the artery, comes in its front in the middle third and finally descends along the lateral side of the artery.

Termination

When crossing in front of the ankle, the anterior tibial artery is continued on the dorsum of the foot as **dorsalis pedis artery** in the midpoint between medial and lateral malleoli.

Branches

The named branches of the anterior tibial artery are the following:
- **Posterior tibial recurrent artery** is an inconstant branch and it arises before the anterior tibial artery reaches the extensor compartment.
- **Anterior tibial recurrent artery** passes through the tibialis anterior muscle. Both the tibial recurrent arteries take part in the anastomosis around the knee joint.
- **Muscular branches** are multiple which supply the muscles of anterior compartment of leg. Some of these branches pierce deep fascia to supply the skin and some pierce interosseous membrane to go to the back of the leg.
- **Perforating branches** are named as the *fasciocutaneous branches* which pierce the deep fascia to supply the skin.
- **Anterior medial malleolar artery** arises 5 cm above the level of ankle and proceeds medially deep to the tendons of extensor hallucis longus and tibialis anterior. It anastomoses with *posterior tibial and medial plantar arteries* to form the *medial malleolar network*.
- **Anterior lateral malleolar artery** runs behind the tendons of extensor digitorum longus and fibularis (peroneus) tertius. On the lateral side of the ankle the artery anastomoses with perforating branch of *peroneal (fibular) artery* and ascending branch of *lateral tarsal artery* to form the *lateral malleolar network*.

Variations

- Anterior tibial artery may be small in size.
- On rare occasion, it is found to be absent. During that case, it is replaced by the perforating branch of posterior tibial artery or the perforating branch of the peroneal (fibular) artery.
- It may be larger in size than the normal, when its continuation in the foot also gives branches to the plantar aspect.

> **LA 16.7** Discuss briefly the muscles of lateral (peroneal) compartment of leg.
>
> *Individual muscle may be asked in the form of short notes*

MUSCLES OF LATERAL (PERONEAL) COMPARTMENT

Fibularis Longus (Fig. 16.8)

Fibularis longus (peroneus longus) is the *more superficial* of the two muscles of the lateral compartment of leg.

Origin
- Head and proximal or upper two-thirds of lateral surface of the fibula.
- Deep surface of the deep fascia of leg (fascia cruris).
- **Rarely**, a few fibers from the **lateral condyle of the tibia**.

Course and Important Relations of the Muscle Tendon

The muscle belly ends in a *long tendon* which runs distally *behind the lateral malleolus* in a groove sharing with the tendon of fibularis brevis which lies in front of the longus tendon with direct contact with the bone.

The groove is converted into a tunnel by a fascial band, the **superior fibular retinaculum**. Here both the tendons are contained in a **common synovial sheath**.

Beyond this level, the tendon of fibularis longus runs obliquely forwards *on the lateral side of the calcaneus* **below the fibular (peroneal) trochlea** and **deep to the inferior fibular retinaculum**. Then it crosses obliquely **over the groove on the plantar aspect of the cuboid bone**. This groove is converted into a tunnel by the long plantar ligament. The tendon crosses obliquely across the sole of foot to approach the site of insertion.

Insertion

At the medial side of the sole of foot the tendon divides into two slips to be inserted into:
- Lateral side of the base of first metatarsal bone
- Lateral aspect of the medial cuneiform
- **Occasionally**, a third slip is inserted into the **base of second metatarsal bone**.

Nerve Supply

Superficial fibular (peroneal) nerve (L_5, S_1).

Actions

- Fibularis longus **causes eversion of foot**
- It is **plantar flexor** of the ankle
- For oblique direction of the tendon across the sole of foot, fibularis longus **supports the longitudinal and transverse arches** of the foot.

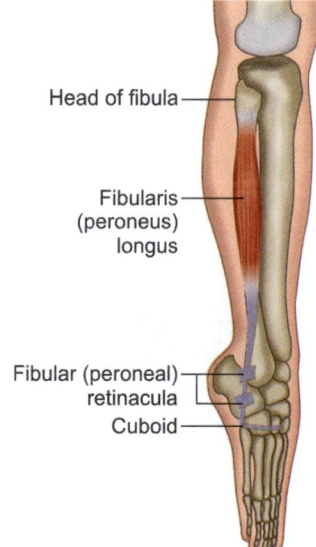

Fig. 16.8: Fibularis (peroneus) longus muscle.

Fibularis Brevis (Fig. 16.9)

Origin

Fibularis brevis (peroneus brevis) arises from:
- Distal two-thirds of the lateral surface of fibula. In the common middle third of the fibula, its origin is anterior to that of fibularis longus.
- Anterior and posterior crural intermuscular septa.

The narrow muscle belly extends vertically downwards and ends in a tendon which passes in relation to the groove on the back of lateral malleolus lying in front of the tendon of fibularis longus.

The two tendons pass deep to the superior fibular (peroneal) retinaculum within a common synovial sheath.

The tendon of fibularis brevis then passes forwards on the lateral aspect of calcaneus superior to the fibular (peroneal) trochlea.

Insertion

To a tubercle on the lateral side of base of fifth metatarsal bone.

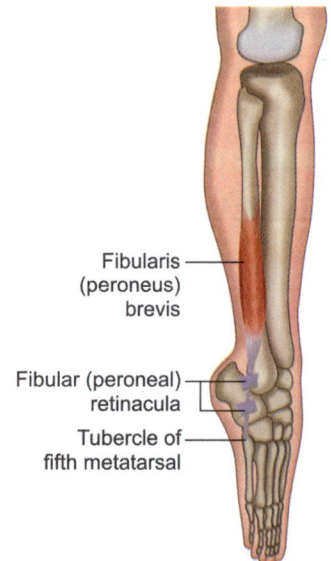

Fig. 16.9: Fibularis (peroneus) brevis.

Nerve Supply
Superficial fibular (peroneal) nerve (L_5, S_1).

Actions
- Fibularis brevis exerts a control over the inversion of foot and thereby it relieves the strain on the ligaments which are tightened by this movement.
- It takes part in eversion of foot.
- It helps to keep the leg steady on the foot in erect posture.

SA 16.8 Write a short note on fibular (peroneal) retinacula.

FIBULAR (PERONEAL) RETINACULA (FIG. 16.10)

Fibular retinacula are two thick bands of deep fascia on the lateral aspect of the ankle. They hold the tendons of fibularis longus and fibularis brevis in position. The retinacula also act as pulley around which the tendons can roll at the sites of their bend on the lateral aspect of foot.

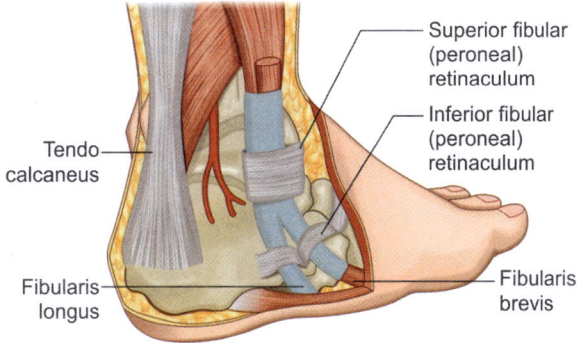

Fig. 16.10: Fibular (peroneal) retinacula.

Superior Fibular (Peroneal) Retinaculum (Fig. 16.10)

It is a condensed band of deep fascia which bridges across the groove on the back of lateral malleolus. It passes from the *back of the lateral malleolus* to the *lateral surface of calcaneus*.

The tendons of fibularis longus and fibularis brevis cross beneath the retinaculum within a common synovial sheath.

Inferior Fibular (Peroneal) Retinaculum (Fig. 16.10)

It is a band of deep fascia attached to the *fibular (peroneal) trochlea* of calcaneus, from which is forms an upper and a lower loop. The upper loop that wraps over the tendon of fibularis brevis is *attached to the superior surface of calcaneus,* where it blends with the common stem of inferior extensor retinaculum. The lower loop covers the tendon of fibularis longus and is attached to the lateral *surface of calcaneus.*

Synovial Sheath

Two tendons are enclosed by a common synovial sheath. It starts from below the level of lateral malleolus as a common sheath for both the tendons up to the fibular trochlea. From this level the sheath splits into two for two tendons which continue independently up to their insertion.

SA 16.9 Discuss briefly the superficial fibular (peroneal) nerve.

SUPERFICIAL FIBULAR (PERONEAL) NERVE

Introduction

Superficial fibular nerve (superficial peroneal nerve) was *previously named musculocutaneous nerve*. It is the nerve of the lateral compartment of leg.

Origin

Superficial fibular nerve begins as bifurcation of the common fibular nerve just beyond the neck of fibula deep to fibularis longus.

Course and Important Relations

Arising close to the neck of fibula, the nerve descends downwards and forwards first between fibularis longus and fibularis brevis, then between fibularis brevis and extensor digitorum longus. It perforates the deep fascia at the junction of middle and lower thirds of the leg and bifurcates into longer medial and shorter lateral terminal branches which reach the dorsum of foot.

Branches

Muscular Branches

To supply fibularis longus and fibularis brevis.

Cutaneous Branches

- **Crural cutaneous (sensory) branches** supply the skin of *lower one-third* of the lateral aspect of the leg.
- **Medial terminal branch** crosses over the ankle and subdivides into two dorsal digital nerves. One supplies *the medial side of the great toe* and other supplies the cutaneous branch to *the second interdigital cleft*.
- **Lateral terminal branch** also bifurcates into two dorsal digital divisions for the skin of the *third and fourth interdigital clefts*.
    Both the terminal branches, while dividing into dorsal digital branches, give cutaneous branches for the skin of adjoining part of the dorsum of foot.

Clinical Anatomy

- **Lesion of superficial fibular nerve** gives rise to following motor and sensory deficits.
    - **Motor loss**: Loss of eversion of foot due to paralysis of fibularis (peroneus) longus and brevis
    - **Sensory loss**: Loss of cutaneous sensation on the lower part of lateral aspect of leg and the dorsum of foot except.
        ◊ Skin of first interdigital cleft—supplied by *deep fibular* nerve
        ◊ Skin of lateral margin of foot and little toe—supplied by *sural nerve*.
- **Compression of superficial fibular nerve**
    There may be entrapment of the nerve at the site where it pierces the deep fascia, it will cause paresthesia of the lower part of the leg and dorsum of foot.

Chapter 17

Back of the Leg and Sole of the Foot

SN 17.1 Write a short note on flexor retinaculum of ankle.

FLEXOR RETINACULUM OF ANKLE (FIG. 17.1)

Introduction

Flexor retinaculum of ankle is an one inch broad condensed part of the deep fascia which bridges over the flexor tendons and the neurovascular bundle on the medial aspect of the ankle as they pass from the back of the leg to the sole of foot.

Attachments

- **Anterosuperior:** Posterior border and tip of medial malleolus.
- **Posteroinferior:** Medial process of the calcaneal tuberosity.
- **Structures passing beneath the retinaculum** (*From anteromedial to posterolateral*)
    - Tendon of tibialis posterior
    - Tendon of flexor digitorum longus
    - Posterior tibial artery with accompanying veins
    - Tibial nerve
    - Tendon of flexor hallucis longus.
- **Structures piercing the retinaculum**
    - *Median calcaneal artery*—branch of posterior tibial artery
    - *Median calcaneal nerve*—branch of tibial nerve.

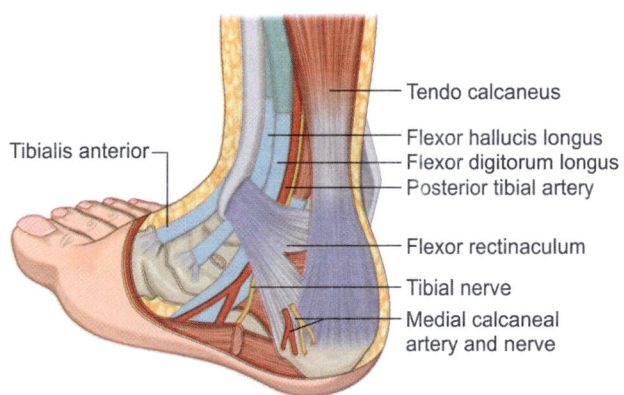

Fig. 17.1: Flexon retinaculum of ankle.

Clinical Anatomy

Osseofibrous tunnel between the back of medial malleolus and the flexor retinaculum is crowded by the flexor tendons and neurovascular bundle. Clinical condition due to compression of the tibial nerve in the tunnel is known as **tarsal tunnel syndrome**. It is characterized by pain in the sole of foot with burning and tingling sensations.

SA 17.2 Write a brief note on the soleus muscle.

SOLEUS MUSCLE (FIG. 17.2)

The muscle arises from:
- The upper one fourth of the back of the fibula extending above up to its head.
- The fibrous arch connecting the lower end of fibular attachment to the upper end of the soleal line.
- The soleal line of the tibia.
- The middle third of the posterior border of the shaft of tibia.

The muscle has dense aponeurotic lamellae on both anterior and posterior surfaces and the muscle fibers slope downwards from the anterior to the posterior lamella. The superficial (posterior) lamella is continued at its lower end into the tendo calcaneus.

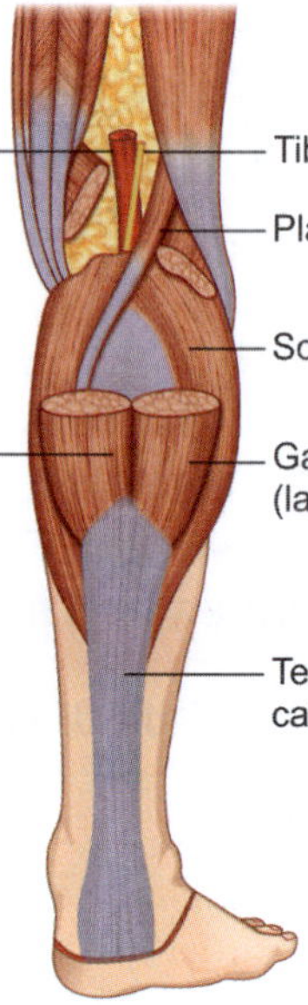

Fig. 17.2: Structures of the back of leg showing soleus muscle.

Soleal Venous Plexus

The soleus muscle contains rich plexus of veins (venous sinuses). The plexus communicates with the deep veins in one side and in another side with the superficial veins through the perforating veins. Soleus is considered as **peripheral heart** because it pumps out the venous blood from the venous plexus through its contraction, thus facilitates venous return.

Stagnation of blood in these veins may lead to the **deep venous thrombosis** that may result in serious complication like pulmonary embolism.

Nerve Supply

The soleus muscle is supplied by two branches of the tibial nerve. One branch originates in the popliteal fossa. Another one supplies from the deep surface in the calf.

Actions

Soleus and gastrocnemius are the **chief plantar flexors** of the foot.

The multipennate soleus is also **a powerful antigravity muscle**. In erect posture, it contracts alternatively with the extensor muscles of the leg to **maintain the balance**. It is a **very strong but slow plantar flexor of the ankle**, due to the obliquity of its multipennate fibers.

For fast walking, running and jumping, rapid contraction of the bellies of gastrocnemius is important. **Slow contraction of soleus** is responsible **for strolling** or quick walking.

SA 17.3 Discuss briefly the Posterior tibial artery.

POSTERIOR TIBIAL ARTERY (FIG. 17.3)

Introduction

Posterior tibial artery is the main artery of the posterior compartment of leg. Its distribution is supplemented by the peroneal (fibular) artery.

Origin

Posterior tibial artery arises at the lower border of popliteus. Here the popliteal artery bifurcates into the anterior and posterior tibial arteries.

Termination

After passing underneath the flexor retinaculum, posterior tibial artery bifurcates deep to the abductor hallucis into **medial** and **lateral plantar arteries**.

Course and Important Relations

From the level of origin, the posterior tibial artery passes deep to the fibrous arch that gives origin to the soleus. Then it runs successively on the tibialis posterior, flexor digitorum longus, tibia and behind the ankle joint. In proximal part, it is covered by gastrocnemius, soleus and deep transverse fascia of leg. But in distal part, the artery lies deep to skin and fascia only. The artery is accompanied by two veins and tibial nerve. The nerve is first medial to the artery but soon it crosses over to become posterolateral in position.

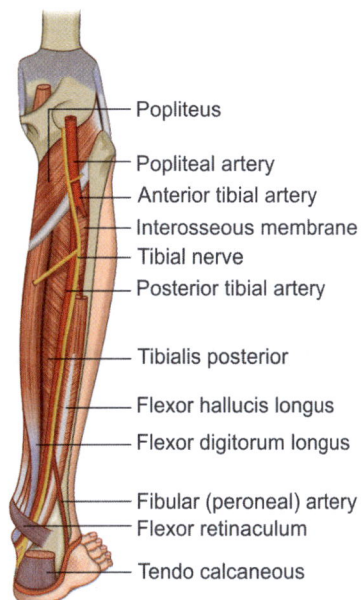

Fig. 17.3: Deep structures of the back of leg (with posterior tibial artery).

Branches

Circumflex fibular artery passes laterally winding round the neck of fibula through the soleus to take part in the anastomosis on the inferior and lateral aspect of the knee joint. It supplies bone and joints of the vicinity.

Nutrient artery of the tibia is one of the largest of the nutrient arteries. After sending a few muscular branches it descends into the bone.

Muscular braches of posterior tibial artery are distributed to the soleus and all the deep flexors of the leg.

Perforating branches are about five fasciocutaneous arteries which come out between flexor digitorum longus and soleus. These arteries run along with the perforating veins. They supply skin, fascia as well as the periosteum.

Communicating branch joins with the communicating branch of fibular (peroneal) artery.

Medial malleolar branch takes part in the medial malleolar network.

Calcaneal branches arise from the posterior tibial artery just before it divides into terminal division. These arteries perforate the flexor retinaculum and supply skin and fascia above the heel and also the muscles on the medial side of the sole of foot.

Medial and lateral plantar arteries arise as bifurcation of the posterior tibial artery under the or just beyond the flexor retinaculum. They are described in the section of the sole of foot (Q 17.6).

Fibular (peroneal) artery: It originates from the posterior tibial artery 2.5 cm distal to the popliteus. Sometimes, the fibular artery is found to arise as the third terminal branch of the popliteal artery along with the origin of the anterior and posterior tibial arteries. Fibular artery descends vertically in a fibrous canal between flexor hallucis longus and tibialis posterior. While descending, it gives **muscular branches**. Some of these muscular branches supply the **calf muscles** and other pierce posterior crural intermuscular septum to supply **fibularis longus and brevis** lying in the lateral compartment of the leg. **Nutrient branch** supplies the fibula. The fibular artery terminates by subdividing into perforating branch and lateral calcaneal branch. **Perforating branch pierces** the interosseous membrane to appear at the anterior compartment of leg. **Lateral calcaneal branch** forms anastomosis with the lateral malleolar and calcaneal branches of posterior tibial artery. *Perforating branch occasionally replaces the dorsalis pedis artery.*

SA 17.4 Write a brief note on the muscles of the second layer of sole of foot.

SECOND LAYER (FIG. 17.4)

This layer presents long flexor tendons and related small muscles of sole of foot.

Tendon of Flexor Hallucis Longus

Disposition of this tendon in the sole is like a bowstring beneath the medial longitudinal arch of the foot. It is crossed inferiorly by the tendon of flexor digitorum longus. While being crossed, it gives two slips for the medial two divisions of tendon of flexor digitorum longus. It passes through the groove between two sesamoid bones beneath the head of first metatarsal bone. Then crossing over the plantar aspect of the proximal phalanx, it is inserted into the base of distal phalanx of the great toe. Throughout the whole course in the sole of foot the tendon of flexor hallucis longus is enclosed by a synovial sheath.

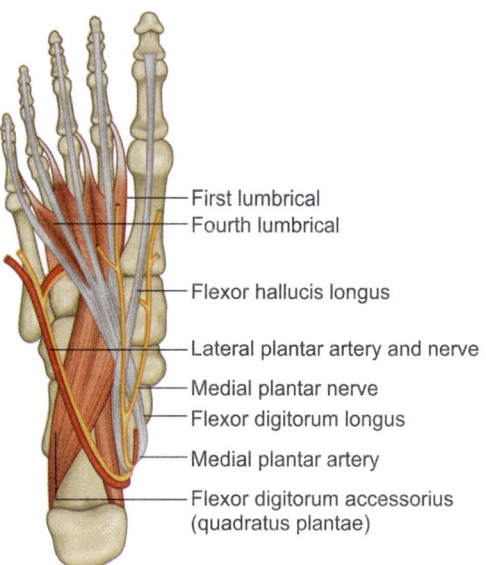

Fig. 17.4: Muscles of second layer of sole of right foot with plantar arteries and nerves.

Tendon of Flexor Digitorum Longus

When the tendon of flexor digitorum longus enters the sole, it lies medial to the tendon of flexor hallucis longus. At the point of division into four slips for lateral four toes, it crosses over the hallucis tendon. The four tendons pass distally in the sole deep to the tendon slips of flexor digitorum brevis. At the site of division into four tendon slips, flexor digitorum longus receives the attachment of *flexor digitorum accessorius (quadratus plantae)* from behind. After giving origin of lumbricals, the tendon slips pass through the fibrous flexor sheaths of the lateral four toes. Each of the tendon is embrassed by the bifurcated tendon slips of flexor digitorum brevis and is inserted into the base of distal phalanx.

Flexor Digitorum Accessorius (Quadratus Plantae)

It is a flat quadrangular muscle which takes origin by two heads. The **large medial head** originates from the medial surface of the calcaneus and the **small lateral head** takes origin from the lateral margin of plantar surface of the calcaneus. The muscular belly formed by union of the two heads is straight in direction and gets inserted into the posterior aspect of obliquely directed tendon of flexor digitorum longus at the site of its division into tendinous slips.

Nerve Supply
The trunk of lateral plantar nerve.

Action
- It helps flexor digitorum longus for flexion of the lateral four toes in any position of the ankle joint.
- It changes oblique pull of flexor digitorum longus into the straight line pull.

Lumbrical Muscles

Lumbrical muscles are four in number and they are numbered serially from medial to lateral side. Lumbricals arise from the four tendinous slips of flexor digitorum longus. First lumbrical is unipennate in origin and takes origin from the medial side of the first tendon slip which goes to the second toe. Other three lumbricals are bipennate in origin which arise from adjacent sides of the four tendons. The muscles end in slender tendons which pass distally on the medial side of metatarsophalangeal joint of the lateral four toes. The tendons pass dorsally to be inserted into the extensor expansions.

Nerve Supply
First lumbrical muscle receives nerve supply from the medial plantar nerve. Lateral three lumbricals are supplied by the lateral plantar nerve.

In palm of the hand, lateral two lumbricals (first and second), being unipennate in origin, are supplied by median nerve. Medial two (third and fourth) having bipennate origin, are supplied by ulnar nerve.

Action
Lumbricals cause extension of the toes at the interphalangeal joints when the flexor digitorum longus tendons flex the toes. So the toes are not buckled or folded below during walking and running.

SA 17.5 Discuss briefly the interosseous muscles of sole of foot.

INTEROSSEOUS MUSCLES

General Plan

Same as palmar and dorsal interossei of the hand, the plantar interossei are adductor and the dorsal interossei are abductors of the toes. In case of hand, it was found that palmar interossei deviate the fingers towards the axis passing through the long axis of the metacarpal and phalanges of the middle finger. Dorsal inerossei, for abduction, deviate the fingers away from the axis. It is important to note that, the axis in case of foot is shifted medially to pass through the long axis of the metatarsal and phalanges of the second toe. As in the hand, the plantar interossei arise from the metatarsal of its own toe through unipennate origin. Bipennate dorsal interossei arise from adjacent metatarsals.

Plantar Interossei (Fig. 17.5)

They are **three in number**. As the great toe has its own adductor, the adductor hallucis, and through the second toe passes the axis, three plantar interossei arises from the plantar aspect of shaft of third, fourth and fifth metatarsal bones. They are inserted by tendons into the medial sides of third, fourth and fifth digits. The three tendons pass dorsal to the deep transverse metatarsal ligament and are inserted into the medial side of the bases of proximal phalanges and into dorsal digital expansion of lateral three toes.

Dorsal Interossei (Fig. 17.6)

Dorsal interossei are four abducting muscles. They deviate the toes away from the axis passing through the second toe. The great toe and the little toe have their abductors. The second toe requires abducting muscles on both sides. The third and fourth toes require one for each, to abduct them laterally away from the axis passing through the second toe. Each arises from the adjacent metatarsals of respective intermetatarsal space. *First dorsal interosseous* is inserted on the *medial side of the second toe*. Second, third and fourth interossei are inserted into the lateral aspect of the second, third and fourth toes. The tendons are inserted mainly into the bases of proximal phalanx and give an extension slip to the respective dorsal digital expansion.

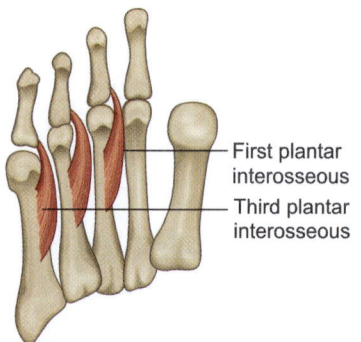

Fig. 17.5: Plantar interossei of right foot.

Nerve Supply

All interossei are supplied by the lateral plantar nerve. Interossei of the fourth space (third plantar and fourth dorsal) are supplied by the superficial branch whereas the others are supplied by the deep branch of the nerve.

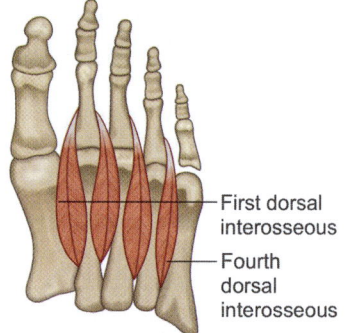

Fig. 17.6: Dorsal interossei of right foot (dorsal view).

Action

Action of the interossei as adductor and abductor is of little significance in case of human foot. Their actions as extensor of interphalangeal joints through extensor expansion and flexor of metatarsophalangeal joint by their attachment in proximal phalanx are important for propagation.

LA 17.6 Discuss briefly the blood vessels and nerves of sole of foot.

BLOOD VESSELS AND NERVES OF SOLE OF FOOT

Blood vessels and nerves of the sole of foot are derived from the posterior tibial neurovascular bundle in the back of the leg. Posterior tibial artery and tibial nerve divide into medial and lateral plantar arteries and nerves deep to the flexor retinaculum. The arteries are more marginal than the nerves on the medial and lateral borders of the foot. Each of the arteries is accompanied by a pair of venae comitantes. **The plantar arteries and nerves lie between the first and the second layer of sole of foot,** below the long flexor tendons.

Medial plantar artery is smaller than the lateral and it does not take part in the formation of the plantar arch. In contrast to the superficial and deep palmar arch in the hand, foot presents one plantar arch formed by the lateral plantar artery. Digital distribution from the medial plantar artery is confined almost to the great toe.

Medial plantar nerve (Fig. 17.4) is initially flanked by the *abductor hallucis* and the *flexor digitorum brevis*, to whom it gives branches. It gives also the branches to the *flexor hallucis brevis* and *first* *lumbrical*. After giving muscular branches, medial plantar nerve divides into digital cutaneous branches which supply skin of medial part of sole and medial three and a half toes. Digital branches are usually four in number to supply medial side of great toe and medial three interdigital clefts.

Lateral plantar artery (Fig. 17.4) passes across the sole obliquely from medial to lateral side between the first and second layers of muscles. Reaching the base of fifth metatarsal, it gives off a branch which accompanies the superficial branch of lateral plantar nerve. But the main artery accompanies the deep branch of the lateral plantar nerve to form the plantar arch.

Plantar arch is the distal curved part of the lateral plantar artery after it gives of the superficial branch. The arch presents the distal convexity and it passes from lateral side across the bases of the fourth, third and second metatarsals successively. Reaching the proximal part of first intermetatarsal space, it is joined by the dorsalis pedis artery reaching sole from the dorsum of foot. Branches from the convex side of the arch are the **plantar metatarsal arteries** which run distally and bifurcate to supply four webs and also the toes. **Perforating branches** arise from the plantar arch as well as its metatarsal branches. They pass dorsally through the intermetatarsal spaces and reinforce the dorsal metatarsal arteries.

Veins of the sole of foot are of two types. Plantar arteries are accompanied by the pair of **venae comitantes**. They converge to the vein accompanying the posterior tibial artery. Another group of veins are **perforating veins**. The perforating veins take most of the blood from the sole, passing through the intermetatarsal space, to the dorsal venous arch. The muscles of the sole of foot act as **'sole pump'** which compress the perforating as well as plantar veins. This helps the *'soleal pump'* for venous drainage in the posterior compartment of leg.

Lateral plantar nerve (Fig. 17.4) presents similarity in course and distribution with the ulnar nerve in the hand. The nerve crosses the sole obliquely form medial to lateral side. It gives branches to *flexor digitorum accessorius (quadratus plantae)* and *abductor digiti minimi*. It sends *cutaneous branches* which pierce the plantar aponeurosis to supply the skin of the lateral side of the sole of foot. Reaching the base of fifth metatarsal bone it subdivides into superficial and deep branches. **The superficial branch** gives medial and lateral divisions. The medial division supplies the skin of the fourth interdigital cleft and communicate with the lateralmost digital branch of the medial plantar nerve. The lateral division innervates the skin of the lateral side of the little toe. These digital nerves also supply the nail beds and adjacent area of the dorsum of the lateral one and a half toes through their short dorsal branches. Unlike the superficial branch of the unlar nerve, the superficial branch of the lateral plantar nerve gives branches to three muscles. These are the *flexor digiti minimi brevis* and the *two interossei of the fourth space* (third plantar and fourth dorsal). **The deep branch** runs from lateral to medial side within the concavity of the plantar arch and ends by passing deep to the oblique head of adductor hallucis. It gives branches to the *remaining interossei* (medial two plantar and medial three dorsal), *adductor hallucis* and *lateral three lumbricals*.

Chapter 18

Joints of Lower Limb

LA 18.1 Describe the hip joint. Add a note on its clinical anatomy.

Short notes/Short answer: Ligaments of hip joint; Bursae around the joint; Movements of the joint; Factors maintaining stability of the joint.

HIP JOINT

Introduction

Hip joint is the **multiaxial ball and socket** variety of **synovial joint** between the deep cup shaped acetabular cavity of hip bone and spherical head of femur.

Configuration of the joint maintains the **stability** for support and transmission of body weight during standing as well as propagation. Parallely, it allows **mobility** in all the axes like the shoulder joint.

In all the joints, the stability is inversely proportional to the mobility. But the hip joint is the exception to provide the high degree of *stability* due to **full congruence of the articular surfaces** and free *mobility* due to presence of **long neck and its angulation with the shaft**.

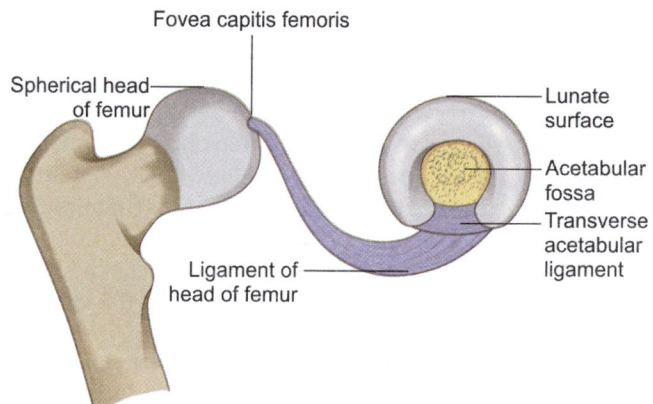

Fig. 18.1: Articular surfaces of hip joint.

Articular Surfaces (Fig. 18.1)

Acetabulum

The cup-shaped acetabulum is formed by fusion of three components of hip bone, ilium, ischium and pubis. The articular surface, covered by hyaline cartilage, does not cover the whole area of the cavity. But it is 'C' shaped with the deficiency inferiorly. This is called **lunate surface.** Central part is deeper and nonarticular. It is called **acetabular fossa** covered by acetabular pad of fat. The interval between the ends of the lunate surface is known as **acetabular notch** which is bridged by the **transverse acetabular ligament**.

Acetabular Labrum

The outline of the acetabular cavity, except the area of acetabular notch gives attachment to a rim of fibrocartilage, called acetabular labrum. The labrum has two kinds of functions for stability of the joint.
1. It deepens the acetabular cavity.
2. It fits as a tight collar around the beginning of neck just beyond the margin of the head.

Head of Femur

It is almost a complete sphere. It is smooth as covered by hyaline cartilage. The center of the head presents a small excavation (depression) called **fovea capitis femoris** which is nonarticular to give attachment to the narrower end of **the ligament of the head of femur**.

Fibrous Capsule (Fig. 18.2)

Proximal Attachment

The capsule is attached proximally to the line of *acetabular labrum* and to the *transverse acetabular ligament*.

Distal Attachment

It is the femoral attachment.
- **Anteriorly,** it is attached to the *intertrochanteric line* beyond the neck of femur and takes the reverse course to extend towards the head wrapping over the anterior surface of the neck. These are known as **retinacular fibers** which carry the blood vessels for the head.
- **Posteriorly,** the fibers of the capsule extends **1cm proximal to the intertrochanteric crest**, where the fibers, instead of being attached, fit as a tight collar over the neck. Posteriorly, deeper predominating circular fibers are known as **zona orbicularis**.

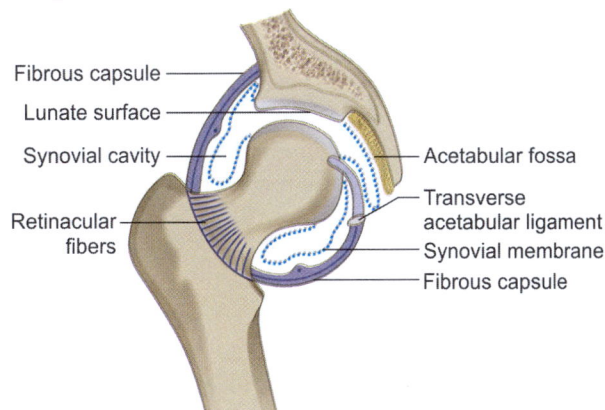

Fig. 18.2: Hip joint in coronal plane to show fibrous capsule and synovial membrane.

Synovial membrane (Fig. 18.2) follows the usual rule for lining and attachment which are as follows:
- It covers the inner surface of capsule
- It gets attached to the margins of both articular surfaces
- It does not cover the articular surfaces anywhere
- It lines the acetabular fossa
- Ligament of head of femur lies outside the synovial cavity.

Ligaments of Hip Joint

These are the following which reinforce the fibrous capsule both in front and behind.

Iliofemoral Ligament (Fig. 18.3)

Iliofemoral ligament is the strongest ligament of the body and is triangular in shape with the apical end directed proximally.

Proximally, the stem of the ligament is attached to:
- Lower part of *anterior inferior iliac spine*
- Adjacent part of *acetabular rim.*

Distally, the base of the ligament is attached to the *intertrochanteric line.* It is inverted 'V' shaped. Sometimes it is referred to be inverted 'Y' shaped. It is composed of *lateral and medial thick bands* and *intermediate thinner part.*

Functions

Iliofemoral ligament *prevents hyperextension* of the hip joint, thereby it *prevents the trunk to lean backwards* in erect posture.

Pubofemoral Ligament (Fig. 18.3)

Pubofemoral ligament is also a triangular ligament but its base is proximal.
Proximally, it is attached to:
- Superior ramus of pubis
- Obturator crest.

The fibers of the ligament are directed inferiorly. **Distally,** the ligament fuses with the fibrous capsule and the medial limb of iliofemoral ligament.

Function

Pubofermoral ligament prevents over abduction of the hip joint.

Ischiofemoral Ligament (Fig. 18.4)

Ischiofemoral ligament reinforces the capsule of the joint posteriorly. **Proximally,** it is attached to the posterior or ischial part of acetabular margin. The fibers spiral in superolateral direction over the back of the neck of femur and it is attached **distally** to the medial aspect of base of greater trochanter of femur.

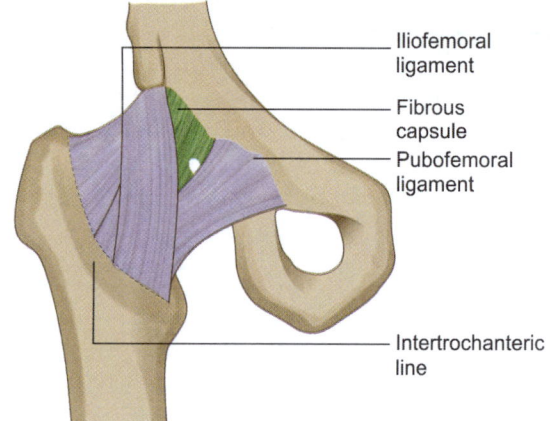

Fig. 18.3: Iliofemoral and pubofemoral ligament.

Function

Ischiofemoral ligament tends to screw the femoral head in medial direction into the acetabulum, *preventing hyperextension of the hip joint.*

Transverse Acetabular Ligament (Fig. 18.1)

It is a fibrous band which bridges across the acetabular notch. The ligament is continuous with the acetabular labrum, the rim of fibrocartilage. But the ligament is made up of collagen fibers only and is devoid of cartilage cells. Acetabular artery and the nerve pass deep to the ligament to the hip joint.

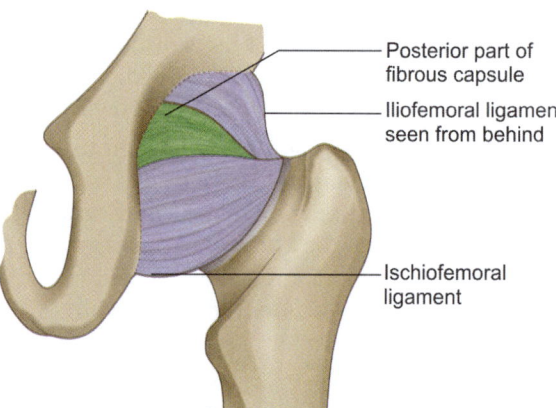

Fig. 18.4: Ischiofemoral ligament of hip joint.

The Ligament of Head of the Femur

It is also called *ligamentum teres femoris* or *round ligament of head of femur*. Its wider end is fixed to the transverse acetabular ligament and the narrower end is attached to the fovea of the head of femur. Usually this intracapsular ligament carries small arteries to the central part of head of femur. These arteries are the branches arising from medial circumflex femoral and obturator arteries.

Morphology

The ligament of head of femur represents the part of the fibrous capsule which has been incorporated within the joint.

Function

This ligament is comparatively week and has little importance to strengthen the hip joint. However, the ligament is stretched in adduction of the joint.

Factors Maintaining the Stability of the Joint

- **Congruence of the articular surfaces**: Cup-shaped acetabular cavity is well adapted with the spherical head of femur.
- **Acetabular labrum** deepens the cavity of acetabulum. The labrum and zona orbicularis of the capsule fit as collar beyond the head.
- **Three strong ligaments** strengthen the capsule
- **Short muscles** all around the joint give additional stability.

Relations of the Joint

Hip joint is surrounded by many structure all around the joint.

Basically, structures of femoral region lie anteriorly. Structures of adductor region and gluteal region are inferior and posterosuperior to the joint respectively. Detail relations are as follows.

Anteriorly

- *Iliopsoas tendon* separated by a *bursa* formed by protrusion of synovial membrane through capsule.
- *Femoral nerve* in the iliopsoas groove
- *Femoral vessels.*

Posteriorly

- Piriformis, obturator internus with gemelli, quadratus femoris, distal end of obturator externus and straight head of rectus femoris.
- Sciatic nerve
- Superior and inferior gluteal vessels and nerves
- All these structures are overlapped by gluteus maximus.

Superiorly

- Reflected head of rectus femoris
- Gluteus medius and gluteus minimus.

Inferiorly

- Pectineus
- Obturator externus.

Bursae Around Hip Joint

Bursae around the hip joint are between the muscles and the capsule of the joint with adjacent bony prominences. Out of the seven bursae, three are related to iliopsoas, gluteus medius and gluteus minimus. Other four bursae are related to gluteus maximus.

The location of the bursae are as follows:
- Most important bursa is deep to iliopsoas tendon, called *subpsoas bursa*. In some of the cases, this bursa communicates with the synovial membrane protruding through the capsular deficiency and the gap between iliofemoral and pubofemoral ligaments.
- Bursa between *gluteus medius* and lateral aspect of *greater trochanter*.
- Bursa between *gluteus minimus* and anterior aspect of *greater trochanter*
- Bursa between gluteus maximus and *the ilium* below the posterior end of outer lip of iliac erect.
- Bursa between gluteus maximus and outer aspect of *greater trochanter*
- Bursa between gluteus maximus and *ischial tuberosity*.
- Bursa between the tendon of gluteus maximus and the *vastus lateralis*.

Arterial Supply

Sources of the arteries for the hip joint are the following:
- Medial and lateral circumflex femoral arteries
- Obturator artery
- Superior and inferior gluteal arteries.

Main blood supply of the hip joint is from the following:
- *Branches form the circumflex femoral (mainly medial) arteries* travel along the course of retinacular fibers of the capsule and run along the neck towards the head of femur. In case of fracture of neck of femur, these *retinacular vessels* may be damaged causing *avascular necrosis* of the femoral head.
- *Artery to the head of femur* is a branch of obturator (and medial circumflex femoral) artery and it accompanies the ligament of head of femur.

Nerve Supply

The nerve supplying the hip joint with their relative positions are following:
- Femoral nerve through the nerve to rectus femoris (anteriorly)
- Accessory obturator nerve, if present (anteriorly)
- Nerve to quadratus femoris (posteriorly)
- Sciatic nerve, occasionally (posteriorly)
- Superior gluteal nerve (superiorly)
- Anterior division of obturator nerve (inferiorly).

Movements

Movements of hip joint are *flexion-extension, abduction-adduction, medial-lateral rotation*, and *circumduction*. As the lower limb moves on hip joint, *movement of the trunk at the hip joint* is also important. This movement occurs, for example, when a person lift the trunk upwards from supine position to sit up.

Axis for all the groups of movement passes through the center of head of femur. Flexion-extension and abduction-adduction movements occur around the transverse and the anteroposterior axis respectively. Rotational movement occurs around vertical axis.

Range of flexion and extension of the hip joint depends upon the position of the knee joint. If the knee is flexed through relaxation of hamstrings, maximum flexion of the hip joint can take place till the thigh touches the anterior abdominal wall. However, this is also combined with the flexion of the vertebral column.

During extension of the hip joint, the iliofemoral ligament along with the capsule becomes tightened. Extension of the joint is possible only up to the range a little beyond the vertical plane of the limb.

Adduction of the hip joint is restricted by the opposite limb. Abduction is somewhat more free. Rotation of the hip joint can be carried out for approximately one-sixth of a circle when the thigh is extended. Range will be increased when it is flexed. Lateral rotation is more powerful than medial rotation of the joint.

Muscles producing the various movements are as follows:
- **Flexion:** Iliopsoas is the strongest flexor. Other flexors are sartorius, rectus femoris and pectineus.
- **Extension**: Hamstring muscles—semitendinosus, semimembranosus and biceps femoris. Gluteus maximus is inactive as extensor in standing position unless forceful extension is required. The muscle acts mostly from the flexed to the straight position, for example, when a person climbs the stairs or rises from a sitting position.
- **Abduction**: Gluteus medius, gluteus minimus and tensor fasciae latae.
- **Adduction:** Adductor longus, adductor brevis, adductor magnus, gracilis, pectineus and obturator externus
- **Medial rotation**: Anterior fibers of gluteus medius, gluteus minimus and tensor fasciae latae.
- **Lateral rotation**: Obturator externus, obturator internus with gemelli, piriformis and quadratus femoris.

Clinical Anatomy

Dislocation of Hip Joint

Congenital dislocation of the hip joint is common, occurring in approximately 1.5 per 1,000 live births. It is bilateral in 50% of cases. Congenital dislocation occurs due to following **reasons**:
- Congenital deficiency of posterosuperior margin of acetabulum, for which **posterior dislocation is more common**.
- Congenital laxity of the capsule of the joint.

The condition is characterized by following **disability** or **deformity**.
- Inability to abduct the thigh
- Shortening of the affected limb
- Lurching gait.

Acquired dislocation of the hip joint is uncommon due to strength and stability of the joint. It occurs in automobile accident when a person is riding a car. Because the knee strikes against the dashboard of the car in flexed, adducted and medially rotated position of the hip. Cause of the dislocation is the rupture of posteroinferior part of the capsule which displaces the head of the femur posteriorly. It may be associated with injury to the sciatic nerve.

Anterior dislocation of the hip joint is less common in which case head of the femur is dislocated anteroinferior to the acetabulum.

Fracture of Neck of Femur

Though the person who are in habit of **contact sports** are frequently exposed to trauma in an around the hip joint, fracture of neck of femur is **not so common** due to following reasons:

1. Persons are younger.
2. Femoral neck is strong.

Fracture of femoral neck is **common in old age groups** and the incidence is further *more common in females due to osteoporosis*.

There are varieties of femoral neck fracture, but broadly it is divided into **extracapsular** and **intracapsular types**. Intracapsular variety is more difficult to manage.

Fracture of femoral neck may cause **injury to the retinacular arteries** which disrupts the blood supply to the femoral head. It causes avascular necrosis of the head of femur.

Diseases of the Hip Joint

Parthe's disease (pseudocoxalgia) is a clinical condition in which case head of the femur shows sign of destruction with flattening of surface. Diagnosis of the disease is confirmed **through radiograph which shows increased joint space**.

Coxa vara is characterized by decrease of the neck shaft angle which may be evident in femoral neck fracture or in Parthe's disease. **Coxa valga** with increase of neck shaft angle is observed in hip dislocations.

Osteoarthritis is the disease of the old age. It is characterized by formation of *bone chips* **(osteophytes)** in and around the articular areas resulting a painful condition.

> **LA 18.2** Describe the knee joint. Add a note on its clinical anatomy.

> Short notes/Short answers: Ligaments of the joint; Semilunar cartilages; Cruciate ligaments; Bursae; Movements of the joint.

KNEE JOINT

Introduction

- Knee joint is a **synovial joint**, the **largest** in the body
- **Functionally**, the knee joint is a **modified hinge** joint primarily allowing flexion and extension movement. This hinge joint is called modified because the **hinge movement** of flexion and extension is **combined with gliding and rolling with rotation** around a vertical axis.
- **Structurally**, the knee joint is a **compound joint** which includes **two condylar joints** between the respective femoral and the tibial condyles and a **saddle joint** between the patella and the femur.
- **The lateral and medial condylar joints** between the femoral and tibial condyles are **partly subdivided by the semilunar cartilages or menisci.**
- Though the knee joint is the largest condylar joint it is **well constructed for its stability.**
- **Stabilizing factors** of the joint are:
  - **Strength and actions of the surrounding muscles** and their tendons.
  - **Both extra-articular as well as intra-articular ligaments** binding strongly the femur and tibia.

Articular Surfaces

Articular Surface of the Femur

Articular surface of the femur is divided into **anterior patellar** and **posteroinferior tibial articular areas.**

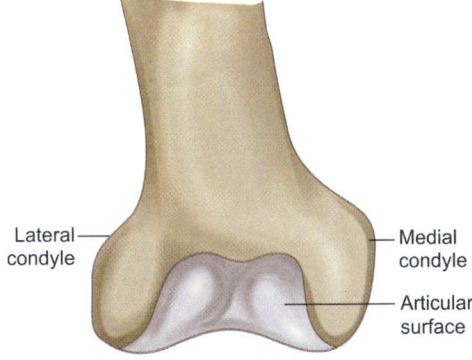

Fig. 18.5A: Patellar articular surface of femur (right).

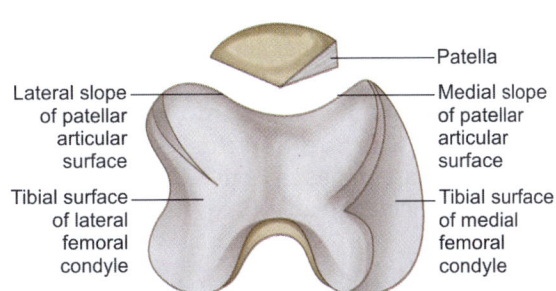

Fig. 18.5B: Femoral condylar articular surfaces (right) for both tibia and patella (inferior view).

Patellar articular area (Fig. 18.5A)

It covers anterior surface of both the condyles, continuous with each other. It is concave from side to side. The articular surface on the lateral condyle is wider and deeper. Inferiorly, the patellar surface is continuous with the tibial articular surface.

Tibial articular surface area (Figs. 18.5B and C)

It covers both inferior as well as posterior surface of both the condyles separated by nonarticular *intercondylar notch*. The tibial condylar articular areas of both condyles of femur are convex anteroposteriorly. Anteroposterior axis of the lateral condyle is straight whereas the long axis of the medial condyle is oblique with convexity on the medial aspect **(Fig. 18.5B)**.

Articular Surface of Patella (Fig. 18.6)

It is primarily divided by a vertical ridge into a *larger lateral* and *smaller medial* areas, which articulate with respective condyles of femur.

On the medial edge of the medial articular area, there is a *'strip-like' articular area* which normally remains free. But *during extreme flexion* of the joint, it comes in contact with the medial condyle of femur. During this position, the medial articular area of the patella comes in relation to the intercondylar notch.

Articular Surface of Tibia (Fig. 18.7)

Articular surface over both the lateral and medial tibial condyles are known as **tibial plateau**.

Lateral and medial condylar articular areas of the tibial plateau are separated by a nonarticular

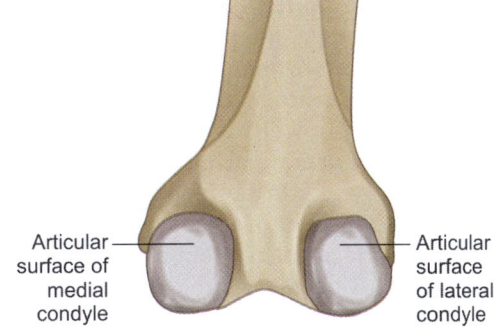

Fig. 18.5C: Tibial articular surface of femoral condyles (posterior view).

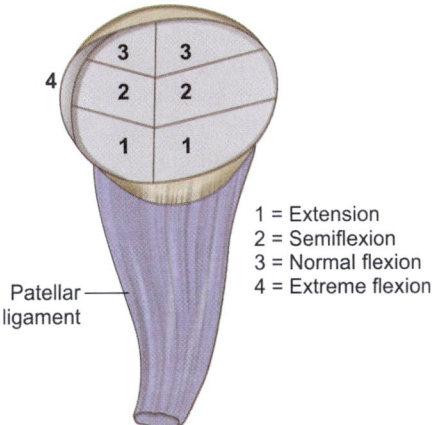

1 = Extension
2 = Semiflexion
3 = Normal flexion
4 = Extreme flexion

Fig. 18.6: Femoral articular surface of right patella.

intercondylar area. The medial tibial articular area is oval with its longer anteroposterior axis. The lateral tibial articular area is almost circular. This difference is reflected on the shapes of the menisci which rest on the peripheral part of the respective condylar articular area.

Fibrous Capsule (Fig. 18.8)

It is the fibrous envelope of variable thinness around the knee joint.

Anteriorly, the fibrous capsule is deficient at the level of lower end of the quadriceps tendon, the patella and the patellar ligament. On either side of the patella, the place of capsule is taken by the patellar retinaculum. Anteriorly, the capsule is only well-defined adjacent to the lateral and medial patellar retinacula. On the middle of superior margin of femoral articular surface, attachment of the capsule is deficient through which the synovial membrane protrudes upwards deep to the quadriceps tendon above the level of patella to form **the suprapatellar bursa (Fig. 18.9).**

Inferiorly, anterior part of the capsule is attached to the margin of the respective condyles of tibia a little beyond the articular surface. In the middle it is strengthened by the patellar ligament attached to the tibial tuberosity.

Posterior Attachment of the Capsule (Fig. 18.10)

Superiorly, from lateral to medial, the fibrous capsule is attached to:
- Upper margin of articular surface of lateral condyle of femur
- Upper margin of intercondylar notch
- Upper margin of articular surface of medial condyle of femur.

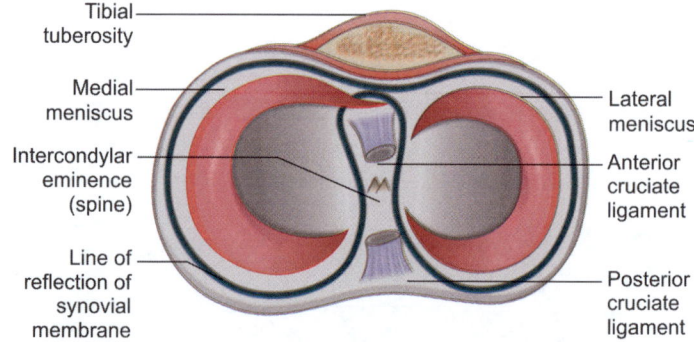

Fig. 18.7: Articular surface of tibial condyles (right).

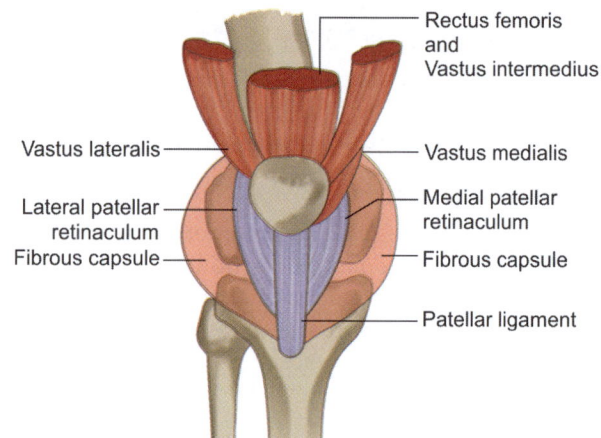

Fig. 18.8: Anterior part of capsule of knee joint (right) related to quadriceps components and patellar retinacula.

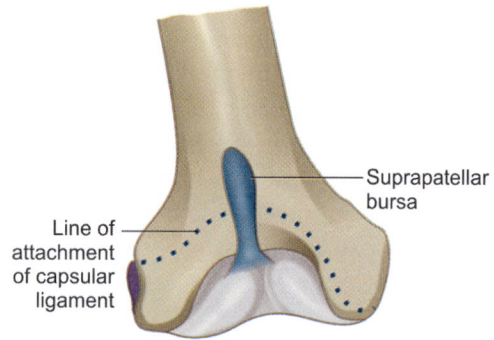

Fig. 18.9: Site of protrusion of suprapatellar bursa.

Inferiorly, lateral to medial, capsule is attached to:
- Posterior margin of lateral condyle of tibia
- Posterior margin of tibial intercondylar area
- Posterior margin of medial condyle of tibia

Posteriorly, the capsule of joint shows a deficiency for exit of the tendon of popliteus.

Capsule Traced on Either Side

On either side, the capsule retreats from the margins of articular surface of femoral condyles to enclose the rough areas of condylar surface. On the lateral side it *includes the groove for origin of tendon of popliteus.*

Below, the capsule is attached on either side to the respective margins of condyle of the tibia.

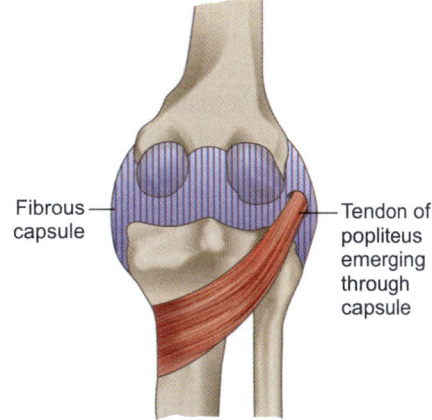

Fig. 18.10: Posterior aspect of right knee joint capsule.

Synovial Membrane

Like other joints, synovial membrane of the knee joint shows following **common characteristics:**
- It covers the inner surface of capsule.
- Usually, it is attached to the margins of the articular surfaces.
- So, it does not cover any articular surface.

But **special characteristics** are the following:
- Anterosuperiorly, it forms suprapatellar bursa.
- In between femoral and tibial condyle, the synovial membrane is attached to the peripheral margin of the semilunar cartilage.
- Cruciate ligaments, anterior and posterior, being intra articular ligaments are intra articular and extrasynovial.

Extra-articular Ligaments

The ligaments reinforce the fibrous capsule to maintain the stability to the joint, as the capsule is loose and thin in some areas for free flexion and extension movements.

Tibial Collateral Ligament (Fig. 18.11)

Tibial collateral ligament of the knee joint is strengthened further, superficially by the *deep fascia* and *expansion of tendon of sartorius* and by the capsular fibers at the deeper plane. Primarily, the tibial collateral ligament is divided into *superficial and deep parts*.
- **Superficial part of the ligament** is inverted 'V' shaped having anterior vertical part and posterior oblique part **(Fig. 18.12).**

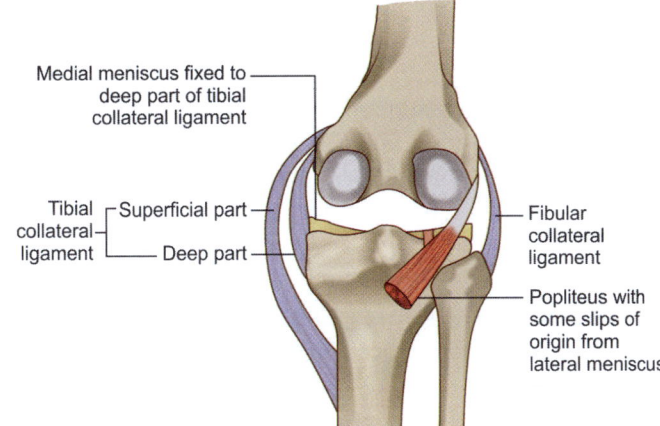

Fig. 18.11: Collateral ligaments of right knee joint (viewed from behind).

- **Anterior vertical limb of the superficial part**, about 10 cm long, extends from medial condyle of the femur, just below the adductor tubercle, to the upper end of the *medial surface of the* **shaft of the tibia**.
- **Posterior oblique limb** of the superficial part passes from medial condyle of femur to the posterior half of the *medial surface of the* **medial condyle of tibia**.
- **Deep part** is shorter and more condensed. It is attached to the medial condyles of the femur and tibia **close to the articular surfaces**. Deep surface of this band is fixed to peripheral margin of medial meniscus through the capsule of the joint. Superficial part of the tibial collateral ligament is joined by an **expansion from the tendon of semimembranosus**.

Morphologically, the tibial collateral ligament of knee joint represents the lowermost part of the tendon of ischial fibers of **adductor magnus distal to the adductor tubercle**.

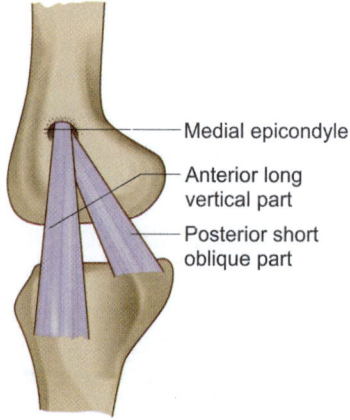

Fig. 18.12: Components of superficial part of tibial collateral ligament.

Fibular Collateral Ligament (Fig. 18.11)

It is a strong cord-like ligament measuring about 5 cm in length. Above it is attached to *the lateral epicondyle of femur* above the groove for origin of the tendon of popliteus. Below, the ligament passes superficial to the tendon of popliteus to be attached to the head of the fibula. Near the lower attachment, the ligament splits up the tendinous insertion of biceps femoris.

Ligaments Reinforcing the Posterolateral Aspect of the Joint

Arcuate Popliteal Ligament (Fig. 18.13)

It is an expansion from the lower end of the fibular collateral ligament. From the head of fibula, these fibers arch round the emerging tendon of popliteus in the medial direction to be attached to the posterior margin of intercondylar area of the tibia.

Popliteofibular Ligament

It extends from the tendon of popliteus downwards and laterally to the head of fibula. It is the most important stabilizer of the posterolateral aspect of the knee joint.

Fabellofibular Ligament

It extends from the sesamoid bone, called **the fabella**, on the tendon of lateral head of gastrocnemius. Distally, it is attached to the styloid process of fibula.

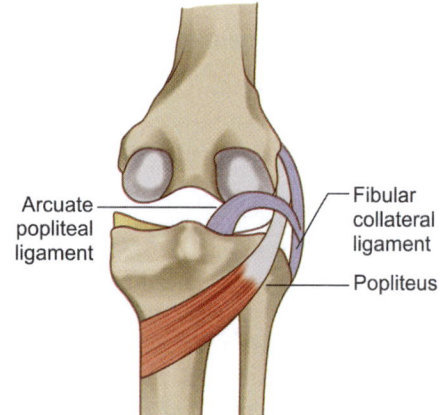

Fig. 18.13: Arcuate popliteal ligament.

Patellar Ligament (Ligamentum Patellae) (Fig. 18.14)

It is also known as **patellar tendon**. It is the band-like central component of the tendon of quadriceps femoris.

Attachments

Proximally, the patellar ligament is attached to:
- Apex of patella
- Adjoining part of the lateral and medial margins of patella
- Rough area on the anterior surface of apex
- Small depression on the lower part of the posterior surface of the bone

Distally, the ligament is attached to *the smooth area on the upper part of the tibial tuberosity.*

Posteriorly, the patellar ligament and the synovial membrane are interposed by *intrapatellar pad of fat.* The ligament is separated from the tibia by a *bursa*.

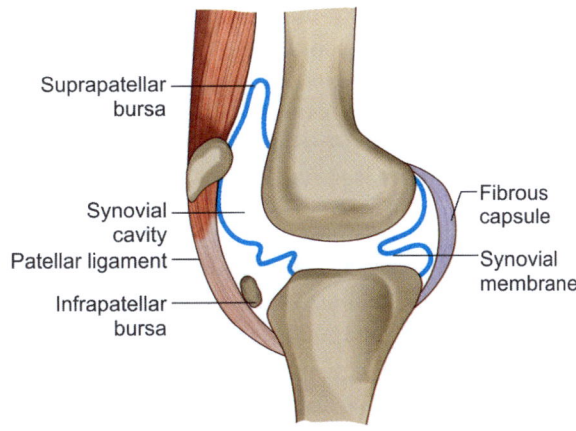

Fig. 18.14: Knee joint in sagittal section to show patellar ligament and vertical reflection of synovial membrane.

Oblique Popliteal Ligament (Fig. 18.15)

It is the superolateral expansion from the insertion of tendon of semimembranosus, reinforcing the posterior part of capsule. The ligament is triangular in shape with its apex attached below, to the tubercle on the medial condyle. The fibers fan out upwards and laterally to be attached to the upper margin of the intercondylar area and the posterosuperior margin of articular surface of the lateral condyle of femur.

Oblique popliteal ligament forms the intermediate part of the floor of popliteal fossa. It is pierced by the *middle genicular vessels and nerves*, and the terminal part of the *posterior division of the obturator nerve.*

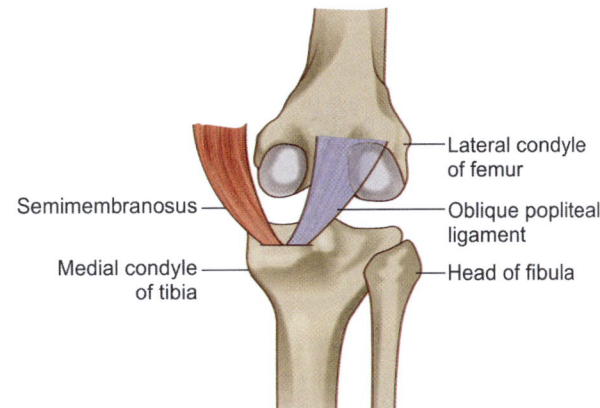

Fig. 18.15: Oblique popliteal ligament of right knee joint.

Intra-articular Cartilages and Ligaments

Semilunar Cartilages (Menisci) (Fig. 18.7)

Fundamental points

Semilunar cartilages or menisci are *two crescentic intracapsular fibrocartilaginous* strips interposed between the condyles of the femur and tibia. They lie in close contact with the peripheral part of the articular surface of the respective tibial condyles.

Features
- **Two ends:** Called *anterior and posterior horns*

- **Two surfaces: Superior surface** is concave for the convexity of the femoral condyles. **Inferior surface** is flat to rest on the tibial condyles.
- **Two margins: The peripheral margin** is thick and convex. This margin is fixed to the deep surface of fibrous capsule. The **central margin** is concave and thin.
- **Two components: Peripheral one-third** is *vascularized* and **central two-thirds** are avascular, whose nutrition is maintained by synovial fluid.

Functions

- The menisci **increase the stability of the knee joint** by improving the congruence of the femoral and tibial condylar articular surfaces
- They act as **shock-absorber** during stress and strain of the joint
- **Total load** carried by the knee is **partially distributed through the menisci**
- Superior sloping surface of the menisci lubricated by synovial fluid **helps in free movement** of femoral condyles on tibial condyles.

Differentiating features of the menisci

- **Medial semilunar cartilage** is more elongated anteroposteriorly and it is *truly semilunar*.
- **Anterior horn** of medial semilunar cartilage is narrower and is divided into *anterior* and *posterior bands*. Posterior band is attached to the peripheral margin of lateral semilunar cartilage. It is called **transverse ligament** of the knee joint.
- **Posterior horn** of the medial semilunar cartilage is broader.
- **Peripheral margin** of the medial cartilage is fixed to the deep surfaces of fibrous capsule as well as tibial collateral ligament of the knee joint. Part of the tibial collateral ligament extending from the peripheral margin of the cartilage to the tibial condyle is known as **coronary ligament**. The abovementioned attachments of medial meniscus make it more fixed or less movable than lateral meniscus.

Lateral Semilunar Cartilage

Though it is called semilunar, its outline *covers four-fifth of a circle*. It is broader than the medial cartilage and its breadth is uniform.

Attachment of lateral semilunar cartilage

- While **the tendon of popliteus** comes out of the joint cavity crossing the posterior margin of lateral meniscus a few fibers of the tendon are attached to the cartilage. This attachment makes the lateral meniscus more mobile during movement of the knee joint, so that it is not crushed between femorotibial condyles.
- **Meniscofemoral ligaments:** From the *posterior horn of the lateral meniscus* two bands of fibers diverge upwards and medially to be attached to the *lateral surface of medial condyle of femur* in front and behind the posterior cruciate ligament (PCL). These are known as *anterior and posterior meniscofemoral ligaments*.

Clinical anatomy

Vide clinical anatomy section at the end of this answer.

Cruciate Ligaments (Fig. 18.16)

Cruciate ligaments are two *strong, intra articular ligaments, anterior and posterior,* which show a *criss cross arrangement*. Strength of these ligaments maintains the stability in erect posture as well as during movements.

Both the cruciate ligaments bind the femoral and tibial condyles. They are called anterior and posterior in view of their relative attachment positions in the tibia.

Cruciate ligaments are intracapsular but extrasynovial. Synovial membrane is reflected forwards from the posterior part of inner surface of the capsule to wind round the cruciate ligaments form both the sides to turn around the anterior aspect of anterior cruciate ligament (ACL) (Fig. 18.7).

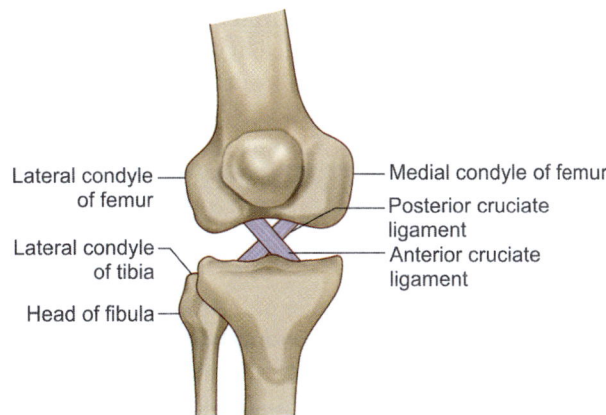

Fig. 18.16: Cruciate ligaments of right knee joint (anterior view).

Anterior Cruciate Ligament

Anterior cruciate ligament (ACL) is termed anterior as because it is **attached to the anterior intercondylar area of the tibia.**

The ligament is directed **upwards, backwards** and **laterally** to be attached to the **posterior part of medial surface of lateral condyle of femur**.

Anterior cruciate ligament is **made stretched in full extension of the knee** and **checks forward displacement of tibial condyles** in hyperextension of the knee joint.

Posterior Cruciate Ligament

Posterior cruciate ligament (PCL) is **stronger** and **thicker** than ACL.

It is called posterior in view of its relative position of attachment in **posterior part of the intercondylar area of the tibia**. From the tibial attachment the ligament is directed **upwards, forwards and medially** to be attached to the **lateral surface of medial condyle of femur.**

Posterior cruciate ligament is **made tense in flexion**. Rupture of PCL is less common than the anterior.

Clinical anatomy

Vide clinical anatomy section at the end of this answer.

Reflection of Synovial Membrane

Sagittal Disposition (Fig. 18.14)

From the upper margin of patella, synovial membrane is reflected upwards behind the quadriceps tendon and then on the lower part of anterior surface of femur. Finally, it is attached to the margin of patellar articular surface of femur. This blind pouch of synovial membrane is known as **suprapatellar bursa**.

Below the level of patella, synovial membrane is separated from the patellar tendon by the **infrapatellar fat pad**. Behind the infrapatellar fat, synovial membrane projects backwards as **infrapatellar fold** or **ligamentum mucosum**.

On the posterior aspect, synovial membrane is attached to the upper margin of the posterior part of articular surface of the femoral condyles. It lines then the inner surface of the capsule. Reaching the level of joint line, the synovial membrane is reflected forwards towards the joint cavity. This occurs because the synovial membrane winds around the cruciate ligaments to keep the ligaments extrasynovial. Finally, it is again reflected back on the lower part of capsule to be attached to the margins of tibial condylar articular surface.

Coronal Disposition

From the lateral and medial sides of the margin of respective femoral condylar articular surface, the synovial membrane lines successively the intracapsular part of femoral condyles and inner surface of the capsule up to the peripheral margin of the meniscus. As the menisci are extrasynovial, originally the synovial membrane used to line the superior surface of the menisci first, then round the central concave margin it covers the lower surface to reach peripheral margin. But the synovial membrane lining the surfaces of the menisci does not have existence. From the peripheral margin of the menisci, synovial membrane lines further the lower part of capsule to be attached to the articular margin of the tibial condyles.

Horizontal Disposition (Fig. 18.7)

Horizontally the synovial membrane lines the inner surface of the capsule from the lateral and medial margins of the patella. In between the condyles of femur and tibia, synovial membrane is reflected forwards from the posterior part of the fibrous capsule to wind around the posterior and anterior cruciate ligaments to keep these structures extrasynovial.

Relations of Knee Joint

- **Anterior:** Tendon of quadriceps femoris, patella, patellar ligament with patellar retinacula. In addition, iliotibial tract on lateral side.
- **Posterior:**
  - Popliteus muscle with its fascia crossing the joint in oblique direction downwards and medially.
  - Popliteal vessels and tibial nerve.
- **Posteromedially:**
  - *In the upper part*: Sartorius, semitendinosus and semimembranosus.
  - *In the lower part*: Medial head of gastrocnemius
- **Posterolateral**:
  - *In the upper part*: Tendon of the biceps femoris and common fibular nerve
  - *In the lower part*: Lateral head of gastrocnemius and plantaris

Bursae Around Knee Joint

Bursae around the knee joint are membranous and arranged in following groups.

Anterior Group

- Large **subcutaneous prepatellar bursa** over the patella. It is also called **housemaid's bursa.**
- **Subcutaneous infrapatellar bursa** over the lower part of the *tibial tuberosity*.
- **Deep infrapatellar bursa** under the lower end of *patellar ligament*
- **Large suprapatellar bursa** is formed by outpouching of synovial membrane between quadriceps tendon and lower end of femur.

Posterolateral Group

- Between lateral head of gastrocnemius and joint capsule
- Between tendon of biceps femoris and fibular collateral ligament.
- Between tendon of popliteus and fibular collateral ligament
- Between tendon of popliteus and lateral condyle of femur.

Posteromedial

- **Semimembranosus bursa** is between insertion of semimembranosus and origin of medial head of gastrocnemius.
- A bursa between semimembranosus and medial condyle of tibia. It may communicate with the abovementioned bursa.
- **Pes bursa** is between the tendons of sartorius, gracilis and semitendinosus, and the tibial collateral ligament.
- A variable number of bursae may be present between the *tibial collateral ligament* and the capsule, femur, tibia, medial meniscus and semimembranosus.

Clinically Important Bursae

- All the bursae of the anterior group
- Semimembranosus bursa
- Pes bursa.

Inflamed prepatellar and infrapatellar bursae are known as **housemaid's knee** and **clergyman's knee** respectively.

In case of degenerative changes of knee in adults, *semimembranosus bursa* may be enlarged. It presents a cystic swelling in the popliteal region.

Inflammation of *pes bursa* is found in athletes.

Arterial Supply

Arteries supplying the knee joint are arranged in following three groups. They form an anastomosing network around the knee joint.

Medial Group

- Descending genicular branch of femoral artery
- Medial superior genicular branch of popliteal artery
- Medial inferior genicular branch of popliteal artery.

Central Group

Middle genicular branch or popliteal artery.

Lateral Group

- Lateral superior genicular branch of popliteal artery
- Lateral inferior genicular branch of popliteal artery
- Recurrent genicular branch of anterior tibial artery
- Circumflex fibular branch of posterior tibial artery.

Nerve Supply

- Femoral nerve through nerve to vastus intermedius
- Terminal end of posterior division of obturator nerve
- Genicular branches of tibial nerve:
  - Medial superior genicular nerve
  - Middle genicular nerve
  - Medial inferior genicular nerve

- Genicular branches of common fibular nerve:
  - Lateral superior genicular nerve
  - Lateral inferior genicular nerve

Movements of Knee Joint

Various groups of muscles surrounding the knee joint indicate that remarkable degree of movements takes place in the joint.

Main movements of the joint are **flexion** and **extension** around a *transverse axis*. In addition, the knee joint enjoys **medial and lateral rotations** around a vertical axis.

Rotational movements are of following two types:
1. **Conjunct rotation**: This rotation movement is *associated with flexion and extension*. When the foot is on the ground in erect posture, *terminal 30° of extension* is associated with the **medial rotation of femoral condyles on tibial condyles**. Again, for initiation of flexion, this twisted position of condyles of femur is corrected by lateral rotation.
2. **Adjunct rotation**: It is **independent rotational movement in partially flexed knee joint**. Range of the adjunct rotation is less than that of the conjunct rotation. This rotational movement takes place in **meniscotibial joint**.

Conjunct Rotation: An Asset of the Knee Joint

Knee joint is not a typical, but **a modified hinge joint** due to following two reasons.
1. Hinge actions of the joint, i.e. flexion-extension are associated with conjunct rotation.
2. Transverse axis of the hinge action is not fixed.

During the position of the **foot off the ground**, when the position is of knee joint is changed from fully flexed position to fully extended position, gliding of the tibial condyles on femoral condyles is associated with lateral rotation of the tibial condyles.

Again, when the foot is on the ground in erect posture, last 30° of extension of knee is associated with medial rotation of femoral condyles on tibia. This medial rotation gives rise to following changes in the knee joint.
1. *'Spirilization'* or *twisting* of the tibial and fibular collateral ligaments and the oblique popliteal ligament with the joint capsule.
2. *Intercondylar spines* (eminences) of the tibia *fit with* the *femoral intercondylar notch*.
3. Menisci are *tightly wedged* between condyles of femur and tibia.

These abovementioned changes in the knee joint in full extension can keep the joint in a secured position on prolonged standing even when the fatigued quadriceps tendon can relax. This is called **locking of the knee joint**.

From the **'locked position'** of the knee joint in erect posture, when an attempt is made for flexion, the movement is not possible by the hamstrings, unless the medial rotation of the femoral condyles is corrected by their lateral rotation first. As the foot is on the ground, insertion end of the popliteus muscle on the tibia is fixed. Contraction of popliteus from below rotates the femoral attachment outwards, causing the lateral rotation of femoral condyles on tibia which correct the medial rotation. This is called **unlocking of the joint** which leads to initiation of flexion by the hamstring muscles.

Muscles for Various Movements

Extension

Quadriceps femoris is the principal muscle which is composed of rectus femoris and three vasti. *Vastus medialis, for its typical fiber direction* near the insertion, plays an important role in terminal stage of extension of knee.

Factor controlling the hyperextension is the tension on the cruciate and collateral ligaments.

Flexion

It is caused by hamstring muscles, namely, biceps femoris, semimembranosus and semitendinosus. Extreme flexion ends when the back of thigh comes in contact with the back of leg.

Rotation

Adjunct rotation is only possible to a limited degree when the knee is partially flexed, as the tibia rotates on femur.

Medial rotation: By popliteus, semitendinosus and partly by semimembranosus. It is restricted by cruciate ligaments.

Lateral rotation: By biceps femoris. This movement is restricted by collateral ligaments.

Conjunct Rotation (For Locking and Unlocking of the Joint)

In full extension, when the foot is on the ground in weight-bearing position, the ligaments are twisted by medial rotation of femoral condyles on the tibia. This movement is **'locking'** of the knee joint caused by the *biceps femoris*. **'Unlocking'** of the joint is the reverse lateral rotation of femoral condyles caused by *the popliteus*.

Clinical Anatomy

Knee Joint Injuries

Knee joint injuries are common because:
- It is a large condylar joint having *incongruent articular surfaces*
- It is the *weight-bearing joint*
- It is *subjected to stress and strain* in daily life from various movements e.g. standing, walking, running, jumping and climbing.
- It is *exposed* to various activities in both *contact and noncontact sports*.

Ligamentous sprains are most common variety of the injuries. These include injuries to the tibial collateral ligaments.

Concomitant injury to the tibial collateral ligament and medial meniscus occurs in case of footballers and athletes, due to sudden twisting of the semiflexed knee. It occurs because the peripheral margin of the medial meniscus is adhered to the inner surface of the tibial collateral ligament along with the capsule. Chance of **lateral meniscus injury is less due to following reasons:**
1. It is separated from the lateral side of the capsule and the fibular collateral ligament.
2. Some fibers of the popliteus attached to the outer margin of lateral meniscus pull the meniscus peripherally to prevent its compression between femoral and tibial condyles.

Types of Menisci Tear

Most common type of menisci tear is the **'bucket handle' type of injury**. In this case, central part of the meniscus is torn in the form of longitudinal split anteroposteriorly. It occurs in young adults, as already mentioned, in sports, due to sudden twist of the joint in semiflexed position.

Transverse injury occurs either in anterior horn or in posterior horn affecting free concave margin of the meniscus. It occurs in old age due to degenerative changes.

Medial meniscus is more commonly injured than the lateral

Menisci or semilunar cartilages are torn due to sudden twisting (rotational) movement of the knee joint in its semiflexed position. This injury is found in footballer and athletes. Injury to the medial meniscus is very often associated with tear of the tibial collateral ligament of the knee joint. Medial meniscus is more commonly injured than the lateral because:
- Medial meniscus is more fixed than the lateral. In addition to the usual attachment of the anterior and posterior horns to the tibial condyle, peripheral margin of the medial meniscus is attached to the inner surface of tibial collateral ligament together with the fibrous capsule. This attachment causes failure of necessary adjustment of the position of the medial meniscus between the femoral and tibial condyles during sudden twisting movement.
- Lateral meniscus is separated from the fibular collateral ligament and also the inner surface of lateral part of the capsule.
- In addition, while the tendon of popliteus emerges through the capsule of the joint, some of its fibers are attached to the posterior part of the peripheral margin of lateral meniscus. Through these fibers, popliteus will pull the lateral meniscus outwards to prevent its compression between lateral condyles of femur and tibia.

Cruciate Ligament Injury

Rupture of anterior cruciate ligament (ACL) may occur when sever force is applied in anterior direction in semiflexed position of the knee. It will cause **forward sliding of the tibia** form the femur. ACL tear is clinically diagnosed by **abnormal forward mobility of the flexed leg.** It is known as **positive anterior drawer sign**.

Rapture of posterior cruciate ligament (PCL) occurs in athletes and players, while **striking suddenly on the tibial tuberosity.** It can also occur in case of head on collision of a car, when the proximal end of the tibia strikes against the dashboard. It is clinically diagnosed by **abnormal posterior mobility of the tibia in flexed leg**. It is known as **positive posterior drawer sign.**

Bursitis Around Knee

Prepatellar bursitis

It is the *friction bursitis of subcutaneous prepatellar bursa* caused by friction between patella and the skin. If the inflammation is chronic, the bursa may be distended with fluid forming a swelling in front of the knee. The condition is known as **housemaid's knee**.

Subcutaneous infrapatellar bursitis

It occurs due to friction of skin against the tibial tuberosity. It is characterized by a swelling over the upper end of the tibia.

Suprapatellar bursitis

Clinically more care should be taken in this condition because infection may spread into the joint cavity and for this reason popliteal group of lymph nodes may be inflamed.

Popliteal Cyst (Baker's Cyst)

This is a fluid filled cystic swelling on the back of the knee which may occur due to:
- Herniation of synovial membrane of knee joint
- Distension of semimembranosus bursa

Popliteal cyst due to the former reason is called Baker's cyst. It may result as a consequence of effusion of the knee joint.

Arthroscopy

Through this clinical device, interior of the joint cavity is approached through the instrumental intervention for the following purposes.
- Diagnosis of any injury or disease within the joint cavity.
- Intra articular surgical management, for example, removal of torn menisci and loose bodies such as bone chips or devitalized articular cartilage.

Effusion of Knee Joint

It is a clinical condition characterized by accumulation of fluid within the joint cavity which occurs *as a consequence of inflammation of suprapatellar bursa*. It can result from any kind of trauma in the lower part of front of thigh. The patient presents a soft cystic swelling above the level of patella.

Osteoarthritis

Degenerative changes are very common in the knee joint because of its weight bearing function throughout the life. It occurs in old age and the incidence is more common in females due to *osteoporosis* as a result of postmenopausal hormonal imbalance. Sometimes articular surfaces may show the growth of small bony spikes *(osteophytes)*.

Knee Deformities

Fracture dislocation and diseases of the knee joint give rise to disfiguration of the joint. Medial deviation of upper end of the tibia from the joint line is known as **genu varum**. Lateral deviation is called **genu valgum**. These deformities cause imbalance in the weight distribution.

Knee Replacement

When the entire knee joint is diseased as in case of osteoarthritis, an artificial knee joint is reconstructed through an operative procedure called **knee replacement arthroplasty**. In this procedure, the femoral articular surface is capped by *metal component* and the tibial condylar articular surface is replaced by *plastic component* with the help of bone cement. These opposing articular surfaces give smoothness of movement like *'ice on ice'* like the natural articular surfaces covered by cartilage.

LA 18.3 Discuss briefly the talocrural (ankle) joint. Write a note on its clinical anatomy.

ANKLE (TALOCRURAL) JOINT

Introduction

Ankle joint is the articulation between the talus (the tarsal bone of forefoot) and the lower ends of tibia and fibula (the crural bones). That is why it is called talocrural joint.

The joint is equally important for support of body weight and for propulsion.

Type

Ankle joint is a **synovial joint of modified hinge variety**. It is modified because the axis of the hinge movement is not fixed but changes in extremes of plantar flexion and dorsiflexion.

Articular Surfaces (Fig. 18.17)

Proximal Articular Surface

Proximal articular surface presents a **mortise** (deep socket) formed by:
- Inferior surface of **lower end of the tibia** which is continuous with the smooth articular area on the lateral surface of **medial malleolus**.
- Triangular articular surface on the medial aspect of the **lateral malleolus**
  Both of the above articular surfaces of the joint are covered by hyaline articular cartilage.
- Transverse component of **inferior tibiofibular ligament**
  The deep socket formed by above structures is known as *tibiofibular mortise*.

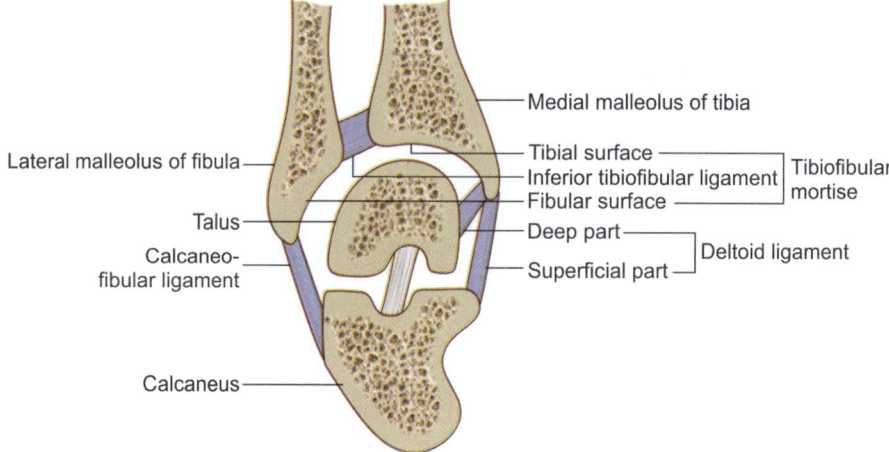

Fig. 18.17: Ankle joint in coronal plane.

Distal Articular Surface

It is formed by following areas of **talus:**
- **Superior trochlear surface**
- **Medial curved articular surface**
- **Lateral triangular articular surface**
  All these surfaces are covered by hyaline cartilage
  Weight-bearing surfaces of the joint are the upper trochlear facet of the talus and the inferior facet of the tibia.

Fibrous Capsule

It invests the joint all around. Its attachments are as follows.
- **Proximally,** it is attached to all around the **margins of articular surface of the tibia** with its **medial malleolus** and **the lateral malleolus of fibula**. In between it is attached to the transverse component of **inferior tibiofibular ligament.**

- **Distally,** it is attached to the margin of **the articular surfaces of the talus.** On the superior surface of the neck, the capsule is prolonged forwards a little beyond the anterior margin trochlear articular surface.

  Fibrous capsule is thin in front and behind to allow free anteroposterior hinge movement of the joint. But it is thicker on either side and strengthened further by the collateral ligaments.

Synovial Membrane

- It is attached everywhere to the margins of the articular surface
- It lines the inner surface of the fibrous capsule
- It covers also the intracapsular part of the superior surface of neck of talus
- A small part of synovial lining protrudes upwards towards the inferior tibiofibular joint.

Medial Ligament (Deltoid Ligament) (Figs. 18.17 and 18.18)

It is a very strong ligament, triangular in appearance and it strengthens the medial side of the capsule. The ligament is divided into superficial and deep part. Both the parts have **identical proximal attachments** to the tip and the margins of medial malleolus. Distal attachments are as follows.

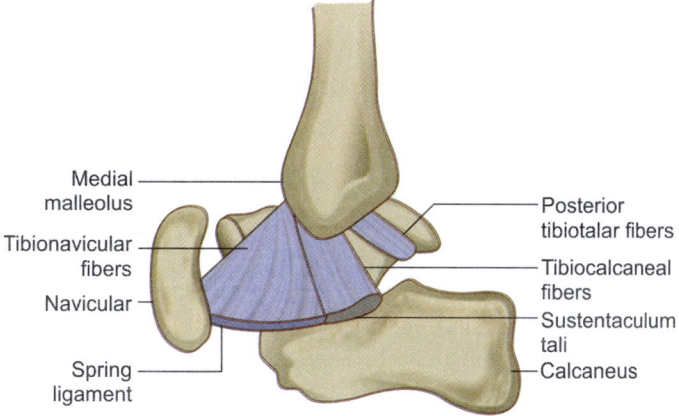

Fig. 18.18: Medial collateral (deltoid) ligament of right ankle joint.

Superficial Part

It is further divided into following three parts.
1. **Anterior tibionavicular band** is attached to the tuberosity of navicular and the medial margin of plantar calcaneonavicular (spring) ligament.
2. **Middle tibiocalcaneal band** is attached to the sustentaculum tali.
3. Posterior band is named as **posterior tibiotalar ligament.** It is attached to the medial tubercle and the adjacent part of medial surface of talus.

   Deep part of the deltoid ligament is called **anterior tibiotalar ligament** which is attached to the anterior area of medial surface of the talus.

   Deltoid ligament is crossed on its superficial aspect by the tendons of tibialis posterior and flexor digitorum longus.

Functions

- Deltoid ligament stabilizes the ankle joint during eversion
- It also prevents subluxation (partial dislocation) of the joint.

Lateral Ligament (Figs. 18.17 and 18.19)

Like the superficial part of the deltoid ligament, the lateral ligament is also divided into three parts. **Anterior and posterior parts connect talus with fibula. Intermediate part connects calcaneus with fibula.**

- **Anterior talofibular ligament** extends from **neck of talus** to the **anterior margin of lateral malleolus** of fibula
- **Posterior talofibular ligament** is a strong band which connects the **posterior tubercle of talus** with the **posterior margin of lateral malleolus of fibula**
- **Calcaneofibular ligament** is longer and cord-like. It extends from the tubercle on the lateral surface of calcaneus to the notch on the **inferior aspect (tip) of lateral malleolus of fibula.**

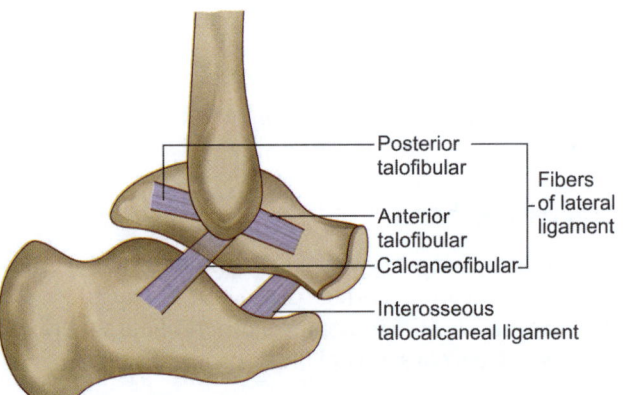

Fig. 18.19: Lateral ligament of right ankle joint.

Lateral ligament is crossed superficially by the tendons of fibularis longus and fibularis brevis. Three components of the lateral ligament possess their independent identity, through their individual names.

Relations of the Ankle Joint

Anterior

From medial to lateral:
- Tendon of tibialis anterior
- Tendon of extensor hallucis longus
- Anterior tibial vessels
- Deep fibular (peroneal) nerve
- Tendon of extensor digitorum longus
- Tendon of fibularis (peroneus) tertius.

Posteromedial

From anteromedial to posterolateral:
- Tendon of tibialis posterior
- Tendon of flexor digitorum longus
- Posterior tibial vessels
- Tibial nerve
- Tendon of flexor hallucis longus.

Posterior

Tendo calcaneus (Ttendo-Achilles').

Posterolateral

Tendons of fibularis brevis and fibularis longus.

Arterial Supply

By the malleolar branches of anterior tibial, posterior tibial and fibular (peroneal) arteries.

Nerve Supply

By the deep fibular and the tibial nerves which carry fibers of L_4, L_5, S_1, S_2 segments.

Factors Maintaining the Stability of Ankle Joint

- **Reciprocal congruence** of the tibiofibular mortise and the trochlear surface of the talus.
- **Increase of the depth of the socket** by the transverse part of **inferior tibiofibular ligament.**
- Strength of the **collateral ligaments.**
- **Tendons** crossing the joint all around.

Grip with the help of the malleoli on the trochlea is strongest during dorsiflexion of the foot because the wider anterior part of the trochlear surface of the talus fits more tightly in the mortise with slight stretching of the collateral ligaments and tibiofibular syndesmosis. **Ankle joint is relatively less stable during plantar flexion** because the trochlea is narrower posteriorly and this part lies relatively loosely within the mortise during plantar flexion of the ankle.

Movements

The main movements are *dorsiflexion* and *plantar flexion*.

When the foot is plantar flexed, some *rotation, adduction* and *abduction* of the ankle joint are possible.

The axis for the hinge movement of dorsiflexion and plantar flexion is not horizontal but it slopes downwards and laterally passing through the points just below the apices of the malleoli. The axis also changes its position anteroposteriorly from the position of dorsiflexion and plantar flexion.

Due to obliquity of the axis downwards and laterally, as stated above, full plantar flexion is associated with the movement like inversion. Reverse movement like slight eversion is found to be associated in dorsiflexion. But these movements are not true inversion and eversion.

From the upright position, with the foot at right angles to the leg, active plantar flexion is produced by gastrocnemius and soleus for about 20°. It is assisted by long flexors and the fibularis muscles. Similarly, active dorsiflexion for about 10° is produced by tibialis anterior, long extensors and fibularis (peroneus) tertius.

Muscles Producing Dorsiflexion

Principal muscle for dorsiflexion is **tibialis anterior**. It is helped by *extensor digitorum longus, extensor hallucis longus and fibularis (peroneus) tertius.*

Dorsiflexion is limited by:
- Passive antagonism by triceps surae (the two heads of gastrocnemius and the soleus)
- Stretching of the collateral ligaments.

Muscles Producing Plantar Flexion

Principal muscles for plantar flexion are **gastrocnemius** and **soleus**. These are supported by *plantaris, tibialis posterior, flexor hallucis longus and flexor digitorum longus.*

Plantar flexion is restricted by stretching of dorsiflexors.

Clinical Anatomy

Ankle Injuries

Among all the major joints of the body, ankle is **most frequently injured. Ankle sprains** (*tear in ligament fibers*) are most common. It occurs due to *inversion injury* which is the effect of twisting of the weight-bearing foot. The foot is forcibly inverted when a person steps on an uneven surface. The lateral ligament is more commonly injured because it is much weaker than the medial ligament. Anterior talofibular ligament fibers are usually torn, resulting instability of the joint. Severe injury may lead to **fracture of lateral malleolus**.

Dislocation of Ankle

Dislocation of the ankle is very rare because of the tibiofibular mortise giving stability to the joint. But it occurs if there is fracture dislocation of the malleoli which disrupts the grip of the mortise.

Pott's Fracture Dislocation of the Ankle

It is the result of **forcible eversion injury** of foot. It will cause **tear in the deltoid ligament and fracture of medial malleolus.** Pressure exerted by the talus on the lateral side may **break the fibular malleolus.** In extreme condition the posterior margin of the lower end of the tibia **(third malleolus) is fractured**. The condition is known as **trimalleolar fracture.**

LA 18.4 Discuss briefly the tarsal joints. Write a note on inversion and eversion of foot.

Short notes: Spring ligament; Inversion and eversion of foot.

TARSAL JOINTS

Most important tarsal joints are:
- Joint between talus, calcaneus and navicular
- Joint between calcaneus and cuboid

On the undersurface of talus there are two separates joints collectively known as **subtalar joint**.
1. **Talocalcanean joint:** It is the posterior joint between upper surface of the calcaneus and undersurface of the talus.
2. **Talocalcaneonavicular joint**: It is a more complicated joint in front with single synovial cavity. This joint is made up of following two parts.
   1. Joint between the inferior surface of head of talus and the superior surface of sustantaculum tali and body of calcaneus, and the spring ligament.
   2. Joint between anterior surface of the head of the talus and the navicular bone.

Talocalcanean Joint

It is a plane synovial joint formed by:
- Concave facet on the inferior surface of body of talus and
- Convex facet on the intermediate part of superior surface of calcaneus.

Fibrous capsule attached to the articular margins is strengthened by **lateral** and **medial talocalcanean ligaments**. Other ligaments of the joint are mentioned below.
- **Interosseous talocalcanean ligament**: It is the thick and strong ligament connecting the talus and calcaneus both of which have very important role in support and transmission of bodyweight.

This ligament occupies the space called *sinus tarsi* and it lies between talocalcanean joint and talocalcaneonavicular joint. Tension of the ligament *restricts the eversion movement*.
- **Cervical ligament**: It is lateral to the interosseous talocalcanean ligament. It extends upwards and medially from superior surface of calcaneus to the inferolateral aspect of the neck of talus. Tension on this ligament *restricts the inversion movement*.

Talocalcaneonavicular Joint (Fig. 18.20)

It is a *ball and socket type of synovial joint*. The ball is the head of talus. The socket is formed by the navicular, calcaneus and the spring ligament.

The male articular surface is formed by smooth convex anterior and inferior aspect of the *head of the talus*. Female articular surface is formed by:
- *Posterior concave surface of the navicular*
- *Anterior end of upper surface of the calcaneus*
- *Fibrocartilaginous upper surface of the spring ligament between the calcaneus and navicular.*

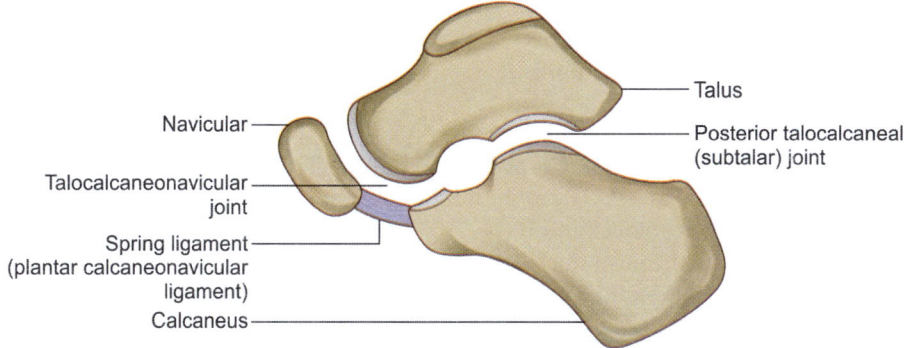

Fig. 18.20: Talocalcanean and talocalcaneonavicular joints.

Spring Ligament (Plantar Calcaneonavicular Ligament) (Figs. 18.20 and 18.21A)

It is a very strong fibrous band which connects the anterior margin of sustentaculum tali to the plantar aspect of the navicular. Its upper surface presents a *fibrocartilaginous facet* which completes the socket for head of the talus between calcaneus and navicular. Lower fibers of the ligament passes transversely across the foot. Like all other ligaments, it is *made up of collagen fibers* and is very strong. Though it is named as 'spring ligament', *it is not elastic*. It is supported by tibialis posterior medially and, flexor hallucis longus and flexor digitorum longus laterally.

Bifurcate Ligament

This ligament bifurcates from a common stem into a medial and lateral limbs. *The stem* is attached to the superior surface of calcaneus under the origin of extensor digitorum brevis. *The medial limb* is attached to the navicular and *the lateral limb* is attached to the cuboid.

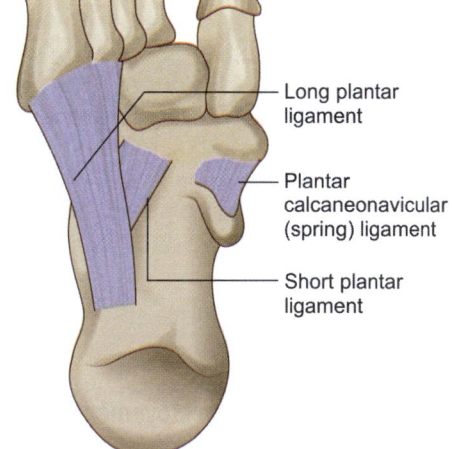

Fig. 18.21A: Ligaments of joints of right foot.

Calcaneocuboid Joint (Fig. 18.21B)

Calcaneocuboid joint is *a saddle type of synovial* joint between reciprocally curved concavoconvex anterior surface of calcaneus and posterior surface of cuboid. The calcaneocuboid joint and the talonavicular part of talocalcaneonavicular joint are together termed as **midtarsal joint**.

Capsular ligament surrounds the margins of articular surfaces. It is *thickened on the dorsal and plantar aspects.* Accessory ligaments are the lateral band of the bifurcate ligament and the long and short plantar ligaments.

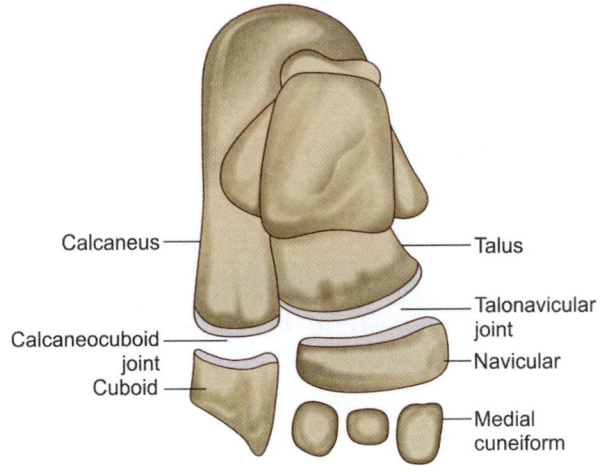

Fig. 18.21B: Midtarsal joints.

- **Short plantar ligament (Fig. 18.21A)** is truly named **plantar calcaneocuboid ligament**. It is a ligament made up of thick bundle of fibers which fill up the concavity between *anterior tubercle of calcaneus* and *posterior ridged margin of cuboid*. It is overlapped by the long plantar ligament.
- **Long plantar ligament (Fig. 18.21B)** extends forwards from the anterior tubercle of the calcaneus and area in front of the tubercle and it *covers the short plantar ligament.* Deeper fibers of the ligament are attached to the posterior ridge of the cuboid. Superficial fibers bridge over the groove of the cuboid, converting it into a tunnel for the passage of the tendon of fibularis (peroneus) longus. The fibers are attached to the anterior ridge of the cuboid and some of the fibers extend forwards to be attached to the bases of the central three (2nd, 3rd and 4th) metatarsal bones. The ligament is covered by flexor digitorum accessorius. Posterior fibers of the long plantar ligament is visible through the gap between two converging heads of the muscle.

INVERSION AND EVERSION OF THE FOOT

Inversion and eversion are the movements which occurs in **the subtalar** and **midtarsal joints**. It involves the subtalar joint more. Inversion leads to **adduction and supination** of the forefoot **raising the medial border of the foot**. Everson is characterized by **abduction and pronation** of the forefoot **raising the lateral border of the foot**. **Plantar flexion** increases the range of inversion. Again, a fully inverted foot is associated with plantar flexion. **Dorsiflexion** is associated with the more restricted movement of **eversion**.

Axis of the inversion—eversion movement is directed **obliquely from the lateral tubercle of calcaneus** upwards forwards and medially through **the neck of talus**. Line of pull of the muscles for these talus—neck movements is at right angle to the line of the axis. Planned movements of the ankle and tarsal joints are the effect of the balanced action of the muscles acting on joints of inversion and eversion.

Muscles Producing the Movements

- **Movement of inversion**, which causes raising of the medial border of foot, is produced by the muscle attached to the medial side of the foot. Muscles leading to inversion are **tibialis anterior** and **tibialis posterior.** This movement is supported by *extensor* and *flexor hallucis longus tendons.*

- **Movement of eversion**, which results in elevation of the lateral border of foot, is produced by the muscle which pulls up or is attached to the lateral side of the foot. These are **fibularis longus, fibularis brevis** and **fibularis tertius**.

Mechanism of Inversion and Eversion

Movements of inversion and eversion occur mainly in the **subtalar** and **talocalcaneonavicular joint** and partly in **the transverse tarsal joint**. During these movements, the foot moves below the talus, medially and laterally. Rotation of talus is restricted, as it is wedged between the malleoli. The calcaneus and navicular move medially or laterally around the oblique axis. For the obliquity of the axis, during inversion *supination of the foot is associated with adduction and plantar flexion*. During eversion, *pronation of foot is associated with abduction and dorsiflexion*.

Chapter 19

Miscellaneous Topics

LA 19.1 Discuss briefly the arches of foot. Write a note on its clinical anatomy.

Short notes/Short answer: Medial/Lateral longitudinal arches; Factors maintaining the arches; Anomalies of arches of foot.

ARCHES OF FOOT

Introduction

In erect posture following parts of the foot touch the ground (Fig. 19.1).
- The heel
- Lateral margin of foot
- Ball of the foot
  (The part under the heads of metatarsals)
- Pads of the distal phalanges.

The medial margin of the foot is arched upwards between the heel and the ball of the great toe, forming a *visible medial longitudinal arch*. But, though the lateral margin of the foot is in contact with the ground, all the bones of this side of the foot do not bear with the equal pressure on the ground. Like the medial longitudinal arch, there is a bony longitudinal arch extending from the calcaneus to the heads of the lateral metatarsals. But the *lateral longitudinal arch* is much flatter than the medial.

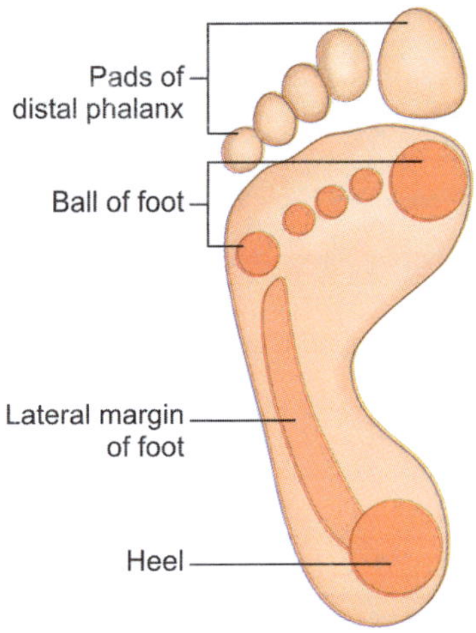

In addition to the longitudinal arches, foot presents *one transverse arch*. The transverse arch, in reality, is only the half of an arch, completed by the same of the opposite foot placed side by side. It is composed of cuboid and three cuneiforms with the bases of the five metatarsals.

There is no existence of transverse arch opposite the level of the heads of the metatarsals, as heads of all the five metatarsals touch on the ground, though the heads of the first and the fifth bear more weight than the others.

Fig. 19.1: Parts of the sole of foot touching the ground in erect posture.

Bony Configuration of the Arches

Medial Longitudinal Arch (Fig. 19.2)
(From behind forwards)
- Calcaneus
- Talus

- Navicular
- Three cuneiforms
- Medial three metatarsals.

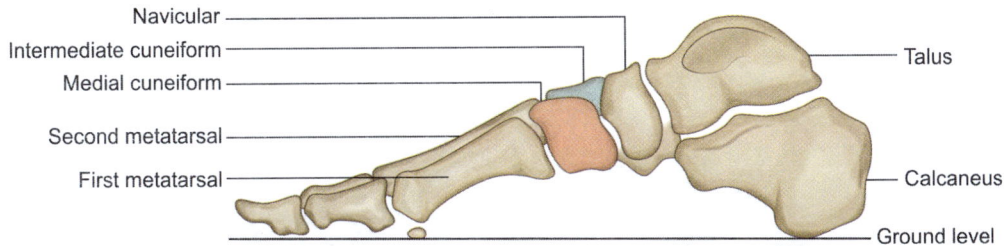

Fig. 19.2: Bony configuration of medial longitudinal arch of right foot.

Lateral Longitudinal Arch (Fig. 19.3)
(From behind forwards)

- Calcaneus
- Cuboid
- Lateral two metatarsals.

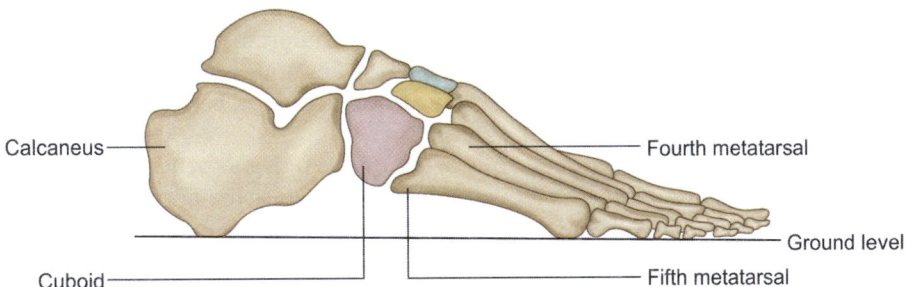

Fig. 19.3: Bony configuation of lateral longitudinal arch of right foot.

Transverse Arch (Fig. 19.4)
(From lateral to medial)

- Cuboid
- Three cuneiform, and in front of these are
- Bases of the metatarsal bones.

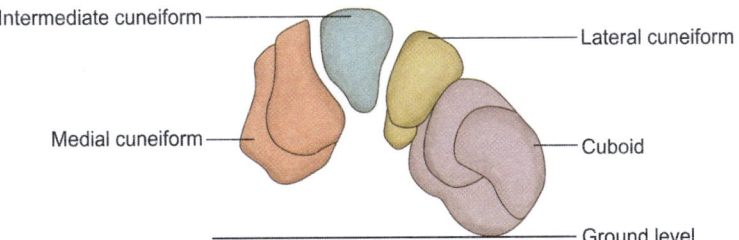

Fig. 19.4: Transverse arch of foot is truely the half of an arch formed by mainly four tarsal bones.

Structural Mechanism of Arch Support (Fig. 19.5)

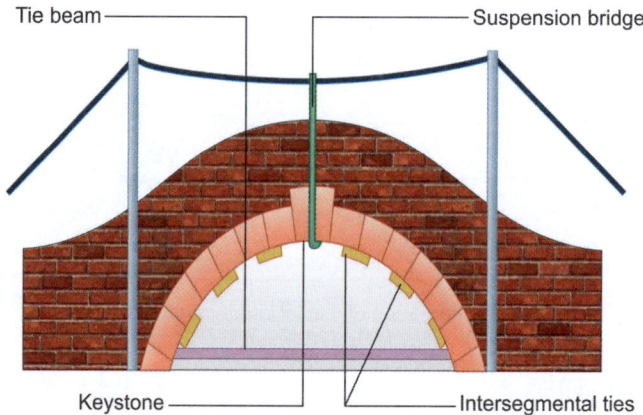

Fig. 19.5: Structural mechanism of arch of foot can be compared with that of an arched bridge.

Load of body weight in erect posture and during propagation is supported and transmitted through the arch of foot in a similar fashion, as it is done by an arched stone bridge carrying heavy traffic load. For this, following architectural mechanisms come into force.
- **Shape of the stones**: *Wedge-shaped stones* will be functioning most effectively. The narrower side of the wedge must be directed inferiorly. The most important stone occupying the center is known as the **'keystone'. Talus** is considered as the keystone of bony arch of foot.
- **Intersegmental ties**: Intertarsal ligaments, like **spring ligament**, act in the similar fashion as the **metal staples** interlock the adjacent stones.
- **Tie beams**: A tie beam connecting the ends of the bridge prevents separation of the pillars at both ends. **Abductor hallucis** on the medial side of foot plays a similar role.
- **Suspension bridge**: It suspends the arch of the bridge from above. Pull of the ligament or long tendon from above acts as the suspension bridge for the arch of foot.

Factors Maintaining the Arches of Foot

Medial Longitudinal Arch (Figs. 19.6A and B)
- **Bony configuration and the keystone**
  - *Posterior pillar*: Medial half of calcaneus
  - *Anterior pillar:* Heads of the medial three metatarsals
  - *Keystone (summit):* Talus.
- **Intersegmental ties (staples)**
  The plantar ligaments of the medial side of the foot, which are stronger than the dorsal ligaments, are intersegmental ties. **Spring ligament** is most important.
- **Tie beams**
  - Medial part of plantar aponeurosis
  - Medial part of flexor digitorum brevis
  - Abductor hallucis
  - Flexor hallucis brevis.
- **Suspension bridge from above**
  - Tibialis anterior
  - Deltoid ligament
  - Flexor hallucis longus.

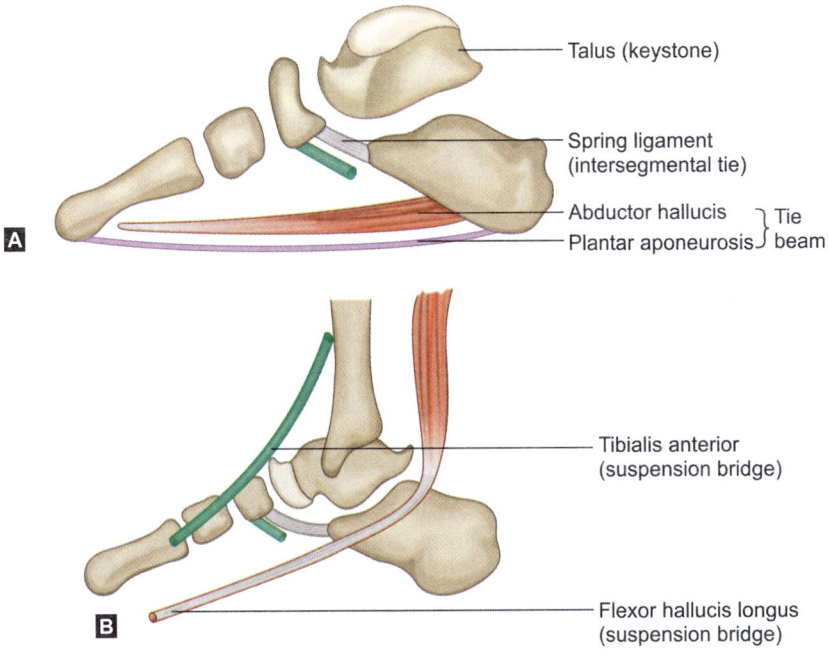

Figs. 19.6A and B: Factors maintaining medial longitudinal arch of foot.

Lateral Longitudinal Arch (Figs. 19.7A and B)

- **Bony configuration and the keystone**
  - *Posterior pillar*: Lateral tubercle of calcaneus
  - *Anterior pillar*: Heads of the lateral two metatarsals
  - *Keystone (Summit)*: Cuboid.
- **Intersegmental ties (staples)**
  - Long and short plantar ligaments
  - Origin of short muscles from adjacent bones.
- **Tie beams**
  - Lateral part of plantar aponeurosis
  - Abductor digiti minimi
  - Lateral part of flexor digitorum brevis.
- **Suspension bridge from above**
  Tendons of fibularis longus and fibularis brevis.

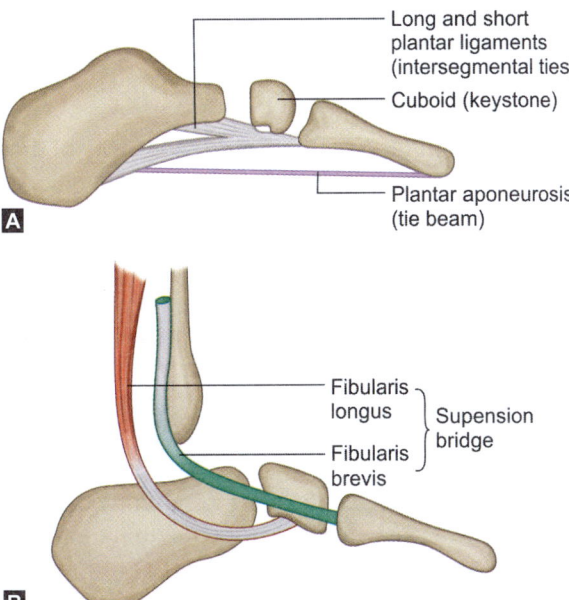

Figs. 19.7A and B: Factors maintaining lateral longitudinal arch of foot.

Transverse Arch

- **Bony configuration**
  As the transverse arch is truly the half of an arch, its lateral pillar is represented by the cuboid and the bases of the lateral two metatarsals.

- **Intersegmental ties (staples)**
  - Dorsal interosseous muscles connecting the bases of adjacent metatarsals.
  - Plantar intertarsal and intermetatarsal ligaments.
- **Tie beams**
  - Adductor hallucis
  - Distal part of the fibularis longus tendon crossing across the sole of foot.
- **Suspension bridge from above**
  Sling action of the tendons of fibularis longus and fibularis brevis.

Functions of the Arches of Foot

- **Distribution of body weight**
  In erect posture, arches of the foot distribute the body weight from its summit through the two pollars. The pillars are in the heel and toes. In case of the anterior (distal) pillar, weight is principally distributed through the great toe and the fifth toe.
- **Propulsive function**
  Powerful propulsive action by the gastrocnemius and soleus during walking, running and jumping is enhanced by arching of foot with flexion of the toes. During propulsion or propagation **spring action of the arch** of foot plays an important role.
  The sequence of events in walking is described as the following four phases:
  Phase I: Heel strike
  Phase II: Standing erect (weight bearing)
  Phase III: Push off through the toes
  Phase IV: Clearance of foot off the ground (swing phase), when the body is supported by the heel strike of the other foot.
- **Shock absorbing function**
  Elasticity of the arch of foot makes it as a mobile and pliable part of the limb which acts as a shock absorber and helps to adjust the foot on uneven surface of the ground.
- **Protective function**
  In addition to the other factors, concavity of the arch protects the soft tissue structures of the sole of foot including the blood vessels and nerves.

Clinical Anatomy

Infant's Feet

Flat appearance of infant's feet is normal and it is due to presence of subcutaneous fat in their sole. Arches of foot are always present since birth in normal babies, but they are not visible. The arches become apparent within a few months when the infants start walking.

Flat Foot (Pes Planus)

The flat foot or pes planus is the condition characterized by absence of the arches, especially the medial one. It may be *congenital* due to fattening of the bony configuration of arches. *Acquired* flat foot may result due to prolonged abnormal stretching or weakness of the ligaments and small muscles of sole of the foot. Flat foot may result *osteoarthritis* due to undue pressure on the bones or *neuralgic pain (metatarsalgia)* due to compression of plantar nerves.

High Arched Foot (Pes Cavus)

This is the clinical condition characterized by increase of the height of the arch of foot. This may result from the shortening or contracture of the plantar ligaments and muscles. It may be associated with the **claw foot** characterized by hyperextension of the metatarsophalangeal joint and hyperflexion of the toes due to deficient function of lumbricals and interossei.

Talipes (Clubfoot)

This is the congenital deformity characterized by *twisting of foot*. These may be of following varieties:
- **Talipes varus**: Foot is inverted and the patient walks on outer border of the foot.
- **Talipes valgus**: The foot is everted and the patient walks on inner border of the foot.
- **Talipes equinus**: The heel is raised with the foot plantarflexed. The patient walks on the toes.
- **Talipes calcaneus**: The foot is raised with dorsiflexed ankle. The patient walks on heel.

Commonest variety of the congenital deformity of the clubfoot is combination of two types, *talipes equinus* and *talipes varus*. It is known as **talipes equinovarus**. This is characterized by *inverted, adducted* and *plantarflexed* position of the foot.

LA 19.2 Give an account of the venous drainage of the lower limb. Add a note on its clinical anatomy.

VENOUS DRAINAGE OF LOWER LIMB

Introduction

Study of venous drainage of the lower limb deserves special attention because the venous system of this limb presents some mechanism which helps to drain the blood centrally *against the gravity*. Incompetence or failure of these mechanism will lead to stagnation of blood. This will result in *engorgement, dilatation* and *tortuosity* of the subcutaneous veins, which is known as **varicose veins**. Stagnation of blood in the deep seated veins may give rise to a serious vascular complication, the **deep vein thrombosis**.

Classification of Veins

The veins of lower limb are classified into three groups:

1. Superficial Veins

These are great saphenous vein and small saphenous vein with their tributaries. They lie on the deep fascia in the plane of superficial fascia. The superficial veins drain their blood to the deep veins *either directly* or *through the communicating veins* passing through the deep fascia and muscles.

Structurally, the superficial veins of lower limb present comparatively *thicker muscular wall* with more elastic fibers. These veins present number of *valves* which direct blood flow towards the deep veins.

2. Perforating Veins

Perforating veins are *communicating vessels* which direct the flow of blood from superficial to deep veins through the unidirection of their valves. These valves are very competent to prevent the reverse flow of blood from deep to superficial veins even against the gravity.

3. Deep Veins

Deep veins are *deep to the deep fascia*. They are the venae comitantes in relation to anterior tibial, posterior tibial and fibular (peroneal) arteries, the popliteal vein and the femoral vein. Return of blood through the deep veins is facilitated by *more number of valves, pulsation of the adjacent artery* and *contraction of the muscles* related closely.

Factors Helping Antigravity Venous Return

- **Soleal pump**: Contraction of soleus and gastrocnemius pumps the venous blood more centrally. This is the most important factor helping venous return against the gravity.
- **Venous valves**: Valves are present in all the three groups of lower limb veins. All of these valves *act as one way traffic*.
- **Arterial pulsation**: Pulsation of the arteries which are adjacent to the veins are transmitted to the venous wall.
- **Negative intrathoracic pressure:** Negative pressure in the thoracic cavity sucks in blood from the lower limb towards the heart. This negative pressure in increased during inspitration.

GREAT SAPHENOUS VEIN (FIG. 19.8)

Introduction

Great saphenous vein (long saphenous vein) is the longest vein of the body extending from the dorsum of foot to the level just below the groin.

Formation

Great saphenous vein is formed as a continuation of the *medial marginal vein* where it joins with the medial end of *dorsal venous arch* of foot.

Termination

Below the inguinal ligament and inferolateral to the pubic tubercle, the great saphenous vein opens into the *femoral vein* passing through the cribriform fascia of saphenous opening.

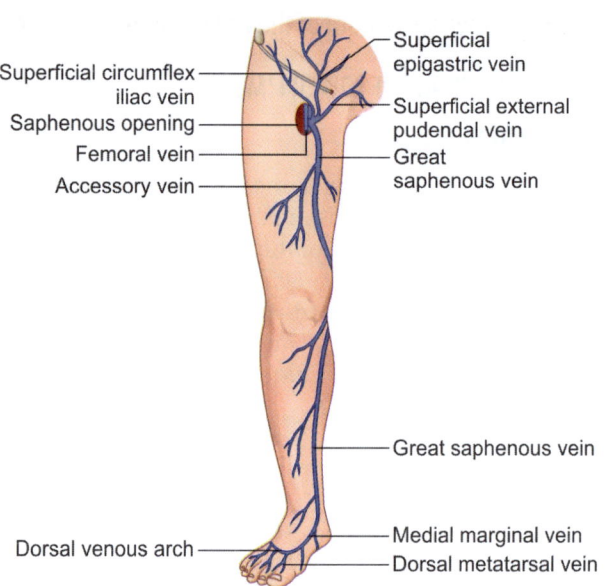

Fig. 19.8: Great saphenous vein.

Course and Important Relations

After formation at the medial border of dorsum of foot, the vein ascends in front of medial malleolus close to the saphenous nerve.

It crosses obliquely the lower third of medial surface of the shaft of tibia and runs obliquely upwards and backwards to the medial border of the bone. It crosses the medial side of the knee *one hand's breadth behind the medial border of patella*.

Then the great saphenous vein ascends along the medial aspect of the thigh *accompanied by the medial femoral cutaneous nerve*.

Finally, it opens into the femoral vein *passing through the saphenous opening*.

The vein is *often duplicated*, especially distal to the knee.

It contains *10–20 valves* which are *more in number in the leg* than in the thigh.

The vein lies entirely in the superficial fascia but is *connected to the deep veins* through channels which perforate the deep fascia and direct the blood flow towards the deep veins.

Tributaries

- **At the ankle**:
  - *Medial marginal vein* draining the sole.
  - *Dorsal venous arch* draining the dorsum.
- **In the leg**:
  - *Short saphenous vein* at the roof of popliteal fossa.
  - A vein from the *tibial malleolar region*.
  - A vein *from the calf.*
- **In the thigh**:
  Here the great saphenous vein receives may tributaries
  - *Posteromedial vein* (may be double): It is sometime known as *accessory saphenous vein*. It may receive communication from short saphenous vein.
  - *Anterolateral vein*: It starts from distal end of front of thigh and opens in the great saphenous vein at the level of upper half of femoral triangle.
  - *Preinguinal veins*: These veins are superficial circumflex iliac, superficial epigastric, superficial external pudendal and deep external pudendal veins.

Communications

The great saphenous vein communicates with the deep veins through the *perforating veins* which perforate the deep fascia. They are as follows:
- *Medial malleolar perforators*: Above the ankle, they are three in number, lower, middle and upper.
- *Below knee perforator*: One in number
- *Adductor canal perforator*: Near adductor canal.

Clinical Anatomy

- Varicose veins
- Great saphenous vein cut down
- Great saphenous vein in coronary bypass surgery.
  (*Vide clinical anatomy section at the end of this answer*).

SHORT SAPHENOUS VEIN (FIG. 19.9)

Short saphenous vein or *small saphenous vein* begins behind the lateral malleolus as a continuation of the *lateral marginal vein* where it joins with the *lateral end of dorsal venous arch* of foot.

In the lower third of the calf, it ascends lateral to the tendo calcaneus over the deep fascia. Then it inclines medially to pass along the midline of the calf. It pierces the deep fascia usually at the junction of upper and middle thirds of the calf to pass between two heads of gastrocnemius. But the vein may pierce the deep fascia anywhere between this point and the roof of popliteal fossa. It terminates in popliteal vein at a point 3 to 7.5 cm above the level of the knee joint. Lower and upper halves of the vein are related to the *sural nerve* and *the posterior cutaneous nerve of the thigh* respectively.

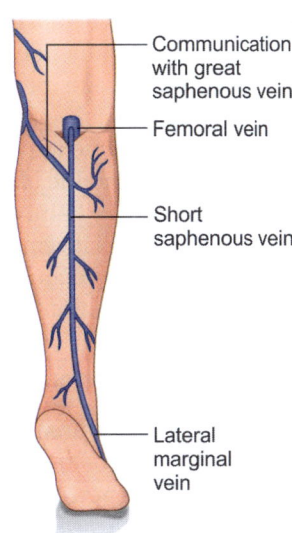

Fig. 19.9: Short saphenous vein.

Tributaries

- *Communicating veins* from deep veins of the foot.
- *Numerous small veins* from the back of the leg.
- *Anastomotic veins*, through which it is connected to the great saphenous vein.

Variations

The main variations are in relation to the termination to the great saphenous vein.
- It may join the great saphenous vein.
- It may split into two. One joins the popliteal vein and the other drains into the great saphenous vein.
- It may give a communicating branch to the accessory saphenous vein.
- It may end in deep muscular vein below the knee.

Perforating Veins

These are short venous channels which perforate deep fascia to connect the superficial veins with the deep veins for unidirectional blood flow.

The perforating veins or **perforators** are of following two types:

1. Direct perforators (Fig. 19.10)
These veins connect superficial veins with the deep veins directly just piercing the deep fascia.

2. Indirect perforators (Fig. 19.11)
They connect superficial veins with the deep veins through the venous network within the muscles.

Indirect perforators have an important role in **calf muscle pump**. This facilitates venous return in the lower limb.

The soleus muscle of the back of leg contains a venous network within it called **soleal venous sinus.** This venous network communicates with the deep veins of the calf directly and with the superficial veins through the indirect perforators. Contraction of soleus squeezes the veins to **pump out** the blood towards the deep veins and consequently **sucks in** the blood from the superficial vein because of one sided direction of all the venous valves. That is why the soleus muscle is considered as **peripheral heart.**

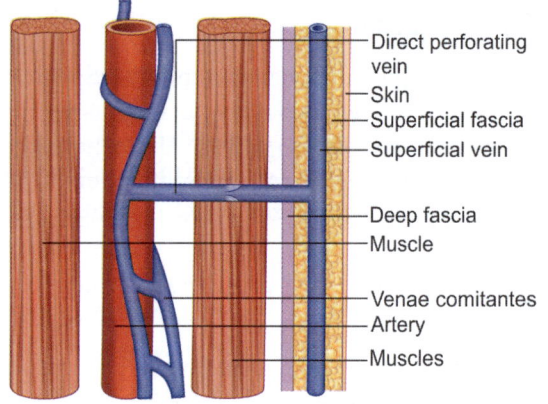

Fig. 19.10: Direct perforating vein.

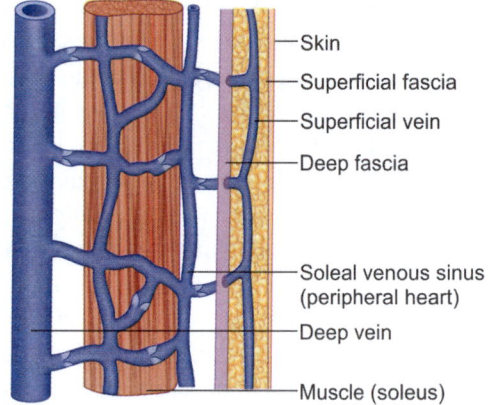

Fig. 19.11: Indirect perforating veins.

Positions of the Perforators

The perforators are *primarily classified* into three groups in reference to the landmark of the knee.
A. **Below knee perforators**
   They are *three* **medial ankle perforators** and *one* **lateral ankle perforator**

1. **Lower medial ankle perforator** is on the posteroinferior aspect of medial malleolus.
2. **Middle medial ankle perforator** is a little above the medial malleolus.
3. **Upper medial ankle perforator** is placed at the junction of middle and lower third of the leg.
   All of the above perforators are situated adjacent to the *lower third of the medial border of tibia* and connect great saphenous vein with the venae comitantes of posterior tibial artery.
4. **Lateral ankle perforator** is situated on the lateral side of the junction of middle third and lower third of the leg. It *communicates the short saphenous vein with the fibular vein.*

B. **Knee level perforator** is *just below the level of knee* close to the medial border of tibia. It connects the great saphenous vein with the posterior tibial vein.

C. **Above knee (Adductor canal) perforator** connects the great saphenous vein with the femoral vein at the level of lower part of adductor canal.

DEEP VEINS

Deep veins accompany various arteries of lower limb and lie underneath the deep fascia in relation to the muscles of lower limb. Their valves are centrally directed. Column of blood from the deep vein is emptied through muscular contraction and arterial pulsation. Once the deep veins are emptied, blood is sucked in from superficial veins through the perforators.

Groups of Deep Veins

A. **Deep veins of sole**: These are venae comitantes of medial and lateral plantar arteries.
B. **Deep veins of the calf**: These are venae comitantes of anterior tibial, posterior tibial and fibular (peroneal) arteries. They are within the tight fascial compartment.
C. **Popliteal vein.**
D. **Femoral vein.**

Clinical Anatomy

Venous Pump of the Lower Limb

Within the tight fascial compartments of lower limb, thin walled, valved venae comitantes (deep veins) related to contractile muscles and pulsatile arteries are *subjected to intermittent compression* at rest as well as during exercise or movements. *Compression of the muscles* and *pulsation of adjacent arteries* are the factors which move the column of the blood up. Emptied deep veins suck in the blood from the superficial (saphenous) veins through the perforators. The superficial veins are therefore emptied through indirect reason, but not due to compression forces, as they are in the plane of superficial fascia.

'Sole Pulp' and 'Soleal Pump'

Veins draining all the layers of sole of foot open into the dorsal metatarsal tributaries of the dorsal venous arch through the perforating veins passing through the intermetatarsal spaces. Contraction of plantar muscles pump out blood from the sole towards the dorsal venous arch following the direction of the valves. This mechanism of pumping of venous blood is known as sole pump.

Soleal pump is the mechanism by which blood is squeezed from the soleal venous plexus towards the deep veins due to contraction of soleus.

Varicose Veins

'Varicose veins' of lower limb is the clinical condition characterized by *dilatation, engorgement* and *tortuosity* of the superficial veins of the limb. This results due to stagnation of blood along with the back pressure from the deep veins and perforating veins. Causes are weakness of venous wall or incompetence of the valves.

Gradual degeneration of the walls the varicosed vein may lead to the formation of **varicose ulcer**.

Great Saphenous Vein 'Cutdown'

It is the procedure for the purpose of intravenous infusion. It is indicated when the subcutaneous veins for infusion are not visualized due to presence of fat or due to collapse of the thin-walled veins. Exposure of the great saphenous vein for cannulation is done above the ankle where the vein crosses over the anterosuperior aspect of medial malleolus. Its close relation with the saphenous nerve is to be remembered while skin incision is made. This venous cutdown is advantageous because it can be done very promptly during emergency and it is also chosen when infusion for a prolonged period is required. This procedure has a disadvantage that phlebitis (inflammation of venous wall) may be the complication.

The Great Saphenous Vein in Coronary Bypass Surgery

In patients with occlusive disorder of coronary artery due to atherosclerosis, atheromatous arterial segment can be bypassed by inserting a graft made up of a segment of the great saphenous vein.

Deep Vein Thrombosis

A rich network of vein is present within the musculature of soleus. It is connected in one side with the deep veins of the calf and in another side with the superficial veins through the perforating veins. Valves are present in the superficial, perforating and deep vein in one direction for flow of blood towards the heart. Network of veins in soleus, which can be considered as **soleal venous sinus** does not present any valve. Drainage is facilitated by calf muscle contraction. During prolonged rest in bed, either after major surgical operation or due to long duration convalescence or serious illness, stagnation of blood in deep veins of leg may lead to formation of thrombus. The dislodged thrombus may cause a serious complication like **pulmonary embolism**.

Chapter 20

Explanatory Notes (Clinical/Embryological/Morphological)

20.1 Coxa vara and coxa valga.

The angle of inclination of the neck of the femur with the long axis of the shaft is known as 'neck-shaft angle'. In adult normal individual, it ranges from 115° to 140° with an average of 126°. The angle is widest at birth and it diminishes gradually until the adult-life angle is reached. The neck shaft angle is lesser in females because the true pelvis is wider and the shaft of the femur is more oblique.

The neck-shaft angle varies due to *congenital defect in ossification of the femoral neck*. It may also show change due to *weakness of the neck* as a result of some *pathological process* like *rickets*. When the angle of inclination is *decreased* the condition is called *coxa vara*. When it is *increased*, the condition is known as *coxa valga*. Coxa vara leads to the following disabilities.
- It causes mild shortening of the limb
- It limits passive abduction of the hip.

20.2 Fracture of the neck of femur is more common in old-aged women.

In normal healthy individual, obliquity of the long axis of shaft of the femur due to neck-shaft angle makes the neck of the femur more vulnerable to fracture. When the knee is locked in erect posture, a rotatory force applied to the foot is greatly amplified or increased at the upper end of femur causing fracture of neck of femur.

In case of young adult, plates of compact bone, called *'calcar femorale*, extending from the linea aspera of the shaft to the posteroinferior part of the neck provide the strength and resists the incidence of fracture.

In older women fracture of neck of femur is more common due to following reasons:
- The calcar femorale becomes thinner and weaker due to postmenopausal osteoporosis as a result of estrogen deficiency.
- The neck-shaft angle is lesser in females as a results of greater breadth of pelvis and more obliquity of the femoral shaft.

20.3 Inguinal lymph nodes may be enlarged for a pathology in a distant area.

Inguinal lymph nodes receive the lymph from the remote areas of the lower limb. So the lymph has to travel a large distance. This is clinically significant. For example, in case of infection of the great toe, the inguinal lymph nodes may be inflamed and enlarged. The lymph vessels pass from the foot to the inguinal region along the direction of the great saphenous vein.

Inguinal lymph nodes not only receive the lymph from the whole lower limb, but also its medial group receives lymph from the following regions of the body.
- External genitalia
- Perineum
- Lower part of anal canal
- Uterus in females.

So in case of any pathological condition (inflammation or malignancy), the medial group of superficial inguinal lymph nodes is affected.

20.4 Femoral hernia is more common in females.

Femoral canal so also the femoral ring is a deficiency at the bottom of anterior abdominal wall at its junction with the front of thigh. Through this deficiency the abdominal contents may bulge downwards with the peritoneal sac to cause **femoral hernia**.

Direction of the femoral hernia: First the herniated mass passes *downwards vertically* through the femoral ring and femoral canal bulging through the femoral septum. Then it bulges *forwards* through the cribriform fascia over the saphenous opening which is the line of minimum resistance. If the herniated mass extends further outwards, it is pushed *upwards and laterally* below and parallel to the lateral half of the inguinal ligament.

Femoral hernia is more common in females because the femoral ring and also the femoral canal are wider in females due to following reasons.
- The lacunar ligament forming the medial boundary of the femoral ring is smaller.
- Other outlines of the femoral ring are wider due to more breadth of the female pelvis.
- The femoral canal, the medial compartment of the femoral sheath is more spacious in females as the femoral vein, lying lateral to the canal is narrower.

20.5 The pubic tubercle acts as a guide to differentiate the clinical diagnosis of the inguinal hernia from the femoral hernia.

Final outlet for protrusion of the inguinal hernia is the superficial inguinal ring. The femoral hernia protrudes through the femoral ring. The base of the *superficial inguinal ring* is formed by the pubic crest which is *medial to the pubic tubercle*. But the *femoral ring* is lateral to the pubic tubercle which gives attachment to the lacunar ligament forming the medial boundary of the ring. So the sac for the *inguinal hernia* protrudes through the superficial inguinal ring *above* and *medial* to the pubic tubercle. But the *femoral hernial sac* protrudes through the femoral ring *below* and *lateral* to the tubercle.

20.6 Special care is to be taken by a surgeon while incising through the base of the lacunar ligament to reduce (release) the strangulated femoral hernia.

The femoral hernia gets strangulated when the neck of the hernial sac is obstructed at the narrow femoral ring jeopardizing the blood supply of the herniated loops.

To release the strangulation, widening of the ring is necessary through surgical operation. The outline of the femoral ring is formed as follows:
- **Anteriorly:** Inguinal ligament
- **Posteriorly:** Fascia covering pectineus
- **Laterally:** Fascia over the femoral vein
- **Medially:** Free base of the triangular lacunar ligament.

So, the free edge of the lacunar ligament needs to be incised to relieve the obstruction of the strangulated hernia. Occasionally, the pubic branch of inferior epigastric artery is very prominent when it is named as *abnormal obturator artery*. This artery passes downwards in close relation to the base of the lacunar ligament. So, while incising through the base of the lacunar ligament to widen the femoral ring, the surgeon must take care of this artery, otherwise there may be the chance of hemorrhage during the operation.

20.7 Increased 'Q angle' more than normal may lead to chance of lateral dislocation of patella.

The 'Q angle' or Quadriceps angle is a narrow angle with the apex directed downwards, between the following two lines:
1. The line joining the anterior superior iliac spine and the center of patella—this line is parallel to the long axis of quadriceps femoris and the long axis of the shaft of femur.
2. Vertically upward extension of the line joining the center of the tibial tuberosity and the center of the patella.

The angle is normally 10° in males and 15° in females. It is slightly more in females due to more obliquity of the shaft of the femur because of greater breadth of the pelvis.

Up to the limit of this angle, dislocation of the patella upwards and laterally due to the oblique pull of the quadriceps is balanced by downwards vertically pull of the patellar ligament. If the angle is more than normal, more oblique pull of quadriceps muscle cannot be resisted by the patellar ligament. It will give rise to upward and lateral dislocation of the patella.

20.8 The tendency of upward and lateral displacement of the patella from the femoral surface is counteracted by the stabilizing factors.

The patella, developed as a sesamoid bone in the quadriceps tendon is mobile from side to side against the patellar surface of the femoral condyles. Though the patellar ligament is vertical in direction, the pull of the quadriceps tendon is obliquely directed upwards and laterally, parallel to the line of the shaft of the femur. So, when the muscle contracts, it tends to pull the patella obliquely upwards and laterally, leading to the chance for lateral dislocation of patella from the patellar surface of the femoral condyle. This is prevented by following three factors.
1. **Ligamentous factor**: It is the vertical direction of the pull by the patellar ligament and the tension of the medial patellar retinaculum.
2. **Bony factor**: It is the more forward projection of the patellar articular surface on the lateral condyle of the femur than that on its medial condyle.
   But unless the muscular factor comes into action, these two factors are not capable to prevent the lateral displacement of patella.
3. **Muscular factor**: The lowest fibers of vastus medialis which are inserted into the medial border of patella, are horizontal in direction at their insertion end. This plays most important role to correct the lateral dislocation.

20.9 The gracilis muscle is commonly used for transplantation in reconstructive surgery.

The gracilis is the long, thin, weak strap like muscle in the adductor (medial) compartment of thigh. It is also superficial in position and extends from the inferior ramus of the pubis to the medial aspect of upper end of the shaft of tibia. The muscle receives a long vascular pedicle from the profunda femoris artery.

The gracilis is used as a muscle transplant in reconstructive surgery for the following reasons.
- The length of the muscle is an advantage for the graft.
- This muscle has a long neurovascular pedicle which can be easily mobilized.
- As the gracilis has a negligible role as adductor muscle, it can be easily spared for transplantation. Gracilis is used for hand, pelvic and perineal reconstructive surgery.

20.10 Paralysis of gluteus medius and mininus leads to positive Trendelenberg's sign.

During walking, when one leg is lifted off the ground, the unsupported side of the pelvis will have a tendency to tilt or sag downwards. This is prevented by contraction of gluteus medius and minimus muscle of the other sided limb which is on the ground. As this limb is fixed on the ground, both the gluteal muscles act from below with their trochanteric attachment (insertion end) remaining fixed. Their contraction will pull the normal side of pelvis downwards thus preventing the sagging or tilting downward of the unsupported side of the pelvis.

So, when the lower limb of the normal side is lifted off the ground, the gluteus medius and minimus muscles of the paralyzed side will fail to prevent the downward tilting of the normal side of the pelvis. This feature is termed as positive Trendelenberg's sign. The condition will lead to *lurching gait.*

The lurching gait due to unsupported condition of one side of pelvis actually results for the following factors:
- If the gluteus medius and minimus muscles are paralyzed.
- If the head of the femur is not properly secured within the socket of the acetabulum.
- If the neck-shaft angle of the femur is not normal.

20.11 As the hip joint needs to be well secured to support the body weight, the stability is the more important factor at the expense of mobility.

Through the evolution of the bipedal animal including the man, polyaxial shoulder joint has become free to enjoy the freedom of wide range of mobility including circumduction. On the other hand, the hip joint is to take more load, as compared to quadrupeds, to support the body weight. For this reason, following stabilizing factors come into action for the hip joint.
- **Congruence of the articular surfaces:** Deep cup-shaped acetabular cavity is well adapted with the spherical head of the femur.
- **Acetabular labrum**: It is the fibrocartilaginous rim attached to the margin of the acetabular cavity. The labrum fits as a tight collar all around just beyond the peripheral margin of the articular surface of the femur head.
- **Zona orbicularis fibers** from the deeper part of the capsule spiral around the posteroinferior aspect of the femoral neck to its anterosuperior aspect to form a cuff.
- **Three strong ligaments**—iliofemoral, pubofemoral and ischiofemoral, strengthen the capsule from outside.
- **Short muscles all around the joint** play also an important role to maintain the stability as both of their origin and insertion attachments are very close to the joint.

20.12 Congenital dislocation of the hip joint is more common than the acquired one.

Congenital dislocation of the hip joint is common, occurring approximately in 1.5 per 1000 live births. It is bilateral in 50% of cases.

Congenital dislocation of the hip occurs due to following reasons:
- Congenital deficiency of the posterosuperior margin of the acetabulum, for which the posterior dislocation is more common.
- Congenital laxity of the capsule of the joint.

Disability and **deformity** are the following:
- Inability to abduct the thigh
- Shortening of the affected limb
- Lurching gait.

Acquired dislocation of the hip joint is less common due to stability of the joint. It occurs in automobile accidents when a person is riding a car, because the knee strikes against the dashboard of the car in flexed, adducted and medially rotated position of the hip. Cause of dislocation is the rupture of the posteroinferior part of the capsule which displaces the head of the femur posteriorly. It may be associated with the injury to the sciatic nerve.

20.13 Fracture of the neck of femur is common in old-aged females. It may lead to avascular necrosis of the head of femur.

Though the persons who are in habit of contract sports are frequently exposed to the trauma in and around the hip joint, the fracture of the neck of femur is not common due to following reason:
- Persons are younger
- Femoral neck is strong.

Neck femur fracture is common in old age groups and the incidence is further more common in females due to osteoporosis.

Broadly, femoral neck fracture are of two types—*extracapsular* and *intracapsular*. Intracapsular fracture is more complicated and it may lead to injury to the following arteries supplying the neck and head of the femur.
- **Nutrient artery**: It ascends towards the neck from the diaphysis along the cancellous bony tissue.
- **Artery of the head of the femur:** It follows the course of the ligament of the head of femur and supplies a small area of the head around the fovea capitis femoris.
- **Retinacular arteries:** These are so called because these arteries run along the **retinacular fibers of capsule** on the anterior surface of the neck. The fibers of the capsular ligament of the hip joint, after being attached to the intertrochanteric line of femur, are prolonged along the surface of the neck towards the peripheral margin of the head. These fibers are called retinacular fibers.

Among the above-mentioned arterial sources, the retinacular arteries are most important as these arteries are not only the main arteries supplying the neck, but also they supply the head of femur.

In case of intracapsular fracture of neck of femur, the retinacular fibers are torn. Tear of the fibers leads to injury to the retinacular arteries. For this reason blood supply to the major peripheral area of the head will be jeopardized resulting in avascular necrosis of the head of the femur.

20.14 Abnormal angulations of the knee joint are known as 'genu valgum and 'genu varum'.

Normal obliquity of the long axis of the shaft of the femur downwards and medially and, the vertical direction of the long axis of the tibia make a normal obtuse angle measuring 170° to 175°. This angle is open on the lateral side of the limb. It does not interfere with the transmission of the body weight because the adjacent articular surfaces of the femoral and tibial condyles are horizontal. This angulation is known as *physiological valgus angle* of the knee joint. If the angle is less than 170°, it is called '**genu valgum**' or '**knock knee**'. Again, if the angulation on the lateral side of the joint is more than 180°, the condition is called **'genu varum'** or **bowleg**. Both these conditions results in distruction of the knee joint cartilage—*arthrosis*.

Children are commonly found bow-legged for 1–2 years after they start to walk. Children of 2–4 years of age present the appearance of the knock-knee. If these abnormal knee angles persist in the late children, these defects require correction otherwise wear and tear of the articular cartilage develops.

20.15 Medical meniscus (semilunar cartilage) is more commonly injured than the lateral.

Menisci or semilunar cartilages are torn due to sudden twisting (rotational) movement of the knee joint in its semiflexed position. This injury is found commonly in footballers and athletes. Injury to the medial meniscus is very often associated with the tear of the tibial collateral ligament of the knee joint.

Medial meniscus is more commonly injured than the lateral because:
1. Medial meniscus is more fixed than the lateral. Beside its usual attachment of the anterior and posterior horns to the tibial condyle, peripheral convex margin of the medial meniscus is attached to the deep surface of the tibial collateral ligament along with the fibrous capsule. This attachment prevents necessary adjustment of the position of the medial meniscus between the femoral and tibial condyles during sudden twisting movement.
2. Lateral meniscus is free from the fibular collateral ligament and also the deep surface of the lateral part of the capsule.
3. In addition, while the tendon of the popliteus emerges through the capsule of the joint, some of its fibers are attached to the posterior part of the peripheral margin of the lateral meniscus. Through these fibers, the popliteus will pull the lateral meniscus outwards to prevent its compression injury between the lateral condyles of the femur and tibia.

12.16 Anterior and posterior drawer signs are positive in rupture of anterior and posterior cruciate ligaments respectively.

The cruciate ligaments are two strong intra-articular ligaments of the knee joint. They are named 'anterior' and 'posterior' in reference to their relative sites of attachment in the intercondylar area of the tibia. The anterior cruciate ligament extends from the anterior intercondylar area upward backward and laterally to be attached to two medial surface of the lateral condyle of femur. The posterior cruciate ligament crosses at right angle the anterior ligament passing upward forward and medially from the posterior intercondylar area of tibia to be attached to the lateral surface of medial condyle of femur.
- **Rupture of anterior cruciate ligament (ACL)** may occur when severe force is applied in anterior direction in semiflexed position of the knee from behind. It will cause forwards sliding of the tibial condyles from the femur. ACL tear is clinically diagnosed by abnormal forward mobility of the flexed leg. It is known as **positive anterior drawer sign**.
- **Rupture of posterior cruciate ligament (PCL)** occurs in athletes and players, while striking suddenly on the tibial tuberosity. It can also occur in case of head-on-collision of a motor vehicle, when the proximal end of the tibia strikes against the dashboard. It is clinically diagnosed by abnormal posterior mobility of the tibia in flexed leg. It is known as **positive posterior drawer sign**.

20.17 Housemaid's knee.

It is a clinical condition characterized by a soft cystic 'fluid-filled' swelling in front of the knee joint. It results from chronic inflammation of the prepatellar bursa lying between the skin and the patella in front of the knee joint. The swelling results due to regular friction of the skin against the patella. It is so called because this chronic prepatellar bursitis is commonly found among the housemaids as occupational hazard. If the inflamed bursa becomes distended with fluid, the swelling drops down below the level of knee. Though it is called housemaid's knee, this kind of bursitis may develop in following cases:
- It may develop following injury to the bursa due to compressive force resulting from a direct blow or falling from a height on a flexed knee.
- It may develop among the people who are in a habit of work with friction on their knee.

20.18 Clergymen's knee.

Clergymen are the Christian priests who are in a habit of kneeling during their prayers. Clergymen's knee is a clinical condition characterized by edematous swelling in front of the tibial tuberosity. It results from inflammation of the infrapatellar bursa which is subcutaneous in position and located in front of the tibial tuberosity and upper part of the patellar ligament. It is caused due to chronic friction of the skin against the tibial tuberosity which occurs regularly among the clergymen during their prayer with the habit of kneeling. However, it is also found among the manual labors with the habit of works for the roof or the floor tiles.

20.19 The popliteus is the unlocking muscle of the knee joint.

The popliteus is called the 'unlocking muscle' of the knee joint because, it corrects the locking position of knee joint which occurs during last 30° of extension of the joint when the lower limb is fully extended in erect posture for weight-bearing condition. The unlocking action of the popliteus is explained as follows.

When the foot is on the ground in erect posture, last 30° of extension of the knee is associated with the medial rotation of the femoral condyles on the tibial condyles. This rotational movement is an example of conjunct rotation of the knee joint and it gives rise to the following changes in the joint.
- 'Spiralization' or 'twisting' of the tibial and fibular collateral ligaments and the oblique popliteal ligament along with the joint capsule
- Intercondylar spines (eminences) of the tibia fit with the femoral intercondylar notch
- Menisci are tightly wedged between the condyles of the femur and tibia.

The above-mentioned changes of the knee joint in full extension can keep the joint in a secured position on prolonged standing even allowing the fatigued quadriceps tendon to relax. This is called locking of the knee joint.

From the 'locked position' of the knee joint in erect posture, when an attempt is made for flexion, the movement is not possible by the hamstring muscles, unless the medial rotation of the femoral condyles is corrected first through their lateral rotation on the tibial condyles. As the foot is on the ground, the insertion end of the popliteus muscle on the tibia is fixed. Contraction of popliteus from below rotates the proximal tendinous femoral attachment of the muscle outwards, causing the lateral rotation of the femoral condyles on the tabia which corrects the medial rotation of locked position of the joint. This action, performed by the popliteus, is called unlocking of the knee joint which leads to initiation of the flexion of the joint by the hamstring muscles.

20.20 The soleus muscle is called the 'peripheral heart'.

The soleus muscle forms the deeper part of the bulk of the calf muscle. The fleshy mass of the muscle contains a rich plexus of veins. This venous plexus is known as soleal venous sinus as these communicating venous channels are devoid of valves. The soleal venous sinuses have both way communications with superficial and deep veins. The superficial vein, e.g. great saphenous vein drain into the soleal venous sinuses through the perforating veins. On the other hand, the soleal sinuses drain blood into the deep veins like posterior tabial vein and fibular (peroneal) vein.

During daily life activities, e.g. in erect posture or while walking or running, contraction of soleus of calf muscle pumps the venous blood through its venous sinuses superiorly against the gravity via the deep veins. Once the soleal venous sinuses are emptied, they suck in the blood from the superficial vein through the perforators. That is why the soleus muscle is called the peripheral heart.

20.21 Fracture of the neck of fibula results in 'foot-drop'.

Foot drop is the muscular deformity of the lower limb manifested by unopposed action of the plantar flexors of the ankle as a result of paralysis of the dorsiflexors which are supplied by the deep fibular (peroneal) division of common fibular (peroneal) nerve.

Fracture of the neck of the fibula may lead to injury to the trunk of common fibular (peroneal) nerve, as it is closely related to the bone at this site. Arising from the popliteal fossa, the common fibular nerve passes downwards and laterally medial to biceps femoris and disappears in the substance of fibularis (peroneus) longus to lie in relation to the neck of fibula. So, due to the fracture of the neck of fibula, if the nerve is damaged, following effects will be observed.

Motor Loss

Main deformity is the foot drop. It is presented as plantar flexed position of the ankle due to unopposed action of the plantar flexors as a result of paralysis of dorsiflexors supplied by fibers of the deep fibular division of the common fibular nerve.

In addition, foot will be in adducted and inverted position due to paralysis of fibularis (peroneus) longus and brevis which are evertors and supplied by the superficial fibular (peroneal) branch of the common fibular (peroneal) nerve.

Sensory Loss

Along with the 'foot drop' and other motor deformities, common fibular (peroneal) nerve lesion at the neck of fibula will cause loss of cutaneous sensation on the lateral aspect of the leg and the dorsum of the foot.

20.22 Ankle sprain is usually common in plantar flexed position of the foot.

Ankle joint is also called the talocrural joint as it is the articulation between the talus of foot and the bones of the cruris (leg)—tibia and fibula. The wedge-shaped trochlea of the talus, being broader in front than behind, fits with the tibiofibular socket (mortis) formed by medial malleolus and inferior surface of lower end of the tibia and the lateral malleolus of the fibula. In addition, the joint is supported by medial collateral ligament (deltoid ligament) and lateral collateral ligament (talofibular and calcaneofibular ligament).

As the trochea of the talus is broader anteriorly, during dorsiflexed position of the ankle, wider anterior part of the trochlea is pushed posteriorly to become tightly packed within the tibiofibular mortise to make the ankle joint more stable. It is called 'close-pack position' of the ankle joint.

On the other hand, during plantar flexion, the trochlea of the talus moves forwards and downwards, so its narrower posterior part comes in relation with the mortise making the grip loose. So the ankle will have a chance of twist through inversion or eversion with stretching of the collateral ligaments causing ankle sprain in plantar-flexed position of the foot.

20.23 Pott's fracture is the most common ankle fracture that occurs when one's foot is caught within the hole of ground (rabbit hole).

When the foot of a person is caught within a ground hole it leads to the following series of injuries.
- First, the affected lower limb with the tibia rotates medially with the foot strongly held within the hole. It leads to *spiral fracture of the lateral malleolus* of the fibula.
- This is followed by an attempt for forceful eversion of foot. It causes avulsion of the tibial collateral (deltoid) ligament with or without *avulsion of the medial malleolus* of the tibia.
- The tibia is carried then forwards. It causes injury to the posterior margin of the lower end of the tibia (third malleolus) by the talus.

This three staged fracture of the ankle is known as *tri-malleolar fracture* or 1st, 2nd and 3rd degree of *Pott's fracture.*

20.24 'Flat foot' and 'clubfoot'.

FLAT FOOT (PES PLANUS)

The flat foot or pes planus is the condition characterized by absence of the longitudinal arches of foot, specially the medial one. It may be *congenital* due to flattening of the bony configuration of the arches. *Acquired* flat foot may result due to prolonged abnormal stretching or weakness of the ligaments and/or small muscles of the foot. Flat foot may result *osteoarthritis* due to undue pressure on the bones or may cause *neuralgic pain (metatarsalgia)* due to compression of the plantar nerves.

CLUBFOOT (TALIPES)

This is the congenital deformity characterized by *twisting of foot*. This may be of following varieties:
- **Talipes varus**: The foot inverted and the patient walks on the outer border of the foot.
- **Talipes valgus:** The foot is everted and the patient walks of the inner border of the foot.
- **Talipes equinus:** The heel is raised with the foot plantar flexed. The patient walks on the toes.
- **Talipes calcaneus:** The foot is raised with the dorsiflexed ankle. The patient walks on the heel.

Commonest variety of the congenital deformity of the clubfoot is combination of two types—*talipes equinus* and *talipes varus*. It is called **talipes equinovarus**. The deformity shows *inverted, adducted* and *plantar-flexed* position of the foot.

20.25 Incompetence of superficial and perforating varicose veins can be diagnosed through positive Tredelenberg test.

Defect or incompetence of the superficial and perforating veins can be confirmed through this test in a patient suffering from varicose veins of the lower limbs. In this clinical condition competence of the valves of these veins is lost or weakened to drain the blood against the gravity.

The clinical test is very simple. First, the patient is asked to lie down on the bed. Then the limb is lifted vertically up and mild stroke is applied from distal to the proximal end of the limb to facilitate the venous return. Next a thumb pressure is applied at the saphenofemoral junction 3–4 cm inferolateral to the pubic tubercle keeping the thumb pressure sustained. The patient is now asked to stand erect on the bed. Incompetence of two different veins are confirmed as follows:

1. If the thumb pressure is released immediately after the patient stand erect, varicose superficial veins will be again tortuous and dilated.
2. If the thumb pressure is sustained for about a minute, gradual filling up of the superficial veins indicates the incompetence of the perforating veins.

Chapter 21

SECTION 3: ABDOMEN AND PELVIS

Anterior Abdominal Wall

SA 21.1 Write a brief note on umbilicus with its embryological and clinical significance.

UMBILICUS

Umbilicus is a round prominent scar placed in a small depression in the middle of anterior median line of anterior abdominal wall.

This scar represents the healed cut end of umbilical cord which is cut to detach the newborn from the placenta after birth.

In normal healthy adult individual, umbilicus is at the level of lower border of body of *third lumbar vertebra*.

Embryological Significance

It represents the site of meeting of four folds (head fold, tail fold and two lateral folds) of embryonic disk.

Anatomical Significance

- Level of umbilicus is considered as '*Water shed line*' of anterior abdominal wall. Superficial veins above umbilicus drain upwards into the axillary vein and those below umbilicus drain into the great saphenous vein. Lymph vessels above and below the umbilicus drain into the axillary and inguinal groups of lymph nodes respectively.
- Belt of skin *(dermatome)* of anterior abdominal wall at the level of umbilicus is supplied by cutaneous nerves arising from anterior ramus of *tenth thoracic (T_{10}) spinal nerve*. Any pathological condition of viscera supplied by autonomic nerve fibers of same spinal cord segment (T_{10}), causes *referred pain* around umbilicus.

Clinical Significance

- Umbilicus is the site of anastomosis between the veins of portal system draining gut with its associated organs and systemic system draining the body wall. In case of diseases due to portal venous obstruction, superficial veins around umbilicus become engorged and tortuous in a radiating fashion which is known as **Caput Medusa (Fig. 21.1)**. It is so called because the dilated veins look like snakes radiating from the head of Greek goddess Medusa.

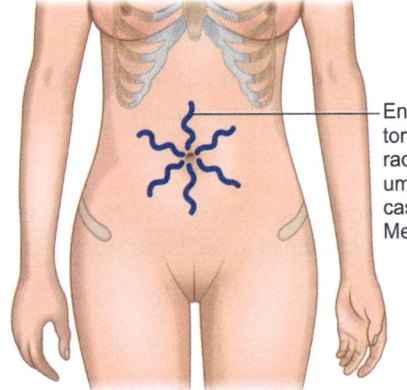

Engorged and tortuous veins radiating from umbilicus in case of Caput Medusa

Fig. 21.1: Caput Medusa.

- Due to *deficiency in closure* of fetal umbilical ring at the site of umbilicus, a newborn presents protrusion of abdominal organ like intestinal loop through umbilicus which becomes visible through transparent layer of amniotic membrane. This condition is known as **exomphalos** or **omphalocele**.
- Due to *weakness or deficiency* of abdominal wall at the site of umbilicus, sometimes there is incidence of **congenital or acquired umbilical hernia**.
- In case of persistence of whole length of vitellointestinal duct extending from midgut loop to umbilicus, the communication may cause **leakage of intestinal content** through umbilicus (Fig. 21.2). The condition is clinically known as Meckel's fistula.
- When the *urachus*, representing the distal part of allantoic diverticulum, remains patent, **leakage of urine** occurs through umbilicus from urinary bladder (Fig. 21.3).

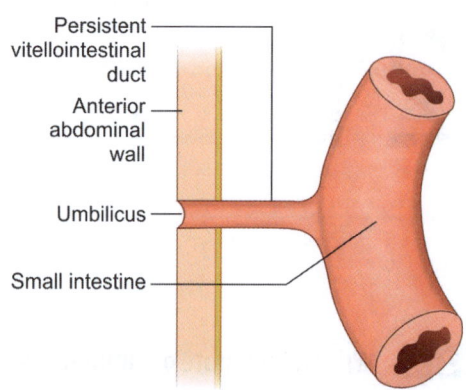

Fig. 21.2: Patent vitellointestinal duct opening at umbilicus.

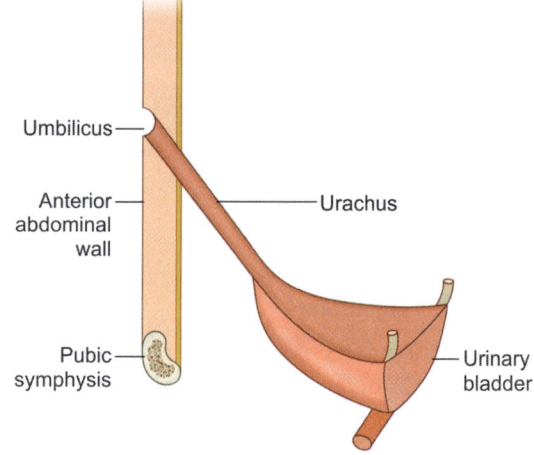

Fig. 21.3: Patent urachus communicating urinary bladder with umbilicus.

SA 21.2 Discuss briefly the external oblique abdominis muscle with a note on its specialized aponeurotic fibers.

Short notes: Inguinal ligament.

EXTERNAL OBLIQUE ABDOMINIS (FIG. 21.4)

It is the outermost sheet like muscle of anterior abdominal wall and the fibers are directed *downwards forwards and medially*.

Origin

The muscle takes origin by eight fleshy slips from the intermediate part of lower border and adjacent area of outer surface of lower eight ribs.

Insertion

1. **Lowest fibers** arising from lowest two (11th and 12th) ribs are fleshy and vertical. These fibers are inserted into *anterior two-thirds* of *outer lip of ventral segment* of iliac crest.

2. **Middle and upper fibers** forming major component become aponeurotic as approaching medially. Reaching midline the fibers intermingle with the fibers of opposite sided muscle and form a *linear and white* fibrous band which extends from the xiphoid process to the pubic symphysis. It is known as **linea alba.**

Specialization of Aponeurotic Fibers

Lowermost fibers of aponeurosis of external oblique are specialized and **condensed** to form following components **(Fig. 21.5).**

Inguinal Ligament

It is the *oblique lower condensed incurved* margin of the aponeurosis of external oblique which extends from anterior superior iliac spine to **pubic tubercle**. Average length is *10 cm*. Lateral half of the ligament is rounded cord like. Medial half is flattened and grooved upwards. Whole length of the ligament presents convexity downwards due to pull of deep fascia (*fascia lata*) of thigh which is attached to inferior aspect of inguinal ligament. Lateral half of inguinal ligament gives origin to the lower fibers of internal oblique and transversus abdominis.

Medial fibers of the inguinal ligament from following specialization.

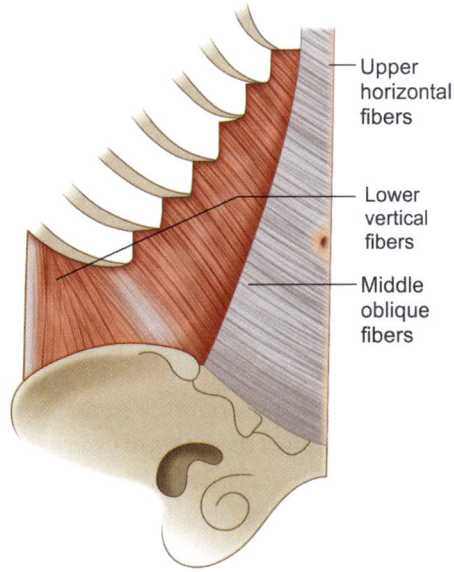

Fig. 21.4: External oblique abdominis muscle.

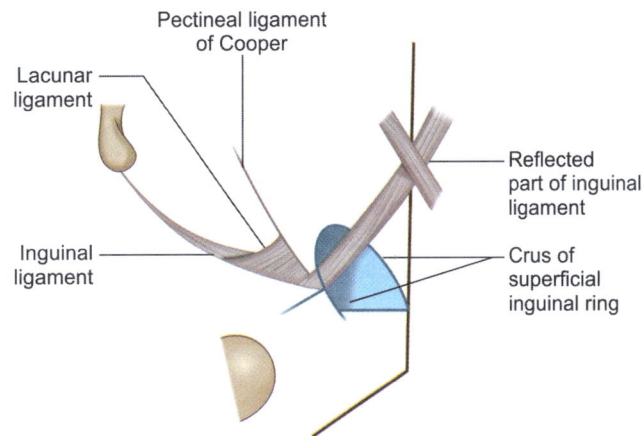

Fig. 21.5: Specialized fibers of external oblique.

- **Lacunar ligament:** It is also called *pectineal part of inguinal ligament*. The ligament is triangular in outline with the two surfaces being superior and inferior. Anterior margin is attached to medial end of inguinal ligament and posterior margin is fixed to pecten pubis. Apex of the ligament is attached to pubic tubercle. Base is free and slightly concave. It forms medial boundary of femoral ring.
- **Pectinate ligament or ligament of Cooper**: This is nothing but extension of aponeurotic fibers from posterior end of base of lacunar ligament. The ligament presents a linear attachment on pecten pubis.
- **Lateral and medial crura of superficial inguinal ring**: Protrusion of spermatic cord in male and round ligament of uterus in female through external oblique aponeurosis form mouth of a pouch above pubic crest known as superficial inguinal ring. Lateral and medial margins of the

ring are known as lateral crus and medial crus respectively which meet above and laterally at the apex of the triangular ring. Base is formed by pubic crest.
- **Reflected part of inguinal ligament**: Actually these are the fibers passing upwards and medially from lateral crus of superficial inguinal ring. The fibers passing behind the superficial ring interlace with the similar fibers of opposite side at lower end of linea alba.

Clinical Anatomy of Inguinal Ligament

- Curved upper surface of the medial half of the inguinal ligament forms the floor of the inguinal canal which is the deficiency or weakness of anterior abdominal wall for occurrence of the inguinal hernia.
- Lateral and medial margins (crura) of the superficial inguinal ring are connected by the intercrural fibers which prevent the protrusion of inguinal hernia through the superficial ring through contraction of the fibers of external oblique.
- Pectineal part of inguinal ligament (lacunar ligament) forms the medial boundary of the femoral ring which is the deficiency (gap) for occurrence of the femoral hernia.

SN 21.3 **Write a short note on linea alba.**

LINEA ALBA

It is a linear white band of collagen fibers extending along anterior median line of anterior abdominal wall. It extends from xiphoid process to pubic symphysis.

Formation

Linea alba is formed by interlacement of aponeurotic fibers of external oblique, internal oblique and transversus abdominis of both sides.

Layers of Fibers of Linea Alba

Before decussation in the midline, fused aponeurotic fibers of the three muscles of each side divide into *superficial and deep lamellae.* Superficial (anterior) lamella of one side decussate with deep (posterior) lamella of other side and vice versa. It provides additional strength to linea alba.

Weakness of Linea Alba

As the blood vessels fail to reach the midline, linea alba in the midline is *comparatively avascular*. Collagen fibers of the aponeurosis along the line of linea alba are *comparatively thinner*. Because of these two reasons, postoperative sutures along this line will have less chance of healing or union. That is why, paramedian incision, which is a little away from the midline is preferred in case of any abdominal operation.

Clinical Anatomy

Weakness or deficiency of broader and thinner supraumbilical part of linea alba may give rise to ventral (epigastric) hernia.

SN 21.4 Write a brief note on the rectus abdominis and pyramidalis muscles.

RECTUS ABDOMINIS MUSCLE (FIG. 21.6)

The muscle is so called because of its straight vertical disposition on either side of midline of anterior abdominal wall.

Origin

Origin of the muscle is **tendinous** by following two heads.
1. **Medial:** From ventral pubic ligament on anterior aspect of pubic symphysis.
2. **Lateral**: From pubic crest

Insertion

Insertion of the muscle is **fleshy** on the front of xiphoid process and on a horizontal lie at the same level on 5th, 6th and 7th costal cartilages.

Adjacent medial borders of the muscle of both sides are free and separated by linea alba.

Important Relations

The rectus abdominis muscle is enclosed by aponeurosis of external oblique, internal oblique and transversus abdominis which forms the **rectus sheath**.

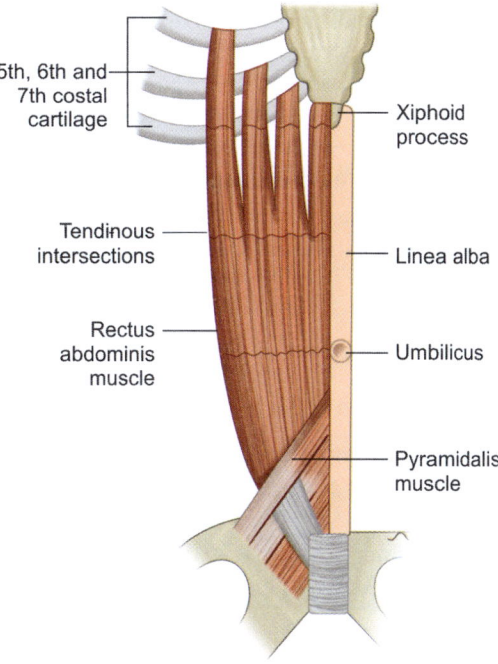

Fig. 21.6: Rectus abdominis and pyramidalis muscles.

Tendinous Intersections

These are 3 to 4 zigzag horizontal fibrous bands on the anterior surface of rectus abdominis muscle. Through these fibrous bands anterior surface of rectus abdominis muscle is fixed to posterior surface of aponeurotic anterior wall of rectus sheath.

Level of the intersections are following:
- At the level of xiphiod process
- At the level of umbilicus
- Midway between xiphoid process and umbilicus
- *Occasionally,* one below the level of umbilicus.

Significance of Intersections
- Tendinous intersections signify that rectus abdominis is embryologically segmental in origin
- The intersections divide the elongated muscle into shorter segments which helps in better force of contraction.

Posterior surface of rectus abdominis is related to *superior and inferior epigastric arteries*. Upper end of posterior surface of the muscle rests directly on *5th, 6th and 7th costal cartilages*.

Posterolateral aspect of the muscle is pierced by entry of terminal part of *lower five intercostal and subcostal nerves*.

Nerve Supply
Lower five intercostal nerves and subcostal nerve.

Actions
- Rectus abdominis muscle along with its sheath formed by aponeurosis of flat muscles supports abdominal viscera.
- Rectus abdominis of both sides acting together is a flexor of vertebral column.

PYRAMIDALIS MUSCLE (FIG. 21.6)
This is a rudimentary triangular muscle, not always found in human body, situated in front of lower end of rectus abdominis.

Origin
It arises through a round tendon from the front of body of pubis.

Insertion
To the lower end of linea alba.

Nerve Supply
Subcostal nerve.

Action
Tensor to linea alba, although significance of this action is not clear.

LA 21.5 **Discuss briefly the rectus sheath with a note on its clinical anatomy.**

RECTUS SHEATH
Definition
It is an aponeurotic covering which encloses the rectus abdominis muscle with pyramidalis if present.

Walls
Rectus sheath presents two walls—*anterior* and *posterior.*

Basic Difference between the Two Walls
- **Anterior wall** is **complete** all through the length but ***not uniform in*** composition. It is *adherent* to rectus abdominis muscle through tendinous intersections.
- **Posterior wall** is **incomplete** at the upper end and below the level of midpoint between umbilicus and symphysis pubis. But it is ***uniform in composition*** where it is present.

Formation of the Sheath
- **Above costal margin (Fig. 21.7A):**
    - Anterior wall is formed by aponeurosis of external oblique only.
    - Posterior wall is deficient. The muscle directly is in contact with 5th, 6th and 7th costal cartilages.

- **Up to the level of midpoint between umbilicus and symphysis pubis (Fig. 21.7B):**
  - Anterior wall is formed by the aponeurosis of external oblique fused with split up anterior lamina of aponeurosis of internal oblique
  - Posterior wall is formed by split up posterior lamina of aponeurosis of internal oblique and the aponeurosis of transversus abdominis.
  - As below this level, aponeurosis of all the three muscles come in front of rectus abdominis, lower margin of posterior wall forms a cresentic margin which is known as **arcuate line of Douglas**.
- **Below the level of arcuate line (Fig. 21.7C):**
  - Anterior wall is formed by fused aponeurosis of all the three flat muscles. Due to the deficiency of posterior wall, rectus abdominis muscle is directly in contact with fascia transversalis posteriorly.
  - Both the walls of rectus sheath meet with each other at the medial margin of rectus muscle and their fibers intermingle with the fibers of opposite side along the line of linea alba.

Contents of Sheath

- Rectus abdominis muscle
- Pyramidalis muscle if present
- Anastomosis between superior and inferior epigastric arteries along with the corresponding veins embedded on posterior surface of the muscle
- Lower five intercostal nerves (T_7 - T_{11}) and subcostal nerve (T_{12}) which enter the sheath from posterolateral aspect.

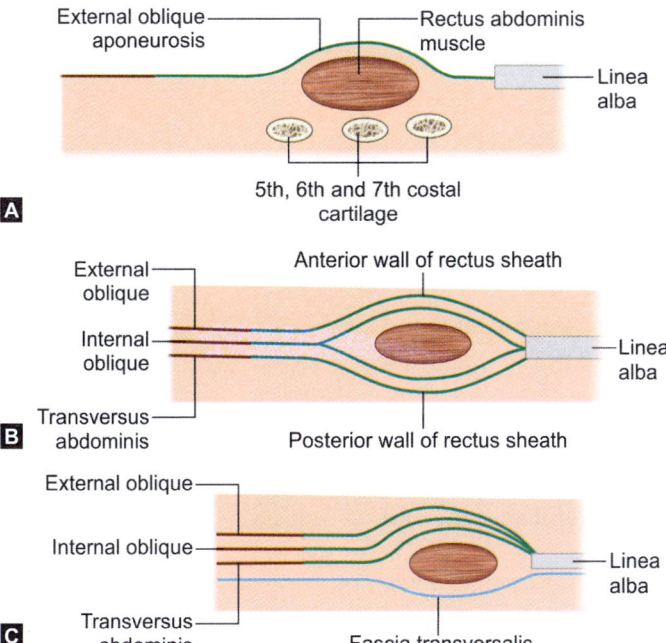

Figs. 21.7A to C: Formation of rectus sheath at different levels: (A) Above the costal margin; (B) From costal margin to the midpoint between umbilicus and pubic symphysis; (C) Below the midpoint between umbilicus and pubic symphysis.

Clinical Anatomy

- Toughness of aponeurotic fibers of rectus sheath acts as additional support of anterior abdominal wall at the plane of rectus abdominis muscle
- **Paramedian incisions are preferred in abdominal operation:** During exploration of abdominal cavity in surgical operation, abdominal wall is incised layer by layer. During these stages, first the skin, superficial fascia and anterior wall of rectus sheath are incised. Rectus abdominis muscle is retracted laterally to prevent undue stretching of nerves which approach from lateral aspect of the muscle. Posterior wall of rectus sheath along with succeeding layers of abdominal wall up to the parietal peritoneum are then incised in similar fashion. *Incision of these layers are preferred along paramedian line*, instead of midline incision because:
    - Along the midline, aponeurotic collagenous fibers show maximum lamellations and interlacement. During closure of incision, these will give less chance of healing of scar.
    - Maximum avascularity of the fibers in the midline will cause more hindrance in repair
    - Fibers of linea alba are thinnest, so weakest in the midline.
    - Postoperative closure line of paramedian incision opposite the line of rectus abdominis muscle will get additional support due to tonicity of rectus muscle.
- **Weakness of supraumbilical part of linea alba may cause epigastric hernia:** Supraumbilical part of the linea alba is 1 cm wide. In case of children with ill health, multiparous women giving birth to multiple children, or in individual with weak postoperative abdominal scar, protrusion of peritoneal sac with omental fat and portion of small bowel loop through the gap between interlacing fibers of linea alba may cause incidence of epigastric hernia.

> **LA 21.6** Discuss in brief the inguinal canal. Mention its shutter mechanism. Add a note on its clinical anatomy.

INGUINAL CANAL (FIG. 21.8)

Introduction

Inguinal canal in an oblique intermuscular passage in lower and medial part of anterior abdominal wall on either side of the midline. The canal is 4 cm long and is situated *above and parallel to the medial half of inguinal ligament.*

Extent

The canal is directed downwards forwards and medially from *deep inguinal ring to superficial inguinal ring* (**Fig. 21.8**).

- **Deep inguinal ring** is an *oval aperture* in the fascia transversalis situated *1.25 cm above the midinguinal point* which is the midpoint between anterior superior iliac spine and pubic symphysis.
- **Superficial inguinal ring** is a *triangular gap* in the aponeurosis of external oblique. It is wider than the deep ring which admits just the tip of a finger. The base of the triangular aperture of superficial ring is formed by

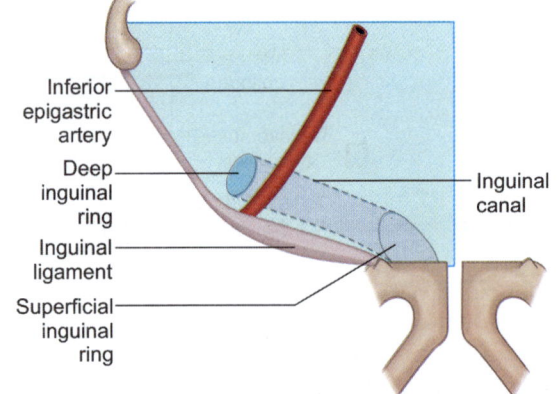

Fig. 21.8: Inguinal canal.

pubic crest. Inferolateral and superomedial margins are formed by condensed aponeurotic fibers of external oblique. These margins are known as *crura*. Near the apex of the ring two margins are linked by *intercrural fibers*.

These two rings are not the rent or deficiencies of respective layers of anterior abdominal wall. These are actually the sites of outpounching developed as a result of protrusion of structures through the canal.

Developmental Background of the Inguinal Canal (Why Inguinal Canal is Formed)

Gonads (testis and ovary) develop in the intermediate cell mass of dorsal body wall. From the caudal pole of the gonads a mesenchymal band extends distally and protrude through the lower part of ventral body wall in fetal life in an oblique fashion to reach up to the pubic region **(Figs. 21.9A and 21.10A)**. This is known as **gubernaculum of testis or ovary**. Distal end of gubernaculum is fixed to pudendal (pubic) region which is the site for labioscrotal swelling. **The course of gubernaculum through anterior abdominal wall explains the development of inguinal canal**.

In case of male, a slip from gonadal end of gubernaculum is attached to proximal end of mesonephric duct. This proximal end of mesonephric duct, connected to upper pole of testis through small ductules, forms epididymis. Continuation from epididymis forms the vas deferens. Contracture or shrinkage of guberbaculum is followed by the descent of the testis with epididymis and vas deferens through the inguinal canal into the scrotal sac. As the testis with epididymis reaches the scrotal sac, the vas deferens with its blood vessels, lymphatics and nerves along with the same for testis form a composite structure known as **spermatic cord**. That is why the spermatic cord becomes the content of male inguinal canal **(Fig. 21.9B)**.

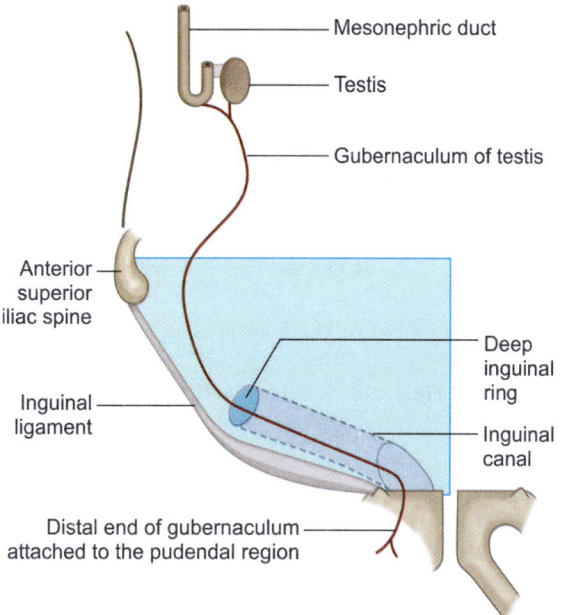

Fig. 21.9A: Gubernaculum of testis protruding to form male inguinal canal.

In case of female, in fetal life the mesonephric duct becomes rudimentary, but the paired paramesonephric duct grows. Its proximal part forms the uterine tube and distal part of both sides fuses to form the uterus. Gubernaculum of ovary extends caudally like that of testis to form inguinal canal of female. But unlike male, it gets attached in the middle at the junction of developing uterine tube and uterus. So, due to mid-attachment of the gubernaculum, ovary becomes unable to complete the journey of its descent unlike the testis. The ovary manages to descend only up to the level of uterus and uterine tube in the pelvis. As a result, shorter proximal part of gubernaculum extending from ovary to the junction of uterus and its tube forms *ligament of ovary*. The distal part extending from lateral angle (cornu) of uterus to pudendal region (labium majus) remains as a content of inguinal canal. This is known as round ligament of uterus **(Fig. 21.10B)**.

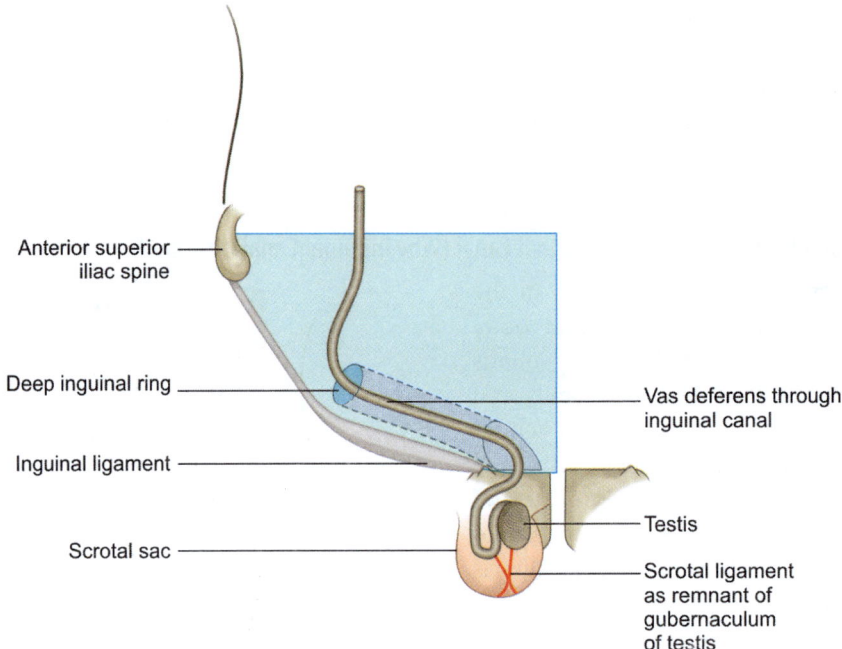

Fig. 21.9B: Spermatic cord becomes content of male inguinal canal due to pull of vas deferens along with descent of the testis through the canal.

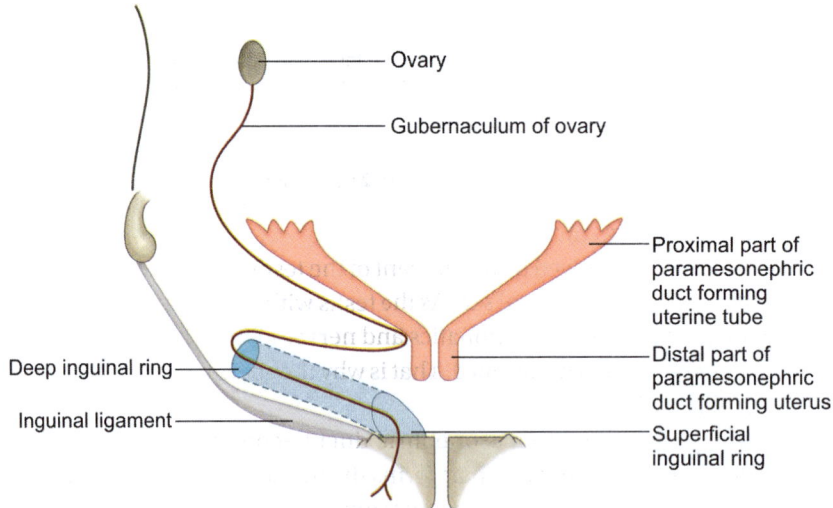

Fig. 21.10A: Gubernaculum of the ovary protruding to form the inguinal canal in female.

This developmental background explains the following:
- Inguinal canal is formed due to protrusion of gubernaculum of gonads from the plane of fascia transversalis (forming deep inguinal ring) to the plane of external oblique (forming superficial inguinal ring). **So the canal is not formed due to descent of testis or ovary**, and it is also very clear from above explanation, the ovary never descends through female inguinal canal.
- **Content of male inguinal canal is the spermatic cord** formed by vas deferens with associated structures, as the testis completes the journey of descent.

- **Content of female inguinal canal is the round ligament of uterus** which is the distal remnant of gubernaculum due to incomplete journey of descent of ovary.

Contents of Inguinal Canal

In Male
- Spermatic cord
- Ilioinguinal nerve (L$_1$)

Spermatic cord is a composite structure which contains the *vas deferens* as main component and associated structures eg. arteries of testis and vas, venous plexus called pampiniform plexus, lymph vessels, sympathetic nerve fibers and its coverings derived as prolongations from fascia transversalis, transversus abdominis, internal oblique and external oblique.

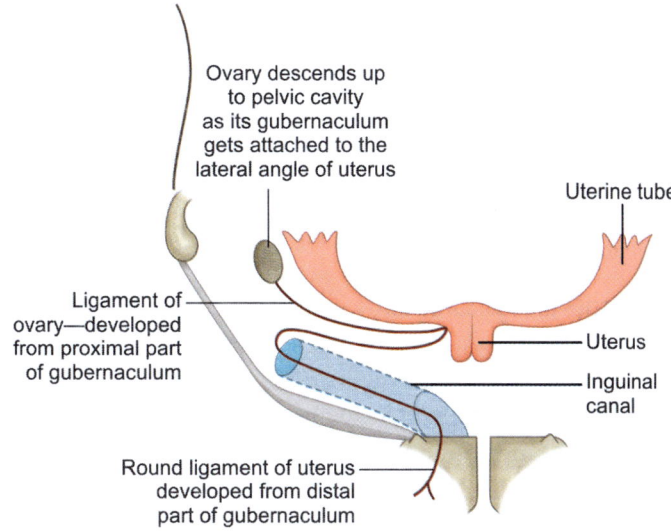

Fig. 21.10B: Round ligament of uterus becoming the content of inguinal canal in female.

Coverings of spermatic cord
- **Internal spermatic fascia (Fig. 21.11):** It is the prolongations of fascia transversalis from the level of deep inguinal ring. Beyond superficial inguinal ring, this fascia forms one of the layers of scrotum.
- **Cremasteric muscle and fascia (Fig. 21.12):** This is formed by fleshy loops of muscle fibers of internal oblique with transversus abdominis. These fibers arise from middle of inguinal ligament. Then the fibers form a loop embedded in a thin layer of fascia. This thin musculofascial layer passes through inguinal canal as a covering of spermatic cord. Finally the fibers, after coming out of superficial inguinal ring, form one of the layer of scrotal bag to hold the testis in male. Beyond superficial inguinal ring, cremasteric muscle fibers, while turn back to form the loop, are inserted into the pubic crest.

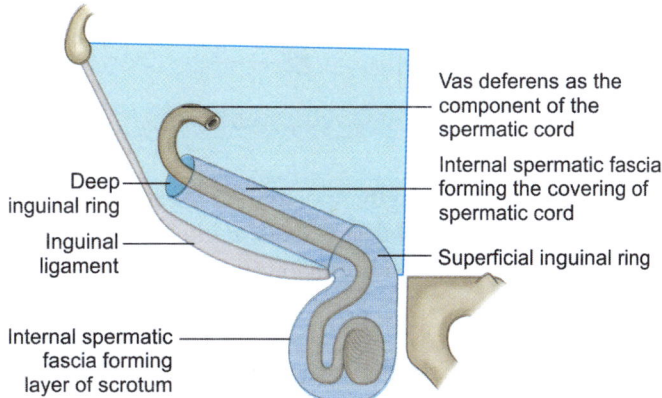

Fig. 21.11: Internal spermatic fascia forming the covering of spermatic cord and the layers of scrotum.

- **External spermatic fascia:** This is formed by prolongation of aponeurotic fibers of external oblique beyond superficial inguinal ring, so it forms the covering of spermatic cord distal to superficial inguinal ring. In addition, it also takes part in formation of layers of scrotum.

In Female

Contents of inguinal canal are:
- Round ligament of uterus
- Ilioinguinal nerve (L_1)

(Reason for difference in the contents of male and female inguinal canal has already been explained in the section of developmental background of this answer).

Boundaries of Inguinal Canal

Inguinal canal presents two ends:
1. Superolateral: Deep inguinal ring
2. Inferomedial: Superficial inguinal ring

The below-mentioned three differences between the two rings are the reason for *obliquity of the canal.*

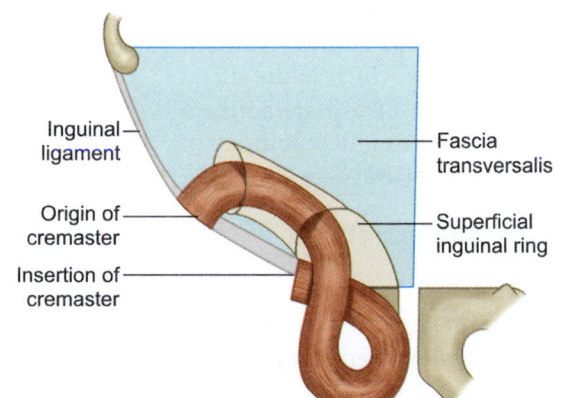

Fig. 21.12: Loop of cremasteric muscle.

- Deep ring is **lateral** to superficial ring
- Deep ring is at a **higher** level than superficial ring
- Deep ring is **in a more posterior plane** than superficial ring.

Walls of the Canal

- Anterior
- Posterior
- Superior (roof)
- Inferior (floor).

Anterior Wall

Muscles

- **Along the whole length**: Aponeurosis of external oblique **(Fig. 21.13A)**
- **Lateral half**: Arched fleshy fibers of *internal oblique and transversus abdominis* arising from lateral part of inguinal ligament **(Fig. 21.13B).**

Superficial to Muscles

Two layers of *superficial fascia* covered by *skin.*

Posterior Wall

- **Along the whole length**: *Fascia transversalis.* Beneath the fascia lie *extraperitoneal fatty tissue* and *parietal peritoneum* **(Fig. 21.13C).**
- **Medial half**: In front of medial half of fascia transversalis, posterior wall is additionally strengthened by a strong flattened tendon known as *conjoint tendon* **(Fig. 21.13B).**
- **Conjoint tendon or falx inguinalis**: It is formed by lower arched fibers of internal oblique and transversus abdominis muscles arising from lateral half of inguinal ligament. These fleshy fibers first form the lateral half of anterior boundary of inguinal canal. Then the arching fibers form the roof of canal and finally becomes tendinous to form posterior boundary of medial half of the canal. Conjoint tendon is attached to pubic crest and medial part of pecten pubis. Conjoint tendon strengthens the anterior abdominal wall at the site of superficial inguinal ring

which is a deficiency or weakness of the wall.

Roof

It is formed by arched fibers of internal oblique and transversus abdominis while these spiral over the canal from its anterior wall to posterior wall **(Fig. 21.13B)**.

Floor (see Fig. 21.14)

- **Whole length** of floor is formed by superior concave surface of *inguinal ligament*.
- **Medial end** of floor is supplemented by superior surface of *lacunar ligament* (*see* **Fig. 21.5**).

Shutter Mechanism of Inguinal Canal

Formation of the inguinal canal is the result of a developmental process. But once formed, it creates a deficiency or weak point in the lower and medial part of anterior abdominal wall. Through this weak point, there is chance of protrusion (herniation) of abdominal contents. These are prevented by following factors which are known as shutter mechanism of inguinal canal.

Obliquity of Canal

Inguinal canal is directed obliquely *downwards, forwards and medially*. Deep and superficial inguinal rings are not in same line horizontally as well as anteroposteriorly. The deep ring is at a higher level and more lateral in comparison to the superficial ring. It is also in deeper plane. Obliquity of the canal prevents protrusion of abdominal contents even when there is rise of intra-abdominal pressure.

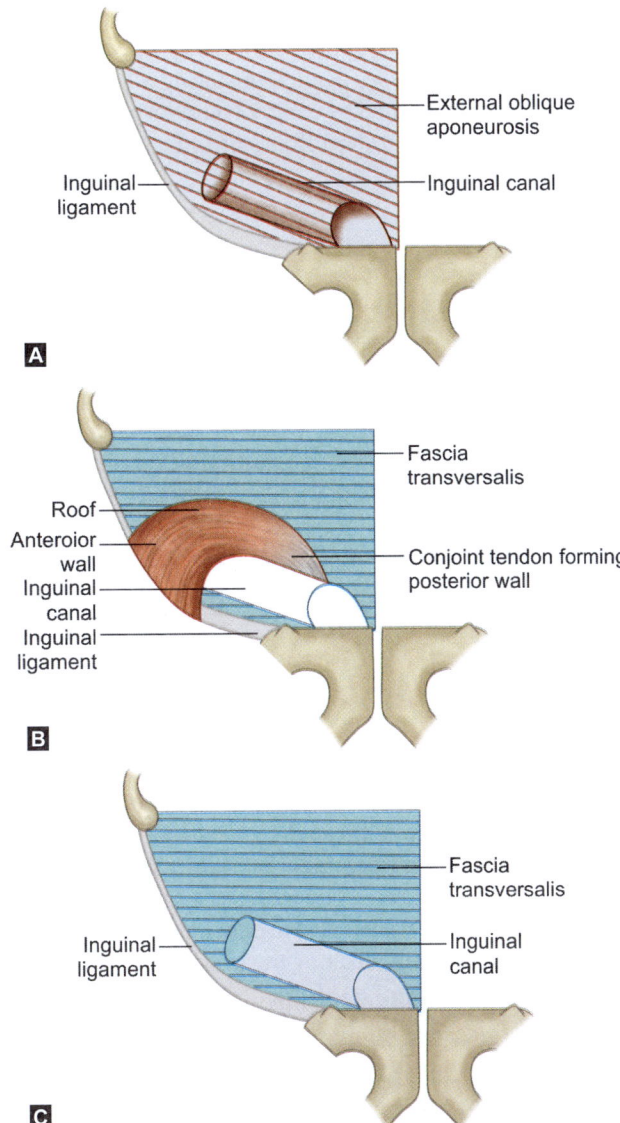

Figs. 21.13A to C: Different wall of inguinal canal: (A) External oblique aponeurosis forming anterior wall of inguinal canal; (B) Internal oblique transversus abdominis forming anterior wall, roof and posterior wall of the canal; (C) Fascia transversalis forming posterior wall of the canal.

Flap Valve Mechanism

Internal oblique and transversus abdominis play an important role in shutter mechanism. These muscles form anterior wall of inguinal canal laterally. But the same muscles, form the roof of the canal through their arched fibers and also form the posterior wall in the medial part of the canal as conjoint tendon. So these muscles, specially the internal oblique, have three fold flap valve action.

During their contraction, when there is rise of intra-abdominal pressure, these two muscles help in shutter mechanism in following three ways.
1. Anterior wall presses against posterior wall of the canal in lateral half.
2. Posterior wall formed by conjoint tendon, presses against anterior wall in medial half of the canal.
3. Roof formed by arched fibers of internal oblique and transversus abdominis presses down against the floor.

Ball Valve Mechanism

This mechanism *comes into action in case of males*. Rise of intra-abdominal pressure causing contraction of internal oblique and transversus abdominis, leads to contraction of loop fibers of cremaster. This contraction pulls up the 'ball of testis' to plug the aperture of the superficial inguinal ring.

Slit Valve Mechanism

Through this mechanism, *the slit of superficial inguinal ring is narrowed* due to shrinkage of intercrural fibers connecting lateral and medial crura of superficial inguinal ring as a result of contraction of external oblique.

Hormonal Mechanism

Tonicity and elasticity of anterior abdominal wall muscles are considered to be maintained under the influence hormones.

Clinical Anatomy of Inguinal Canal

Inguinal Hernia

An inguinal hernia is a protrusion of parietal peritoneum (sac) and mobile structures of abdominal cavity as contents (bowel loops and/or omentum) **through inguinal canal**. The protrusion of inguinal hernia may be through:
- *Normal opening*: Deep inguinal ring
or
- *Abnormal opening*: It is due to deficiency or weakness in the posterior wall of the canal formed by fascia transversalis all along the wall and in addition, conjoint tendon in its medial part.

Contents of the inguinal hernia may be:
- *Loop if intestine*: Bubonocele
- *Greater omentum*: Omentocele.

Complete and incomplete inguinal hernia

Inguinal hernia is called *complete*, when the herniated mass *protrudes through superficial inguinal ring*. When the contents of the hernia *do not cross superficial ring*, it is called incomplete inguinal hernia. So incomplete inguinal hernia is confined within inguinal canal.

Most of the inguinal herniae are reducible
- In most of the cases, contents of inguinal hernia can be returned back or pushed back to their normal position inside the abdominal cavity through proper manual manipulation or when the patient is in lying down position. In some cases, the hernia becomes irreducible, when it is clinically termed as **obstructed inguinal hernia**.
- When the loop of intestine of obstructed inguinal hernia becomes distended, ring or neck of the hernia seems to be further narrow in comparison to the distended loop. Then the hernia is termed as **strangulated inguinal hernia**. Compression of blood vessels of the strangulated loop at the site of neck may lead to *gangrenous change*.
- Out of different varieties of abdominal herniae, incidence of inguinal hernia is 90%.

Indirect inguinal hernia (Fig. 21.14)

Indirect inguinal hernia is the **commonest form** of abdominal hernia. In this variety of inguinal hernia, herniation occurs through deep inguinal ring lateral to inferior epigastric vessels.

Hernial sac protrudes through the inguinal canal. It is called *complete hernia* when it extends beyond superficial inguinal ring to reach scrotum or base of labium majus. While extending beyond superficial ring, inguinal hernia is *above and medial to pubic tubercle*.

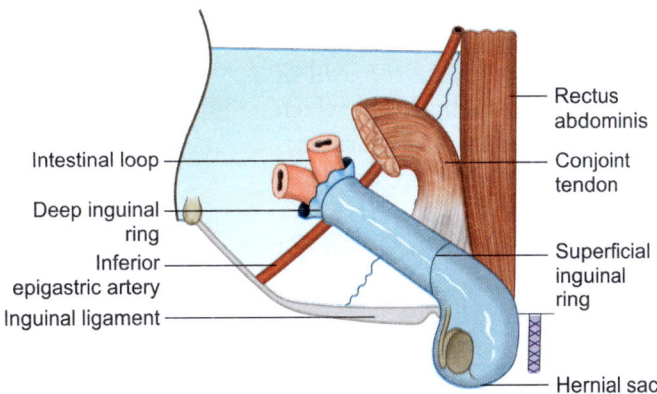

Fig. 21.14: Indirect inguinal hernia protrudes through the deep ring lateral to inferior epigastric artery.

Predisposing factor

Incidence of indirect inguinal hernia is because of congenital reason. In fetal life formation of inguinal canal is associated with prolongation (outpouching) of a part of peritoneal cavity which is pulled by a slip of gubernaculum of the gonad through the length of inguinal canal. This is called **processus vaginalis (Fig. 21.14).**

Normally the processus vaginalis extending through the inguinal canal gets obliterated beyond deep inguinal ring. In case of male, the part of processus vaginalis beyond superficial inguinal ring persist and gets invaginated by testis to form **tunica vaginalis.**

If the proximal part of processus vaginalis remains patent, it will maintain communication with main peritoneal cavity through deep inguinal ring. In female this is known as *canal of Nuck*. In both the sexes persistent part of processus vaginalis, which is prolonged from peritoneal cavity, beyond deep ring, through the inguinal canal and the superficial ring, *acts as a potential sac* for development of indirect inguinal hernia.

Important points related to indirect inguinal hernia

- Indirect inguinal hernia is more evident in case of childhood and young adults because of congenital reason behind
- It is 20 times more common in males than females
- Hernia sac is formed by persistent proximal part of processus vaginalis
- Coverings are formed by all the layers of anterior abdominal wall
- Neck of the sac is narrow at the site of deep inguinal ring lateral to inferior epigastric vessels
- Indirect inguinal hernia is more common in incidence than direct inguinal hernia
- Hernia sac extending through superficial inguinal ring is positioned *above and medial to the pubic tubercle*. It is an important point for differential diagnosis from *femoral hernia*, in which case the sac is *below and lateral to the pubic tubercle*.
- Hernia sac may extend down to the scrotum or labium majus.

Important points related to direct inguinal hernia (Fig. 21.15)

- It is so called as this type of inguinal hernia occurs directly pushing through the weak or deficient posterior wall of inguinal canal
- 15% of inguinal hernia is of direct type

- Unlike the indirect type, predisposing factor is not congenital. It is the weakness or laxity of posterior wall of inguinal canal in old age which is the reason for its occurrence
- Hernia pushes the anterior abdominal wall directly horizontally forwards, so not in oblique direction unlike the indirect one which is also called oblique inguinal hernia
- In most of the cases, it is bilateral
- It is rare in females
- Direct inguinal hernia bulges out medial to deep inguinal ring pushing through a triangular area of anterior abdominal wall called **triangle of Hesselbach**. The triangle is bounded as follows **(Fig. 21.15)**:
  - Laterally: Inferior epigastric artery
  - Medially: Lateral border of rectus abdominis muscle
  - Inferiorly: Medial half of inguinal ligament (base of the triangle)
- Triangle of Hesselbach is divided into lateral and medial half by the course of obliterated umbilical artery. These two halves are the areas of protrusion of **lateral direct** and **medial direct** inguinal herniae respectively
- Direct inguinal hernia does not traverse through the whole length of inguinal canal, but it bulges through the medial part of inguinal canal
- Sac of the hernia is not derived from processus vaginalis, but it is a protrusion from peritoneal lining which comes out through the gap between the fibers of conjoint tendon (falx inguinalis) of insertion of internal oblique and transversus abdominis
- As the direct hernia finds some degree of resistance to push through strong tendinous fibers of insertion of falx inguinalis, the hernia, even on both sides appears as a simple bulge on lower part of anterior abdominal wall
- Coverings of hernial sac is formed by fascia transversalis in both lateral as well as medial types, but in case of medial type, falx inguinalis or conjoint tendon is superadded
- In males, in most of the cases, it does not extend beyond superficial ring to scrotum.

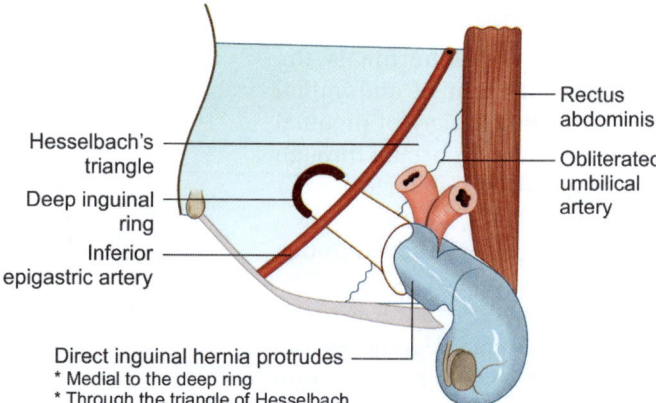

Fig. 21.15: Direct inguinal hernia protrudes through the Hesselbach's triangle.

Short notes:	Superficial inguinal ring; Deep inguinal ring; Conjoint tendon
Short answers:	Boundaries and contents of inguinal canal; Shutter mechanism of inguinal canal; Anatomical concept of inguinal hernia.

Chapter 22

Peritoneum

SA 22.1 Write a brief note on the primitive ventral and dorsal mesogastria.

PRIMITIVE VENTRAL AND DORSAL MESENTERIES OF GUT

Nature of splitting of lateral plate of mesoderm into somatopleuric and splanchnopleuric mesoderm and fusion of the corresponding components from two sides is something different in case foregut, as compared with midgut and hindgut. As a result, foregut is connected to both dorsal as well as ventral walls of body by double layers of splanchnopleuric mesoderm, known as primitive dorsal and ventral mesenteries. As because stomach (gastrium) is a part of foregut, these two folds of the foregut are actually named as **dorsal mesogastrium** and **ventral mesogastrium (Fig. 22.1A)**. Midgut and hindgut are suspended from dorsal body wall only by **dorsal mesentery of midgut and hindgut (Fig. 22.1B)**.

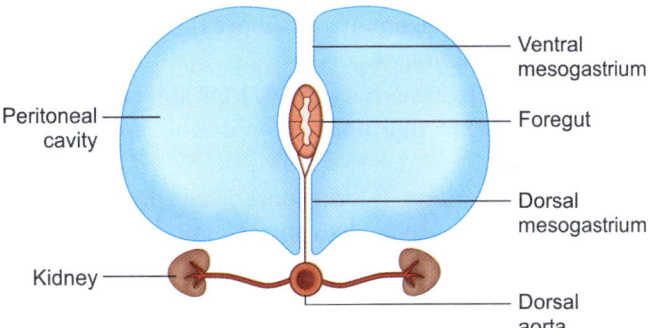

Fig. 22.1A: Developing foregut is connected to the body wall by both dorsal and ventral mesenteries.

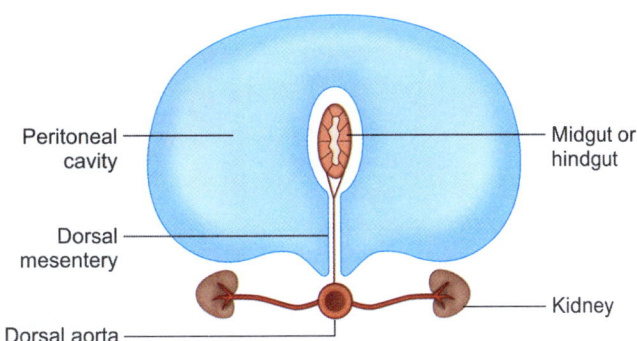

Fig. 22.1B: Developing midgut and hindgut are connected to the dorsal body wall by dorsal mesentery.

Further Subdivision of Dorsal and Ventral Mesogastria (Fig. 22.2)

Dorsal mesogastrium: Buds of mesodermal tissue develops in *left layer of dorsal mesogastrium*. These aggregate to form the *spleen*. Dorsal part of dorsal mesogastrium from spleen to kidney in dorsal body wall will form **lienorenal ligament**. Ventral part from stomach of the foregut to the spleen will form **gastrosplenic ligament**. Actually, dorsal mesogastrium is divided into following four parts **(Fig. 22.3)**.

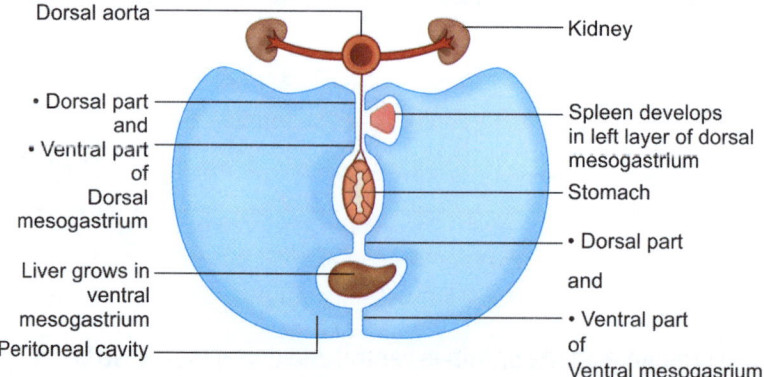

Fig. 22.2: Further subdivision of primitive dorsal and ventral mesenteries (mesogastria) of foregut.

1. **Gastrophrenic ligament**: It is above the level of developing spleen, extending from stomach of foregut to diaphragm.
2. **Lienorenal ligament:** It extends from spleen to kidney on dorsal body wall.
3. **Gastrosplenic ligament**: It is double fold of dorsal mesogastrium from stomach to spleen.
4. **Greater omentum**: It is the most distal part of dorsal mesogastrium, below the level of spleen, extending from stomach to dorsal body wall.

Ventral mesogastrium: A diverticulum, called b*iliary diverticulum* grows in between two layers of ventral mesogastrium from the junction of foregut and midgut. From this diverticulum, biliary duct system with gallbladder will be formed. End of diverticulum is capped by mesodermal tissue of septum transversum. It is called hepatic bud to form the liver **(Fig. 22.3)**.

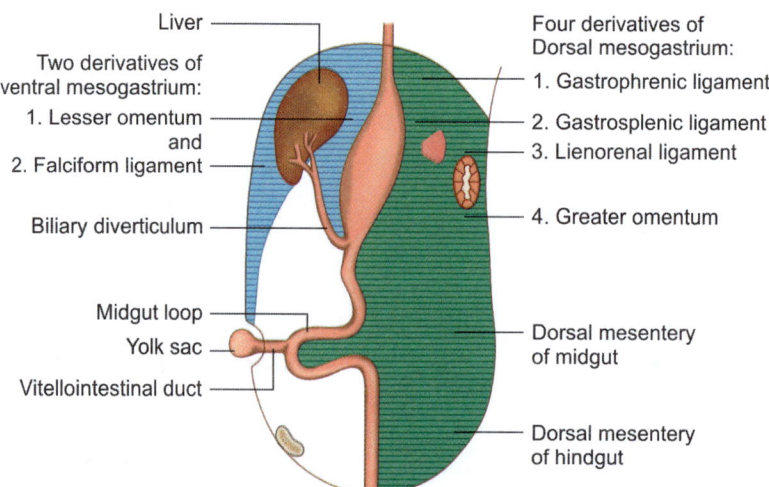

Fig. 22.3: Derivatives of dorsal and ventral mesenteries in sagittal plane.

Developing liver along with biliary diverticulum between the two layers of ventral mesogastrium divides it into two parts **(Figs. 22.2 and 22.3)**.
1. **Lesser omentum**: It extends from ventral border of stomach to liver.

2. **Falciform ligament**: It extends from liver to anterior part of under surface of the diaphragm and anterior abdominal wall up to umbilicus.

SN 22.2 Write a short note on the functions of peritoneum.

FUNCTIONS OF PERITONEUM

- **Facilitates free movement of viscera:** Visceral peritoneum covering the surface of the viscera is smooth and glistening. It *prevents undue friction of one viscera against another one.*
- **Lubrication of visceral surface:** Normal quantity of thin watery fluid (peritoneal fluid) in the peritoneal cavity constantly lubricates the surfaces of viscera.
- **Defensive function:** Peritoneum presents number of phagocytic cells. These cells possess the power to engulf (digest) microorganisms, so prevent infection. Besides, the lymphocytes present in peritoneal fluid helps for immunity or body defense mechanism.
- **Facilitates motility of the gut:** Peritoneal folds connecting some parts of small and large intestines, helps in free movement of those parts of the gut.
- **Carries blood vessels:** Peritoneal folds carry blood vessels in between two layers for the corresponding viscera.
- **Healing of wounds**: For example, after suturing of abdominal incision for surgical operation, fibroblasts are formed in the sutured peritoneal lining. It helps in healing of wound.
  Again, in case of inflammation of vermiform appendix, the greater omentum, a free peritoneal fold of stomach, is localized at the site of inflammation to seal the wound.
- **Peritoneal dialysis**: In case of impaired function of kidney (renal failure), toxic nitrogenous substances are filtered out through peritoneum as an alternative way of kidney filtration.

LA 22.3 Discuss briefly the changes in the foregut and peritoneum for development of lesser sac.

CHANGES IN THE FOREGUT MAKING PERITONEAL CAVITY COMPLEX

Changes in Borders of Stomach (Figs. 22.4A to C)

Fusiform dilated part of the foregut forming the stomach presents dorsal and ventral borders during initial phase of development. Surfaces are right and left. The borders of stomach shows following two changes:
- Ventral border of stomach undergoes almost 90° rotation to the right. Due to the rotation, ventral border becomes right border, so dorsal border becomes left border.
- Length of both the borders increases at a differential rate. Left border (original dorsal border) grows more rapidly than the right (original ventral border). So larger left (dorsal) border bulges out to become convex and called **greater curvature**. Right (ventral) border becomes shorter and concave. It is called **lesser curvature**.

Changes in Relationship between Stomach and Liver (Fig. 22.5)

Even after rotation of the stomach, the liver, growing in ventral mesogastrium, shows still ventrodorsal relation with the stomach. But finally this relationship is altered. Liver, growing in anterior plane, is pushed *upwards and to the right* mainly under the right dome of the diaphragm. The stomach, though in more posterior plane, is pushed *downwards and to the left*. So, section at the level of stomach will show cross section through lesser omentum which is a double fold of peritoneum extending from lesser curvature of the stomach to the liver.

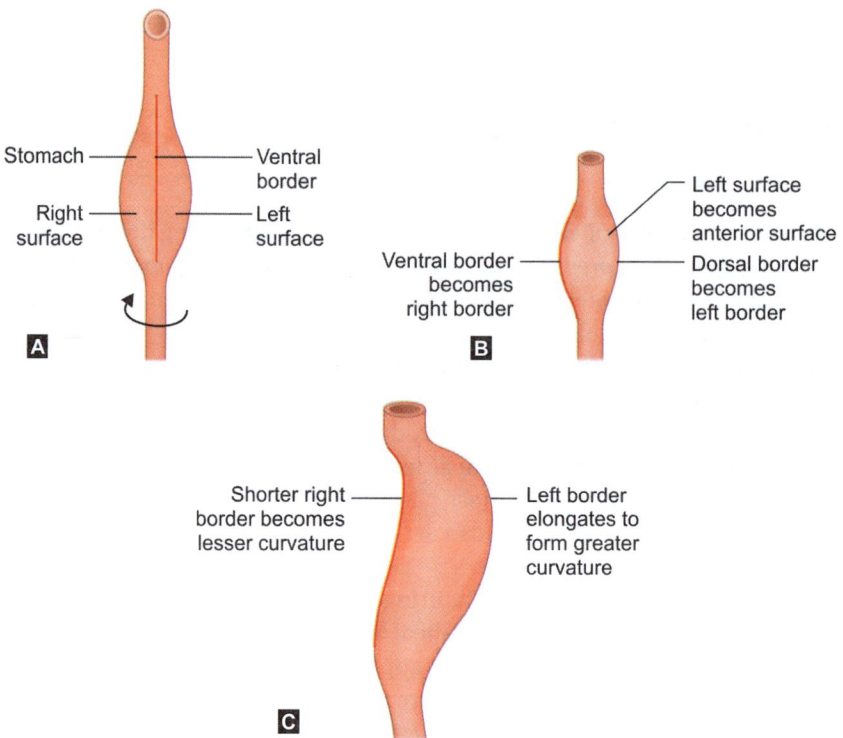

Figs. 22.4A to C: Changes in borders and surfaces of stomach due to rotation of foregut to the right: (A) Before rotation; (B) After rotation: (C) After rotation the left border elongates more than right.

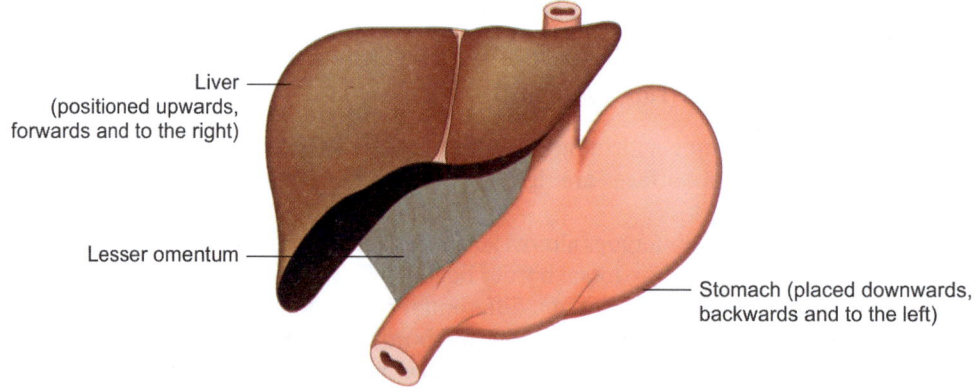

Fig. 22.5: Anteroposterior relation of liver and stomach is altered.

Spleen Pushed to the Left Growing in Left Layer of Dorsal Mesogastrium (Fig. 22.6)

As the spleen grows more and more in left layer of dorsal mesogastrium, it pulls the dorsal mesogastrium more to the left side. Due to this change, a part of peritoneal cavity falls behind the stomach which has already rotated to the right. This pocket of peritoneal cavity is known as **lesser sac of peritoneum (Fig. 22.6).** Towards the right, the lesser sac communicates with main peritoneal sac called **greater sac of peritoneum**. The part of greater sac with which the lesser sac

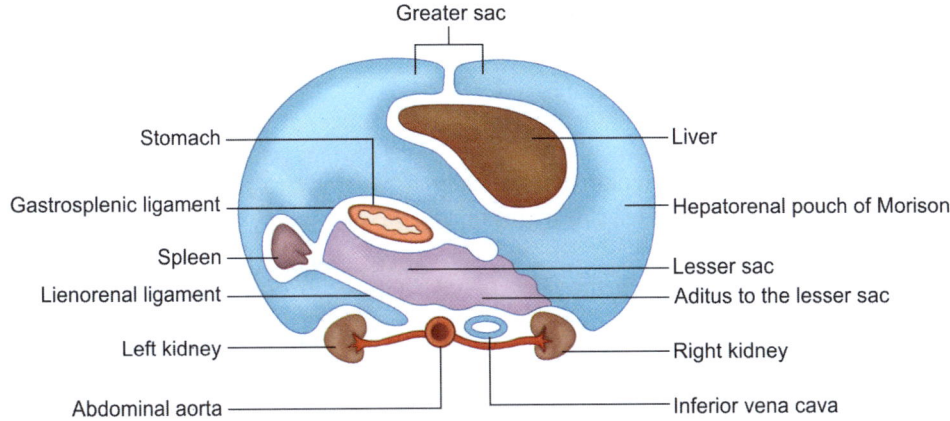

Fig. 22.6: Horizontal disposition of peritoneal cavity showing deviation of dorsal mesogastrium with spleen to the left and formation of lesser sac.

communicates is known as **hepatorenal pouch of Morison**. This pouch of greater sac is bounded by right lobe of liver in front and right kidney behind. The slit like space connecting lesser sac with greater sac is bounded in front by right free margin of lesser omentum and behind by posterior abdominal wall opposite the inferior vena cava. This slit possesses following three names:
1. Epiploic foramen,
2. Aditus to lesser sac
3. Foramen of Winslow.

Lesser sac of peritoneum is a peritoneal pocket between the hollow organ like stomach in front and rigid posterior abdominal wall behind. The sac acts as a cushion like bursa during distension of stomach. That is why the lesser sac is called **omental bursa**.

Factors Playing Role in Formation of the Lesser Sac
- Stomach rotates to the right
- Lesser omentum comes at the level of stomach
- Liver is pushed upwards and to the right, so stomach deviates downwards and to the left.
- Spleen growing in left layer of dorsal mesogastrium is pushed to the left along with the gastrosplenic and lienorenal ligaments.
- A small space, known as *pneumoenteric recess* appearing in right layer of dorsal mesogastrium ruptures in main peritoneal cavity.

Changes in the Midgut and Hindgut Making Peritoneal Cavity Complex

Originally, the midgut so also the hindgut remain suspended from dorsal body wall by only dorsal mesentery. So both right and left halves of peritoneal cavity becomes freely communicating in front of the gut. But peritoneal cavity becomes more complex due to following change of midgut in fetal life:
- 'U' shaped loop of midgut with proximal and distal limb herniates through umbilical ring.
- The loop rotates to the right side for 90°. The proximal limb of the loop rotates to the right. So the distal limb turns to the left.
- Then the loop reenters the abdominal cavity.
- Within the abdominal cavity, the loop again rotates from left to right for another 180°.
- Part of the midgut forming small intestine is placed centrally.

- As a result of rotation of midgut, part of midgut and whole of hindgut forming large intestine change into following positions (**Fig. 22.7**).
  - Transverse colon is transversely disposed across abdominal cavity.
  - Ascending and descending colon are vertically oriented along the right and left side of posterior abdominal wall respectively.
  - 'S' shaped sigmoid colon takes the place of left side of pelvis.
  - Rectum lies straight in the midline of pelvis along with the anal canal.

Selective Persistence of Dorsal Mesentery of Midgut and Hindgut (Fig. 22.7)

In some part of midgut and hindgut primitive dorsal mesentery persists as follows:

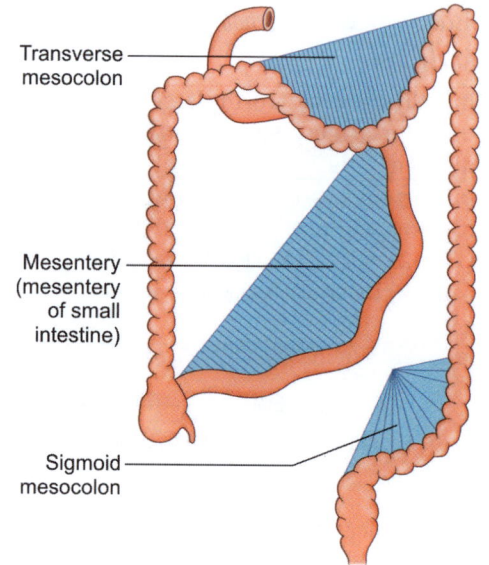

Fig. 22.7: Selective persistence of dorsal mesenteries of some portions of the gut.

- **Jejunum and ileum of small intestine**: Dorsal mesentery persists as double fold of peritoneum connecting these two parts of small intestine to the dorsal abdominal wall along the oblique line extending from left side of the lower border 1st lumbar vertebra to the right sacroiliac joint. This peritoneal fold is known as **the mesentery.**
- **Transverse colon:** Dorsal mesentery persists as double fold of peritoneum connecting transverse colon to the dorsal abdominal wall. This is knowns as **transverse mesocolon**.
- **Sigmoid (pelvic) colon:** Dorsal mesentery persists as double fold of peritoneum connecting sigmoid (pelvic) colon to the left side of posterior wall of pelvic cavity. This is known as **sigmoid (pelvic) mesocolon.**

Selective Absorption of Dorsal Mesentery of the Gut

Duodenum

Small intestine starts as duodenum next to stomach. Duodenum is initially suspended from dorsal body wall by its mesentery *(mesoduodenum)* (**Fig. 22.8A**). Due to rotation of stomach, duodenum, being the next part, also rotates to the right. Due to the rotation, mesoduodenum gets fused with the peritoneum of dorsal body wall (**Fig. 22.8B**) and finally it gets absorbed. Due to loss of mesoduodenum, the duodenum becomes a retroperitoneal part of the gut. This process is known as **zygosis (Fig. 22.8C).**

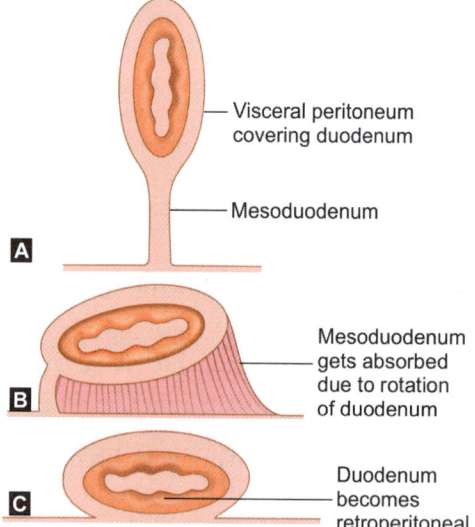

Figs. 22.8A to C: Selective absorption of dorsal mesentery of duodenum of zygosis.

Ascending Colon, Descending Colon, Rectum and Anal Canal

Initially, these parts of the large gut used to have their dorsal mesentery **(Fig. 22.9A)**. Growth of different viscera inside the abdominal cavity, pushes these guts further backwards against the corresponding part of dorsal body wall **(Fig. 22.9B)**. Their mesentery gets pressed against the body wall peritoneum and finally gets absorbed **(Fig. 22.9C)**. So these parts of large gut finally become retroperitoneal.

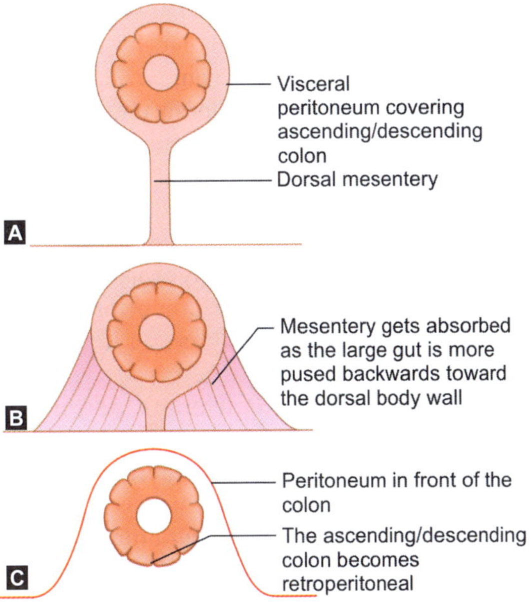

LA 22.4 Discuss briefly the vertical and horizontal disposition of the peritoneal cavity.

DISPOSITION OF PERITONEAL MEMBRANE IN ABDOMINAL CAVITY

The lining of parietal peritoneum of body wall is reflected on viscera as visceral peritoneum from where it may be reflected as same on another viscera or it may be reflected back on body wall as parietal peritoneum **(Fig. 22.10)**.

Due to alteration in disposition of different parts of the gut and also other viscera, reflection of peritoneal membrane appears to be somewhat complicated. Peritoneal reflection is studied through following two dispositions:
1. **Vertical disposition**
2. **Horizontal disposition**

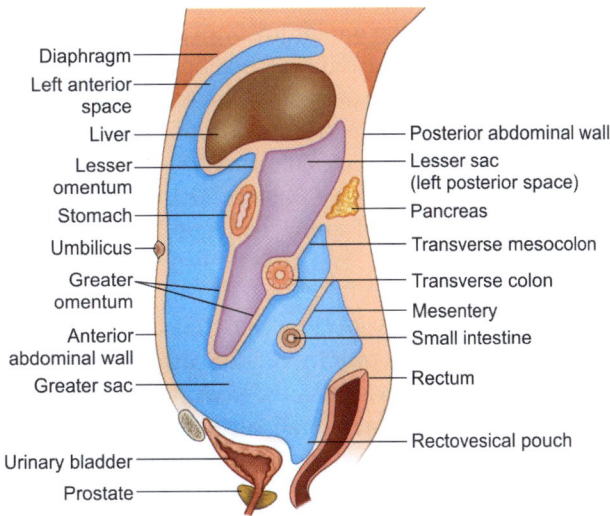

Figs. 22.9A to C: Selective absorption of dorsal mesentery of ascending/descending colon.

Vertical (Sagittal) Disposition (Fig. 22.10)

- From the level of umbilicus, peritoneum passes upwards to line the inner surface of anterior abdominal wall and then to the under surface of the diaphragm.
- From under surface of the diaphragm, peritoneum is reflected on posterosuperior aspect of liver. Covering round superior, anterior and inferior surface of liver, peritoneal membrane dips into the fissure for the ligamentum venosum on posterior surface between left lobe and caudate lobe.
- From the floor of fissure for the ligamentum venosum, peritoneum returns down as anterior layer of

Fig. 22.10: Vertical disposition of peritoneal cavity (in male).

lesser omentum to be attached to lesser curvature of stomach.
- Posterior layer of lesser omentum ascends up to the floor of fissure for ligamentum venosum from where it returns back, covers round caudate lobe of liver and reflected on under surface of diaphragm and then to the posterior abdominal wall up to anterior surface of body of pancreas.
- Posterior layer of lesser omentum, as it extends down, reaches the lesser curvature of stomach.
- Two layers of lesser omentum covering respective surfaces of stomach, extend as 1st and 2nd layer of greater omentum from greater curvature of stomach.
- 1st and 2nd layers of greater omentum descend for some distance and turn upwards and backwards from a free border. These two layers ascend as 3rd and 4th layers of greater omentum upto the anterior border of body of pancreas.
- 3rd layer is then continuous over the anterior surface of body of pancreas. With this reflection, a part of peritoneal cavity

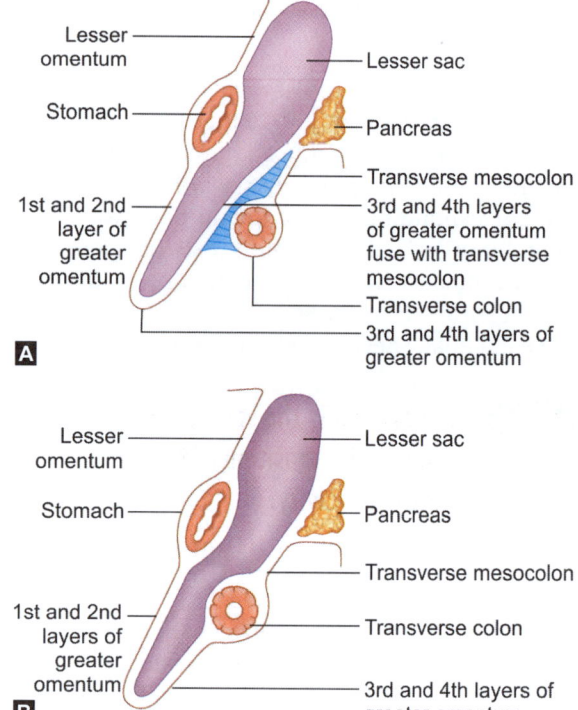

Figs. 22.11A and B: Reorientation of greater omentum and transverse mesocolon.

is bounded anteriorly by lesser omentum, posterior surface of stomach and 1st and 2nd layers of greater omentum. Posteriorly, it is bounded by peritoneum lining posterior abdominal wall from the level of caudate lobe to the anterior surface of body of pancreas. Below the pancreas posterior boundary of the space is formed by 3rd and 4th layers of greater omentum. This peritoneal space is *lesser sac of peritoneum.*
- 4th layer of greater omentum, from anterior border of body of pancreas, comes downwards and forwards to enclose transverse colon and goes back to same anterior border of body of pancreas. Thus, the two folds of peritoneum extending from transverse colon upwards and backwards to the anterior border of pancreas from *transverse mesocolon,* as middle two layers of peritoneum between the transverse colon and the pancreas fuse and disappear **(Figs. 22.11A and B).**
- It will be clear from the **Figures 22.11A and B** that greater omentum ultimately extends from greater curvature of stomach (1st and 2nd layers) to anteroinferior aspect of transverse colon (3rd and 4th layers). Transverse mesocolon extends from transverse colon to the anterior border of body of pancreas.
- Posteroinferior layer of transverse mesocolon, after being attached to anterior border of body of pancreas, sweeps over its inferior surface in the posterior abdominal wall.
- Then peritoneum is reflected from posterior abdominal wall as double fold to enclose coils of jejunum and ileum of small intestine as *the mesentery.*
- Peritoneum descends from posterior abdominal wall to left side of posterior pelvic wall from where it forms the *sigmoid (pelvic) mesocolon* (not shown in **Figure 22.10**)
- Reaching the posterior wall of pelvic cavity peritoneum covers the upper two thirds of anterior surface of rectum. From this level of rectum, when peritoneal membrane is reflected to the other

pelvic viscera, it differs in male and female as follows:

- *In Case of Male (Fig. 22.10)*
  From the junction of upper two thirds and lower one third of anterior surface of rectum, peritoneum is reflected forwards to the *upper part of posterior surface of urinary bladder*. A peritoneal pouch is thus formed between rectum and urinary bladder called **rectovesical pouch**. Form upper part of posterior surface of urinary bladder, peritoneum extends forward over the superior surface of urinary bladder.

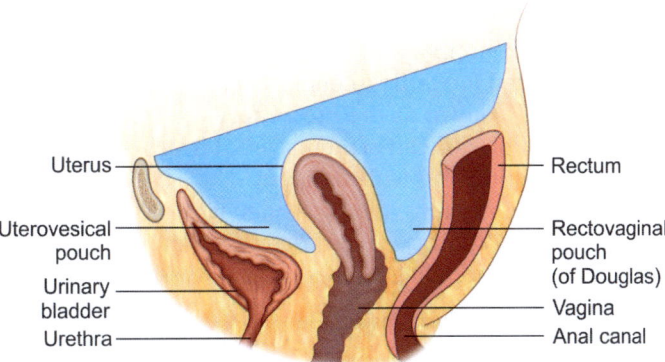

Fig. 22.12: Vertical disposition of peritoneum in female pelvic cavity.

- *In Case of Female (Fig. 22.12)*
  From the junction for upper two thirds and lower one third of anterior surface of rectum, peritoneum is reflected forwards to the upper end of posterior surface of vagina and then covers the posterior surface of uterus. A peritoneal pouch is thus formed between rectum behind and the upper end of vagina and the uterus in front. This is called **rectovaginal pouch** or **rectouterine pouch**. It is also known as **pouch of Douglas**. Peritoneum, covering around the fundus of uterus, it comes in front to cover anterior surface of its body. Form the junction of body and cervix, peritoneum is reflected on to the *superior surface of urinary bladder* to form **uterovesical pouch**. Peritoneum is then continued forward to cover the superior surface of urinary bladder.
- Further forwards, in both male and female, peritoneum is reflected from superior surface of urinary bladder to the posterior surface of anterior abdominal wall.

Horizontal (Transverse) Disposition in Abdomen

Horizontal disposition of peritoneum shows different pictures above and below the level of transverse colon, which are described as supracolic and infracolic disposition.

Horizontal Disposition at Supracolic Compartment (Fig. 22.6)

Double fold of peritoneum extends forwards and to the left from either side of midline as **lienorenal ligament** as it extends from the front of the left kidney to the hilum of spleen. Left layer, wrapping around spleen joins right layer at the anterior end of hilum. Double fold of peritoneum extends forwards and to right (medially) to the greater curvature of stomach to form **gastrosplenic ligament.** Two folds of this ligament passing in front and behind the stomach is extended further medially as two layers of **lesser omentum.** A pocket of main peritoneal cavity (greater sac) falls behind stomach and lesser omentum. It is known as **lesser sac** or **omental bursa**. Right free margin of lesser omentum forms anterior boundary of a slit known as **epiploic foramen**. Its posterior boundary is formed by the parietal peritoneum of posterior abdominal wall opposite the inferior vena cava. In front and to the right of stomach and lesser omentum, cross section of liver is found to be covered by peritoneum. From anterior aspect of liver a double fold of peritoneum extends forwards to the anterior abdominal wall. It is known as **falciform ligament**. Right and left layers of falciform ligament, falling on respective sides of anterior abdominal wall, line the respective sides of anterolateral wall of abdomen. Parietal peritoneum of respective side is continuous at posterior abdominal wall in front of kidney of respective side.

Horizontal Disposition at Infracolic Compartment (Fig. 22.13)

In posterior abdominal wall, the peritoneum from the front of abdominal aorta and inferior vena cava is reflected forwards to enclose jejunum and ileum of small intestine. This double fold of peritoneum in known as **the mesentery**. In front of coils of small intestine, **4 layers of greater omentum** are placed. Out of the 4 layers, 1st and 4th layers are continuous with each other whereas 2nd layer is continuous with 3rd layer.

Parietal peritoneum, when extended laterally in the posterior abdominal wall, on either side of vertebral column, it forms a vertical depression known as **paravertebral gutter**. Further laterally, lateral to ascending and descending colon, similar depression lined by peritoneum is known as **paracolic gutter**.

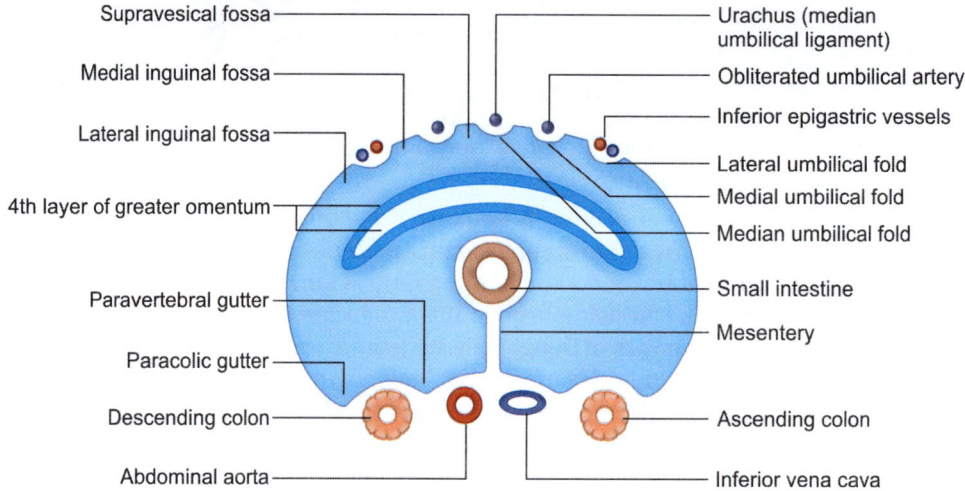

Fig. 22.13: Horizontal disposition of peritoneum (infracolic compartment of abdomen).

Lateral to the paracolic gutter, pearietal peritoneum lining lateral wall of abdomen, presents following characteristics while lining the inner surface of anterior abdominal wall.

From midline of anterior abdominal wall, on either side, peritoneum raises following three peritoneal folds in relation to three linear structures inclining towards umbilicus.

1. **Median umbilical fold**: Raised due to *urachus* or *median umbilical ligament* extending from apex of urinary bladder to umbilicus.
2. **Medial umbilical fold**: Raised by *obliterated umbilical artery*.
3. **Lateral umbilical fold**: Raised by *inferior epigastric vessels*.

On the posterior surface of anterior abdominal wall, as above-mentioned peritoneal folds are formed, following peritoneal fossae are formed in between these folds.

1. **Supravesical fossa**: It is on either side of midline, between median and medial umbilical folds.
2. **Medial inguinal fossa**: It is between medial and lateral umbilical fold.
3. **Lateral inguinal fossa**: It is lateral to the lateral umbilical fold.

Horizontal Disposition at the Level of Pelvis

- It will be difficult for a student to follow horizontal disposition of pelvic peritoneum at this stage.
- It will be better understood when pelvic viscera are studied. That is why, it is discussed with the chapter of male and female pelvic viscera.

Short note: Epiploic foramen.

LA 22.5 Give an account of the important peritoneal spaces with the lesser sac (omental bursa). Add a note on the clinical anatomy.

IMPORTANT PERITONEAL SPACES

The parietal peritoneum lining body wall is continuous with the visceral peritoneum covering the viscera. Peritoneum is reflected from the body wall to the viscera, one viscera to another viscera or from the viscera again to the body wall. Due to these reflections, within the abdominal cavity some peritoneal spaces, fossae or pouches are formed which are as follows:

Spaces around Liver (Spaces under the Diaphragm)

Right-sided Spaces (Fig. 22.14)

- **Right anterior space:** It is in front of right lobe of liver (**Fig. 22.14**).
- **Right posterior space:** It is comparatively more prominent space between right lobe of liver and right kidney below right dome of diaphragm. It is called **hepatorenal pouch of Morison.** Towards the left side, it communicates with lesser sac through epiploic foramen.

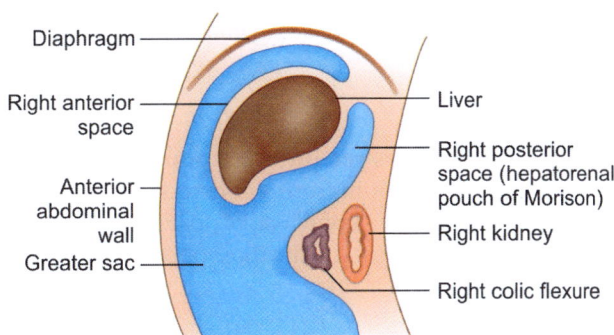

Fig. 22.14: Right-sided subphrenic peritoneal spaces.

Left-sided Spaces (Fig. 22.10)

- **Left anterior space**: It is a narrow space above and in front of left lobe of liver under the left dome of diaphragm.
- **Left posterior space**: This is the **lesser sa**c of peritoneal cavity. It is posteroinferior to left lobe and caudate lobe of liver. It is a pocket of general peritoneal cavity (greater sac) lying mainly behind the stomach and in front of posterior abdominal wall. The space is bounded in front, from above downwards, by posterior layer of lesser omentum, posterior surface of stomach and 2nd layer of greater omentum. From below upwards, posterior boundary is formed by 3rd layer of greater omentum, transverse colon, transverse mesocolon, peritoneum over anterosuperior surface of body of pancreas and parietal peritoneum lining upper part of posterior abdominal wall.
- **Lower end of lesser sac** between 2nd and 3rd layers of greater omentum is obliterated, as these two layers fuse with each other.
- **Superior recess of lesser sac** is between caudate lobe of liver and under surface of the diaphragm.
- **Communication with greater sac** is through epiploic foramen which is bounded in front by right free margin of lesser omentum and behind by peritoneum in front of inferior vena cava.

Spaces in infracolic compartment (Fig. 22.13)

- Right and left paravertebral gutters
- Right and left paracolic gutters.

These have been discussed above in connection with horizontal disposition of peritoneum at infracolic compartment of abdomen (Question No. 22.4).

Spaces in pelvic cavity (Figs. 22.10 and 22.12)

In male

Rectovesical pouch

This pouch is formed due to reflection of peritoneum from junction of upper two thirds and lower one third of anterior surface of rectum to upper part of posterior surface of urinary bladder. It is the most dependent part of peritoneal cavity in male. It is 7.5 cm deep to the plane of perineal body as well as anal orifice.

Clinical importance

- As it is the most dependent part of peritoneal cavity, in pathological conditions, accumulation of peritoneal fluid starts from this pouch.
- This pouch and condition of adjacent viscera like prostate or urinary bladder can be clinically assessed through per rectal digital examination.

In female

Rectovaginal pouch

This is also known as **rectouterine pouch** or ***pouch of Douglas***. This pouch is formed due to reflection of peritoneum from the junction of upper two thirds and lower one third of anterior surface of rectum to the upper end of posterior surface of vagina from where peritoneum is reflected on to the back of uterus. It is the most dependent part of peritoneal cavity in female. It is 5 cm deep to the plane of perineal body.

Clinical importance

- In some pathological conditions, accumulation of peritoneal fluid starts in this space.
- Conditions of this pouch and the viscera adjacent to it, e.g. uterus, uterine tube, ovary can be clinically assessed through per vaginal digital examination.

Uterovesical pouch

This pouch is shallower and is formed due to reflection of peritoneum from the junction of anterior surface of the body and cervix of the uterus to the superior surface of urinary bladder.

The above-mentioned pouches in both male and female normally contain coils of ileum.

Clinical Anatomy of Peritoneum

- In case of male, peritoneal cavity is a closed sac within abdominal cavity. In case of female peritoneal cavity communicates with uterine tube at its lateral end, so through the uterus and vagina the peritoneal cavity opens to the exterior. That is why, the **chance of infection of peritoneal cavity in female is more common.**
- Infection of peritoneal cavity is known as **peritonitis**. It is commonest due to intra-abdominal injury of any organ.
- Accumulation of fluid in the peritoneal cavity is known as **ascitis**. In case of ascitis, peritoneal fluid may be required to be drained out through a clinical procedure, known as **paracentesis abdominis**.
- When the peritoneal fluid starts accumulating in peritoneal cavity, first it fills up to **most dependent part of the cavity**. In supine position, **rectovesical pouch** in male and **rectovaginal pouch (pouch of Douglas)** in female along with the **hepatorenal pouch** are the most dependent parts.

- Fluid-filled rectovesical pouch or rectovaginal pouch and the conditions of the viscera adjacent to the pouches can be clinically felt through **per-rectal** or **per-vaginal digital examinations.**
- Through the narrow neck of peritoneal cavity at epiploic foramen, mobile small gut loops **may herniate into the lesser sac**. This is called internal abdominal hernia. When blood vessels of the herniated loops at epiploic foramen is obstructed, the hernia will be called **strangulated hernia**.
- The peritoneal cavity so also the abdominal cavity with its viscera are directly visualized through an instrument called **laparoscope**. The clinical procedure is known as **laparoscopy**.

Short note: Hepatorenal pouch; Pouch of Douglas.

Chapter 23

Stomach and Small Intestine

LA 23.1 Discuss briefly the gross anatomy of stomach.
(*Important for viva voce and practical*)

STOMACH

Introduction

Stomach is known by a term '*gaster*'. That is why, the adjective terminology, *gastric* is used in anatomy.

Stomach is *most dilated and distensible* part of alimentary tract having a thick muscular wall.

It is the part between esophagus proximally and duodenum component of small intestine distally.

Stomach is situated in upper and left part of abdominal cavity occupying the areas of *left hypochondrium* and *epigastrium*. To a variable extent it may extend into *umbilical region* (**Fig. 23.1**).

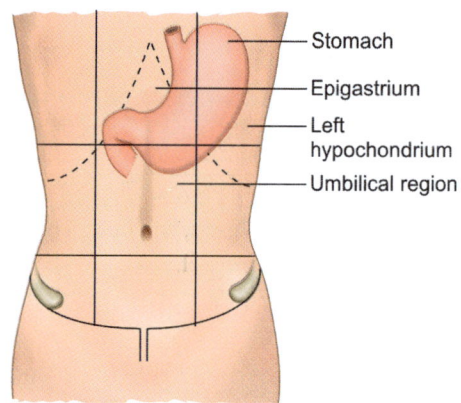

Fig. 23.1: Situation of stomach in relation to areas of abdomen.

Functions

- **Reservoir of food:** Following swallowing, stomach initially acts as the reservoir of food.
- **Grinding and mixing of food:** Due to contraction of thick muscular wall, stomach grinds or breaks down the food material and mixes it with gastric juice to make it ready for digestion.
- **Digestion of food:** *Pepsin* and *hydrochloric acid* secreted by gastric mucosa, helps in digestion of food.
- **Absorption:** Some substances, e.g. salt, water, alcohol and some drugs are absorbed from stomach. Vitamin B_{12} is absorbed from the stomach by the intrinsic factor of Castle produced by stomach.
- **Protection:** **Mucus** secreted from the gastric mucosa, forms a protective layer on mucous membrane of stomach.
  Hydrochloric acid liberated by the stomach kills bacteria ingested in gastrointestinal tract.

Features of Stomach (Fig. 23.2)

Stomach presents 2 ends (orifices), 2 borders and 2 surfaces.

Orifices

Cardiac (esophageal) orifice of stomach is the proximal end which is thinner when palpated between two fingers.

Pyloric orifice is the distal intestinal end of stomach which is felt thicker, when palpated, due to presence of sphincter formed by condensation of circular muscle fibers.

Margins

Both the margins are curved for which they are also termed **curvatures** of stomach.

Lesser curvature: It is the *shorter* and *concave right border* of stomach.

Greater curvature: It is *longer* and *convex left border* of stomach.

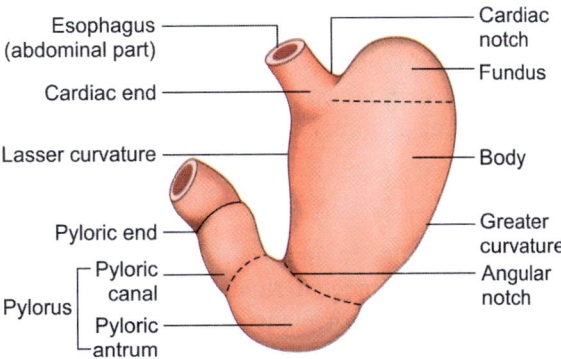

Fig. 23.2: External features of stomach (anterior view).

Surfaces

Anterior surface: It is the **anterosuperior surface** facing *forwards and upwards*.

Posterior surface: It is the **posteroinferior surface** facing *backwards and downwards*.

Anatomical Position of Stomach

Instruction for the Students

- First, differentiate cardiac and pyloric orifices. Comparatively thin-walled cardiac orifice, which is the esophageal end, will be at a higher level. Thick-walled pyloric orifice guarded by sphincter will be at a lower level.
- Then, identify two borders (curvatures) of stomach. Lesser curvature is shorter and more or less concave. Greater curvature is the longer convex border.
- Anterior and posterior surfaces are clearly identified in empty collapsed stomach.
- Place the stomach on the *palm of your left hand* in such a way that:
  - Cardiac orifice is at a higher level and facing upwards. Pyloric orifice is at a lower level and facing to the right.
  - Shorter concave lesser curvature is directed to the right side and longer convex greater curvature is directed to the left side.
- Finally extend the wrist joint of the left hand to make the anterior surface anterosuperior in direction.
  (For oral and practical only)

Shape and Size

Stomach looks like a muscular bag. When empty, stomach is J shaped. But variation in shape of the stomach depends upon degree of distension of the organ and adjacent viscera.

In average, length of stomach of an adult is 25 cm.

Capacity

30 mL	=	at birth
1000 mL	=	at puberty
1500–2000 mL	=	in adults

External Features

Stomach has two orifices (**Fig. 23.2**):
1. **Cardiac orifice** is at the junction of lower end of esophagus and beginning of stomach.
   Level: Lower border of body of 11th thoracic vertebra, but behind the left 7th costal cartilage.
   Physiological sphincter: Cardiac orifice *does not present any anatomical sphincter*. But tonicity of the orifice is relaxed at the end of 3rd stage of deglutition for passage of food bolus into stomach.
2. **Pyloric orifice** connects cavity of stomach with that of duodenum of small intestine. This orifice is directed from left to right in a horizontal plane.
   Level: Transpyloric plane (L_1 vertebra) 1.25 cm to the right of midline.

Surface Landmark

- **Pyloric constriction:** A circular groove opposite the pyloric sphincter formed by condensed circular muscle.
- **Prepyloric vein:** It runs in front of the sphincter.

Curvatures

Stomach has two curvatures (**Fig. 23.2**).

1. Lesser curvature

Lesser curvature is the shorter, concave right border of stomach. Embryologically, it is the ventral border which falls to the right due to rotation of stomach to the right.

Towards the lower end, the curvature presents a notch which is known as **angular notch**.

A double fold of peritoneum, called **lesser omentum**, extends from liver to the lesser curvature of stomach (**Fig. 23.3**).

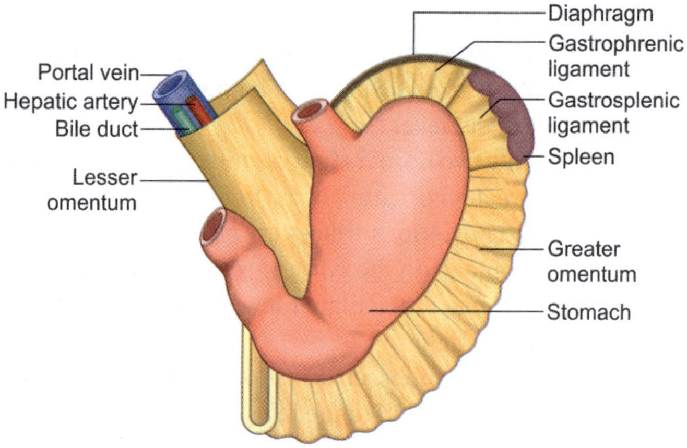

2. Greater curvature

Fig. 23.3: Peritoneal folds attached to stomach.

Greater curvature is the longer, convex left border of stomach starting from left margin of esophagus. At this site, an acute angular notch is present. It is called *cardiac notch*. During distended condition of stomach, the notch becomes more acute which prevents regurgitation of food into esophagus.

From proximal to distal end, greater curvature gives attachment to following double fold of peritoneum (**Fig. 23.3**).
1. **Gastrophrenic ligament**—to undersurface of diaphragm
2. **Gastrosplenic ligament**—to spleen
3. **Greater omentum**—two layers of greater omentum, hanging freely, turn upwards to be attached to transverse colon (**Fig. 23.3**).

Surfaces

- *Anterior surface* is truly is **anterosuperior surface** as it faces forwards and upwards.
- *Posterior surface*, as facing backwards and downwards, is known as **posteroinferior surface**.

Parts of Stomach (Fig. 23.2)

Upper cardiac part and **lower pyloric part** is divided by an oblique line extending from the angular notch of lesser curvature to the greater curvature.

Cardiac Part

Upper larger cardiac part is subdivided into *fundus* and *body*.
- **Fundus** of the stomach is uppermost dome-shaped part of the organ which is above the horizontal line passing through cardiac notch.
  In erect posture, fundus is filled up with gas which can be identified through radiograph (X-ray). Black shadow of the gas becomes visible under left dome of diaphragm.
- **Body** of the stomach is the larger component of cardiac part. It is the part which is distended to a maximum limit.
  Gastric glands are present in both fundus and body of stomach. The glands present following types of cells which liberate different substances.
- **Mucus secreting cells**
- **Peptic, chief or zymogenic cells**—secrete digestive enzymes
- **Parietal or oxyntic cells** which liberate hydrochloric acid.

Pyloric Part

It is subdivided into *pyloric antrum* and *pyloric canal*:
- **Pyloric antrum** is the proximal dilated component of pyloric part. It is 3 inches in length and separated from pyloric canal by a less defined sulcus called *sulcus intermedius*.
  Gastric glands of pyloric antrum are **mucus secreting glands.**
- **Pyloric canal** is the narrower and short component of pyloric part of stomach. It is 1 inch long. At its right end, it communicates with the beginning of duodenum.

Relations of Stomach

Peritoneal Relations

Both anterosuperior and posteroinferior surfaces of stomach are covered by peritoneum. Only a **small triangular area** of posteroinferior surface near cardiac notch is nonperitoneal as it is in direct contact with left crus of diaphragms. This area is called **bare area of stomach**.

Lesser curvature gives attachment to **lesser omentum**, a double fold of peritoneum extending from liver.

Greater curvature gives attachment to following peritoneal folds from above downwards:
- Gastrophrenic ligament
- Gastrosplenic ligament
- Greater omentum

Visceral and Parietal Relations

Anterosuperior surface
- Left lobe of liver
- Anterior part of left dome of the diaphragm
- Anterior abdominal wall.

Posteroinferior surface

A pocket or diverticulum of general peritoneal cavity, called **lesser sac** lies just behind the posteroinferior surface of stomach. This peritoneal recess separates stomach from the following structures which lie further behind in the posterior abdominal wall.
- Left crus of diaphragm
- Left suprarenal gland
- Splenic artery
- Left kidney
- Body of pancreas
- Left colic flexure
- Transverse mesocolon.

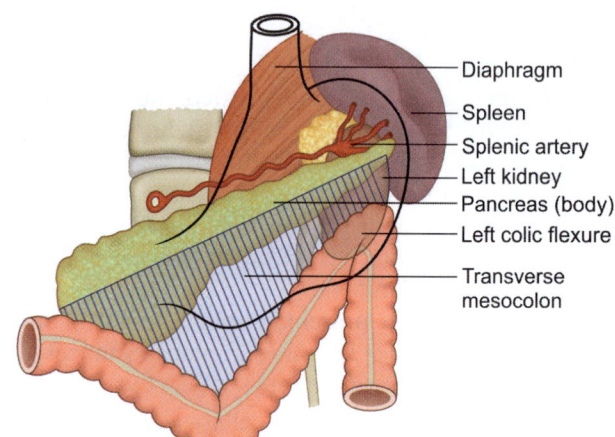

Fig. 23.4: Structures forming 'stomach bed'.

These structures form an area on posterior abdominal wall on which the stomach rests in supine position. That is why it is called **stomach bed (Fig. 23.4)**.

Important Points Related to Structures of Stomach

Like other parts of gut, stomach wall is made up of following layers from within outwards:
1. Mucous coat
2. Submucous coat
3. Muscular coat
4. Serous coat

Mucosal surface of empty stomach is thrown into number of folds called *rugae*. These folds are longitudinal along the lesser curvature and irregular in appearance everywhere.

Submucous coat is made up of connective tissue with finer ramifications of blood vessels and nerves.

Muscular coat is made up of three layers which are superficial longitudinal, middle circular and *inner oblique*. Middle circular fibers are condensed at pyloric end to form the **pyloric sphincter**. Oblique muscle fibers loop around greater curvature from anterior to posterior surface. But on both the surfaces, fibers do not reach upto lesser curvature. Due to this reason, part of the gastric lumen along the lesser curvature shows a separate identity known as **gastric canal**. During swallowing of liquid, it passes more rapidly through the gastric canal to the lower part of stomach.

Serous coat is made up of visceral layer of peritoneum.

SA 23.2 Discuss briefly the blood supply of stomach.

ARTERIAL SUPPLY OF STOMACH (FIG. 23.5)

Stomach, being the part of foregut, is supplied by the **branches of celiac trunk, the artery of foregut.**

The arteries are mainly distributed along the lesser and greater curvatures of stomach.

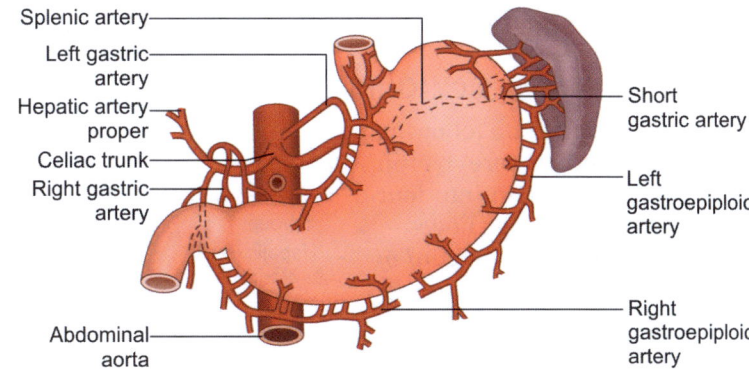

Fig. 23.5: Arterial supply of stomach.

Along the lesser curvature the arteries are
1. *Left gastric artery*: The direct branch of celiac trunk.
2. *Right gastric artery*: It arises from the hepatic branch of celiac trunk.

The two arteries anastomose freely and lie in between two layers of lesser omentum.

Along the greater curvature the arteries are
1. *Right gastroepiploic artery*: The branch of gastroduodenal artery which is a branch of hepatic artery.
2. *Left gastroepiploic artery*: The branch of splenic artery which is a branch of celiac trunk.

Both the gastroepiploic arteries anastomose lying in between two layers of greater omentum.

Near the fundus of stomach, *short gastric arteries* are short multiple branches arising from terminal part of splenic artery.

VENOUS DRAINAGE OF STOMACH (FIG. 23.6)

Stomach, being part of gut is drained by the veins, all of which drain in portal venous system. Some of the veins directly drain into portal vein and some drain into its tributaries.

- **Right and left gastric veins** drain into portal vein.
- **Right gastroepiploic vein** drains into superior mesenteric vein.
- **Left gastroepiploic vein** drains into splenic vein.

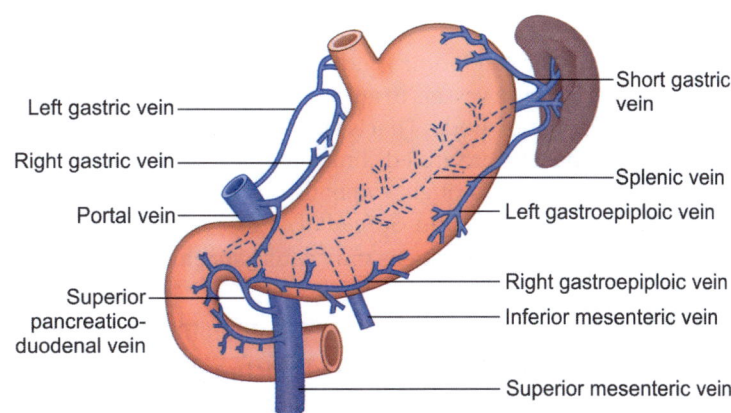

Fig. 23.6: Venous drainage of stomach.

- **Short gastric veins** from fundal area of stomach drain into splenic vein.

Gastroesophageal junction is one of the important sites of communication between portal and systemic veins. Here the esophageal tributaries of left gastric vein (portal system) and those of hemiazygos vein (systemic system) communicate freely. In case of diseases of portal venous obstruction, these veins dilate leading to a condition called *esophageal varices*. Rupture of these engorged veins causes vomiting of blood (*hematemesis*).

SA 23.3 Write a brief note on lymphatic drainage of stomach.

LYMPHATIC DRAINAGE OF STOMACH (FIG. 23.7)

Stomach is divided into following four areas from where lymph vessels primarily drain into four different groups of lymph nodes.

1. *Upper part of left one third of stomach adjacent to greater curvature*: Lymph vessels drain into the **pancreaticosplenic lymph nodes** related to splenic artery.
2. *Lower part of left one third of stomach*: Lymph vessels drain into the **right gastroepiploic lymph nodes** related to corresponding artery. From this group of nodes, lymph vessels pass to the **hepatic group of lymph nodes**.
3. *Pyloric part of stomach*: Lymph vessels from this area of stomach drain into the **pyloric group of lymph nodes** which send lymph vessels to the **hepatic group**.
4. *Right two-thirds of stomach towards the lesser curvature*: Lymph vessels from this area drain into the **left gastric group of lymph nodes** lying in relation to corresponding vessels.

Final drainage: Finally lymph vessels from all the above-mentioned groups of lymph nodes drain into the **celiac group of lymph nodes**.

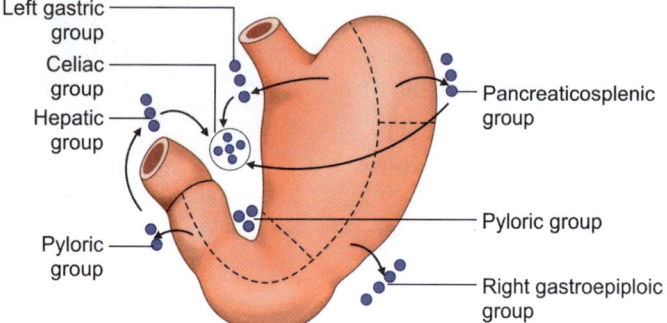

Fig. 23.7: Lymphatic drainage of stomach.

Clinical Anatomy

Incidence of gastric carcinoma is not uncommon. Metastasis (secondary spread) of gastric cancer occurs through lymph vessels to adjacent lymph nodes and also to the distant lymph node, the left supraclavicular lymph node. That is why, when gastric carcinoma is suspected, left supraclavicular lymph nodes must be examined clinically.

Besides metastasis through lymphatics, carcinoma of stomach may spread to adjacent structures like liver, pancreas and colon. Spread of cancer cells in peritoneal cavity causes ascites.

Transperitoneal metastasis may cause spread in ovary in females (*Krukenberg's tumor*).

SA 23.4 Discuss the surface features and anatomical position of duodenum.
(*Important for viva voce and practical*)

DUODENUM
Introduction

Duodenum is the *most proximal, widest, shortest* and *fixed* part of the small intestine commencing at the pyloric end of the stomach. Being mostly retroperitoneal in position, it is fixed over the structures of posterior abdominal wall to the right side of the midline.

Nomenclature

Duodenum is the Latin terminology of the Greek word, *'duo-deka-daktulos'* which literally means twelve fingers. Roughly the duodenum measures equal to the breadth of twelve fingers.

Functions

Duodenum receives the openings of the bile duct and the pancreatic ducts. The main function of the duodenum is **digestion of food**. The *chyme* prepared from the food within the stomach, is received in the duodenum. Further, it is mixed with bile and pancreatic enzymes for digestion.

Location

Duodenum is 'C' shaped with the concavity directed towards the left to accommodate the globular head end of the pancreas.

The curve of the duodenum is flattened anteroposteriorly in the **umbilical region** with its proximal end lying in the **epigastric region (Fig. 23.8)**.

Duodenum lies opposite the level of the bodies of 1st to 3rd lumbar vertebrae to the right side of midline.

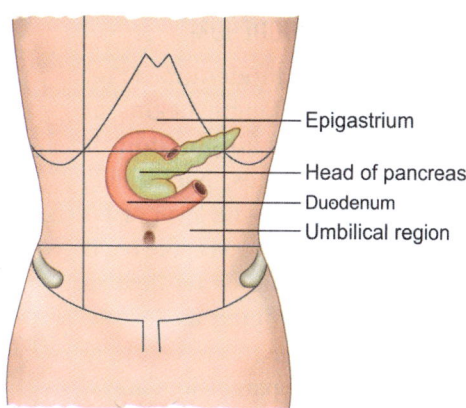

Fig. 23.8: Location of duodenum.

Length

About 25 cm (10 inches).

Parts

Duodenum presents following four parts from the proximal to the distal ends.

1st part : Superior part : 2 inches
2nd part : Descending part : 3 inches
3rd part : Horizontal part : 4 inches
4th part : Ascending part : 1 inch

Reasons for Fixation and Curvature of the Duodenum

In fetal life, the distal end of the duodenum is connected to the dorsal body wall by a band of mesoderm called *superior retention band*. It leads to formation of the bend of duodenojejunal flexure. Subsequent elongation of duodenum gives rise to the formation of its C shaped curve with its convexity directed ventrally. Rotation of the stomach becomes associated with rotation of the duodenum also to the right. This rotation results in the following two changes in the duodenum.
1. Mesentery of the duodenum (mesoduodenum) is lost through the process of zygosis. So the duodenum becomes retroperitoneal.
2. Convexity of the duodenum is directed to the right.

Peritoneal Relation in General

In general, the duodenum, being retroperitoneal in position, is covered by the peritoneum in its anterior surface. Posterior surface is nonperitoneal, but the following two parts of the duodenum is covered by peritoneum all around.
1. **First one inch** of the first part
2. Fourth part of duodenum which is the **last one inch**.

Anatomical Position

- Anterior surface of the duodenum is to be identified first by its smooth glistening appearance, as it is covered by peritoneum.
- Posterior surface, recognized by its raw (non-shining) appearance, is to be placed over the left palm with hyperextension of the wrist, so that the anterior surface faces forwards.
- The concavity of the duodenum must be directed towards the left.
  (Head of pancreas, if present with duodenum, is accommodated within the concavity).

SN 23.5 **Write a short note on the first part of duodenum.**

FIRST PART OF DUODENUM

First part of duodenum (**Fig. 23.9**), 5 cm in length begins at the **pyloroduodenal junction**. It is directed **upwards, backwards** and **to the right** at the level of 1st lumbar vertebra. It ends at the bend called **superior duodenal flexure** where it is continued as second part of duodenum to run vertically downwards. First part of duodenum is divided into two equal halves. First one inch is covered by peritoneum on both surfaces. Upper and lower borders give attachment to the right ends of lesser and greater omentum respectively. Second one inch is covered by peritoneum on its anterior surface only.

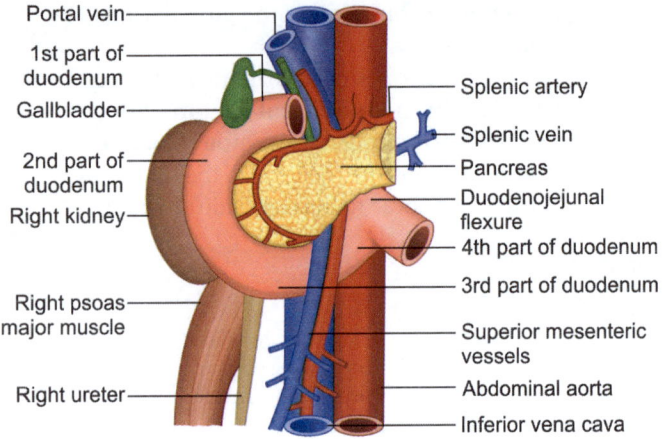

Fig. 23.9: Duodenum with related structures.

First part duodenum is related to the following structures:
- **Anteriorly: Gallbladder** and **quadrate lobe** of liver.
- **Posteriorly: Portal vein, bile duct** and **gastroduodenal artery**
- **Superiorly:** It forms lower boundary of the **epiploic foramen**.
- **Inferiorly: Head of pancreas.**

Interior of the first part of duodenum does not show semicircular mucous folds unlike the other parts.

Clinical Importance

Ulceration of duodenal mucosa due to acid peptic disease is called **duodenal ulcer**. It is common in the first part.

First one inch of the first part is known as **duodenal cap.** When radiograph (X-ray) is taken after swallowing a radiopaque dye, e.g. barium sulfate, duodenal cap normally shows a triangular opaque shadow. Barium metal X-ray shows **deformed duodenal cap** in a case of duodenal ulcer.

LA 23.6 Describe the second part of duodenum with a note on clinical anatomy.

SECOND PART OF DUODENUM

Introduction

Second part of duodenum is known as the **descending part of duodenum** as it descends vertically in front of the medial marginal part of anterior surface of right kidney along the right side of the bodies of 1st to 3rd lumbar vertebrae.

Special Function

Second part of duodenum is different from the other parts as it receives the openings of the common bile duct with the pancreatic ducts which carry bile and pancreatic juice for digestion of food.

Length

7.5 cm (3 inches)

Extent

From **superior duodenal flexure** at the level of right side of lower border of 1st lumbar vertebra to **inferior duodenal flexure** at the level of right side of lower border of 3rd lumbar vertebra. At the lower end, it is continuous with the third part of duodenum.

Features

- **Two surfaces**: Anterior and posterior
- **Two borders**: Lateral convex and medial concave borders.

Peritoneal Relations

Anterior surface is covered by the peritoneum except at its middle where it is crossed by the right end of transverse colon separated by loose areolar tissue.

Posterior surface is nonperitoneal.

Relations

Anteriorly (Fig. 23.10)

- *Above:* **Gallbladder** with right lobe of **liver.**
- *In the middle:* It is crossed by right end of **transverse colon** with **transverse mesocolon.**
- *Below:* **Coils of small intestine.**

Posteriorly (Fig. 23.11)

- Anterior surface of **right kidney** adjacent to its medial border with structures at the hilum.
- **Inferior vena cava.**
- **Right psoas major muscle.**

Medially

- **Head of pancreas.**

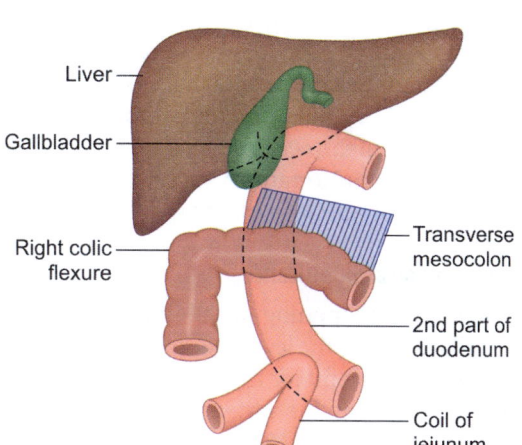

Fig. 23.10: Anterior relation of 2nd part of duodenum.

- Anastomosis between **superior and inferior pancreaticoduodenal arteries** in the groove between pancreas and duodenum.
- Terminal ends of **bile duct and pancreatic ducts**.

Laterally

Right colic flexure with the terminal end of ascending colon.

Interior (Fig. 23.12)

Mucosal surface of second part of duodenum presents following features:
- **Plicae circulares**: These are circular or semicircular mucous folds arranged parallelly at right angle to the long axis of the gut. These are also known as **valves of Kerckring**. These folds are absent in the first part of the duodenum, but present in other parts of duodenum and also jejunum and ileum. They are more crowed in the lower half of the second part.
- **Major duodenal papilla**: It is a prominent mucosal elevation on the *posteromedial wall* of second part of duodenum *10 cm distal to the pyloric end of stomach*. The summit of the papilla presents the common opening of the bile duct and the main pancreatic duct through a dilated end known as **ampulla of Vater** (hepatopancreatic ampulla). A semilunar arch of mucous fold lies over the major duodenal papilla. It looks like, so it is called **monk's hood.**
- **Minor duodenal papilla**: It is a small conical projection *on the medial margin* of mucosal surface of the second part of duodenum *2 cm proximal* to the major papilla. Its summit presents the opening of the accessory pancreatic duct.
- **Plica longitudinalis**: A small, vertical and tortuous mucous fold extending downwards from the major duodenal papilla.

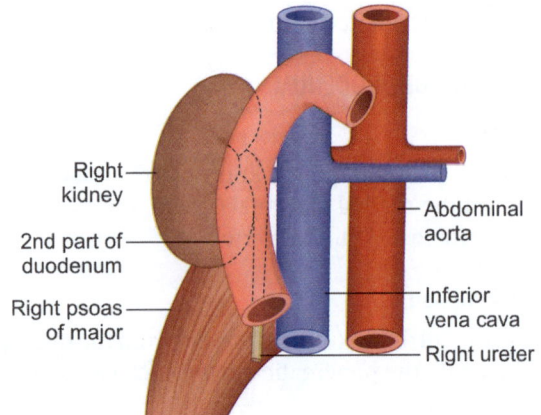

Fig. 23.11: Posterior relation of 2nd part of duodenum.

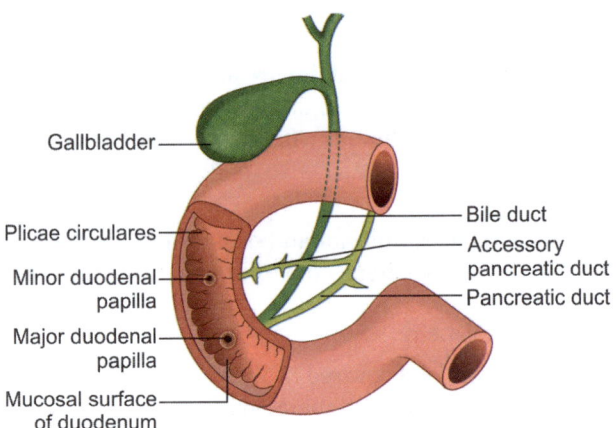

Fig. 23.12: Interior of duodenum showing plicae circulares and duodenal papillae.

Embryological Significance

The common opening of the bile duct and the main pancreatic duct through major duodenal papilla indicates the level of junction between foregut and midgut. So, the second part of duodenum proximal to the major duodenal papilla is supplied by the artery of the foregut, i.e. celiac trunk. The part distal to the major papilla is supplied by branches of the superior mesenteric artery, the artery of the midgut. The venous drainage, lymphatic drainage and nerve supply are also different for the two components of second part of duodenum.

Vascular Supply, Lymphatic Drainage and Nerve Supply

	Proximal to major duodenal papilla (foregut)	Distal to major duodenal papilla (midgut)
Arterial supply	Superior pancreaticoduodenal artery branch of gastroduodenal artery	Inferior pancreaticoduodenal artery— branch of superior mesenteric artery
Venous drainage	Superior pancreaticoduodenal vein which drains into the portal vein directly	Inferior pancreaticoduodenal vein which drains into the superior mesenteric vein
Lymphatic drainage	To the celiac group of lymph nodes	To the superior mesenteric group of lymph nodes
Nerve supply	* Via celiac plexus	* Via superior mesenteric plexus

* For both the components of second part of duodenum, the sympathetic fibers are derived from T_6 to T_9 segments of spinal cord and the parasympathetic fibers are derived from the vagus nerve.

Clinical Anatomy

Duodenal Diverticula

Second part of duodenum is the commonest site for congenital duodenal diverticula. These are outpouching of duodenal mucosal lining through the congenital deficiency in the duodenal muscular wall, which is commonly found at the site of entry of the bile duct and the pancreatic ducts.

Duodenal Compression

It may result from the incidence of **annular pancreas** which is a congenital error. In this case, pancreatic tissue encircles the second part of duodenum. **Carcinoma of the head of pancreas** may lead to pressure effect on the duodenum.

ERCP

Catheterization through major duodenal papilla is done for injection of a radiopaque material through the duodenal papilla to visualize the bile duct and pancreatic ducts. This procedure is known as endoscopic retrograde cholangiopancreatography (ERCP).

SN 23.7 Write a short note on the suspensory muscle of duodenum (ligament of Treitz).

SUSPENSORY MUSCLE OF DUODENUM (LIGAMENT OF TREITZ) (FIG. 23.13)

Introduction

It is a fibromuscular band which suspends the duodenojejunal flexure from the right crus of the diaphragm at the posterior abdominal wall.

Attachments
- **Upper end:** To the right crus of the diaphragm
- **Lower end:** To posterosuperior aspect of duodenojejunal flexure.

Components
- **Upper part: Striated muscle fibers,** fused with those of the diaphragm
- **Intermediate part:** Connective tissue **(elastic fibers)**
- **Lower part: Nonstriated muscle fibers** fused with those of the gut.

Morphology

In fetal life, proximal and distal ends of the 'U' shaped midgut loop used to be connected to the dorsal body wall by the superior and inferior retention bands respectively. Duodenojejunal flexure is the site of the proximal end the midgut loop. The ligament of Treitz represents the **superior retention band**.

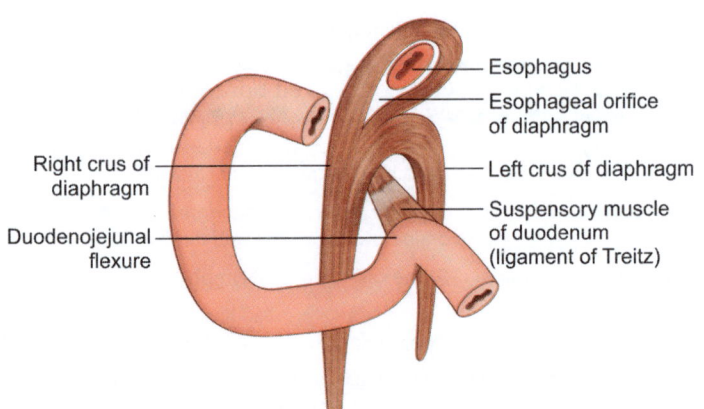

Fig. 23.13: Suspensory muscle of duodenum.

Functions
- Upward pull of the ligament of Treitz prevents the mobile loops of small intestine to be dragged down by the weight.
- The ligament of Treitz maintains the position of the duodenojejunal flexure which acts as a landmark in radiological diagnosis of abnormal rotation of the gut.

Clinical Anatomy

Shortening of the ligament of Treitz may cause partial intestinal obstruction due to abnormal kink of the duodenojejunal flexure.

SN 23.8 Discuss the general characteristics of the jejunum and ileum.
(Important for viva voce and practical)

JEJUNUM AND ILEUM

General Plan (Fig. 23.14)
- Jejunum and ileum are the **longest compoment** of the gastrointestinal tract.
- These parts of the gut are **most mobile** as suspended by a double fold of peritoneum called **the mesentery**.
- The length of jejunum and ileum is **6 meters** or **20 feet**.
- **Proximal two fifth** is jejunum and **distal three fifth** is ileum. But there is no clear line of demarcation between the two.
- The great length of jejunum and ileum is to provide a **very large mucosal surface area** which helps in aborption of nutrients.
- This part of the gut begins at the **duodenojejunal flexure** located at the left side of lower border of body of 1st lumbar vertebra.

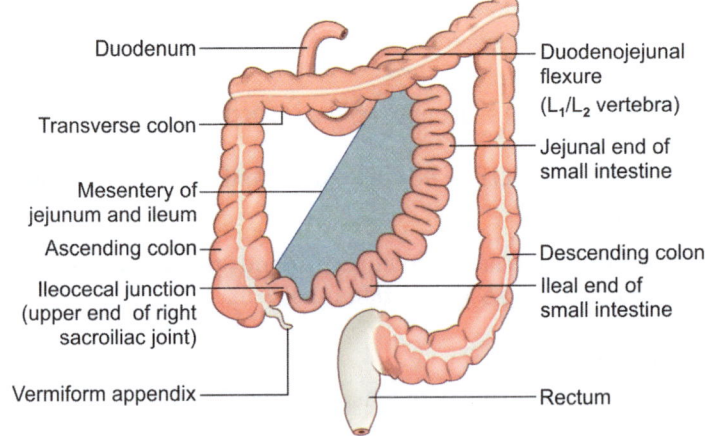

Fig. 23.14: Extent of jejunum and ileum.

- Ileal end terminates at the **ileocecal junction** at the upper end of right sacroiliac joint.
- Double fold of the mesentery connects jejunum and ileum to the posterior abdominal wall through its oblique posterior fixed border which extends from the left side of upper border of 2nd lumbar vertebra to the upper end of right sacroiliac joint.

Salient Points Related to the Structures

Layers

Jejunum and ileum, being parts of gastrointestinal tract, are made up of four layers which are following from within outwards:
1. Mucosa (mucous membrane)
2. Submucous coat
3. Muscular coat made up of outer longitudinal and inner circular layers.
4. Serous coat made up of lining of visceral layer of peritoneum.

Borders and Surfaces

Jejunum and ileum represents the borders and surfaces of the fetal life. The border giving attachment to the mesentery is called **mesenteric border**. The border opposite to it is known as **antemesenteric border**. These are original fetal dorsal and ventral borders respectively. Original fetal surface of the jejunum and ileum, like other parts of the gut are **right and left**. But these are not maintained as the loops or coils of this part of intestine are irregularly placed within the abdominal cavity.

Mucosal surface

Total surface area of mucosal lining of jejunum and ileum is **200 sq mtrs** to facilitate absorption of nutrients. This extensive surface area for absorption is due to the following factors in addition to the 20 feet length of this part of the gut.

Plicae circulares *(sing: plica circularis)* (Fig. 23.15) are complete or incomplete circular folds arranged parallelly on the surface of entire length of mucous membrane. These are also known as **Valves of Kerckring**. These mucous folds are oriented transversely or slightly obliquely to the long axis of the gut. Most of them extend round *half or two thirds of the luminal circumference*. Some are complete circles and some of them bifurcate.

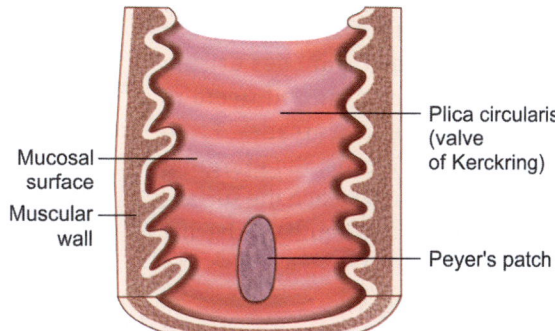

Fig. 23.15: Plica circularis and Peyer's patch.

The folds begin in the duodenum, 5 cm distal to the pyloroduodenal junction. They are most crowded in distal duodenum and proximal jejunum. Beyond this, they diminish in size as well as number and disappear completely at the terminal end of ileum. Unlike the folds of gastric mucosa, plicae circulares do not disappear during physiological distension of the intestine. These circular folds increase the absorptive surface area of the intestinal mucosa.

Intestinal villi are highly vascularized projection from the mucosal surface, just visible to the naked eye. They lead to **seven times increase** of the surface area of the mucous membrane. Villi are large and numerous in jejunum (also duodenum). They are smaller and less in number in ileum. Height of the villi are **0.5 mm to 1 mm**. Their density varies from **10 to 40 per sq mtrs**.

Microvilli are ultramicroscopic finger-like projections from the free surface of the intestinal columnar epithelium called **enterocytes.** Each of the cells presents about 300 microvilli. They **greatly increase the surface area for absorption**.

Infolding of the mucosal surface from the base of the villi for a short distance in the lamina propria of mucous membrane forms intestinal glands. They are called **crypts of Lieberkuhn.** These glands liberate digestive enzymes.

Peyer's patches are specialized variety of mucosa associated lymphoid tissue **(MALT)** underneath the intestinal epithelium. They are oval patchy areas of aggregated lymphoid tissue scattered **along the antemesenteric border** of jejunum and ileum. The long axis of these oval follicles is oriented along the long axis of the intestine. Peyer's patches are **more in number** and larger in size **towards the ileal end**. Here, they extend deeper in submucous plane.

SN 23.9 Write a short note on arterial supply of jejunum and ileum.

ARTERIAL SUPPLY OF JEJUNUM AND ILEUM (FIGS. 23.16A AND B)

Parallelly arranged series of **jejunal and ileal branches** arise from the convex left side of the **superior mesenteric artery** while it runs obliquely downwards and to the right along the root or posterior fixed border of the mesentery.

Jejunal and ileal arteries, while running between the two layers of mesentery, bifurcate in an arched fashion. Bifurcated branches anastomose with each other and form **arterial arcade**. Branches arising from the arcade again bifurcate to form the successive arcades. From the final stage arcade, the **marginal arteries** ultimately reach the surface of the jejunum and ileum. For having straight course, these arteries are called **arteria recta**.

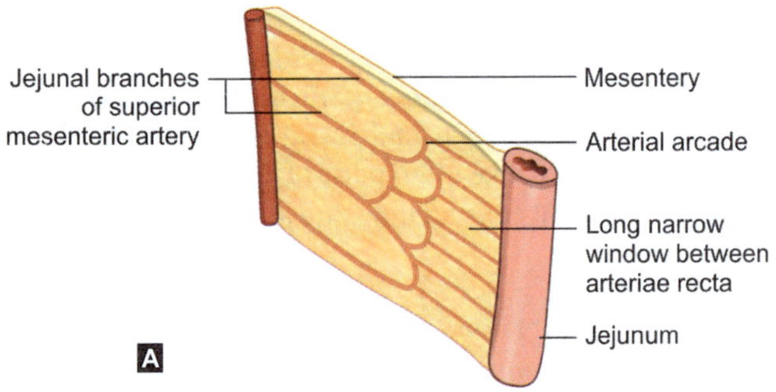

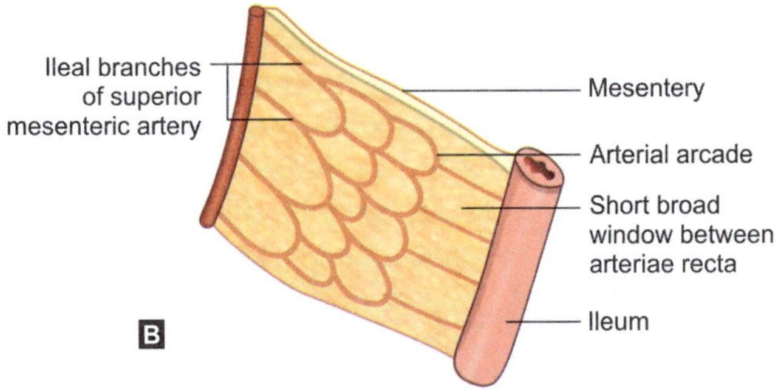

Jejunal arteries are **4–6 branches**. They are distributed to the jejunum via **1 to 3 arterial arcades**. The most distal arcade gives rise to straight arteries (arteriae recta) which are distributed alternately to the either side of the jejunum.

Figs. 23.16A and B: Arterial arcades and arteriae recta of jejunum and ileum: (A) Jejumum: Less number of arcades and long narrow windows; (B) Ileum: More number of arcades and short broad windows.

Small branches from the jejunal arteries supply **mesenteric lymph nodes**.

Ileal arteries are **more numerous (8 to 10)**. They form as many as **6 arterial arcades** before giving rise to multiple straight arteries which appear to be shorter than those of the jejunum.

Because of the abundance of fat in the ileal end of the mesentery, the arterial arcades and the straight arteries are less clearly visible at the ileal end. Due to more number of arterial arcades, arteriae recta are shorter at the ileal end of the small intestine.

SA 23.10 Write a brief note on the mesentery of small intestine.

THE MESENTERY (MESENTERY OF SMALL INTESTINE)

Introduction
The mesentery is the double fold of peritoneum by which mobile loops of jejunum and ileum are connected to the posterior abdominal wall.

Morphology
The mesentery is one of the persistent component of primitive dorsal mesentery of the gut of fetal life.

Features
- **2 layers:** Right and left.
- **2 ends:** Proximal (jejunal) and distal (ileal).
- **2 borders:** Ventral (intestinal) and dorsal (vertebral).
- Dorsal border of the mesentery, fixed to the posterior abdominal wall is known as the *root of the mesentery.*
- Anteroposterior breadth of the mesentery is 8 inches at the middle.
- **Proximal end** of the mesentery is at the level of **duodenojejunal flexure**.
- **Distal end** is at the level of **ileocecal junction**.

Root of the Mesentery (Fig. 23.17)
- **Introduction:** Root of the mesentery is the posterior, fixed vertebral border of the mesentery.
- **Direction:** Obliquely directed downwards and to the right.
- **Length:** 6 inches.
- **Extent:** Root of the mesentery begins at the left side of upper border of body of **L$_2$ vertebra** at the level of **duodenojejunal flexure**. It ends at the upper end of **right sacroiliac joint** at the level of **ileocecal junction**.
- **Structures crossed by the root:** The followig structures are crossed by the root of the mesentery from above downwards and to the right in the posterior abdominal wall **(Fig. 23.17)**.
  - Abdominal aorta
  - Inferior vena cava
  - Right gonadal (testicular or ovarian) vessels
  - Right ureter
  - Right psoas major muscle.
- **Structures present in the root:** Superior mesenteric vessels and lymph nodes.

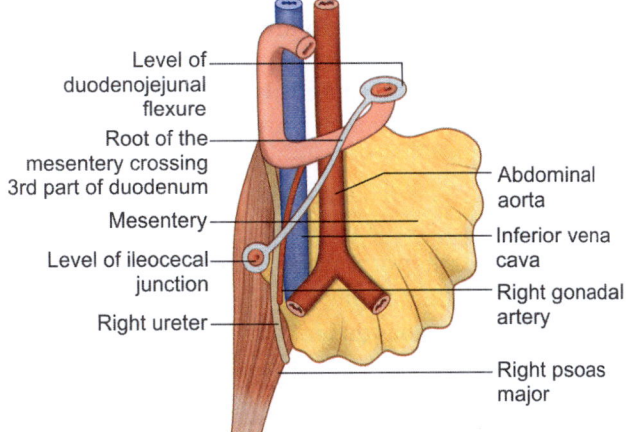

Fig. 23.17: Mesentery of small intestine.

Intestinal Border of the Mesentery
It is the **anterior free border** of the mesentery. Along this line double folds of the mesentery are continuous with each other around the jejunum and ileum. Length of this border is **6 meters** or **20 feet**, i.e. equal to the length of the jejunum and ileum. This border is thrown into pleats or folds like those of a folded cloth.

Contents of the Mesentery
- **Superior mesentery vessels** along the root or posterior fixed border. The vein is to the right of the artery.
- **Jejunum and ileum**: Enclosed by the mesentery at its anterior free border.
- Jejunal and ileal branches of superior mesenteric artery with the corresponding veins. The arterial arcades and arteriae recta (*sing: arteria recti*) are also the contents.
- Mesenteric lymph nodes, as many as 200 in number
- Lymph vessles
- Autonomic nerves forming superior mesenteric plexus
- Variable amount of mesenteric fat.

Functions
- The mesentery carries the blood vessels, nerves and lymphatics to and from the jejunum and ileum.
- It allows mobility of this part of the gut.

Clinical Anatomy
- The freely mobile folds of the mesentery acts as a **facilitating factor for herniation** of mobile loops of small intestine.
- Large number of **mesenteric lymph nodes** are the **common sites for various kinds of infection.** Tuberculous infection is known as Tabes mesenterica. In abdominal tuberculosis, pain is felt along the line of root of mesentery on clinical examination.
- A **tumor or cyst** of the mesentery may be detected along the line of the root of the mesentery.
- **Mesenteric arterial occlusion** may occur in cases of air embolism or thrombosis of superior mesenteric artery or any of its branches. It will cause avascular necrosis (cellular death) of affected segment of the intestine.
- **Mesenteric venous thrombosis** may occur due to stasis or stagnation of the venous blood within the mesentery. Cirrhosis of liver leading to portal hypertension may predispose this condition.

SA 23.11 Mention the differences between jejunum and ileum.
(*For viva voce and practical*)

DIFFERENCES BETWEEN JEJUNUM AND ILEUM
External Character
- **Relative length: Proximal two fifth** is jejunum. **Distal three fifth** of total length is ileum.
- **Location**: Jejunum is placed in upper and left part of abdominal cavity. Ileum is located in lower and right part.
- **Vascularity**: Surface of jejunum looks more vascular, so more pinkish in color.

- **Wall:** Wall of the jejunum is thicker than that of ileum.
- **Lumen:** Lumen of the jejunum is wider.

Mucosal Surface

- **Plicae circulares** are more prominent and more closely arranged in jejunum. They gradually become lesser in number in ileum and finally disappear in the terminal end.
- **Peyer's patches** are found in the ileum.
- **Villi** are longer and thicker, and more crowded in the jejunum.

Mesentery

- More **quantity of fat** is present within the mesentery at the ileal end.
- **Arterial arcades** are 2 to 3 at the jejunal end of the mesentery. These are 3 to 6 at the ileal end.
- **Arteriae recta** are longer at the jejunal end of the mesentery. They are shorter at the ileal end.
- **Arterial windows** in between the arteriae recta are more clearly visible at the jejunal end due to less amount of fat.

SN 23.12 Write a short note on the Meckel's diverticulum.

MECKEL'S DIVERTICULUM (FIG. 23.18A)

Introduction
Meckel's diverticulum is the persistent proximal part of embryonic vitello intestinal duct. In fetal life, the vitellointestinal duct extends from the summit of the 'U' shaped midgut loop to the yolk sac.

Incidence
In 2–3% of individuals.

Location
At the antemesenteric border of the ileum 2 feet proximal to the ileocecal junction.

Length
About 2–5 cm in adults.

Caliber of the Lumen
Similar to that of ileum.

Blood Supply
Meckel's diverticulum is supplied by the branch from the terminal end of the superior mesenteric artery lying in a small *'mesentery'* of adipose tissue. This vessel represents the terminal end of the *vitellointestinal artery*.

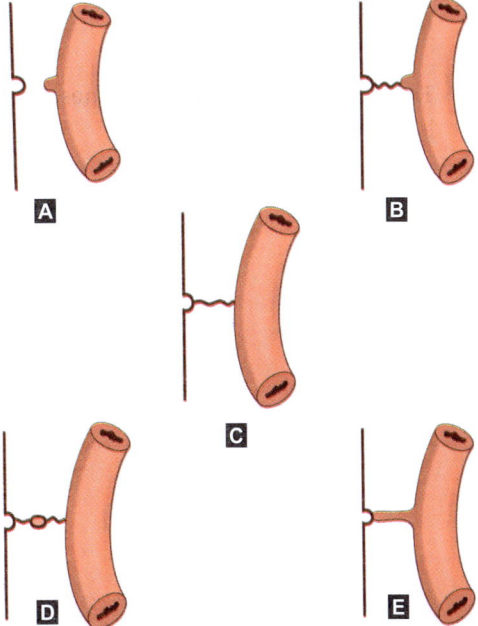

Figs. 23.18A to E: Anomalies of vitellointestinal duct: (A) Meckel's diverticulum; (B) Diverticulum with fibrous band; (C) Vitellointestinal duct persisting as fibrous band; (D) Meckel's cyst; (E) Meckel's fistula.

Mucosa

The mucous membrane of the Mackel's diverticulum is typically like that of ileum. But it presents some **heterotopic areas**. These are **gastric body type epithelium** and, may be **pancreatic** and **colonic types**.

Clinical Anatomy

Variations

- Meckel's diverticulum may be connected through a **fibrous band** to the umbilicus **(Fig. 23.18B)**. The diverticulum may be absent but the whole of the vitellointestinal duct is represented by a fibrous band extending from ileum to the umbilicus **(Fig. 23.18C)**. In these cases, a loop of small gut may be twisted around the band to cause **intestinal obstruction**.
- **Meckel's cyst**: In this case, intermediate part of the vitellointestinal duct persists in the form of a cyst which is connected by both sided fibrous bands to the ileum and umbilicus **(Fig. 23.18D)**.
- **Meckel's fistula**: It occurs due to patency of the whole of the vitellointestinal duct which communicates ileum with umbilicus **(Fig. 23.18E)**. Because of this anomaly, a newborn presents discharge of intestinal contents through umbilicus.

Mucosal Ulceration and Bleeding

- **Unopposed acid secretion** by the gastric type of epithelium may lead to ulceration of the mucosa and subsequent bleeding.
- **Inflammation** of the Meckel's diverticulum (*diverticulitis*) may give rise to pain in abdomen which may be confused with that of **appendicitis.**
- **Calculi** (stone formation), **tumor** and **perforation** of the diverticulum are rare complications.

Chapter 24

Liver and Biliary Apparatus

LA 24.1 Mention the gross features and anatomical position of the liver.
(For viva voce and practical in general)

LIVER

Introduction
- Liver is the *largest organ* of the body. It is reddish, very vascular, soft and friable in nature in living state. In adults, liver is roughly 1500 g in weight and 1500 mL of blood passes through it per minute.
- Liver is a wedge-shaped organ with 5 surfaces **(Fig. 24.1).**

Position
- Liver is situated in right side of upper abdomen *under right dome* and *central part* of the thoracoabdominal diaphragm.
- Liver is mainly in *right hypochondrium* and *epigastrium* extending into *left hypochondrium*.

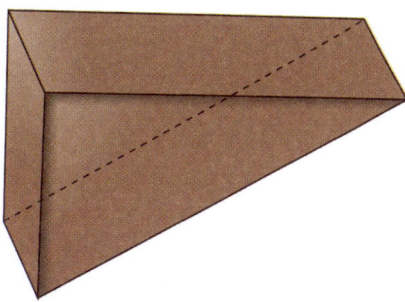

Fig. 24.1: Liver is a wedge-shaped organ having 5 surfaces.

Functions
Liver has three basic functions:
1. **Glandular:** Liver is the *largest gland* in the body having both exocrine and endocrine components
   - **Exocrine component** is concerned with **synthesis of bile** which is transported in the intestine for digestion *of fat.*
   - **Endocrine component** liberates **heparin** which is an *anticoagulant* of blood.
2. **Metabolic:** Liver is involved in various metabolic functions concerned with carbohydrate, protein and fat metabolism.
3. **Detoxication:** Liver is concerned with detoxication of body through filtration of blood, thus removing bacteria and other toxic substances which enter the blood from the lumen of gastrointestinal tract.

Gross Features
Liver is known also as **hepar**. Both the terms liver as well as hepar are made up of **5 letters**. The number 5 is important because the organ has:
1. 5 surfaces
2. 5 borders

3. 5 lobes
4. 5 peritoneal folds
5. 5 nonperitoneal areas called bare areas.

5 Surfaces

1. Right lateral ⎫
2. Anterior   ⎬ **Diaphragmatic surfaces**
3. Posterior   ⎪
4. Superior   ⎭
5. Inferior   = **Visceral surface**

Out of these, first four surfaces are commonly called **diaphragmatic surfaces** as related to under surface of the diaphragm. Inferior surface of liver related to different abdominal organs, is called **visceral surface**.

5 Borders

Geometrically wedge of the liver is supposed to have many borders **(Fig. 24.2A)**. But primarily liver shows five (5) borders as follows.

1. **Anterior border:** Separates anterior from superior surface.
2. **Posterior border:** Separates superior from posterior surface.
3. **Right inferior border:** Separates right lateral surface from inferior surface.
4. **Anteroinferior border:** Separates anterior from inferior surface.
5. **Left superior border:** Separates left end of superior surface from inferior surface.

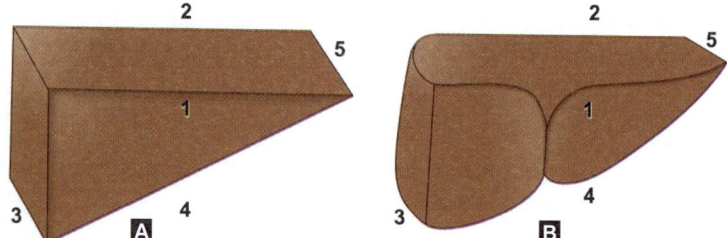

Figs. 24.2A and B: 5 borders (No. 1 to 5) of wedge-shaped liver form 3 prominent borders of the organ: (1) Anterior border—separates anterior from superior surfaces; (2) Posterior border—separates superior form posterior surfaces; (3 to 5) Inferor border—separates inferior surface from right lateral, anterior and left end of superior surfaces.

But liver presents only **one sharp and prominent inferior border** which is made up of the borders 3, 4 and 5 **(Figs. 24.2A and B)** which separates inferior visceral surface from right lateral surface, anterior surface and left end of superior surface.

5 Lobes (Fig. 24.3)

2 major lobes:
1. Right lobe
2. Left lobe

3 minor lobes:
3. Caudate lobe—on posterior surface
4. Quadrate lobe—on inferior surface
5. Riedel's lobe—occasional, projecting as a small tongue-shaped process from the inferior border on the right side of gallbladder.

Anatomical Position of Liver

As the liver is an unilateral organ lying almost to the right side of midline, question of side determination does not arise.

First, 5 Surfaces are to be Identified as follows:
- **Right lateral surface** is more or less flat and *vertically oriented*.
- **Anterior surface** is recognized by a peritoneal fold called *falciform ligament* which is vertically directed.
- **Superior surface** is slightly *depressed in the middle*, where two layers of falciform ligament diverge.
- **Posterior surface** is known by a *segment of inferior vena cava which* is connected to the surface as hepatic veins just coming out from posterior surface of liver open in inferior vena cava. *The groove lodging the vena cava is vertically directed.*
- **Inferior surface** is identified by presence of gallbladder on its bed (fossa) on right lobe of liver and various other visceral impressions.

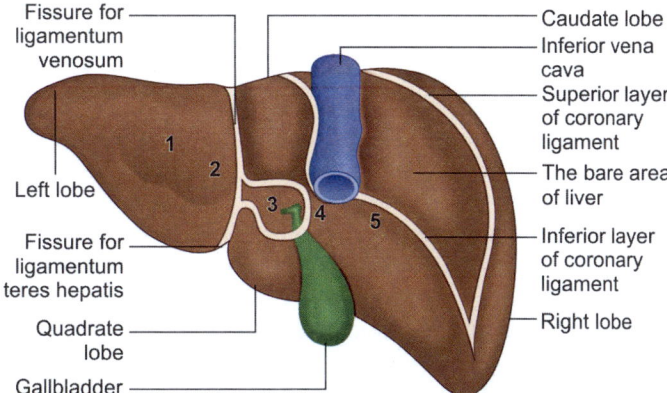

Fig. 24.3: Posterior surface is demarcated from inferior surface by: (1) A ridge on left lobe; (2) Fissure for ligamentum venosum; (3) Porta hepatis; (4) Caudate process; (5) Inferior layer of coronary ligament.

Sharp inferior border is identified by following points:
- It is **cut by the fissure for ligamentum teres hepatis**
- It is **crossed by gallbladder** usually.

Points for Anatomical Position

If above-mentioned points are clear, following two points are sufficient for anatomical position of liver.
1. **Groove for inferior vena cava** lodging a segment of the vein is **vertically directed** on posterior surface of liver which faces backwards.
2. **Inferior surface**, lodging gallbladder in its fossa, **faces downwards, backwards and to the left.**
   Automatically other 3 surfaces, anterior, superior and right lateral, face to the corresponding aspects.

Hepatic Lobes (Fig. 24.3)

Liver is primarily divided into **large right lobe (five sixth)** and smaller **left lobe (one sixth).** On the surface, right and left lobes are demarcated as follows.
- *On anterior and superior surface*: By the line of attachment of **falciform ligament**
- *On the posterior surface*: By the fissure for the **ligamentum venosum** lodging the ligament of same name.
- *On the inferior surface*: By the fissure for the **ligamentum teres hepatis** lodging the ligament of same name.

Posterior and inferior surfaces of right lobe of liver shows well demarcated small rectangular caudate lobe and quadrate lobe respectively.
- **Caudate lobe** is a small rectangular well-bounded area of posterior surface of right lobe of liver. It is demarcated on the right by *groove for inferior vena cava*, on the left *by fissure for the ligamentum venosum* and inferiorly by the hilum of liver called *porta hepatis*.

- **Caudate process** is a narrow conical projection from the *right end* of lower margin of caudate lobe.
- **Papillary process** is a small round projection from the *left end* of lower margin of caudate lobe.
- **Quadrate lobe** is the similar small rectangular well-demarcated portion of right lobe of liver on its inferior surface. It is bounded to the right by the *fossa for gallbladder*, to the left by the *fissure for ligamentum teres hepatis* and posteriorly by the *porta hepatis*.
    - **Riedel's lobe**: It is an occasional lobe of liver. Riedel's lobe is a small tongue-shaped projection *from inferior margin* of right lobe of liver to the right side of fossa for gallbladder.

Physiological Subdivision of Hepatic Lobes

Physiological right and left lobes are the two halves of liver which receive ramifications from right and left division hepatic artery, portal vein and bile duct respectively. Venous blood from right and left physiological lobes are drained by tributaries of right and left hepatic veins respectively.

As per this consideration caudate and quadrate lobes are parts of left lobe of liver. Actually, the caudate lobe receives blood from both right and left divisions of hepatic artery and portal vein.

Porta Hepatis—the Hilum of Liver (Fig. 24.3)

Porta hepatis is the gateway or hilum of liver for transmission of structures in to-and-fro direction. It is a transverse fissure of 5 cm length situated at the junction of posterior and inferior surfaces, between caudate and quadrate lobes of liver.

Structures passing through the porta hepatis are the following

Structures Entering
- Right and left divisions of hepatic artery
- Right and left divisions of portal vein
- Sympathetic and parasympathetic nerve fibers for the liver.

Structures Leaving
- Right and left hepatic ducts
- Lymph vessels draining liver.

Lymph nodes at the porta hepatis receive lymph vessels from *liver and gallbladder*. Efferent vessels from these nodes drain into *celiac lymph nodes*.

Glisson's Capsule

Liver is enclosed all around by a fibroconnective tissue capsule which surrounds the margin of porta hepatis. This is known as Glisson's capsule.

Hepatic Pedicle

These are bunch of structures which pass through porta hepatis and surrounded by continuation of Glisson's capsule from liver. In the hepatic pedicle two divisions of hepatic duct, hepatic artery and portal vein lie in anteroposterior relation.

Peritoneal Folds of Porta Hepatis

A double fold of peritoneum called *lesser omentum* extends from the porta hepatis and fissure for ligamentum venosum to the lesser curvature of stomach and first one inch of the duodenum. Part of the lesser omentum extending from the porta hepatis to the duodenum is known as hepatoduodenal part forming right free margin of lesser omentum.

Supports of Liver

Large sized liver needs supports to maintain its position. In order of importance supports of liver are following.
- **Hepatic veins**—3 hepatic veins (right, middle and left) are the most important support of liver. They are very short and immediately *coming out from posterior surface* they drain into inferior vena cava.
- Surrounding viscera—packing all around.
- Peritoneal folds attached to liver.

Segments of Liver (Fig. 24.4)

Liver is divided into eight (8) segments which are numbered from Segment I to Segment VIII. Out of these segments, right and left lobe of liver contain four (4) segments each, of which *segments I to IV belong to left lobe and segments V to VIII are in right lobe of liver.*

Each of the segments receives an independent division of hepatic artery and portal vein and from each of them independent unit of hepatic duct comes out. When independent branch of hepatic artery lies within one hepatic segment (intrasegmental), a tributary of hepatic vein is intersegmental in position receiving venous blood from adjacent segments.

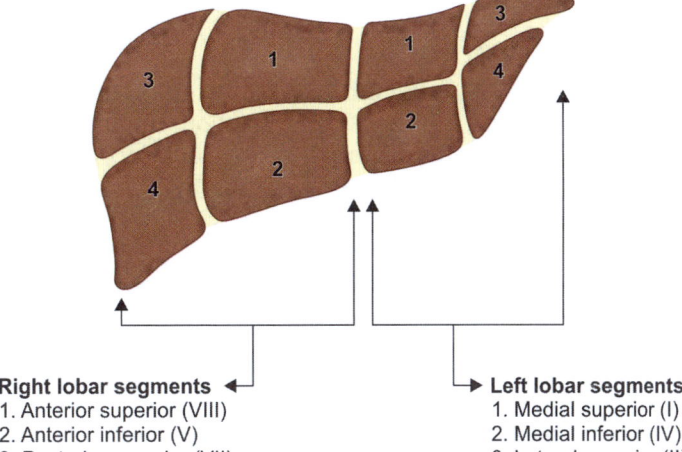

Right lobar segments
1. Anterior superior (VIII)
2. Anterior inferior (V)
3. Posterior superior (VII)
4. Posterior inferior (VI)

Left lobar segments
1. Medial superior (I)
2. Medial inferior (IV)
3. Lateral superior (II)
4. Lateral inferior (III)

Fig. 24.4: Segments of liver (Roman numerals are segment numbers).

Subdivisions of Hepatic Segments

Left lobe segments (segments I to IV)
Medial: 1. Medial superior = segment I
2. Medial inferior = segment IV
Lateral: 3. Lateral superior = segment II
4. Lateral inferior = segment III

Right lobe segments (segments V to VIII)
Anterior: 1. Anterior superior = segment VIII
2. Anterior inferior = segment V
Posterior: 3. Posterior superior = segment VII
4. Posterior inferior = segment VI

Importance of Segment I

- Segment I, though belong to left lobe, consists of caudate lobe, which anatomically belong to the right lobe of liver.
- Segment I or caudate lobe segment receives blood from both right and left branches of hepatic artery and portal vein.
- This segment drains blood neither to right nor to the left hepatic vein. Blood drains directly to inferior vena cava.
- The caudate lobe segment drains bile to the biliary channels of both right and left sides.

Importance of Intersegmental Plane

Inter segmental planes are detected by position of tributaries of hepatic veins. These tributaries act as a guide to find out the planes for segmental resection of liver which is required to remove only the diseased segment of liver. Replacement of an adequate part of liver is compensated by great regenerating power hepatocytes (liver cells) from normal liver tissue left behind.

Peritoneal Relation of Liver

As peritoneum is reflected from body wall to the liver and again from the liver back to the body wall, following points are to be noted in connection with the peritoneal relation of the organ.
- Most of the area of surfaces of liver is covered by peritoneum.
- Some areas are nonperitoneal for being directly in contact with some structures (**Fig. 24.3**), e.g.
    - Fossa for gallbladder
    - Groove for inferior vena cava
- **Porta hepatis**, transmitting the structures of hepatic pedicle, is the area not covered by peritoneum (**Fig. 24.3**).
- As peritoneum is reflected from upper and lower margin of posterior surface of right lobe of liver to the undersurface of diaphragm and to the anterior surface of right kidney respectively (**Fig. 24.5**), an area of posterior surface of right lobe of liver, triangular in outline, bounded above and below by superior and inferior layers of coronary ligament respectively is nonperitoneal (**Figs. 24.3 and 24.5**). This nonperitoneal area of liver is called **the bare area of liver**. Base of the bare area is formed by groove for inferior vena cava and apex is formed by meeting of upper and lower layers of coronary ligament at right triangular ligament (**Fig. 24.3**).

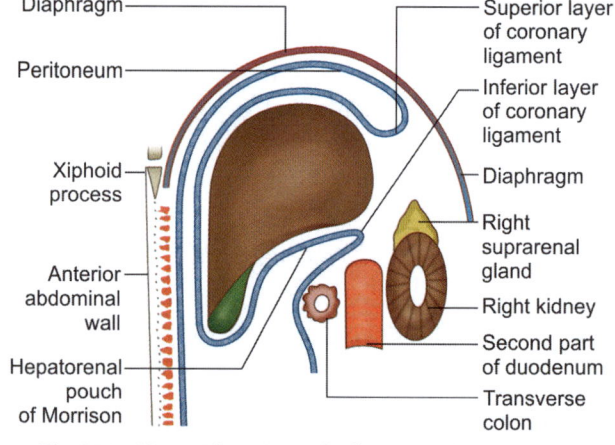

Fig. 24.5: Liver with peritoneal reflection and its important anterior, superior and posterior relations.

- When double layer (right and left) of falciform ligament fall from undersurface of anterior part of diaphragm and supraumbilical part of anterior abdominal wall on to the anterior and superior surfaces of liver, two layers diverge from each other on superior surface. For this reason, a triangular area on superior surface with apex directed downwards and forwards (**Fig. 24.6**) becomes devoid of peritoneal lining.

Bare Areas (Nonperitoneal Areas) of Liver (Figs. 24.3 and 24.6)

Bare areas of the liver are the area which are not covered by the visceral peritoneum.
- Fossa for the gallbladder—on inferior surface
- Groove for inferior vena cava—on posterior surface
- Porta hepatis—at the junction of posterior surface and inferior surface, between caudate and quadrate lobes
- The bare area of liver—on posterior surface of right lobe of liver it is a triangular area.
  Boundary of the bare area:
  - *Base* (to the left)—groove for inferior vena cava
  - *Apex* (to the right)—right triangular ligament
  - *Upper margin*—superior layer of coronary ligament
  - *Lower margin*—inferior layer of coronary ligament.
- A triangular area, with the apex directed downwards, is on superior surface of liver. This area is bounded by divergent right and left layers of the falciform ligament (**Fig. 24.6**).
  Besides the above five wide bare areas of liver, following narrow areas are also nonperitoneal areas.
- Floor of fissure for ligamentum venosum—between left lobe and caudate lobe of liver (**Fig. 24.3**).
- Floor of fissure for ligamentum teres between left and quadrate lobe of liver (**Fig. 24.3**).
- Small area **between anterosuperior and posteroinferior layers of right triangular ligament** as continuation of two layers of coronary ligament (**Fig. 24.3**).
- Small area **between anterior and posterior layers of left triangular ligament** on superior surface of left lobe of liver (**Fig. 24.6**).

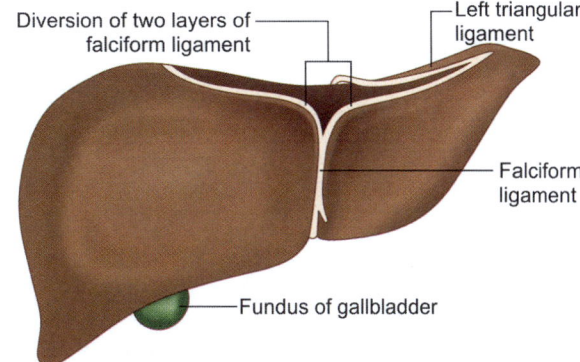

Fig. 24.6: Line of reflection of falciform ligament.

Ligaments of Liver

Peritoneal Ligaments (False Ligaments)

Falciform ligament (Fig. 24.7)

It is a sickle-shaped double fold of peritoneum which extends from anterior part of undersurface of diaphragm and supraumbilical part of anterior abdominal wall, to the superior and anterior surfaces of liver. The ligament presents following three borders.

1. **Anterior convex border:** Attached to diaphragm and anterior abdominal wall.
2. **Posterior concave border:** Attached to superior and anterior surfaces of liver.
3. **Inferior free border:** Extends from umbilicus to the notch on inferior border of liver.

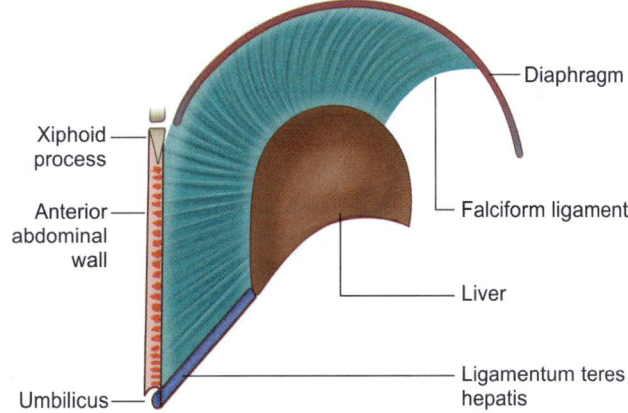

Fig. 24.7: Outlines of falciform ligament.

Right and left layers of falciform ligament are continuous with each other at the inferior free border which contains ligamentum teres hepatis and paraumbilical vein.

Coronary ligament

This peritoneal ligament of liver is composed of *superior and inferior layers*. Superior layer is reflected from the right end of the junction of superior and posterior surfaces of liver to the undersurface of diaphragm (**Fig. 24.5**). Inferior layer is reflected from the right end of the junction of posterior and inferior surfaces of liver to the front of right kidney to form a peritoneal recess called **hepatorenal pouch of Morison (Fig. 24.5)**. Two layers of coronary ligament converge at the right triangular ligament **(Fig. 24.3)**.

Right triangular ligament (Fig. 24.3)

This is a double layered angular peritoneal fold extending from apex of coronary ligament on *posterior surface* of liver to the undersurface of diaphragm. Layers of the ligament are anterosuperior and posteroinferior.

Left triangular ligament

This is a double layered angular peritoneal fold extending from *superior surface* of left lobe of liver to the undersurface of left dome of diaphragm (**Fig. 24.6**). Two layers converge at the left end.

Lesser omentum (Fig. 24.8)

Lesser omentum is included in the list of peritoneal folds of both stomach as well as liver. This is a double fold of peritoneum which extends from fissure for ligamentum venosum and porta hepatis to lesser curvature of stomach and upper border of first one inch of 2 inches length of 1st part of the duodenum.

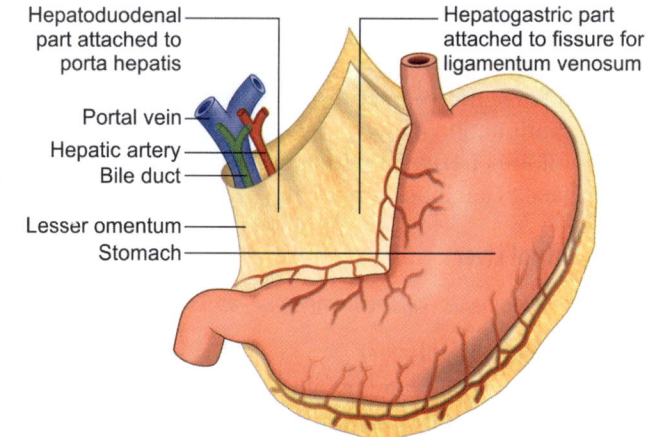

Fig. 24.8: Lesser omentum of stomach is also a peritoneal fold attached to the liver.

Parts of lesser omentum

- **Hepatogastric part**: It extends from fissure for ligamentum venosum of liver to lesser curvature of stomach. This part contains left and right gastric vessels.
- **Hepatoduodenal part**: It extends from the porta hepatis of liver to the upper border of 1st one inch of 1st part of duodenum. This part forms right free border of lesser omentum and contains portal vein, bile duct and hepatic artery. Hepatoduodenal part of lesser omentum forms anterior boundary of epiploic foramen.

Nonperitoneal (True) Ligaments

Ligamentum teres hepatis

This is a band of embryological remnant which passes along the inferior free margin of falciform ligament and extends from umbilicus to left division of portal vein at porta hepatis. This ligament represents the *obliterated left umbilical vein*.

Ligamentum venosum

This cord like structure is also another embryological remnant which represents *obliterated ductus venosus*. It used to connect the left division of portal vein with the hepatic vein draining into inferior vena cava or the inferior vena cava itself.

Visceral Relations of Liver

Only those visceral relations are discussed here which are anatomically and clinically important.

Visceral relations of liver are discussed in reference the five surfaces. It is already known that the surfaces are *anterior, posterior, superior, inferior* and *right lateral*. But for visceral relations surfaces are better discussed as per following order.

1. **Posterior** } merge with each other
2. **Inferior**
3. **Anterior** } merge with each other
4. **Superior**
5. **Right lateral**—has independent relations

Posterior Surface (Fig. 24.9)

First, it is to be known that the posterior surface is demarcated from the inferior surface by the following from left to right **(Fig. 24.3)**.
1. A slight bulge on posteroinferior aspect of left lobe called omental tuberosity related to lesser omentum of stomach
2. Fissure for ligamentum venosum
3. Porta hepatis
4. Caudate process
5. Inferior layer of coronary ligament.

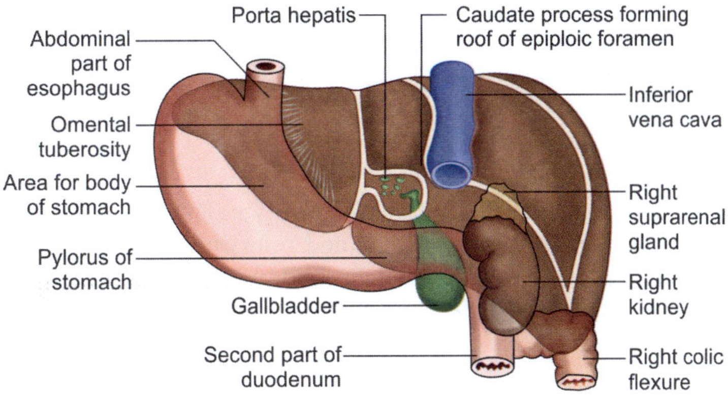

Fig. 24.9: Visceral relations of posterior and inferior surfaces of liver.

Middle of posterior surface presents a backward concavity to adapt convexity of body of vertebra.

Posterior surface of liver presents following relations *from left to right* **(Fig. 24.9)**:
- Posterior surface of narrow left lobe of liver presents a shallow vertical depression as this is related to **abdominal part of esophagus**.
- **Fissure for ligamentum venosum** is in between left lobe and caudate lobe. It is very deep fissure to extend from left margin to anterior surface of the caudate lobe. It lodges the ligamentum venosum.
- **Caudate lobe** is posteriorly related to **superior recess of lesser sac**. Caudate process forms the upper boundary of epiploic foramen.
- **Groove for inferior vena cava** is not only related to inferior vena cava, but also connected with a segment of this large venous channel because the hepatic veins, just emerging from posterior surface of liver drain into it.
- **The bare area of liver** lies at the right end of posterior surface. It is directly related to undersurface of **right dome of diaphragm** separated by loose connective tissue. It is

also related to **right suprarenal gland**. The bare area of liver is also an important **site for portocaval anastomosis** for communication between veins of portal system and systemic system.

Inferior Surface (Figs. 24.3 and 24.9)

Inferior surface is directed *downwards, backwards and to the left.*

from left to right, it bears following relations.
- **gastric impression**: Inferior surface of left lobe presents a concavity which is related to anterosuperior surface of stomach.
- **Tuber omentale**: It is a small bulge above and to the right of gastric impression. It is related to lesser omentum of stomach.
- **Fissure for ligamentum teres**: It extends from the inferior border of the liver to left end of porta hepatis. It lodges the ligamentum teres hepatis.
- **Quadrate lobe**: It is related to **pylorus of stomach** and **1st part of duodenum**.
- **Fossa for gall bladder**: It is the nonperitoneal bed for gallbladder lodging usually the neck and body of gallbladder, as the fundus projects beyond inferior border.
- Lateral end of inferior surface of right lobe of liver is related to following structures.
    - **Second part of duodenum**
    - **Anterior surface of right kidney**
    - **Right colic flexure.**

Anterior Surface (Fig. 24.5)

- Major part of anterior surface of liver is under cover of **costal margin**.
- Upper part of the surface is related to **forward slope of right dome of diaphragm**.
- Lower part is related to **anterior abdominal wall** with **xiphoid process**.
- Posterior margin of **falciform ligament** is attached to the anterior surface of liver (**Fig. 24.7**).

Superior Surface (Fig. 24.10)

Superior surface of liver presents a **central concavity** with bulge on either side. **Central tendon of diaphragm** separates the central depressed part of superior surface of liver from the **diaphragmatic surface of heart**.

Right and left dome of **diaphragm** separates the bulge of superior surface of corresponding lobe of liver from the **base of the lung** of respective side and the **diaphragmatic pleura**.

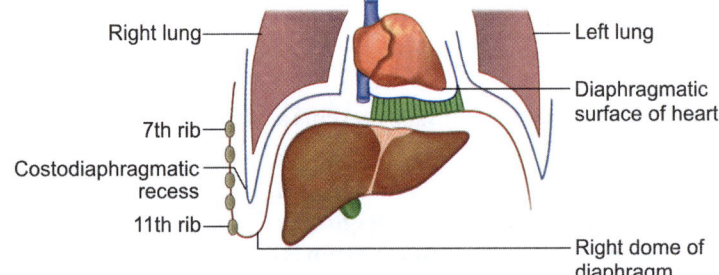

Fig. 24.10: Relations of superior and right lateral surfaces of liver.

Right Lateral Surface (Fig. 24.10)

Right lateral surface is quadrangular in outline. It is flattened from above downwards and convex in anteroposterior direction.

Right dome of the diaphragm separates this surface of liver form **right lateral body wall** at the level of **7th rib to 11th rib**. In the midaxillary line, right lateral surface of liver is related to **costodiaphragmatic recess of right pleura** *up to 10th rib* and **base of right lung** *up to 8th rib* between the diaphragm and lateral chest wall.

Short notes: **Porta hepatis; Segments of liver; Bare areas of liver; Ligaments of the liver**

SN 24.2 Write a short note on the basic architecture of liver.

BASIC ARCHITECTURE OF LIVER (FIG. 24.11)

- Liver cells are named **hepatocytes**.
- Hepatocytes in rows radiate peripherally from the smallest tributary of hepatic veins, called **central vein**.
- Rows of hepatocytes, called **hepatic laminae** radiating from the central vein form hexagonal histological units called **hepatic lobules**.
- Spaces between the hepatic laminae of hepatic lobule are alternatively occupied by minute vascular and biliary channels called **sinusoids** and **bile canaliculi**.

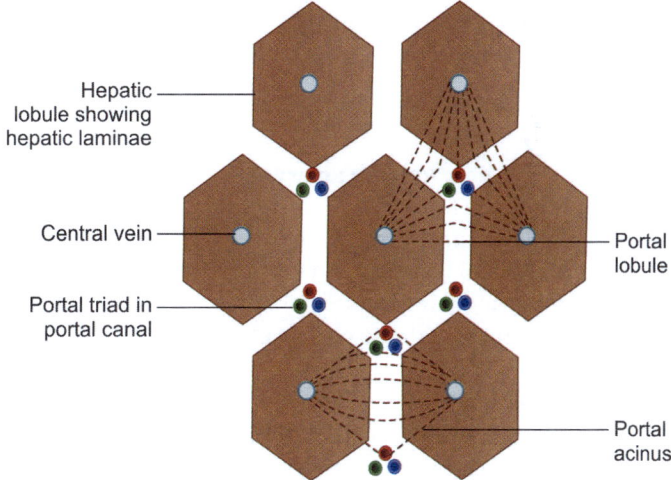

Fig. 24.11: Architecture of liver.

- Space bounded by three adjacent hepatic lobules is known as **portal canal** which contains final branch of hepatic artery, final division of portal vein and initial radical of biliary duct. These three channels are collectively called **portal triad**.
- Sinusoids extend from central canal of hepatic lobule containing central vein to portal canal containing divisions of hepatic artery and portal vein. Sinusoids are lined by **fenestrated endothelial cells** which are related to **Kupfer cells** possessing phagocytic activity.
- Space between wall of sinusoid and hepatic lamina is known as **space of Disse** which contain **Ito (perisinusoidal) cells**. These cells liberate substances which are required for regeneration of hepatocytes. Space of Disse opens into **space of Mall** at the portal canal.
- Bile synthesized by hepatocytes are poured into bile canaliculi which open into **bile ductule** in portal canal.

Triangular area outlined by the lines joining the central vein of *three adjacent hepatic lobulse* is known as **portal lobule** which is fed by ultimate division of hepatic artery and portal vein.

Portal acinus is the diamond-shaped area of two side by side hepatic lobules. Its two diagonally opposite angles are formed by central veins. Another two opposite angles are formed by divisions of hepatic artery lying in two portal canals. Portal acinus is divided into following three zones.

Zone I: Peripheral zone
- Close to hepatic artery
- Hepatocytes are richly supplied by oxygen
- So suffer least from cell damage

Zone II: Intermediate zone

Zone III: Central zone
- Farthest form branch of hepatic artery
- Receive minimum supply of oxygen
- So hepatocytes suffer maximum from cell damage.

SA 24.3 Mention the blood supply, nerve supply, lymphatic drainage and clinical anatomy of liver. (For viva voce and practical).

LIVER

Arterial Supply

Artery for the liver is **hepatic artery**. But out of total amount of blood received by the liver, **80% of blood** is carried from gastrointestinal tract **through portal vein**. This blood carries nutrients, metabolites and toxins for respective use. **Hepatic artery carries 20% of total blood.** Right and left divisions of the hepatic artery and the portal vein for corresponding lobes divide into segmental and finally into interlobular branches which lie in portal canal. Finally in the hepatic sinusoids hepatic arterial blood mixes with the portal venous blood.

Venous Drainage

Veins draining the liver are hepatic veins. Venous channels start from **hepatic sinusoids** located between hepatic laminae. Venous blood from sinusoids reaches first in the **central veins** of hepatic lobules. These unite to form **interlobular veins** which join to form **sub-lobular veins**. Sub-lobular veins form multiple hepatic veins.

Hepatic veins are divided into two groups—upper and lower. **Upper hepatic veins** are three in number—**right, middle and left**. These come out from upper part of groove for inferior vena cava and drain into inferior vena cava. **Lower hepatic veins** are **narrower** and variable in number. These **come out from right lobe and caudate lobe** and drain into inferior vena cava.

Lymphatic Drainage

Knowledge of lymphatic drainage of liver is important from clinical point of view, because the liver is the organ for primary as well as secondary carcinoma.

Lymph vessels start as **minute blind channels in the space of Mall** of portal canal. Then the lymph vessels are divided into superficial and deep groups.

Superficial lymph vessels come out from all round the surfaces of liver and drain into following lymph nodes in different directions.
- **Hepatic nodes** at porta hepatis
- **Para-cardiac nodes** related to lower end of oesophagus, adjacent to heart, and receive lymph vessels from left lobe.
- **Celiac nodes** receive direct lymph vessels from right lobe.
- **Retrosternal, phrenic** and **mediastinal** group of lymph nodes of thorax.

Deep lymph vessels finally come out to form two trunks. **Upper trunk** enters thorax through vena caval orifice and drains into *lymph nodes related to terminal part of inferior vena cava*. **Lower trunk** drains into *hepatic nodes related to porta hepatis*.

Nerve Supply

Main source of autonomic innervation of liver is **celiac plexus**. Sympatheic fibers are derived **from the greater splanchnic nerve (T_5 to T_9)** and the **vagus nerve** supplies parasympathetic fibers. Fibers are distributed through the hepatic artery and its branches.

Autonomic nerve fibers also reach the liver **through its peritoneal folds.**

Clinical Anatomy

Viral Hepatitis

It is an inflammatory disease of liver due to some viral infection. Commonest varieties are hepatitis A and hepatitis B viruses. **Hepatitis A** is caused by contaminated drinking water. **Hepatitis B** virus is carried through infected needle used for any injection or because of transfusion of infected blood.

Fatty Liver

This condition is characterized by accumulation of lipid droplets in the cytoplasm of hepatocytes. This occurs due to toxic effects of some ingested substances or some drugs. This is followed by degeneration of hepatocytes and subsequent fibrosis of liver, called **cirrhosis of liver**. Commonest causative agent for cirrhosis is alcohol. Cirrhosis of liver is complicated by **portal venous obstruction** and **portal hypertension**.

Malignant Disease of Liver

Liver is the organ for **primary origin** of cancer. Again it is the common site for **metastasis** or secondary deposit from the cancer anywhere in the gastrointestinal tract. This spread occurs through portal vein.

Malignant cells from other organs, e.g. from the lungs, breast or any pelvic organ may be deposited in the liver.

Liver Biopsy

Liver biopsy is a common procedure for diagnosis of some liver diseases. A small quantity of liver tissue is taken out through a needle for histopathological study. The needle is introduced through right midaxillary line at the level of 9th intercostal space. The needle passes through intercostal muscles, costodiaphragmatic recess of pleura, right dome of diaphragm and subphrenic space to reach the liver.

LA 24.4 **Give an account of the extrahepatic part of biliary apparatus.**

BILIARY APPARATUS

Introduction

Biliary apparatus is made up of series of channels which are concerned with *synthesis, transport, storage* and *concentration* of bile and its *time to time discharge* into the intestine for digestion of fat in the food.
- **Intrahepatic part,** within the liver is concerned with *synthesis* of bile.

- **Extrahepatic part** of biliary apparatus is composed of the parts which are concerned with *release of bile outside the liver*, its *storage and concentration* in the reservoir and *discharge into the small intestine*.

Components (Fig. 24.12)
- Right and left hepatic ducts
- Common hepatic duct
- Gallbladder with cystic duct
- Bile duct.

Brief Notes on the Components (Fig. 24.13)

Hepatic Ducts

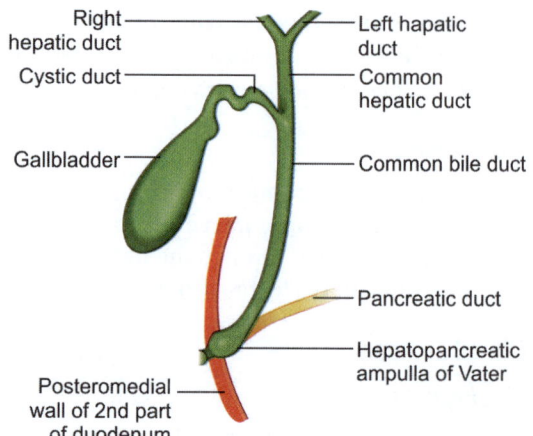

Fig. 24.12: Extrahepatic part of biliary apparatus.

Right and left hepatic ducts emerge from respective (right and left) lobes of the liver at its hilum, the **porta hepatis**. At the porta hepatis, right and left hepatic ducts are interrelated with following structures *from anterior two posterior*.
- Right and left hepatic ducts
- Right and left branches of hepatic artery
- Right and left divisions of portal vein.

All these structures form the hepatic pedicle which is enclosed by hepatobiliary capsule or Glisson's capsule.

Common Hepatic Duct

Formation of common hepatic duct is through union of right and left hepatic ducts at the right end of porta hepatis.

Common hepatic duct, being joined by the cystic duct as continuation of gallbladder at its right side, **ends** as bile duct *3 cm below the level of porta hepatis*.

Accessory Hepatic Ducts

These are additional ducts arising from right lobe of liver and may open in any of the following sites **(Fig. 24.13)**.
- Common hepatic duct
- Cystic duct
- Gallbladder
- Bile duct.

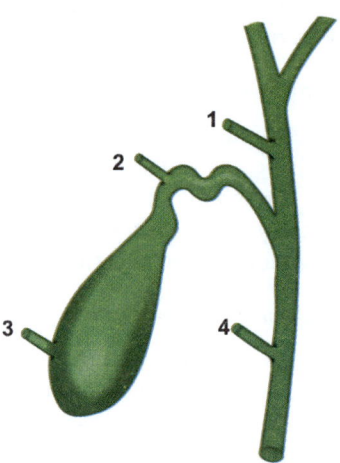

Fig. 24.13: Sites of opening of accessory hepatic duct at: (1) Common hepatic duct; (2) Cystic duct; (3) Gallbladder; (4) Common bile duct.

Clinical importance

During the steps of gall ladder operation (cholecystectomy) surgeon must search for this accessory duct and if present, must ligate it. Otherwise there is chance of postoperative oozing of bile from the operation field during the postoperative period.

Gallbladder

Gallbladder is a **pear-shaped** sac of biliary tract which is connected through its duct called cystic duct to the common hepatic duct 3 cm below the level of porta hepaits.

Dimensions of gallbladder are as such:
- Length—*7 cm*
- Breadth—*3 cm* at its widest part

Capacity – is *30 to 50 mL*

Function:
- Storage of bile
- Concentration of bile (10 times)
- Discharge of bile through its contraction into duodenum when fat containing food enters the alimentary canal.

Situation: Gallbladder is adhered to the fossa for gallbladder on the inferior surface of liver. Because of the slope of inferior surface of liver, long axis of gallbladder is directed downwards and forwards with slight inclination to the right.

Parts:
- **Fundus**—anteroinferior blind end
- **Body**—intermediate part
- **Neck**—posterosuperior narrow end which is continuous with the cystic duct, the duct from gallbladder.

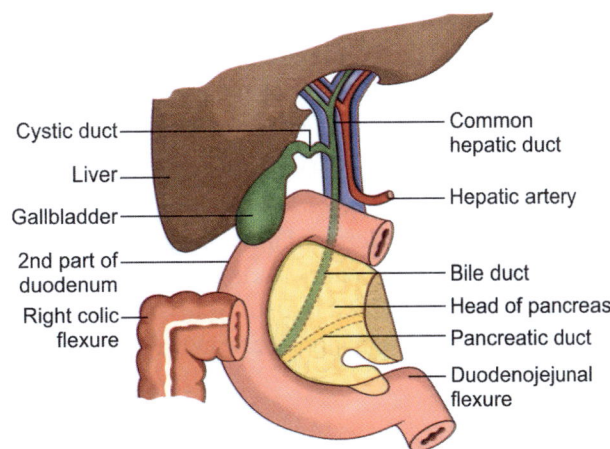

Fig. 24.14: Relations of extrahepatic part of biliary apparatus.

Peritoneal relation (Fig. 24.15)

- **Fundus**: As this part of gallbladder *usually* projects beyond inferior margin of liver, fundus is covered by *peritoneum all around*.
- **Body and neck**: *Inferior surface* is covered by peritoneum. *Superior surface* is embedded in gallbladder fossa of liver, connected by loose connective tissue which lodges superior branch of *cystic artery* and *cystic lymph node*. Occasionally the body and neck of gallbladder may be suspended from the liver-bed by a fold of mesentery.

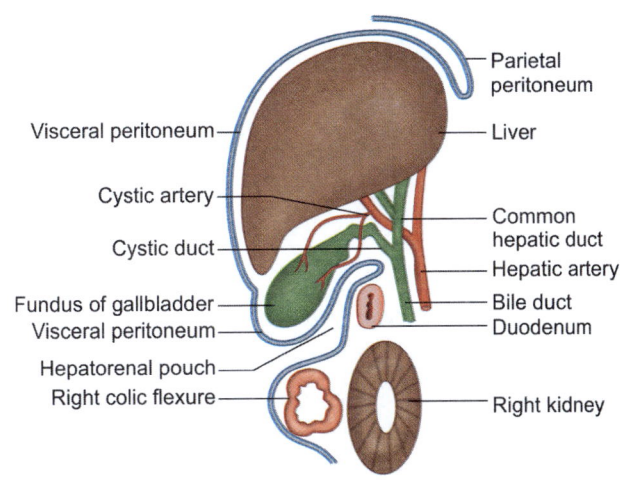

Fig. 24.15: Relations of gallbladder seen from left side.

Visceral relations (Figs. 24.14 and 24.15)

Fundus is related to anterior abdominal wall at the junction of lateral border of rectus abdominis muscle and ninth costal cartilage of the right side.

Body and neck

Superior surface: It is related to *fossa for gallbladder* on inferior surface of right lobe of liver. Loose connective tissue intervening contains *superior division of cystic artery* and *cystic group of lymph node*.

Inferior surface:
- Beginning of transverse colon
- Superior duodenal flexure with junction of 1st and 2nd part of duodenum.

Characteristic features of the neck:
- **Direction**: Neck of gallbladder presents a bend. First it is directed *upwards forwards and medially*. Then it passes *downwards backwards and medially* to become continuous with cystic duct.
- **Mucosal folds**: Interior of neck of gallbladder presents *spiral folds* of mucosa. It maintains the patency of lumen of neck during contraction of gallbladder.
- **Hartmann's pouch**: It is an outward bulge from the posteromedial wall of neck of gallbladder. If it is present, stagnation of bile in the pouch may cause formation of gallstones.

Cystic Duct

- **Introduction**: Cystic duct is the continuation of the neck gallbladder.
- **Length**: 4 cm
- **Direction**: *Downwards, backwards* and *medially (to the left)*
- **Termination**: Cystic duct joins at an acute angle at the right side of common hepatic duct *3 cm below the porta hepatis* to form *bile duct*.
- **Lumen of duct**: Mucosal lining of the cystic duct presents number of crescentic spiral folds called **valve of Heister (Fig. 24.16)**. These folds of the valve maintain the patency of lumen of the duct during contraction of the wall of the duct.

Calot's triangle (Fig. 24.16)

It a small triangle **bounded** as follows:
- **Above (base):** Inferior surface of liver
- **Right:** Cystic duct
- **Left:** Common hepatic duct.

Contents
- Cystic artery
- Cystic lymph node.

Clinical importance
- In case of cholecystectomy (removal of gallbladder), surgeon identifies the cystic artery at Calot's triangle for ligation.
- Enlarged cystic lymph node at the triangle draws attention for pathology of gallbladder or liver.

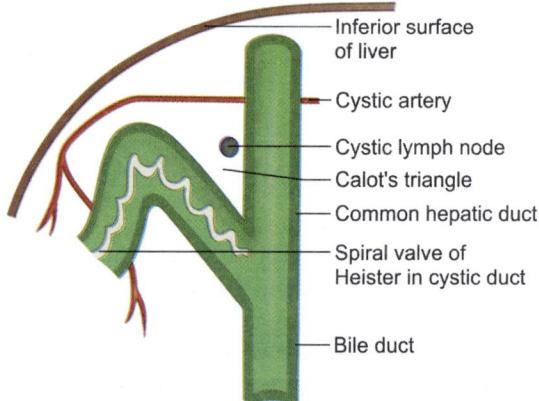

Fig. 24.16: Calot's triangle and spiral valve of Heister.

Bile Duct

Introduction: This is the biliary channel formed by union of the common hepatic duct and the cystic duct 3 cm bellow the porta hepatis.

Length: 8 cm

Parts:
- Supraduodenal
- Retroduodenal

- Infraduodenal
- Intraduodenal.

Termination: End of the bile duct joins with pancreatic duct in the posteromedial wall of second part of duodeneum, 10 cm distal to the pyloric end of stomach. Within the muscular wall of duodenum, two ducts unite to form a dilated end known as **hepatopancreatic ampulla or ampulla of Vater**. The summit or tip of the opening is narrow and is known as **major duodenal papilla.** Sometimes the bile duct and the pancreatic duct may open independently.

Course and relations

- **Supraduodenal part:** This part is above the first part of duodenum and lies in the right free margin of lesser omentum. Here the duct is related to hepatic artery to the left, and the portal vein behind. Supraduodenal part of bile duct is directed downwards and backwards.
- **Retroduodenal part** lies behind first part of duodenum and in front of inferior vena cava.
- **Infraduodenal part** is below first part of duodenum. This part inclines downwards and to the right towards the left side of second part of duodenum, being embedded in posterior surface of head of pancreas.
- **Intraduodenal part (Fig. 24.17):** This part is so called because it is situated within the wall of second part of duodenum 10 cm distal to pyloric end of stomach. Intraduodenal part is dilated and called **ampulla of Vater.** Ampullated end of the bile duct opens on mucosal surface of duodenum on its posteromedial wall through a narrow aperture called **major duodenal papilla** in reference to *minor duodenal papilla,* 2 cm proximally, through which the accessory pancreatic duct opens. Main pancreatic duct joins with the bile duct before formation of ampulla **(Fig. 24.17)**. Ampulla of Vater is encircled by a sphincter made up of smooth muscle fibers derived from the following three sources.

  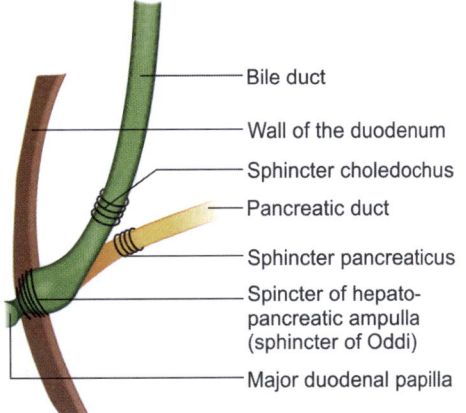

  Fig. 24.17: Sphincters of bile duct and pancreatic duct.

  1. Circular muscle fibers of bile duct
  2. Circular muscle fibers of pancreatic duct
  3. Circular muscle fibers of wall of duodenum

  This sphincter is known **as sphincter of Oddi (Fig. 24.17).**

Besides the sphincter of Oddi, terminal end of bile duct and pancreatic ducts, before their union, are guarded independently by their respective sphincters. They are named **sphincter choledochus** and **sphincter pancreaticus (Fig. 24.17).**

Arterial Supply of Biliary Apparatus

The cystic artery, artery for the gallbladder, is the chief source of arterial supply of biliary tract. The artery, usually arises from right heptic artery and *passes sequentially* as follows.
- Behind the common hepatic duct
- Across the Calot's triangle
- On the superior surface of gallbladder, where it divides into superior and inferior branches.

Other sources of arterial supply
- Branch from the superior pancreaticoduodenal artery
- Branch from the hepatic artery proper
- Branch from the right hepatic artery.

Venous Drainage of Biliary Tract
- Veins from the superior surface of gallbladder—enter the liver through fossa for gallbladder to drain into tributaries of hepatic vein.
- **Cystic vein** draining the gallbladder opens usually in **right division of portal vein**.
- Veins from bile duct drain into **portal vein** directly.

Lymphatic Drainage of Biliary Tract
Most of the lymph vessels of biliary tract, i.e. from *gallbladder, cystic duct, hepatic duct* and *upper part of the bile duct* drain into constantly placed **cystic node** lodged in Calot's triangle. Cystic node is always enlarged in any gallbladder pathology (inflammatory or neoplastic).

Lymph vessels from *lower part of the bile duct* drain into **hepatic** and **pancreaticosplenic groups of lymph nodes.**

Nerve Supply of Biliary Tract with Gallbladder
Sources of nerve supply are:
- **Parasympathetic:** Both **right as well as left vagus nerve—autonomic**
- **Sympathetic**: From **7th, 8th and 9th thoracic segments of spinal cord—autonomic**
- **Phrenic nerve (right): Somatic**
  All these nerves reach the gallbladder and the biliary tract from the **celiac plexus**. From this nerve plexus, fibers pass along the hepatic artery and then cystic artery.
- *Parasympathetic* (vagal) fibers are for **contraction of musculature** of gallbladder and biliary tract wall.
- *Sympathetic* fibers cause **vasoconstriction** and **contraction of sphincters**.
- *Phrenic nerve* carries **sensory fibers.**

Pain fibers are carried through vagus, sympathetic and also phrenic nerve fibers. **Referred pain** from gallbladder is felt in following areas.
- Epigastrium (lodging stomach)—due to vagus nerve
- Inferior angle of scapula—due to sympathetic nerve
- Tip of right shoulder—due to right phrenic nerve.

Clinical Anatomy

Cholelithiasis (Gallstone)
- Inflammation of gallbladder is known as **cholecystitis**. Chronic or recurrent cholecystitis may cause *impairment of absorption of bile salt cholesterol complex.* It will cause formation gallstones due to precipitation of cholesterol.
- Impaction of gallstone in gallbladder neck, cystic duct or biliary tract causes spasmodic pain known as **biliary colic**.
- **Referred pain** due to gallbladder pathology is felt in epigastrium, inferior angle of scapula and tip of right shoulder due to the reasons as stated above.

Murphy's Sign

Through this clinical sign, sharpness of gallbladder pain is detected clinically. On palpation of abdominal wall, when fingers are placed just below the right costal margin and the patient is asked for deep inspiration, due to sharp feeling of pain, the patient suddenly catches his/her breath.

Exogenous Obstruction of Bile Duct

Besides impaction of gallstones, the common bile duct may be obstructed due to exogenous causes, which are carcinoma of head of pancreas, enlarged lymph nodes at porta hepatis or neoplastic growth of adjacent structures. Obstruction of flow of bile will cause **obstructive jaundice**.

Courvoisier's Law

This law helps *to detect the cause of obstructive jaundice*. If the jaundice is due to obstruction of common bile duct because of either impacted stone or carcinoma of head of pancreas, gallbladder is clinically found distended and palpable. If the jaundice is due to cholelithiasis, contracted gallbladder is not palpable on clinical examination.

Clinical Importance of Calot's Triangle

- Calot's triangle is bounded above by *inferior surface of liver*, medially by *common hepatic duct* and inferolaterally by *cystic duct*. The triangle contains cystic lymph node, cystic artery and right hepatic artery. During gallbladder operation (cholecystectomy), cystic artery is identified for ligation as it lies behind the lymph node.
- Accidental injury to the cystic artery, which is a serious operative hazard, is not uncommon. If surgeon faces it, bleeding is immediately arrested through application of pressure on hepatic artery at right free margin of lesser omentum.

Care for Variations

Biliary tract and related blood vessels very often show variations. During operation, a surgeon must take into considerations about these anatomical variations. Otherwise postoperative leakage through *accessory hepatic duct* will cause *postoperative biliary fistula* or injury to *anomalous arterial branch* will cause *postoperative bleeding*.

> *Short notes/short answer:* **Gallbladder; Cystic duct** with **Calot's triangle; Bile duct (Common bile duct)**

Chapter 25

Pancreas, Spleen and Celiac Trunk

LA 25.1 Discuss the gross anatomy of pancreas with anatomical position and clinical anatomy. *(For viva-voce and practical)*

Long answer: Head of pancreas.
Short notes: Neck of pancreas; Relations of body of pancreas; Tail of pancreas; Pancreatic duct.

PANCREAS

Introduction

Pancreas is an elongated, soft, lobulated gland fixed to the posterior abdominal wall.

The term 'pancreas' is derived from the Greek terminology, '*pan*=all, '*kreas*'=flesh. It is so called because of its soft fleshy appearance.

Functional Components

Functionally, the pancreas is made up of following two types of glandular components:
1. **Exocrine part**: It liberates pancreatic juice containing **pancreatic enzymes**. The enzymes promotes digestion of proteins, lipids and carbohydrates.
2. **Endocrine part**: It is made up of **pancreatic islets (islets of Langerhans)** which produce the hormones **insulin** and **glucagon** having a key role in carbohydrate metabolism.

Location

The pancreas, elongated from side to side, presents enlarged globular end at the right side and tapering narrower end at the left side. It crosses the front the bodies of upper lumbar vertebrae.

It is located in the epigastrium and left hypochondrium **(Fig. 25.1)**.

It is behind the peritoneum of lesser sac.

Its right globular end (head) is received within the concavity of the duodenum. Its left end, the tail, slightly inclined upwards remains in contact with the spleen.

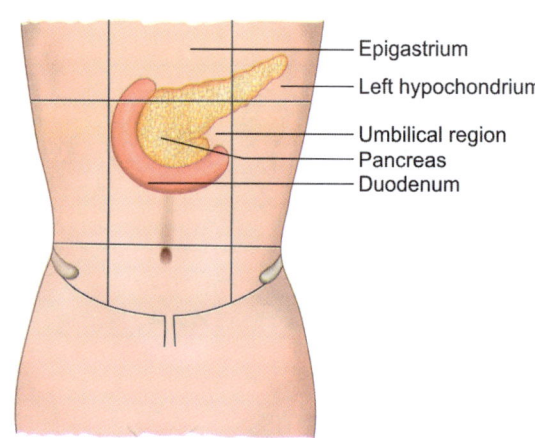

Fig. 25.1: Location of pancreas.

Shape

Pancreas looks like a *retort*. Right globular end represents the bowl of the retort.

Parts (Fig. 25.2)

From right to the left, the pancreas possesses the following parts:
- **Head:** Right globular flattened end; from the left side of inferior margin of the head, a conical projection extends downwards and to the left. It is called **uncinate process**.
- **Neck:** Shorter segment.
- **Body:** Prismoid on cross section; right end of upper margin of the body of the pancreas presents a small elevation called **tuber omentale** or **omental tuberosity**.
- **Tail:** Left narrower end.

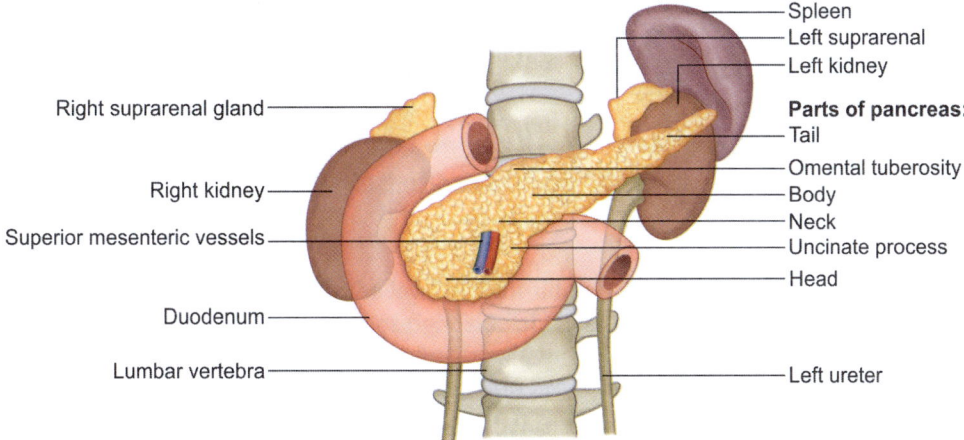

Fig. 25.2: Parts of pancreas related to surrounding structures.

Measurement
- **Length:** 12 cm
- **Breadth:** 4 cm (at its widest head end)
- **Thickness:** 2 cm.

Anatomical Position

The specimen of pancreas may be available as single viscera or along with the duodenum and/or spleen. The organ can be held in anatomical position with the help of its own features only.

The points for anatomical position are the following:
- The organ must be held in transverse position, extending from side to side, with the help of two hands.
- Rounded/globular head end lying on the right side is to be held with the help of right hand. It will be found to be accommodated in the curve of the duodenum, when present.
- Narrower tail end of pancreas is to be held with the help of left hand along with the spleen if present.
- Posterior surface of the body is known by the course of the splenic vein which is embedded in this surface running along the long axis of the viscera.
- Superior border is identified by the presence of the tortuous splenic artery along its course.
- Most prominent border of the body of pancreas is anterior border.
- Finally, the left hand with the tail end of the pancreas is to be held at a higher level than the right hand holding the head.

[Raw (non-shining) posterior surface can be differentiated from the anterior and inferior surface of the body which are shining (peritoneal)]

Head of Pancreas (Fig. 25.3)

Introduction

Head of the pancreas is the expanded, globular and anteroposteriorly flattened right end of the organ.

Situation

- In front of the posterior abdominal wall
- Within the curve of the duodenum
- At the level of bodies of 1st and 2nd lumbar vertebra.

Surface Features

- **Surfaces**: Anterior and posterior
- **Borders**: Superior, inferior and right borders which merge with each other *Forwards and to the left*, the head is continuous with the neck of pancreas.
- **Uncinate process**: It is a projection from the lower and left side of the head of pancreas.

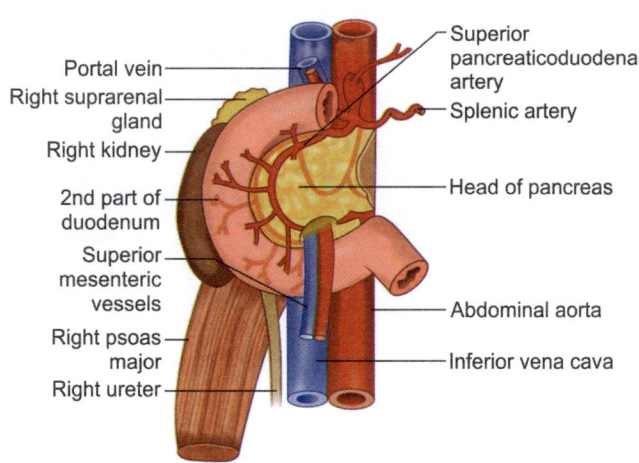

Fig. 25.3: Head of pancreas with related structures.

Peritoneal Relation

- **Anterior surface**: Middle of the anterior surface, crossed by beginning (right end) of the transverse colon, is nonperitoneal. Areas above and below this, are covered by the peritoneum.
- **Posterior surface**: Completely non-peritoneal, as in direct contact with the posterior abdominal wall.

Important Relations (Fig. 25.3)

Anterior surface

Middle of the surface is crossed horizontally by the beginning of the **transverse colon**, connected by loose connective tissue which contains the **right division of middle colic artery**. Area above the level of transverse colon is overlapped by the **1st part of duodenum**. Area below is in contact with the **coils of jejunum**.

Posterior surface

Bile duct and **inferior vena cava** are in direct relation of the posterior surface.

Further behind: Posterior surface of the head of pancreas is related to the following structures:
- Right crus of the diaphragm
- Right psoas major muscle
- Right sympathetic trunk
- Right middle suprarenal and right renal arteries
- Right half of the celiac ganglion
- Right side of the bodies of L_1 and L_2 vertebrae.

Superior border
- First part of duodenum
- Superior pancreaticoduodenal vessels.

Inferior border
- Third part of duodenum
- Inferior pancreaticoduodenal vessels.

Right border
- Second part of duodenum
- Anterior and posterior arterial arcades formed by the corresponding divisions of superior and inferior pancreaticoduodenal arteries.
- Pancreaticoduodenal lymph nodes.

Uncinate process: Posteriorly lies the *abdominal aorta*. Anteriorly, it is crossed by the superior mesenteric vessels, the vein lying to the right side of the artery.

Ducts Related to the Head
- **Main pancreatic duct**, receiving smaller ducts from almost whole of pancreas proceeds towards the right end of the head of pancreas and joins with the bile duct to open into the second part of the duodenum at major duodenal papilla, 10 cm distal to the pyloric end of stomach.
- **Accessory pancreatic duct** drains lower part of the head of pancreas and the uncinate process. It ascends upwards and to the right and crosses the main pancreatic duct to open into the second part of duodenum through the minor duodenal papilla, 2 cm proximal to the major duodenal papilla.

Arterial Supply
- **Superior pancreaticoduodenal artery**—branch of gastroduodenal artery.
- **Inferior pancreaticoduodenal artery**—branch of superior mesenteric artery.

The anterior and posterior divisions of the above-mentioned arteries anastomose to form **anterior** and **posterior arterial arcades** in the pancreaticoduodenal groove. Multiple short branches arising from the arcades supply the head of pancreas.

Venous Drainage
Veins from the head of pancreas drain into portal vein via following two routes:
1. **Superior pancreaticoduodenal vein** drains directly into the portal vein.
2. **Inferior pancreaticoduodenal vein** drains into the superior mesenteric vein, a tributary of the portal vein.

Lymphatic Drainage
Lymph vessels from the head of the pancreas drain primarily into the **pancreaticoduodenal lymph nodes** which finally drain into the **celiac** and **superior mesenteric group** of lymph nodes.

Nerve Supply
Sympathetic fibers are derived from the **greater splanchnic nerve (T_5-T_9)**. Parasympathetic supply is derived from the **vagus (10th cranial) nerve**. Both the fibers proceed through the **celiac** and **superior mesenteric plexuses**.

Clinical Anatomy

Carcinoma (cancer) of the head of pancreas is not an uncommon neoplastic disease. It may lead to pressure effect on the bile duct and the portal vein which are closely related to the head. Compression of the duct by the growth leads to **obstructive jaundice**. It may lead also to the feature of **portal venous obstruction**.

Annular pancreas is a congenital anomaly which occurs due to defect in the normal fusion of ventral and dorsal pancreatic diverticula. In this case, a mass of pancreatic tissue encircles the second part of duodenum. Obstruction to the duodenum results in vomiting in newborns within a few hours after birth.

Neck of the Pancreas

Neck of the pancreas is the anteroposteriorly flattened narrow band of pancreatic tissue lying in front of the formation of portal vein. It is continuous with the head of the pancreas to the right side. Towards the left, it merges with the body of the gland. The neck is **2.5 cm in length** having anterior and posterior surface demarcated by superior and inferior borders. **Anterior surface** is related to the **pylorus of stomach**. **Posterior surface** is in relation to the **formation of the portal vein** by union of the superior mesenteric vein and splenic vein **(Fig. 25.4)**. **Transverse mesocolon** is attached to the lower part of the anterior surface. **Inferior margin** of the neck is separated from the **uncinate process** by a gap through which passes the **superior mesenteric vessels**.

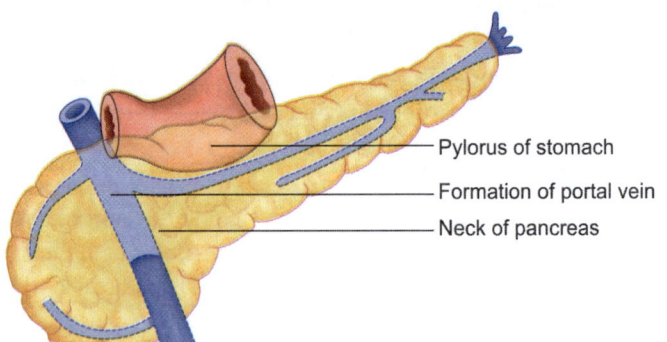

Fig. 25.4: Neck of pancreas with anterior and posterior relations.

Body of the Pancreas

Introduction

Body of the pancreas is the elongated part of the organ which extends from the neck towards the left. It presents **slight upward inclination** towards the hilum of the spleen. It also presents **slight forward convexity** for the curvature of the lumbar vertebrae. **Left end** of the body tapers to from the **tail of pancreas**.

External Features (Fig. 25.5)

Body of the pancreas is triangular on cross section having three surfaces and three borders. Surfaces are anterior (anterosuperior), posterior and inferior. Borders are superior, inferior and anterior.

Peritoneal Relations (Fig. 25.5)

Anterior and inferior surfaces of the body are covered by peritoneum of lesser and greater sacs respectively. Posterior surface is nonperitoneal.

Relations

Anterior surface

Anterior surface presents slight concavity in vertical direction. It forms the 'stomach bed' as it is related to the **posteroinferior surface of stomach** separated by **lesser sac** of peritoneum **(Figs. 25.5 and 25.6)**.

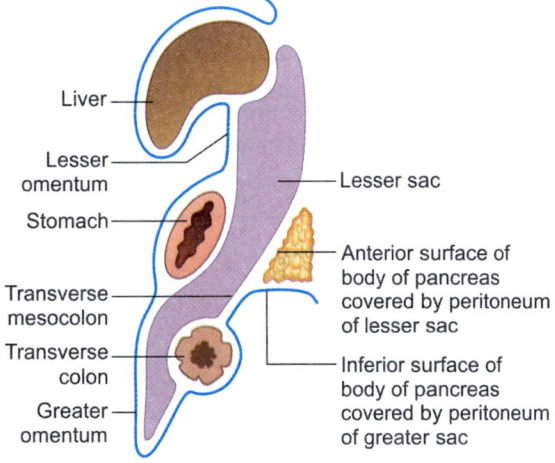

Fig. 25.5: Peritoneal relation and anterior relations of body of pancreas.

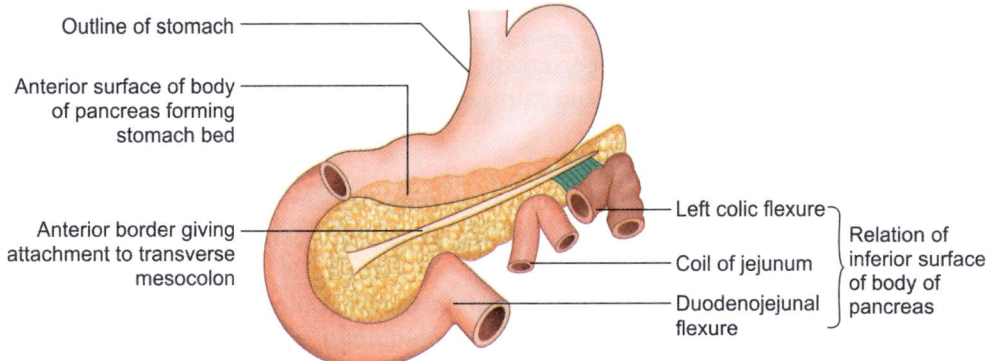

Fig. 25.6: Relations of anterior and inferior surfaces of body of pancreas.

Posterior surface (Fig. 25.7)

Splenic vein runs from left to right along the linear groove on the posterior surface of the body. It is connected to the gland by small multiple pancreatic veins. In addition, the posterior surface of the body is related to the following structures:
- Abdominal aorta with origin of superior mesenteric artery
- Left kidney with left renal vessels
- Left suprarenal gland
- Left crus of diaphragm.

Inferior surface (Fig. 25.6)
- **Duodenojejunal flexure:** At the right end
- **Left colic flexure:** At the left end
- **Coils of jejunum:** At the middle.

Superior border

Splenic artery with its tortuous course runs from right to the left along this border. Right end of the border presents an elevation called **tuber omentale** which is related to the celiac trunk.

Inferior border

Superior mesenteric vessels are related to the right end of this border.

Anterior border

It gives attachment to the **root of transverse mesocolon**.

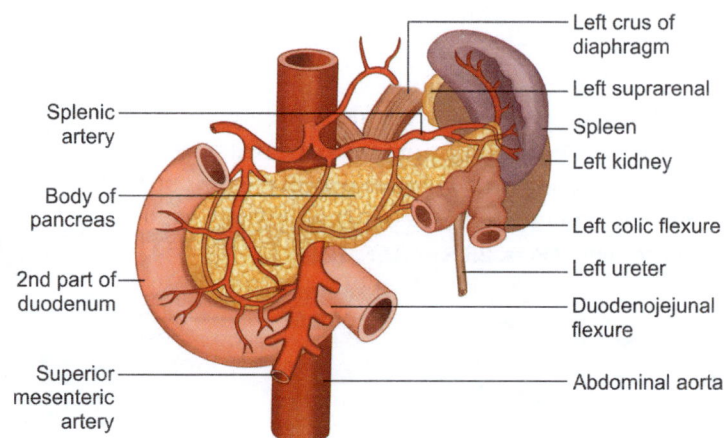

Fig. 25.7: Relations of pancreas.

Tail of the Pancreas

- Tail of the pancreas is the narrow left end of the gland
- It passes upwards and to the left in front of the left kidney
- It is contained within the two layers of **lienorenal ligament** along with the splenic vessels.
- It comes in relation to the **visceral surface of the spleen** in front of hilum
- Tail of the pancreas has immense structural importance as it contains, maximum population of **'islets of Langerhans'** which are clusters of cells concerned with liberation of **insulin** that lowers the blood glucose level.

Clinical anatomy: In splenectomy operation, tail of the pancreas may be accidentally removed as it lies within lienorenal ligament. It may cause diabetes melitus due to loss of remarkable number of islet cells.

Ducts of the Pancreas (Fig. 25.8)

The exocrine component of the pancreas transports its secretion through following two ducts:

1. **Main pancreatic duct (of Wirsung)** is elongated and extends throughout the whole length of the gland from its tail end. It extends from left to right lying very close to the posterior surface. At the level of the neck, it presents a bend to pass *downwards, to the right* and *slightly backwards*. The main duct receives many smaller ducts from both sides of whole length of the gland. 60° angulation of the smaller ducts from directions with the main duct gives an appearance like the herring fish-bone. So, it is called **"herring bone pattern".**

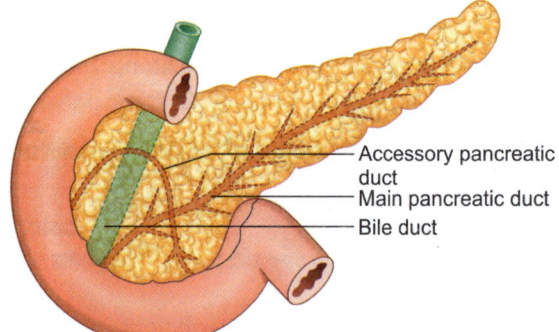

Fig. 25.8: Ducts related to pancreas.

The main pancreatic duct, at its terminal end, joins with the bile duct within the muscular wall of the posteromedial aspect of second part of duodenum to form a dilated end called **hepatopancreatic ampulla of Vater**. The opening of the ampulla, called **major duodenal papilla** is 10 cm distal to the pyloroduodenal junction.

2. **Accessory pancreatic duct (of Santorini)** drains the glandular secretion from the **lower part of the head and the uncinate process.** It runs upwards and to the right and **crosses in front of the main pancreatic duct**. It opens into the second part of the duodenum 2 cm proximal to the opening of the major duodenal papilla. It is called **minor duodenal papilla.** In 40% of cases, the minor pancreatic duct communicates with the major duct at the head-end of the gland.

Vascular Supply, Lymphatic Drainage and Innervation of the Pancreas

Arterial Supply (Fig. 25.9)

As the pancreas develops at the level of the junction of foregut and midgut, it derives its arterial supply from both the celiac and superior mesenteric arteries. The arteries are the following:

- **Pancreatic branches of splenic artery** are multiple short branches which arise while the splenic artery runs along the superior margin of the body of pancreas. One long pancreatic branch, called **arteria pancreatica magna** arises from the splenic artery near the tail and proceeds towards the neck. Another branch, called **arteria cauda pancreatica** supplies the tail-end of the gland.
- **Superior pancreaticoduodenal artery** is a branch of gastroduodenal artery. It descends along the upper part of pancreaticoduodenal sulcus and divides into anterior and posterior divisions.
- **Inferior pancreaticoduodenal artery** is a branch of superior mesenteric artery. It ascends along the lower part of pancreaticoduodenal sulcus. It also divides into anterior and posterior branches which anastomose with the corresponding division of superior pancreaticoduodenal artery to form anterior and posterior arterial arcades.

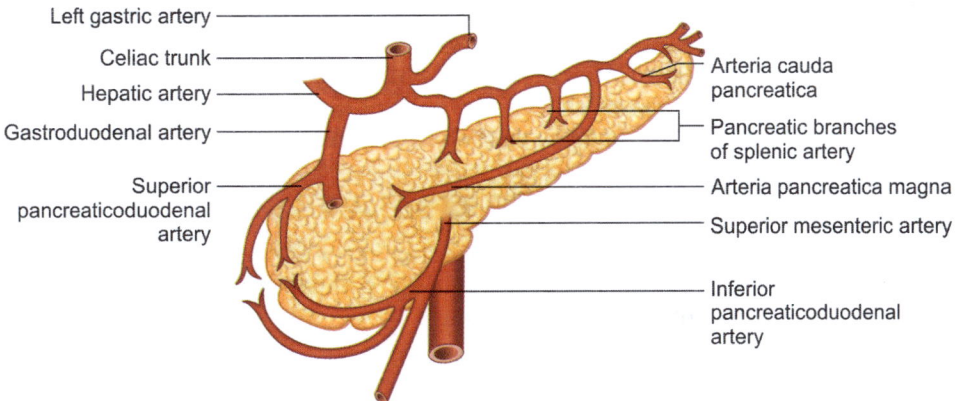

Fig. 25.9: Anteries of the pancreas.

Venous Drainage

Veins correspond to the arteries though their destination shows some difference.
- **Pancreatic veins** emerges in row from the posterior surface and drain into the **splenic vein.**
- **Superior pancreaticoduodenal vein** drains into the **portal vein** directly.
- **Inferior pancreaticoduodenal vein** drains into the **superior mesenteric vein**.

Lymphatic Drainage

Lymph vessels from the pancreas follow the reverse course of the arteries and drain into:
- Pancreaticosplenic group (from the tail end of the gland)
- Coeliac lymph nodes
- Superior mesenteric nodes.

Nerve Supply

Pancreas is supplied by both parasympathetic as well as sympathetic nerves through **celiac** and **superior mesenteric plexuses**. Parasympathetic fibers are derived from the **vagus nerve**. It **stimulates glandular secretion**. But the **hormonal control is more important**. Sympathetic fibers are derived from **greater** and **lesser splanchnic nerves (T_6–T_{10})**. These fibers are **vasoconstrictor** in nature. Pain fibers are also carried through the sympathetic nerves. **Pancreatic pain** is referred to T_6 to T_{10} **dermatomes**.

Clinical Anatomy

Congenital anomalies

Ectopic pancreas is a condition in which pancreatic tissue may be found in the submucosal layer of **stomach, small intestine, Meckel's diverticulum, gallbladder** and **spleen.**

Annular pancreas is a congenital anomaly, in which case a mass of pancreatic tissue encircles the second part of duodenum. It has been discussed in the section of head of pancreas.

Congenital pancreatic fibrocystic disease is caused by abnormal secretion of the mucus. **Thick mucus** obstructs the pancreatic duct and causes **pancreatitis** with **subsequent fibrosis**. Of course, this condition involves lungs, kidneys and liver.

Diagnosis of pancreatic disease

As the pancreas is deeply located in posterior abdominal wall, diagnosis of any disease of pancreas becomes difficult due to following reasons:
- Pain from the pancreas is usually referred to back.
- Disease of the pancreas may be confused with that of stomach and transverse colon as these two organs are related to the front of the pancreas.
- Inflammation of pancreas (pancreatitis) may spread to the lesser sac in front leading to formation of **pseudocyst.**

Malignancy of pancreas

Carcinoma of the head of pancreas causes pressure effect on bile duct leading to persistent **obstructive jaundice**. Portal vein related close to the head of pancreas may also be compressed leading to the clinical feature of **portal hypertension**.

Trauma of the pancreas

As pancreas is well protected for its deep-seated position, injury to this organ is rare. But it may be injured in sports injury or in gunshot/stab wounds. Damaged pancreatic tissue releases activated pancreatic enzymes which produces clinical manifestations of **acute peritonitis**.

Tail of pancreas and splenectomy

Tail of pancreas may be accidentally damaged in splenectomy operation, because the tail is lodged in lienorenal ligament of spleen. It leads to the following complications:
- The damaged pancreatic tissue releases pancreatic enzymes which may digest the surrounding tissue leading to a serious complication.

- As the tail of pancreas contains maximum population of islets of Langerhans, accidental removal of this part of the gland may increase the blood glucose level.

LA 25.2 Give an account of the gross anatomy of the spleen. Add a note on clinical anatomy.

SPLEEN

Introduction

The spleen is the largest lymphoid organ of the body. Classically, the spleen is defined as **hemolymphoid organ**, because it is not only composed of lymphoid tissue but also it is an important storehouse of red blood cells. It is concerned with both lymphoid system as well as hemopoietic system.

Synonyms of spleen are splen (Greek) and lien (Latin).

Functions of Spleen

- Spleen is the organ which **manufactures lymphocytes** (both B and T lymphocytes)
- Plasma cells of the spleen produce immunoglobulin M (IgM) which **provides immunity** of the body to enhance body defense mechanism.
- Spleen is the important **storehouse of RBC** which are released from the spleen as and when required.
- **Old (aged) and abnormal RBC are destroyed** by the phagocytic cells (macrophages) of the spleen.
- **Disintegrated RBC and microorganisms** are **removed by the macrophages** of the spleen.
- **In fetal life, RBC are also manufactured** in the spleen.

Location

- **Normal spleen** is situated in the left hypochondrium. Its posteromedial end extends in the epigastrium.
- **Enlarge spleen** extends downwards and medially to the umbilical region.
- **Hugely enlarged spleen** following some diseases may reach up to the right iliac fossa: Spleen is situated in relation to the fundus of stomach, superolateral to the anterior surface of left kidney under the left dome of the diaphragm.

External Features (Fig. 25.10)

Spleen is **wedge shaped** and **reddish purple** in color.

It presents **2 surfaces**—diaphragmatic and visceral; **2 borders**—superior and inferior and **2 ends**—posteromedial and anterolateral.

Dimensions and Level (Fig. 25.10)

It is interesting to note that the odd numbers 1,3,5,7,9 and 11 indicate the splenic statistics which are as follows:

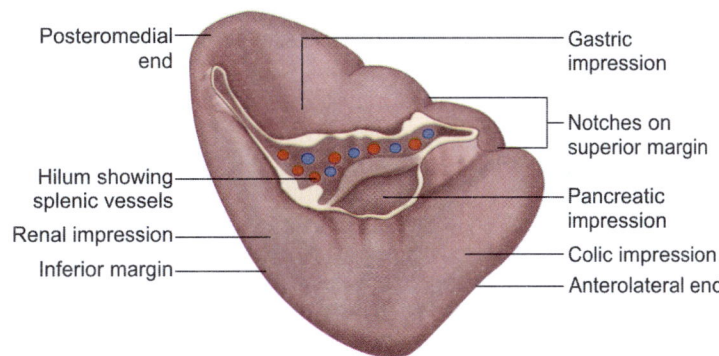

Fig. 25.10: Spleen seen from visceral surface.

Dimensions = 1 × 3 × 5 inches
      = Thickness × breadth × length
Weight   = 7 oz
Level   = 9th to 11th ribs of left side

Anatomical Position (*For Viva Voce and Practical*)

- Visceral surface with the hilum of spleen and the depressions for visceral impression is to be differentiated from the smooth convex diaphragmatic surface.
- Smooth convex diaphragmatic surface is to be kept in contact with the left palm with deeper concave gastric impression towards the thumb and shallower concave renal impression below the hilum towards the little finger.
- While holding the organ in such way, broader anterolateral end must be towards the tips of the fingers with the narrower posteromedial end towards the wrist.
- With this position, usually the superior border presents the notches. But the notches never help to identify the superior border. Sometimes, the inferior border may show notches instead of or in addition to the superior border.
- Finally, the palm of the hand with the organ must face forwards and medially through hyperextension of the wrist.

Ends (Figs. 25.10 and 25.11)

- **Anterolateral end** is broad to look like a margin. It is directed forward, to the left and slightly downward. It is related to the **phrenicocolic ligament**.
- **Posteromedial end** is rounded. It is directed backward, medially and slightly upwards, towards the vertebral column.

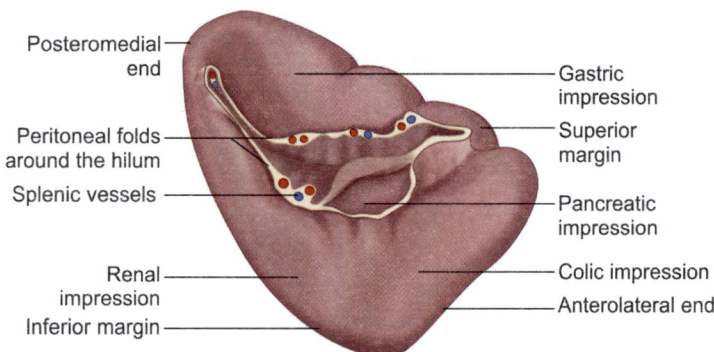

Fig. 25.11: Visceral surface of spleen.

Margins (Figs. 25.1 and 25.2)

- **Superior margin** is thin and it shows a gentle convexity upwards. It separates the visceral surface from the diaphragmatic surface. Usually, the superior margin presents one to two notches near its anterior end. These notches indicate that the spleen is lobulated in origin.
- **Inferior margin** separates the lower part of visceral surface (renal impression) from the diaphragmatic surface. It is comparatively rounded and corresponds to the lower border of the 11th rib.
- **Intermediate margin** is shorter and straighter. It extends from the hilum backwards and it separates the upper gastric impression from the lower renal impression.

Surfaces

Visceral Surface (Fig. 25.11)

It shows the hilum of spleen and some visceral impressions.

Hilum is the porta or the getaway for the spleen. It is a triangular anteroposteriorly elongated slit at the middle of the visceral surface. It presents entry and exit of multiple radicals of splenic artery and splenic vein respectively. The margins of the hilum is surrounded by peritoneal folds which are continuous with the lienorenal ligament backwards and the gastrosplenic ligament forwards.

Visceral impressions

- **Gastric impression** is the deepest impression on the visceral surface. It is situated below the superior margin and above the intermediate margin and the hilum. It is related to the fundus of stomach.
- **Renal impression** is between the intermediate margin and inferior margin of spleen posteroinferior to the hilum. It is related to upper and lateral part of the anterior surface of left kidney.
- **Pancreatic impression** is the small area just in front of the hilum and related to the tail of the pancreas.
- **Colic impression** is a triangular depression just adjacent to the anterolateral end of the spleen. This area is related to the left colic flexure.

Diaphragmatic surface (Fig. 25.12)

The diaphragmatic surface is smooth and convex. It is directed upwards, backwards and to the left lying opposite the level of 9th, 10th and 11th ribs underneath the left dome of the diaphragm. This surface is separated from the costodiaphragmatic recess of pleura by the diaphragm. So, the relations of the diaphragmatic surface of spleen are the following from below upwards and laterally:

- Visceral peritoneum covering the diaphragmatic surface of spleen.
- Parietal peritoneum over undersurface of the diaphragm
- Left dome of the diaphragm
- Costodiaphragmatic recess of pleura of the left side with the corresponding intercostal spaces.

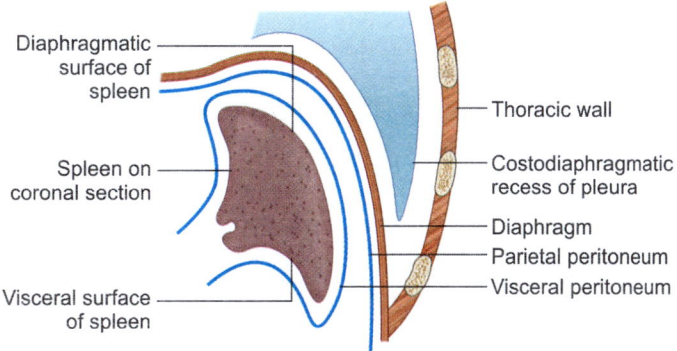

Fig. 25.12 Relations of diaphragmatic surface of spleen (in coronal section).

Peritoneal Relations (Fig. 25.13)

Spleen is completely covered by the peritoneum all around except the following two areas:

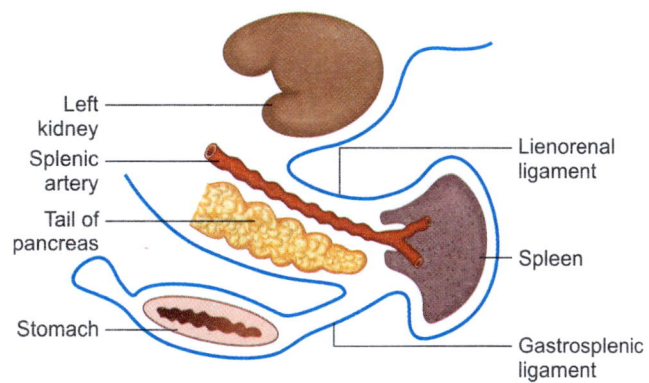

Fig. 25.13 Peritoneal relations and ligaments of spleen.

1. Hilum, through which the structures of splenic pedicle passes in to and fro directions.
2. Pancreatic impression, which is in direct contact with the tail of pancreas.

Ligaments of Spleen

Ligaments related to the spleen are classified in following two groups:
1. **Peritoneal ligaments** are gastrosplenic and lienorenal ligaments which are *attached to the spleen.*
2. **Nonperitoneal ligament** is phrenicocolic ligament which is *related to the spleen*

Gastrosplenic ligament extends from the upper part of greater curvature of stomach near the fundus to the anterior margin of hilum of spleen. It contains the *short gastric vessels.*

Lienorenal ligament is a double fold of peritoneum which extends from the posterior margin of hilum of the spleen to the posterior abdominal wall near the left kidney. It contains the following structures:
- Splenic vessels
- Tail of pancreas
- Pancreaticosplenic lymph nodes.

Morphology: Both the peritoneal ligaments of the spleen are developed from the *dorsal mesogastrium.*

Phrenicocolic ligament is not attached but related to anterolateral end of the spleen. It extends from the left colic flexure to the undersurface of left dome of the diaphragm.

Morphology: It represents the *inferior retention band* of the fetal midgut loop.

Supernumerary Spleen in Splenic Ligaments

Single or multiple supernumerary spleen may be present either in gastrosplenic ligament or in lienorenal ligament.

Clinical importance of this splenic mass is that, they may be hypertrophied after removal of the spleen and they may lead to recurrence of clinical picture of the disease for which the splenectomy operation was performed.

Arterial Supply

Spleen is supplied by the splenic artery which is the largest branch of celiac trunk. To reach the spleen it passes along the *superior border* of body of pancreas. The artery presents a tortuous course which allows free movement of the spleen along with the movement of the diaphragm. It reaches the hilum of spleen through the lienorenal ligament. It divides into five to six branches.

Venous Drainage

Splenic vein is formed by five or more number of tributaries coming out of the hilum. It runs from left to right along the *posterior surface* of the body of pancreas. Behind the neck of the pancreas it joins with the superior mesenteric vein to form the portal vein.

Clinical Anatomy

Clinical Palpation of the Spleen

Normal spleen under the left dome of the diaphragm, covered by the left costal margin is not palpable. Enlarged spleen is palpable only when its size becomes the double.

Splenomegaly

It is the clinical condition presenting enlargement of spleen. A pathologically enlarged spleen **extends in downward and medial direction**. Left colic flexure and phrenicocolic ligament prevent a direct downward enlargement. Hugely enlarged spleen may reach up to the right iliac fossa.

Splenic Trauma (Rupture)

As the spleen is well protected by the left-sided ribcage, it is usually not injured. But the **crushing injury** or **rupture** of the spleen may occur in **road traffic accident.** It needs splenectomy operation.

Splenectomy

Surgical removal of the spleen is not only indicated in case of rupture of spleen, but also in various medical diseases of the organ. Precaution must be taken to avoid accidental removal of the tail of pancreas as it is contained in the lienorenal ligament. Tail of the pancreas contains maximum population of islets of Langerhans.

Splenic Puncture

It is a clinical investigation procedure through which a pinch of splenic tissue is drawn out for cytological study for diagnosis of some diseases.

Short notes: **Visceral relations of the spleen; Ligaments of the spleen.**

SA 25.3 Write a brief note on splenic circulation.

SPLENIC CIRCULATION (FIG. 25.14)

While the blood percolates through the splenic tissue, it is filtered. Macrophages of the splenic tissue bed coming in contact with the circulating blood in the splenic tissue remove the abnormal and effete (exhausted) cells, blood cell particles with old RBC, bacteria, parasites and foreign antigen.

Segmental arteries of the spleen, 5 to 6 in number, run along the **connective tissue trabeculae** and divide

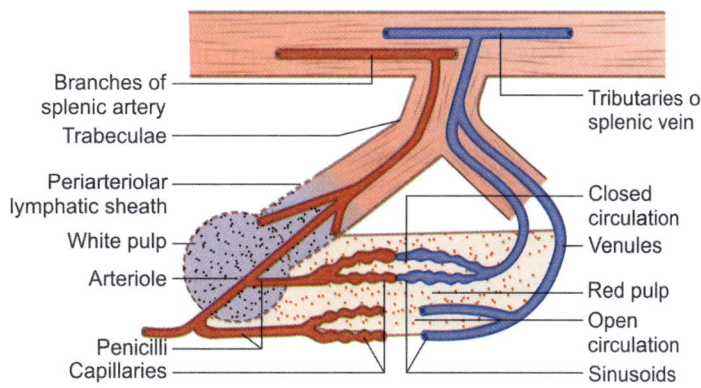

Fig. 25.14: Splenic circulation.

repeatedly to form the **arterioles**. Finally, the connective tissue adventitia is replaced by the **periarteriolar lymphatic sheath (PALS)** made up of aggregations of **T-lymphocytes**. This is expanded in some place to form rounded lymphoid follicles made up of B-lymphocytes. These follicles 0.25 to 1 mm in diameter are visible through the naked eye on the freshly cut surface of spleen as *white semi opaque dots* named as **white pulp** in contrast to the surrounding 80 to 90% reddish purple splenic tissue called **red pulp**. The arterioles, while passing through the white pulp, are eccentrically placed. Arterioles branch into series of parallel divisions called **penicillar arterioles**.

The red pulp forming 80 to 90% of the total splenic volume is the **unique filtration device** which helps the spleen to remove the particulate material from the blood. The red pulp is basically composed of large number of **venous sinusoids**, ovoid vessels which are parallelly arranged and interposed by **small bundles of collagen fibers, network of reticular cells** and **splenic macrophages**. The intersinusoidal areas appear as strips of **splenic cords**.

Blood from the **open ends of the capillaries** which originate from the penicillar arterioles percolates through the reticular spaces of the splenic cords. Macrophages in the space remove blood-borne particulate material including exhausted cell debris, damaged and aging RBC microorganisms and foreign antigens.

Through the venous sinusoids purified blood is collected from the **open tissue bed of splenic cords** into **the venules**. **Small veins** formed by union of the venules run within the trabeculae and drain in the **segmental splenic veins**. Segmental veins come out of the hilum of the spleen to form the splenic vein.

Some amount of the blood **probably** takes an **alternative 'close route'** and enter the venous sinusoids directly from the penicillar arterioles and capillaries. However, either way, the blood is exposed to the splenic macrophages and the filtration mechanism of the splenic tissue.

SA 25.4 Write a brief note on the celiac trunk (Important for viva voce and practical).

CELIAC TRUNK

Introduction

Celiac trunk is the first **unpaired ventral splanchnic branch** of the abdominal aorta. It is principally the **artery of the foregut**. This arterial trunk supplies the following structures:
- Abdominal part of the foregut extending from abdominal part of esophagus to the 2nd part of duodenum up to level 10 cm distal to the pyloric end.
- Liver
- Gallbladder with biliary tree
- Major part of pancreas
- Spleen.

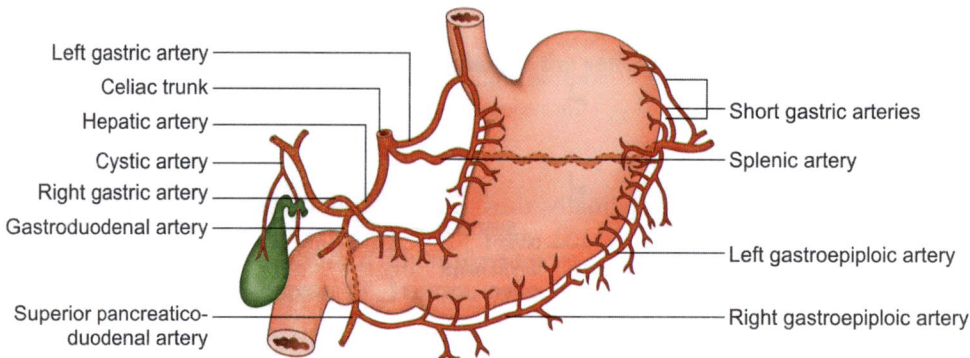

Fig. 25.15: Distribution (branches) of celiac trunk.

Origin

Celiac trunk arises from the front of upper end of abdominal aorta at the level of lower border of body of T_{12} vertebra, just below the aortic opening of the diaphragm. It is 1.25 cm in length with its longer transverse measurement.

(Structures having longer transverse measurement than long axis measurement in the body are the following:
- **Hypophysis cerebri (Pituitary gland):** In the head.
- **Isthmus of thyroid gland:** In the neck.
- **Celiac trunk:** In the upper abdomen.
- **Cecum:** In the lower abdomen.
- **Prostate gland (in males):** In the pelvis.

Relations

- **Anteriorly:** Lesser sac with lesser omentum
- **Posteriorly:** Intervertebral disk between T_{12} and L_1 vertebrae
- **To the right:** Right crus of diaphragm, right celiac ganglion and *caudate process of liver*
- **To the left:** Left crus of diaphragm, left celiac ganglion and *cardiac end of stomach*
- **Inferiorly:** Tuber omentale of the body of pancreas

Celiac trunk is surrounded by the *nerves of celiac plexus* all around.

BRANCHES (FIG. 25.15)

Left Gastric Artery

It is the smallest of the three branches of the celiac trunk and is divided into two parts:
1. **First part** of the artery ascends upwards and to the left to reach the cardiac end of the stomach lying **behind the lesser sac**.
2. **Second part** runs forwards and to the right along the left half of lesser curvature of stomach **within the lesser omentum**. It ends by anastomosing with the right gastric artery.

Branches

- **Esophageal branches:** for abdominal part of esophagus.
- **Gastric branches:** for stomach.
- **Omental branches:** for lesser omentum.

Hepatic Artery

Like left gastric artery, the hepatic artery is also divided into two parts:
1. **First part** is known as **common hepatic artery.** It is so called because it is common for distribution of blood to the liver with gallbladder as well as stomach, duodenum and pancreas. It runs *downwards, forwards* and *to the right* to reach the upper border of first part of duodenum where it is continued as second part of the artery entering the right free margin of lesser omentum.
2. **Second part** is known as **proper hepatic artery** beyond the origin of gastroduodenal artery. It runs along the right free margin of lesser omentum in front of the portal vein and to the left of the bile duct. At the porta hepatis of liver the proper hepatic artery divides into right and left hepatic branches.

Branches

Gastroduodenal artery is a large branch arising from the junction of two parts of hepatic artery at the upper border of the first part of duodenum. Running behind the first part of the duodenum, it divides at its lower border into following two branches:

1. **Superior pancreaticoduodenal artery** runs downwards in the pancreaticoduodenal groove to divide into anterior and posterior divisions. These two divisions form anterior and posterior arcades by anastomosing with anterior and posterior divisions of inferior pancreaticoduodenal branch of superior mesenteric artery. From these arcades, short branches are distributed to the duodenum and head of pancreas.
2. **Right gastroepiploic artery** enters the greater omentum and turns to the left to follow the right half of greater curvature of stomach and anastomoses with the left gastroepiploic branch of the splenic artery. It gives out multiple **gastric** and **epiploic branches** to supply the stomach and greater omentum respectively.

Right gastric artery is a small branch which arises from the proper heptic artery, i.e. *distal to the origin of gastroduodenal artery*. It runs to the left along the right half of lesser curvature of stomach and ends by anatomosing with the left gastric artery. It sends branches to the stomach and the lesser omentum.

Supraduodenal artery is an *occasional branch* of the hepatic artery. It may arise from gastroduodenal artery or any other branch. It supplies the first part of the duodenum.

Right and left hepatic arteries are the terminal branches of the proper hepatic artery. Arising at the porta hepatis, these arteries are interposed between two hepatic ducts in front and two divisions of the portal veins behind. Entering the respective lobes of liver, each of the hepatic artery divides primarily into **segmental branches**.

Cystic artery arises usually from the right hepatic artery. It reaches the triangular interval called **Calot's triangle** bounded by inferior surface of liver, cystic duct and hepatic duct. Reaching the upper surface of neck of gallbladder it divides into **superior** and **inferior branches** for the respective surface of the gallbladder.

Splenic Artery

Splenic artery is the largest branch of the celiac trunk. In addition to the spleen, it is the important source of blood supply to the pancreas and fundus of stomach. Splenic artery runs almost horizontally to the left along the upper border of the body of the pancreas, behind the lesser sac and stomach. Crossing in front of left suprarenal gland and upper part of left kidney, it passes through the lienorenal ligament along with the tail end of the pancreas. At the hilum of the spleen, the splenic artery divides into 5 to 6 terminal branches. The splenic artery presents a tortuous course.

Branches

Pancreatic arteries are multiple short branches arising from the whole length of the splenic artery. They supply body and tail of pancreas. One long pancreatic branch is known as **arteria pancreatica magna** which arises from the left end of the splenic artery and runs to the head end of the pancreas. This artery passes behind the pancreas and anastomoses with a dorsal branch of hepatic artery, superior mesenteric or celiac trunk. One elongated pancreatic branch arising near the tail is called **arteria cauda pancreatica**.

Short gastric arteries are multiple (5 to 7) short branches arising from the terminal end of the splenic artery. These branches pass through the gastrosplenic ligament and supply the fundus of stomach.

Left gastroepiploic artery also arises from the terminal end of the splenic artery. But it is a single long branch which enters into the greater omentum and runs along the left half of greater curvature of stomach. It supplies multiple branches to the stomach and greater omentum.

Chapter 26

Abdominal Part of Large Gut, Mesenteric Arteries and Portal Vein

> **SA 26.1** General consideration of the abdominal part of large gut.
> *(For viva voce and practical examination)*

LARGE INTESTINE

Introduction

In comparison to the small intestine, the large intestine or the large gut is so called because of its *wider caliber*. Large gut begins from the ileocecal junction and ends to the exterior at anus. Its total length is *1.5 meters*.

Components (Fig. 26.1)

From proximal to distal ends, the large gut is composed of following parts:
- Cecum with a vestigial part called vermiform appendix
- Ascending colon
- Transverse colon
- Descending colon
- Sigmoid colon
- Rectum
- Anal canal.

Abdominal part of the large gut extends up to the descending colon, beyond which it is continued in the pelvic cavity.

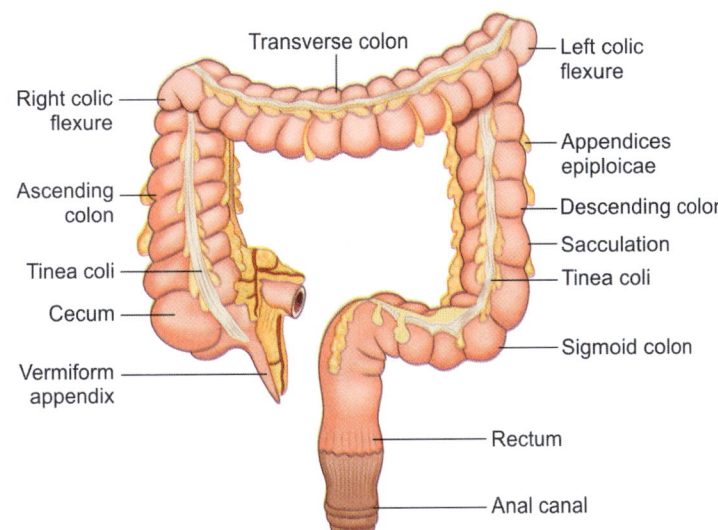

Fig. 26.1: Components of large intestine.

Functions of Large Intestine

- A good amount of water along with salts and solutes is absorbed through the mucosa of large intestine. This absorption of water is the factor for the maintenance of normal consistency of the feces (stool).
- Normal bacterial flora of the intestinal mucosa facilitates synthesis of vitamin B complex.
- Mucosal secretion of the large intestine is rich in antibodies which prevents the attack by microorganisms.

Cardinal Features of Large Gut (Fig. 26.1)

Following are the cardinal features of the large gut, in general, by which it can be distinguished from the small gut.

Teniae Coli

These are three condensed linear bands of longitudinal muscle fibers running along the subserosal surface of whole length of the large intestine except the distal part of sigmoid colon, rectum and anal canal. These three muscular bands, condensed on the outer surface of the longitudinal muscle coat come closer proximally at the base of the vermiform appendix. Distally, the teniae diverge and spread out to blend with the outer longitudinal muscular layer of rectum.

Sacculations (Haustrations)

These are series of puckering or bulging of the wall of the large intestine. These are formed due to the shorter length of the teniae than that of the circular muscle layer of the gut wall so also the length of the gut.

Appendices Epiploicae

These are small outpouchings (pockets) or evaginations of visceral peritoneum of large intestine filled with small amount of fat. They are attached adjacent to the teniae coli, so absent in vermiform appendix, rectum and anal canal. The appendices epiploicae are maximum in number in transverse colon and sigmoid colon.

The above mentioned cardinal features differentiate the large gut from the small gut where they are absent.

SA 26.2 **Write a brief note on the cecum.**

> Short notes: Ileocecal orifice (Ileocecal valve

CECUM

Introduction

The term 'caecum' is a Latin word which means blind. Cecum is the first part of the large intestine which presents the proximal (lower) blind end. So the terminal end of ileum (small intestine) opens on the medial side of caecum.

Morphology (Figs. 26.2A to F)

Caecum, the proximal dilated end of the large intestine is developed from the **cecal diverticulum** of the proximal end of the distal limb of the primitive midgut loop. **In herbivorous animal** caecum is considered as the **'second stomach'** as it is concerned with **digestion of cellulose** of the herbs. In humans, its distal part becomes rudimentary to form the vermiform appendix.

Situation

Cecum is situated on the right iliac fossa.

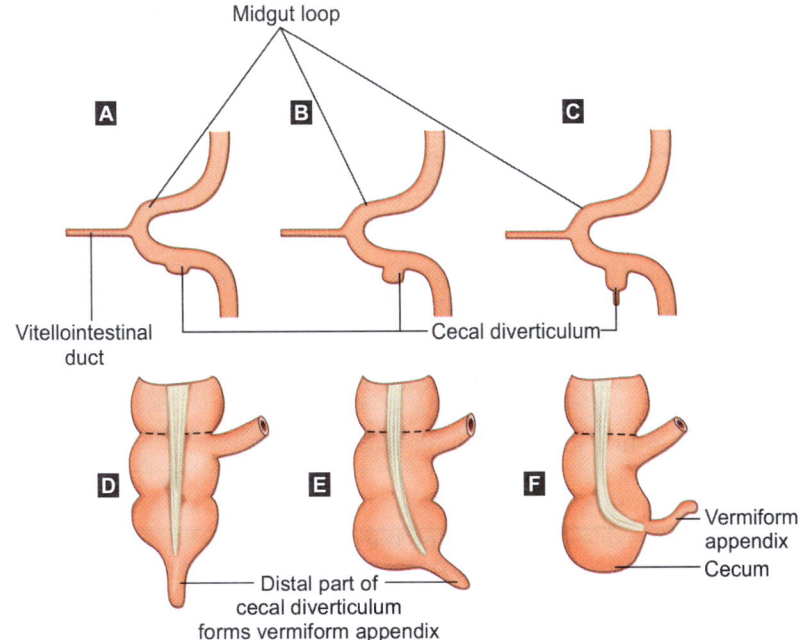

Figs. 26.2A to F: Cecum and vermiform appendix develop from diverticulum of midgut loop.

Shape and Size

Cecum is like a sac with its blind end directed downwards. Its upper end communicates with the ascending colon. Terminal end of ileum opens in the cecum on its medial side.

Vertical measurement of the cecum is **6 cm (2.5 inches)**. *Transverse measurement* is **7.5 cm (3 inches)**.

Extent

Beginning is at the ileocecal orifice on the posteromedial aspect of cecum at the level of junction between the transtubercular plane and right lateral plane.

Termination of the cecum is at its upper end where it is continuous with the ascending colon. It is a little above the level of ileocecal orifice.

Types of the Cecum

The cecum shows various types due to following reasons:
- Relative length of right and left wall of the cecum
- The nature of the walls
- Position of the appendix in relation to the wall
- Distance of the appendicular orifice from the ileocecal orifice.

Types of the cecum are depicted in **Figure 26.3**.

A. **Fetal type (conical type):** It is very rare and found in **2% of cases.** Vermiform appendix is joined at the apex of the conical cecum. Right and left borders of the cecum are oblique, straight and of equal length forming two sides of the cone.
B. **Infantile type (3%):** Right and left walls of equal length show bulging due to overgrowth. The bulgings are known as *saccules*. Appendix is attached to the depression at the junction of two saccules.
C. **Normal type (90%):** In this type, the normal development of the cecum is completed, as *the right wall grows more than the left* forming the **normal cecal pouch** at the lower blind end. So the left cecal wall becomes shorter and the base of appendix shifts towards the left. The appendicular orifice lies **2 cm below the ileocecal orifice.**
D. **Exaggerated type (5%):** In this type, elongation of the right cecal wall is exaggerated forming **the large saccule**. The left wall is almost absent, so the appendicular orifice is very close to the ileocecal orifice.

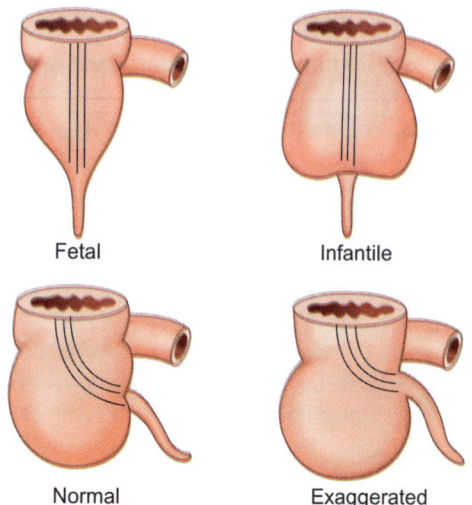

Fig. 26.3: Types of cecum.

Peritoneal Relation (Fig. 26.4)

In most of the individuals, the visceral peritoneum covering anterior surface of the cecum winds round the lower blind end to cover its posterior surface upto its junction with ascending colon. Then the peritoneum is reflected over the iliac fascia as parietal layer. Because of this reason, a peritoneal pocket is formed behind the cecum, called **retrocecal recess**. Sometimes, the vermiform appendix takes its position in this recess. This is called **retrocecal position of appendix**. The other cecal recesses are the following:
- Superior ileocecal recess
- Inferior ileocecal recess.

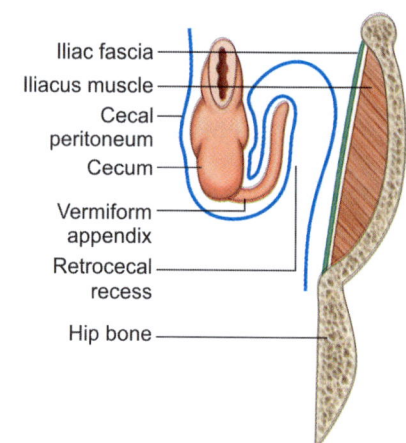

Fig. 26.4: Peritoneal relation of cecum.

Relations of Cecum

Posterior Relations (Fig. 26.5)

Posterior relations of the cecum is important as it lies on the right iliac fossa of the false pelvis. The structures related are the following:
- *Iliacus* and *psoas major* muscles on the right iliac fossa. The muscles are covered by *iliopsoas fascia*.
- *Femoral nerve* in the iliopsoas groove (right)
- *Lateral femoral cutaneous nerve* (right)
- *Right gonadal vessels*
- Sometimes *vermiform appendix* in retrocecal recess.

Anterior Relations

Anterior abdominal wall, interposed by:
- Greater omentum and
- Coils of ileum.

Medial Side

Medial side of the cecum presents *ileocecal junction*.

Inferolmedial Aspect

Inferomedial aspect joins with the base of *vermiform appendix*.

Special Features of the Interior

Interior of the cecum presents following two orifices **(Fig. 26.6)**.

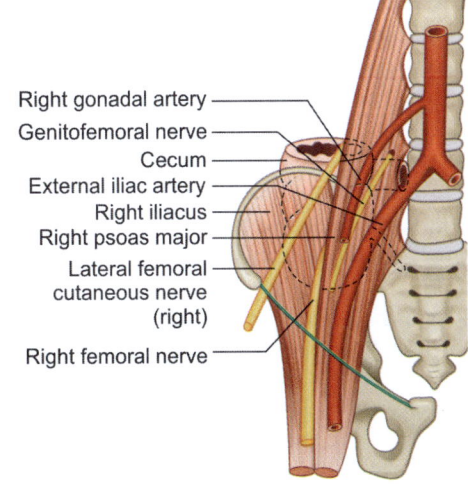

Fig. 26.5: Cecum in right iliac fossa with its posterior relations.

Ileocecal Orifice

Through this orifice the terminal part of ileum opens into the cecum. It is situated on the posteromedial wall of the junction between the cecum and the ascending colon. From the lumen of the cecum, the orifice is found to be directed forwards and laterally. **Landmark** of the ileocecal orifice is at the point of intersection of transtubercular plane and right lateral plane. **Measurement** of the orifice is 2.5 cm horizontally. It is **oval in outline** and guarded by the ileocecal valve bounded by upper and lower lips.

Ileocecal valve (valve of Tulpius) is guarded by two lips which meet with each other at both ends. **Upper lip** is more or less horizontal and is situated at the level of ileocolic junction. **Lower lip** is longer and curved with the convexity downwards. It is located at the level of ileocecal junction. Ends of the lips meet on either side to form the **frenulum** *(pl. frenula)*. The frenula are formed due to mucosal ridges. **Right posterior frenulum** is *pointed* and **left anterior frenulum** is *rounded*.

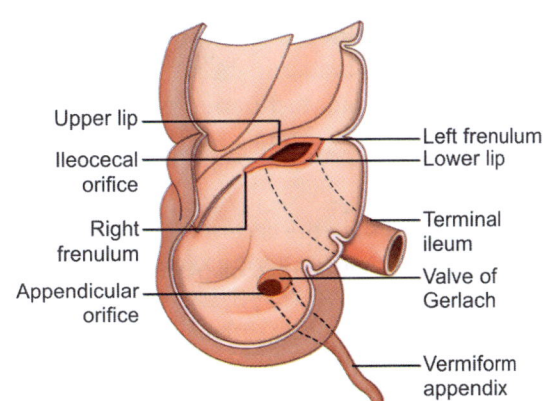

Fig. 26.6: Interior of cecum showing ileocecal orifice and appendicular orifice.

Nowadays, the ileocecal valve is known as **ileal papilla**. The lips guarding the papilla are known as **superior** and **inferior labial folds**. The labial folds are formed by the mucosa, submucosa and muscular layer of the ileocecal wall. Ileal and colonic surfaces of the papilla show the lining epithelia of small and large bowel respectively.

Ileocecal sphincter

Previously muscle fibers of ileal papilla used to be considered as a **physiological sphincter**. But nowadays it is believed that condensed muscle fibers at the base of the ileal papilla form **anatomical**

sphincter. The sphincter gets tonically contracted when cecum gets distended preventing cecoileal reflux. When food bolus is received in stomach, liberation of the hormone, **gastrin** makes the ileocecal sphincter relaxed.

Functions of ileocecal valve
- It regulates antegrade small bowel transit from ileum to cecum.
- During distended condition of cecum, tonic contraction of ileocecal sphincter prevents cecoileal reflux.
- Gastroileal reflex action following release of gastrin in the stomach, relaxes the ileocecal sphincter.
- It gives rise to mechanical and functional separation of luminal environment of small and large intestines which show variation in their content, pH and bacterial content.

Appendicular Orifice

It is a small circular opening 2 cm below the ileocecal orifice lying in a little posterior plane. It represents the position of the base of vermiform appendix. However, its position vary according to the position of the appendix. The appendicular orifice is guarded by a small semilunar fold of mucous membrane called **valve of Gerlach**. It does not have any significance.

Blood supply

Arterial supply of the cecum is derived from **anterior** and **posterior cecal branches** of the **ileocolic artery** which is a branch of the superior mesenteric artery.

Vein corresponds to the artery and finally drains into the superior mesenteric vein which forms the portal vein.

Lymphatic drainage

Lymph vessels from the cecum drain into the **ileocolic group** of lymph nodes which finally drain into the superior mesenteric group of **preaortic lymph nodes**.

Nerve supply

Parasympathetic innervation is derived from the **vagus nerve**. Sympathetic fibers are derived from the T_{11} to L_2 segments of spinal cord. Distension of the cecum stimulates the sensory fibers. Impulse carried centrally leads to tonic contraction of the ileocecal sphincter.

Clinical Anatomy

Abnormal Position of Cecum

Due to arrest of rotation of midgut loop anywhere between left iliac fossa—left hypochondrium—right hypochondrium after the reentry into the abdominal cavity, the cecum may be in abnormal position anywhere between these areas.

Cecum may be undescended with the vermiform appendix from the right hypochondrium. In this case, inflammation of the appendix may give rise to pain in the right hypochondrium which may be confused as inflamed gallbladder.

Cecal Distension in Large Bowel Obstruction

In case of longstanding obstruction of large bowel, distension of cecum may cause failure of relaxation of ileocecal sphincter.

Cecal Distension to Differentiate Large Bowel and Small Bowel Obstruction

During operation of intestinal obstruction, cecum acts as a guide to find out the site of the obstruction. If the cecum is distended, obstruction is in large gut. If the cecum is empty, obstruction is in small gut.

Ileocecal Tuberculosis

Ileocecal region is the common site for intestinal tuberculosis. If it leads to the obstruction, barium meal X-ray will show delayed emptying through the ileocecal orifice.

LA 26.3 Describe the vermiform appendix. Add a node on its clinical anatomy.

VERMIFORM APPENDIX

Introduction

Vermiform appendix is a narrow vestigial muscular tube with large amount of lymphoid tissue in its wall. Though it presents a narrow lumen, it communicates through its orifice with the cecum at its posteromedial aspect 2 cm below the ileocecal orifice.

The term *'vermiform'* comes from the Latin word *'vermis'* which means *'worm'*. It is so called as it looks like a worm.

Morphology

Vermiform appendix is a vestigial structure of the body. This rudiment represents the atrophied distal part of the original cecal diverticulum.

Dimension and Ends

Vermiform appendix, termed simply as appendix is variable in length from **6 to 10 cm** in adult.

Two ends of the appendix are known as the base and tip. The position of the base of the normal appendix is more or less constant on the posteromedial wall of the cecum 2 cm below the level of the ileocecal orifice.

On the surface of the right iliac quadrant of anterior abdominal wall, position of the **base of the appendix** is the **McBurney's point** which is located at the point at the junction of lateral one-third and medial two-thirds of the line extending from right anterosuperior iliac spine to the umbilicus **(right spinoumbilical line).** McBurney's point is clinically important because in case of appendicitis, it is the point of maximum tenderness (perception of pain). In surgical operation, the base of the appendix is identified with the help of teniae coli of the cecum which converge at the base of the appendix.

Tip of the appendix is variable in direction due to variable position of the appendix as a whole, which is discussed below.

Body of the appendix is between the base and the tip.

Mesentery of the Appendix (Mesoappendix) (Fig. 26.7)

The vermiform appendix has a short triangular peritoneal fold, the **mesoappendix**. This peritoneal fold is derived from the posterior layer of the mesentery of the terminal part of ileum. The mesoappendix is attached from the cecum to the proximal part of the appendix, and it *does not extend upto its tip*. It contains the appendicular artery, a branch of ileocolic artery with corresponding vein.

Positions of the Appendix

- **Variable positions of tip, when the appendix with cecum is in right iliac fossa.**
  These positions are following as related to the hour-hand of a clock **(Figs. 26.8A and B)**
  - *Paracolic (11 O'clock):* The appendix is placed to the right side of the beginning of ascending colon and its tip is directed *upwards and to the right*.

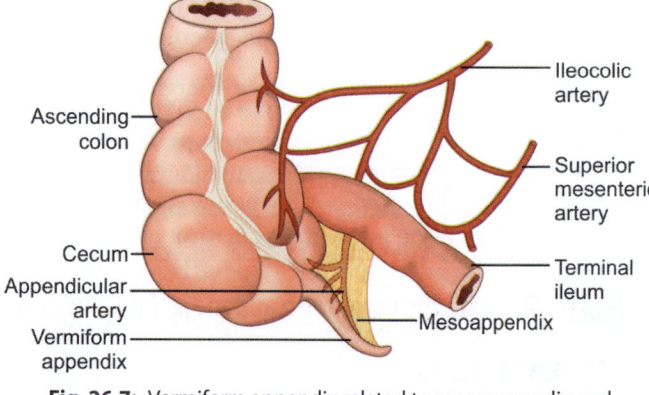

Fig. 26.7: Vermiform appendix related to mesoappendix and appendicular artery.

  - *Retrocecal/retrocolic (12 O'clock):* The tip of the appendix is directed *vertically upwards* behind the cecum. It is the commonest position. The appendix may be longer to extend behind the ascending colon.
  - *Splenic (2 O'clock):* The tip of the appendix is directed *upwards and to the left* towards the spleen. It may cross in front **(preileal)** or behind **(postileal)** the terminal ileum.
  - *Promontoric (3 O'clock):* The tip of the appendix is directed horizontally to the left side pointing towards the sacral promontory. The incidence is very rare.
  - *Pelvic (4 O'clock):* Tip of the appendix is directed downwards and to the left towards the pelvic cavity. In this case, the appendix is related to the ovary and uterine tube in female.
  - *Midinguinal (6 O'clock):* This is also known as **subcecal** position. Tip of the appendix is directed *vertically downwards* towards the inguinal ligament.
- **Variable positions due to arrest in rotation of midgut loop**
  After the fetal midgut loop reenters into the abdominal cavity, it rotates for 180° in anticlockwise direction. For this rotation, the cecal diverticulum with the vermiform appendix follows the path of a semicircle along left iliac fossa, left hypochondrium, right hypochondrium and finally to the right iliac fossa. So, arrest in rotation anywhere in this path, may show **anomalous position** of appendix as follows:
  - Left iliac

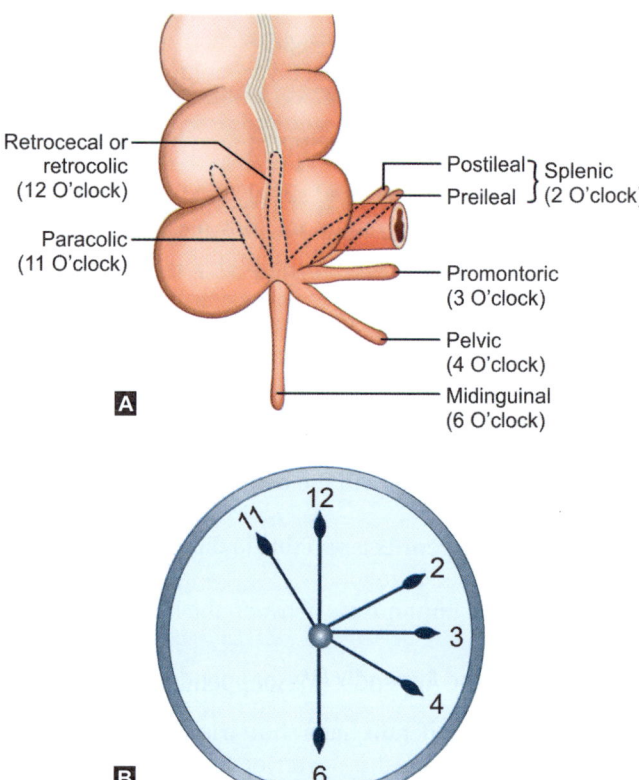

Figs. 26.8A and B: Positions of vermiform appendix.

- Splenic (left hypochondriac)
- Anywhere between left iliac and splenic
- Subhepatic
- Anywhere between subhepatic and right iliac.

Subhepatic position of vermiform appendix is clinically significant, because inflammation of appendix in this case may give rise to pain in right upper abdomen which may be confused with the pain due to gallbladder inflammation.

Blood Supply

Vermiform appendix is supplied by the appendicular artery which normally arises from the **inferior division of ileocolic artery**. It may occasionally arise from the **posterior cecal artery**. The appendicular artery passes behind the terminal end of ileum to enter the mesoappendix. The artery ends a little proximal to the tip where the mesoappendix usually ends. The tip of the appendix is the least vascular part of the organ.

The vein corresponds similar to the artery and drain finally into the superior mesenteric vein which forms the portal vein.

Lymphatic Drainage

Lymph vessels from the appendix drain initially into the **appendicular lymph node** lying within the mesoappendix. Finally, the lymph drain into the **ileocolic lymph nodes**.

Nerve Supply

Both the parasympathetic and sympathetic nerves reach the appendix through the **superior mesenteric plexus**. Parasympathetic fibers derived from the vagus nerve are motor in function and less significant for this vestigial organ. Sympathetic fibers, derived from T_{10} (and T_9) segment of spinal cord are vasoconstrictor and sensory for pain.

Clinical Anatomy

Predisposition of Appendix to Infection

Inflammation of vermiform appendix is known as appendicitis. The appendix is predisposed to infection due to following reasons:
- It is a **long, narrow, blind-ended tube** which predisposes stagnation of large bowel contents.
- The narrow lumen of the organ has the chance to be occluded by the hardened intestinal contents called **enteroliths**.
- The wall of the appendix presents **remarkable amount of lymphoid tissue**.

Reason for Perforation in Appendicitis

The narrow elongated appendicular artery supplying the vermiform appendix does not anastomose with any other arteries. The distal blind end of the appendix is supplied by the terminal branches of the appendicular artery. Edema of the wall due to appendicitis compresses the blood vessel and very often leads to thrombosis of the artery. This condition may lead to a complication like necrosis of the appendicular wall which is followed by perforation.

Pain of Appendicitis

Initially, the **visceral pain** for appendicitis is felt due to *distension* of the wall or *spasm* of the muscle. Afferent pain fibers enter the *10th thoracic segment* of spinal cord. That is why, initially a **vague referred pain** is felt *in the region of umbilicus*. Later on, when the parietal peritoneum *over the right iliac fossa* gets inflamed and irritated, **parietal (somatic) pain** is felt. It is clinically detected through **maximum tenderness at McBurney's point**. This pain is **precise, severe** and **localized**.

SA 26.4 **Write a brief note on transverse colon.**

TRANSVERSE COLON (FIG. 26.9)

Introduction

Transverse colon is the part of large gut which extends horizontally across the abdomen from right to the left. It is the most mobile part of the large intestine having its mesentery called *transverse mesocolon*.
- **Length**: 18 inches (45 cm)
- **Situation**: These colon lies mostly in the umbilical region. Its right end extents in the right lumbar region and left end reaches the left hypochondrium.
- **Extent:** Right end of the transverse colon presents almost a right angle bend at its junction with the ascending colon, called right colic flexure.
  Left end presents an acute bend at its junction with the descending colon called left colic flexure.

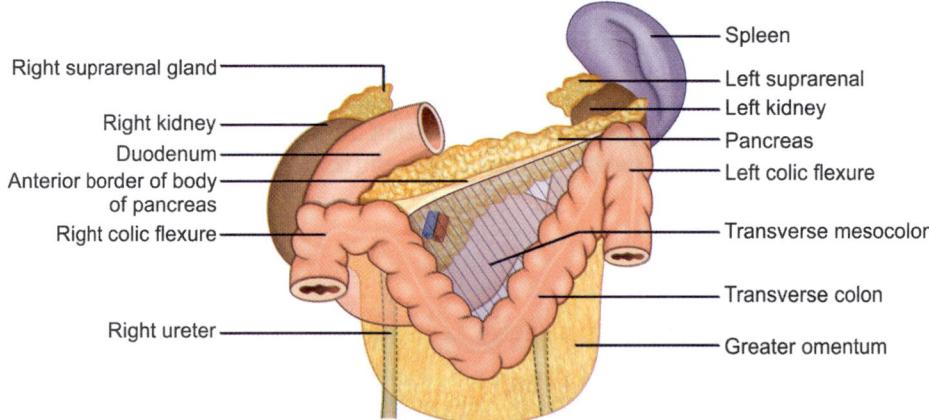

Fig. 26.9: Transverse colon with related structures.

Right Colic Flexure (Fig. 26.9)

Right colic flexure is almost a right angle bend at the junction of ascending colon and transverse colon. It is located **1 inch below the transpyloric plane** and 4 inches to the right of the midline. At this site, transverse colon starts and is directed downwards, forwards and to the left. The flexure lies in front of the lower part of the right kidney. Anterosuperiorly, it is related to the inferior surface of the right lobe of liver. Right colic flexure is also known as **hepatic flexure**.

Left Colic Flexure (Fig. 26.9)

Left colic flexure is an acute bend at the junction of transverse colon and descending colon. It is located **1 inch above the transpyloric plane** and 4 inches to the left side of the midline. At this flexure, the colon descends downwards and backwards. The angulation of this flexure is maintained by a peritoneal band called **phrenicocolic ligament** extending to the undersurface of diaphragm.

The flexure is related to the anterolateral end of the spleen. It is located in front of lower part of anterior surface of left kidney and behind the stomach. Left colic flexure is also known as **splenic flexure** of the colon.

Course of Transverse Colon (Fig. 26.9)

From the right colic flexure, transverse colon extends for a short distance horizontally in front of the second part of duodenum and the head of pancreas. Then it runs downwards and medially towards the midline up to the level of umbilicus and finally passes upwards and laterally to the left presenting a 'V' shaped appearance to end at the colic flexure.

Peritoneal Relation and Peritoneal Folds (Figs. 26.9 and 26.10)

Transverse colon is enclosed by peritoneum all round except the lines of attachment of the transverse mesocolon and the greater omentum which extend from side to side.
Transverse mesocolon: It is mesentery of the transverse colon. This double fold of peritoneum suspends the transverse colon from the posterior abdominal wall.

Attachments

Posterosuperior

- Middle of anterior surfaces of second part of duodenum and head of pancreas.
- Anterior border of the body of pancreas.
- Anterior surface of left kidney.

Anteroinferior

Posterosuperior aspect of the transverse colon along the line of *tenia mesocolica*.

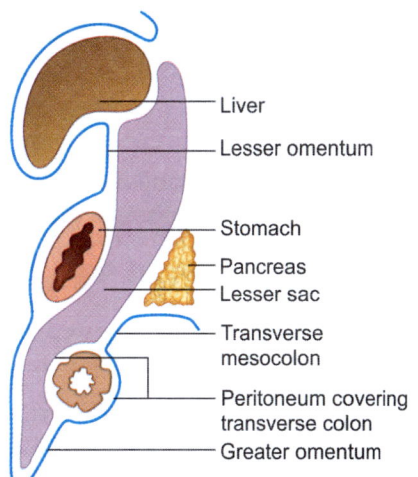

Fig. 26.10: Peritoneal relation and peritoneal folds of transverse colon.

Contents

- Middle colic vessels.
- Ascending divisions of the right colic and the (superior) left colic vessels.
- Lymph vessels, lymph nodes and the nerve plexus embedded in variable amount of fat.

Greater omentum: It is actually the peritoneal fold extending from the greater curvature of stomach. Its 1st and 2nd layers hang freely and are continued upwards and backwards as 3rd and 4th layers which are attached to the anteroinferior aspect of transverse colon along the line of the *tenia omentalis*.

Relations

- **Anteriorly**: Greater omentum of stomach and anterior abdominal wall.
- **Posteriorly**: Second part of duodenum, head of pancreas, coils of small intestine.

Morphological Importance

Right two-thirds and left one-third of the transverse colon are developed from the primitive midgut and hindgut respectively. So, the blood supply, lymphatic drainage and nerve supply of these two components of transverse colon are from two different groups.

Blood Supply

Arteries

- **Proximal (right) two thirds:** Middle colic artery, a branch of superior mesenteric artery.
- **Distal (left) one third:** Left colic artery, a branch of inferior mesenteric artery.

Veins

The veins correspond to the same as the arteries and they drain into superior and inferior mesenteric veins respectively.

Lymphatic Drainage

Lymph vessels from the proximal two-thirds and distal one-third follow the direction of the corresponding veins and drain into the superior mesenteric and the inferior mesenteric group of preaortic lymph nodes respectively.

Nerve Supply

Both the parasympathetic as well as sympathetic nerve fibers supply the transverse colon through superior as well as inferior mesenteric plexuses. Parasympathetic fibers for proximal two-thirds are derived from the vagus nerves and those for distal one-third reach through the pelvic splanchnic nerves.

Clinical Anatomy

Agenesis of Transverse Colon

Though the incidence is rare, the transverse colon may be absent congenitally due to arrest of rotation of the midgut loop beyond left hypochondrium. In this case, cecum with appendix will lie in the left hypochondrium.

Colostomy

To relieve large bowel obstruction beyond the transverse colon, this part of the gut may be brought to the surface of anterior abdominal wall through a small opening. The bowel content is then allowed to drain through this route.

> *Short notes*: **Blood supply, lymphatics** and **nerve supply; Right and left colic flexures; Peritoneal folds.**

SA 26.5 Write a brief note on superior mesenteric artery.

SUPERIOR MESENTERIC ARTERY (FIG. 26.11)

Introduction

Superior mesenteric artery is the ventral midline branch of abdominal aorta to supply the midgut and related organs.

Origin

Superior mesenteric artery takes origin:
- From the anterior aspect of abdominal aorta
- Behind the body of pancreas near its neck
- Just below the level of origin of the celiac trunk
- At the level of 1st lumbar vertebra.

Direction and Position

The artery descends downwards and to the right along the posterior abdominal wall. It runs in between two layers of the root of the mesentery showing a slight convexity to the left.

Termination

Superior mesenteric artery terminates at the upper end of right sacroiliac joint by anastomosing with a branch of ileocolic artery, which is its own branch.

Course and Relations

The superior mesenteric artery, at the site of its origin, crosses the uncinate process of pancreas and the third part of duodenum to enter the root of mesentery. Origin of the artery is overlapped by the pancreas.

While descending downwards and to the right, the artery crosses over the inferior vena cava, right psoas major and right ureter. To the right side, the artery is related to superior mesenteric vein.

Branches (Fig. 26.11)

Jejunal and Ileal Arteries

These are **12 to 15 in number arising from the left side** of the superior mesenteric artery. These branches run parallelly between the two layers of the mesentery of jejunum and ileum. Within the mesentery the branches bifurcate. Adjacent bifurcated branches anastomose to form an **arterial arcade**. Next set of branches arising from the arcade bifurcate, and anastomose to form next arterial arcade. The number of arcades are less (2 to 3) towards the jejunal end and more at the ileal end (3 to 5). From the final arcade, straight branches called **arteriae rectae (vasa recti)** arise to supply both the sides of the intestine in a more or less alternative fashion. Arteriae rectae are longer at the jejunal end and shorter at the ileal end.

All the branches mentioned below **arise from the right side** of superior mesenteric artery.

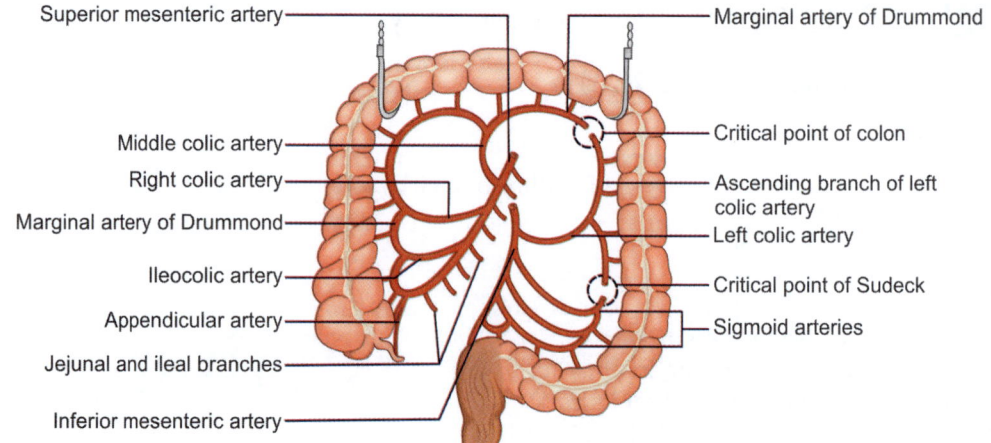

Fig. 26.11: Superior and inferior mesenteric arteries with manginal artery of Drummond.

Inferior Pancreaticoduodenal Artery

It arises from the right side of the superior mesenteric artery at the level of upper border of the third part of duodenum. It may arise from the first jejunal branch. The artery divides into anterior and posterior divisions which run upwards along the groove between the head of the pancreas and the curve of the duodenum. They anastomose with the anterior and posterior divisions of superior pancreaticoduodenal artery to form the arterial arcades.

Middle Colic Artery

Middle colic artery arises from the right side of superior mesenteric artery just below the level of pancreas. The artery follow the plane of transverse mesocolon and is **directed downwards and forwards.** In between the layers of transverse mesocolon, the middle colic artery divides into right and left branches which run in the respective sides parallel to the line of transverse colon. The right division anastomoses with the ascending branch of right colic artery. The left branch anastomoses with the ascending branch of the left colic artery.

Right Colic Artery

Right colic artery usually arises from the middle of the right concave side of the superior mesenteric artery. It may arise through a common trunk either with middle colic artery above or with ileocolic artery below. It passes horizontally towards the right behind the peritoneum of posterior abdominal wall. Near the upper end of the ascending colon, it divides into ascending and descending branches. The ascending branch anastomoses with the right branch of middle colic artery and the descending branch joins with the superior branch of ileocolic artery.

Ileocolic Artery

It is the lowest branch from the right side of the superior mesenteric artery. It runs downwards and to the right behind the peritoneum of right paravertebral gutter of posterior abdominal wall and divides into ascending and descending branches. The ascending branch, as mentioned above, anastomoses with the descending branch of right colic artery. The descending branch gives rise to following arteries and ends by anastomosing with terminal end of superior mesenteric artery:

- Anterior and posterior cecal arteries
- Appendicular artery, which may arise from the posterior cecal artery
- Ileal branch for terminal part of ileum.

SA 26.6 Write a brief note on inferior mesenteric artery.

INFERIOR MESENTERIC ARTERY (FIG. 26.11)

Introduction

Inferior mesenteric artery is the ventral midline branch of abdominal aorta to supply the hindgut.

Origin

Inferior mesenteric artery originates:
- From the anterior aspect of abdominal aorta
- Behind the third part of duodenum and,
- In front of the body of 3rd lumbar vertebra.

Course and Relation

Inferior mesenteric artery passes downwards and to the left behind the parietal peritoneum of left side of posterior abdominal wall to reach the pelvic brim (pelvic inlet).

Termination

At the level of pelvic brim, while the inferior mesenteric artery crosses in front of the left common iliac artery on the medial aspect of the left ureter, it is continued as the **superior rectal artery**.

Branches (Fig. 26.11)

Left Colic Artery (Superior Left Colic Artery)

It is the first branch arising from the inferior mesenteric artery which passes upwards and to the left behind the peritoneum of left side of infracolic compartment of abdomen. After a short course, the left colic artery bifurcates into ascending and descending branches. The ascending branch enters inside the transverse mesocolon and anastomoses with the left branch of middle colic artery. The descending branch anastomoses with the uppermost sigmoid artery which is also branch arising from inferior mesenteric artery.

Sigmoid Arteries (Inferior Left Colic Arteries)

Sigmoid arteries are 3 to 4 in number. Their adjacent bifurcated branches anastomose with each other and their highest branch anastomoses with the descending branch of the superior left colic artery as stated earlier.

Marginal Artery of Drummond (Fig. 26.11)

Adjacent bifurcated divisions of colic branches of superior and inferior mesenteric arteries starting from the ileocecal junction to the rectosigmoid junction form an arterial chain **3 cm away** form the inner margin of the colon. This is called **marginal artery of Drummond**. It is formed by union of the bifurcating branches of:

- Ileocolic, right colic and middle colic branches of superior mesenteric artery
- Left colic and sigmoid branches of inferior mesenteric artery.

From this marginal artery, short parallel branches (arteries rectae or vasa recta) arise to supply the wall of large gut.

Critical point of colon

It is the point which presents the gap or deficiency in anastomosis between adjacent colic arteries. Previously, it was thought that no anastomosis exists between inferior or descending branch of the left colic and the uppermost sigmoid artery. This used to be known as **critical point of Sudeck**. According to the recent concept, the critical point of colon is at the level of splenic flexure because the ascending division of the left colic artery very often fails to communicate with the left branch of the middle colic artery.

This will deprive the splenic flexure from getting the advantage of collateral circulation.

> *Short note*: Marginal artery of Drummond.

LA 26.7 Describe the portal vein. Write a note on the sites of the collateral portocaval (portosystemic) anastomosis.

PORTAL VEIN

Introduction

Portal vein forms an important venous system which carries venous blood from:
- Abdominal part of gastrointestinal tract except lower end of anal canal
- Gallbladder with biliary tract
- Pancreas
- Spleen.

Significance of the Name 'Portal'

Portal vein carries venous blood from:
- Digestive tract transporting products of digestion with nutrients to the liver.
- Spleen to liver transporting products of hemoglobin catabolism.

In case of arteries, finer terminal branches terminate in tissue level as capillary bed. Veins are formed at the beginning in the form of capillary (sinusoids) bed at tissue level and at other end they form bigger veins. Portal system of blood vessels (both vein and artery) present capillary at both ends for which they are termed portal. In case of the portal vein, it starts from capillary bed of the gut and again ends inside the liver in the form of venous sinusoids.

Formation (Fig. 26.12)

Portal vein is formed by union of *superior mesenteric vein* and *splenic vein behind neck of pancreas* at the level of *transpyloric plane* (L_1).

Termination (Fig. 26.12)

The vein ends at the level of porta hepatis by dividing into right and left divisions which enter the liver.

Bifurcation of portal vein occurs at the right end of porta hepatis from where right and left divisions enter corresponding lobes of liver. Right vein is shorter, wider and more straight than the left.

Course with Relations (Fig. 26.12)

From the level of origin, the portal vein passes upwards and to the right having following three parts:

1st part (Infraduodenal): It is behind neck of pancreas.

2nd part (Retroduodenal): It is behind 1st part of duodenum.

3rd part (Supraduodenal): It is the longer part passing upward with slight inclination to the right in right free margin of lesser omentum. This part is more important because:
- It lies in right free margin of lesser omentum.
- Here portal vein is related anteriorly to bile duct to the right and hepatic artery to the left.

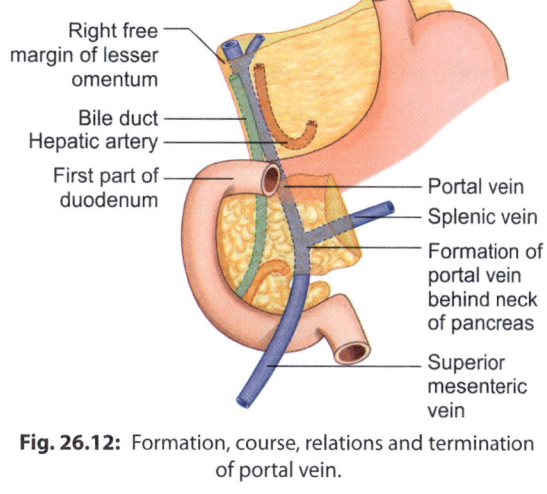

Fig. 26.12: Formation, course, relations and termination of portal vein.

Intrahepatic Part

Right and left division of portal vein, beyond porta hepatis, continue as intrahepatic part. Right division gives branches to right lobe of liver. Left division, after sending branches to caudate and quadrate lobe of liver, ramifies in the left lobe. Terminal radicals of portal vein, lying in the portal canal, end in hepatic sinusoids in between rows of liver cells called hepatic laminae. Portal venous blood in hepatic sinusoids is characterized by following:
- Blood mixes up with hepatic arterial blood.
- Blood comes in contact with liver cells of hepatic laminae
- Finally blood drains into central veins which are most peripheral tributaries of the hepatic vein.

Tributaries (Fig. 26.13)

It is better to classify the tributaries of portal vein in following groups:

A. Tributaries of formation
- Superior mesenteric vein—which drains the midgut
- Splenic vein—which receives blood from
  ◊ Spleen
  ◊ Pancreas
  ◊ Hindgut through its tributary—inferior mesenteric vein.

B. Tributaries of trunk
- Superior pancreaticoduodenal vein

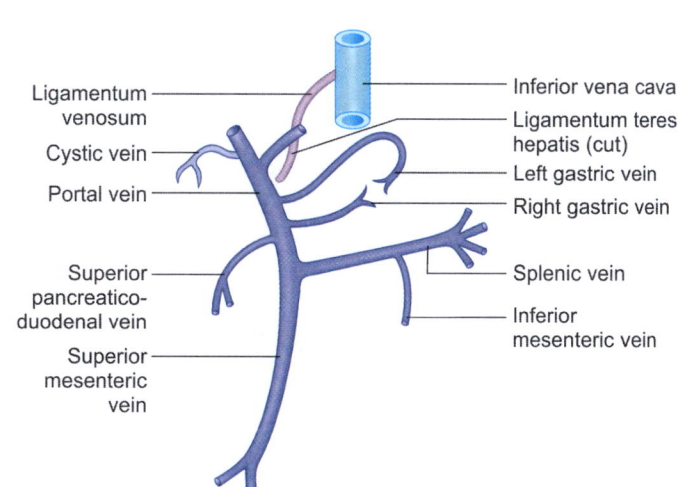

Fig. 26.13: Tributaries of portal vein.

- Right gastric vein } which drain abdominal part of foregut
- Left gastric vein.
C. **Tributary of right division**—cystic vein—which drains gallbladder.
D. **Tributaries of left division**
   - Paraumbilical veins—the veins accompany the ligamentum teres hepatis to pass between the layers of falciform ligament. The veins extend from anterior abdominal wall around the umbilicus to the left division of portal vein.
   - Ligamentum teres hepatis—a remnant of left umbilical vein of fetal life
   - Ligamentum venosum—a remnant of ductus venosus which connects left division of portal vein with inferior vena cava in fetal life.

Ligamentum teres hepatis and ligamentum venosum are the embryological remnants which exist as fibrous cord without patency, as they are obliterated after birth.

Clinical Anatomy

Blood Stream in Portal Vein

Portal vein formed by union of the superior mesenteric vein and the splenic vein (receiving inferior mesenteric vein) present two parallel streams passing side by side. Right-sided stream receives blood from small and large intestines up to the right two-thirds of transverse colon. It carries blood to the right lobe of liver. Left stream receives blood from stomach, spleen, pancreas and hindgut to distribute blood to left lobe of liver along with caudate and quadrate lobe. So metastasis from cancer of two different groups of primarily affected areas occurs in right and left lobe respectively.

Portal Pressure and Portal Hypertension

Normal pressure in portal vein is *15 mm of Hg*. It is measured through recording intrasplenic pressure with the help of splenic puncture.

Portal hypertension is characterized by rise of pressure to *40 mm of Hg*. Common causes of portal hypertension are **cirrhosis of liver** and **portal venous thrombosis**.

For management of portal hypertension, a surgical intervention, portosystemic venous shunt is done. In this operation, portal vein in right free margin of lesser omentum is anastomosed with the inferior vena cava.

Sites of Collateral Portocaval Anastomosis (Fig. 26.14)

In case of obstruction to the normal portal venous blood flow through the liver to the inferior vena cava, portal venous blood is reshunted through following sites of communication between tributaries of portal and systemic veins. These anastomoses are called portosystemic anastomoses. It is also to be noted that engorgement of collateral venous circulation in these areas may give rise to various clinical manifestations.

- **At umbilicus**: *Paraumbilical veins* will shunt portal venous blood from *left division of portal vein* to the veins radiating from

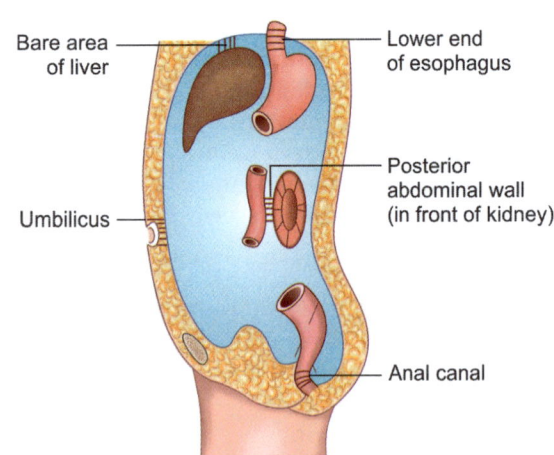

Fig. 26.14: Sites of portosystemic (portocaval) anastomosis.

umbilicus *at anterior abdominal wall*. Engorged tortuous veins radiating around the umbilicus is termed as **Caput Medusa** as these resemble the snakes radiating from head of Greek goddess Medusa.
- **At lower end of esophagus**: *Esophageal tributaries of left gastric vein (portal system)* communicate with *esophageal tributaries of inferior hemiazygos vein* at lower end of esophagus. Engorgement of these veins due to portal obstruction may cause their rupture. It will be manifested by vomiting of blood known as **hematemesis.**
- **At anal canal**: *Superior rectal vein of portal system* communicates with *middle and inferior rectal veins of systemic system*. Engorged and tortuous veins at this site lead to development of **hemorrhoids (piles)**.
- **At the bare area of liver**: *Minute veins draining the liver (portal system)* communicate with *veins draining the diaphragm (systemic system)*.
- **At posterior abdominal wall**
  - Veins which drain the retroperitoneal part of gut, e.g. duodenum, ascending colon and descending colon (portal system) communicate with the parietal *veins of posterior abdominal wall and kidney* (systemic system).
  - *Splenic vein of portal system* sometimes communicates with *renal vein of systemic system.*
- **Persistent ductus venosus**: Very rarely the ductus venosus may be patent after birth connecting the *left division of portal vein (portal system)* with the *inferior vena cava (systemic system)*.

Short note: Sites of collateral portocaval anastomosis.

Chapter 27

Posterior Abdominal Wall

SN 27.1 Write a short note on cisterna chyli.

CISTERNA CHYLI (FIG. 27.1)

It is a short linear lymphatic sac whose lower end is blind. It is situated in front of the bodies of upper two lumbar (L_1 and L_2) vertebrae to the right side of abdominal aorta. Length of cisterna chyli is 5 to 7 cm.

At the level of aortic opening, cisterna chyli is continuous as thoracic duct in posterior thoracic wall.

Afferent channels: Through following three lymphatic channels, cisterna chyli receives lymph from the part of the body below the level of the diaphragm.
- Two lumbar lymph trunks (right and left)—they carry lymph from:
  - Lower limbs
  - Pelvic wall
  - Pelvic viscera
  - Posterior abdominal wall
- One intestinal lymph trunk: This channel carries lymph from abdominal viscera.

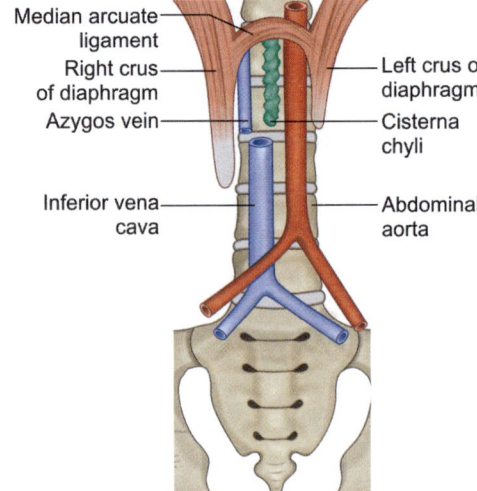

Fig. 27.1: Important midline structures of posterior abdominal wall.

Variations of Cisterna Chyli

Cisterna chyli may be absent with following variations:
- One anastomotic channel may receive both lumbar lymph trunk
- Two lumbar lymph trunks may unite to form the thoracic duct directly.

SA 22.2 Write a brief note on psoas major and quadratus lumborum.

Individual muscle may be asked as short note.

PSOAS MAJOR MUSCLE (FIG. 27.2)

Psoas major is the medial-most muscle of the posterior abdominal wall. It is tubular in shape. The muscle extends:
- In paravertebral region of posterior abdominal wall
- In greater pelvis or false pelvis lateral to pelvic brim
- Beyond inguinal ligament in femoral region where it forms the floor of femoral triangle
- Upper end of the muscle extends in posterior thoracic wall.

Origin

The muscle arises from 3 × 5 sources:
1. From the sides of 5 intervertebral disks between T_{12} to L_5 vertebrae, and the sides of adjacent vertebrae.
2. From the deeper aspect of 5 tendinous arches, called psoas arches, each of which are attached by two ends at the upper and lower ends of sides of 5 lumbar vertebrae.
3. From the medial half of the anterior surface of transverse processes of 5 lumbar vertebrae.

Fleshy ship arising from all the sources fuse to form a tubular muscle.

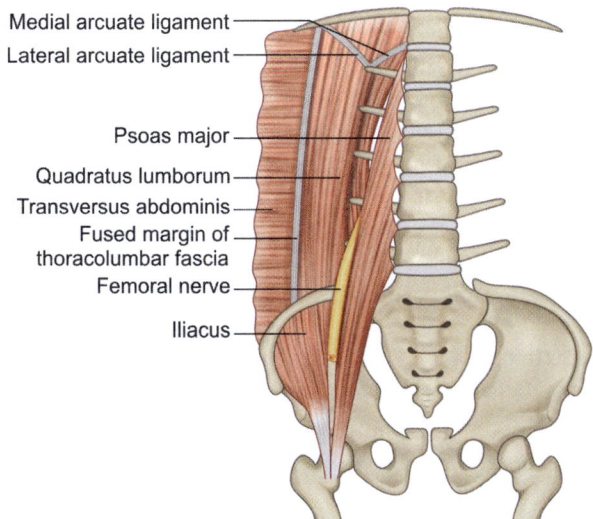

Fig. 27.2: Muscles of posterior abdominal wall.

Insertion

Beyond the inguinal ligament, in the femoral region tendon of psoas major is joined by tendon of iliacus muscle on its lateral side. Conjoint iliopsoas tendon is inserted to the tip and medial part of anterior surface of lesser trochanter of femur.

ILIACUS MUSCLE (FIG. 27.2)

Iliacus is not truly the muscle of posterior abdominal wall, but also closely related to psoas major muscle. This muscle is fan shaped occupying iliac fossa of greater pelvis or false pelvis.

Origin
- From upper two thirds of iliac fossa of hip bone
- Superior surface of lateral mass of sacrum.

Insertion

The fibers of fan-shaped muscle end in a tendon which blends with the tendon of psoas major lying medial to it. The conjoint tendon is inserted into tip and medial part of anterior surface of lesser trochanter of femur.

PSOAS MINOR MUSCLE

Psoas minor is a thin and long muscle lying in front of psoas major. It is not always present.

Origin

It arises from side of the intervertebral disk between T_{12} and L_1 vertebrae and adjoining parts of both of these vertebrae.

Insertion

Long, thin and flat tendon of the muscle is inserted into the iliopubic eminence.

QUADRATUS LUMBORUM MUSCLE
- Quadratus lumborum is so called because it is a quadrangular muscle in the lumbar region.
- It is lateral to psoas major muscle.
- It extends between iliac crest and 12th rib with its origin below and insertion above.

Origin
- **Medial fibers:** From lateral part of anterior surface of transverse process of lower 3–4 lumbar vertebrae
- **Intermediate fibers:** Iliolumbar ligament
- **Lateral fibers:** Posterior 5 cm of inner lip of ventral segment of iliac crest.

Insertion
- Medial fibers are inserted into lateral part of anterior surface of transverse process of upper 3–4 lumbar vertebrae
- Lateral fibers are inserted into medial half of lower border and adjacent part of anterior surface of the 12th rib.

Nerve Supply of Posterior Abdominal Wall Muscles
Muscles of posterior abdominal wall are composite in nature, developed by fusion of multiple segments. So they are supplied by roots of multiple spinal nerve.
Psoas major: From the root of upper four lumbar (L_1-L_4) nerves
Psoas minor: Being developed from single segment, it is supplied by only root of 1st lumbar (L_1) nerve.
Iliacus: It receives fibers from the femoral nerve (L_2, L_3)
Quadratus lumborum: From the subcostal nerve (T_{12}) and upper four (L_1 - L_4) lumbar nerves.

Actions of Posterior Abdominal Wall Muscles

Psoas Major
- As the muscle crosses in front of the hip joint, it is a **flexor of hip joint**. This action is more important as **flexor of the trunk** on hip while a person **sits up from supine position**
- Psoas major is **medial rotator of thigh**. *But the same muscle causes lateral rotation of thigh as deformity of lower limb in fracture of neck of femur.*

Psoas Minor
Being a thin muscle, it is a **weak flexor** of the trunk.

Iliacus
Along with psoas major, it **helps in flexion** of hip joint.

Quadratus Lumborum
- Quadratus lumborum is an important muscle **acting during inspiration**. It **fixes the 12th rib** of the thoracic cage, so that the diaphragm can contract and descend during inspiration
- When the **muscle of one side** contracts, it causes **lateral flexion of vertebral column**
- When the **muscles of both sides** act together, it causes **extension of vertebral column**.

SA 27.3 Write a brief note on psoas sheath.

PSOAS SHEATH

It is also called iliopsoas sheath, as this common fascial sheath covers both iliacus and psoas major muscles. The sheath is composed of two parts.

Part in posterior abdominal wall: It is tubular in shape and extends as follows:
- *Medially*: The sheath presents five concave-free margins called psoas arches. Each of the five arches are free in the middle, but attached by their both upper and lower ends to the sides of intervertebral disks and adjoining vertebral bodies. Deep surfaces of psoas arches gives origin to the muscular slips of psoas major.
- *Laterally*: The sheath is attached to:
  - Middle of anterior surface of transverse processes of five lumbar vertebra
  - Intertransverse ligament
- *Superiorly*: The psoas sheaths present a condensed crescentic margin which extends from the side of intervertebral disk between T_{12} and L_1 vertebrae to the front of transverse process of 1st lumbar vertebra. This arched thickened upper margin of the sheath is known as **medial arcuate ligament** or **medial lumbocostal arch**. Deep to this, the **sympathetic trunk** and the **least splanchnic nerve** pass form the thorax to the abdomen.
- *Inferiorly*: The sheath crosses the iliac crest to reach the false pelvis lateral to the pelvic brim.

Part beyond iliac crest: In the greater pelvis or false pelvis, it becomes truly iliopsoas sheath, as it is the seath also covering the iliacus muscle lying laterally in the iliac fossa. Superolaterally the sheath is attached to the margin of iliac fossa beyond iliacus. Medially it is attached to pelvic brim. Inferiorly iliopsoas sheath passes deep to inguinal ligament over the muscles in femoral triangle and extends up to the lesser trochanter of femur.

Clinical Anatomy of Psoas Sheath

Psoas sheath presents free margin medially in the form of 5 psoas arches. Medially this deficiency of margin is related to bodies of lumbar vertebrae.

In case of tuberculosis of vertebrae (Caries spine), necrotic or dead bony tissue from the damaged infected vertebrae forms a softened substance called caseous material, which looks like thickened pus. As it is noninflammatory and painless, it is called **cold abscess**. This accumulated cold abscess, entering through the deficient psoas arch, lie deep to psoas sheath. Getting resistance against the spread of the abscess on all the aspects, it finds the path to trickle down beyond inguinal ligament, in the femoral region of front of thigh up to the lesser trochanter of femur.

SA 27.4 Write a note on thoracolumbar fascia.

THORACOLUMBAR FASCIA (FIG. 27.3)

Introduction

It is trilaminar fascia which encloses muscles of posterior abdominal wall. The fascia is called thoracolumbar because, its posterior layer extends upwards over the muscles of back of thorax.

Disposition of Three Layers

Posterior Layer

Medially

Attached to spines of lumbar vertebrae and supraspinous ligament.

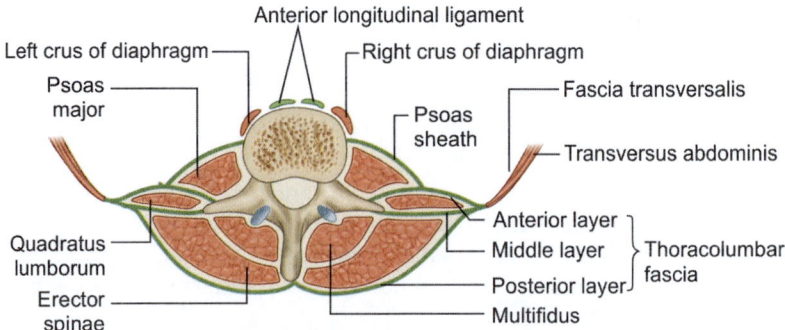

Fig. 27.3: Thoracolumbar fascia in relation to lumbar vertebra.

Laterally
Covering the back of erector spinae, the fascia fuses with middle layer at lateral margin of the muscle.

Superiorly
The fascia covers the muscles of back of thorax and, attached medially to the thoracic spines and laterally to the angle of ribs.

Inferiorly
The fascia is attached to the most posterior part of outer lip of iliac crest and is continued below with the fascia on the back of sacrum.

Middle Layer

Medially
Attached to tip of transverse processes of lumbar vertebrae and to the intertransverse ligaments.

Laterally
Fuses with posterior layer of the fascia at the lateral border of erector spinae muscle.

Superiorly
It is attached to lower border of 12th rib.

Inferiorly
The fascia is attached to posteriormost part of intermediate area of iliac crest.

Anterior Layer

It covers the front of quadratus lumborum muscle and medially it blends with lateral margin of psoas sheath. Extent of this layer is as follows:

Medially
Attached to the middle of anterior surface of transverse process of lumbar vertabrae.

Laterally
It blends with the fused middle and posterior layer of the fascia at the lateral border of quadratus lumborum muscle.

Superiorly

Anterior layer of thoracolumbar fascia becomes condensed and extends medio-laterally as a fascial ridge from transverse process of 1st lumbar vertebra to the middle of lower border of 12th rib. This is called **lateral arcuate ligament** or **lateral lumbocostal arch**. Following structures pass deep to the ligament or fascial arch from above downwards and laterally.
- Subcostal vein
- Subcostal artery
- Subcostal nerve

Inferiorly

The fascia is attached to:
- Iliolumbar ligament
- Posterior one-third of inner lip of iliac crest.

LA 27.5 Describe briefly the abdominal aorta with its branches. *(Important for viva voce and practical)*

ABDOMINAL AORTA (FIG. 27.4)

Introduction

Abdominal aorta is the main arterial trunk of abdomen. It runs vertically downwards in front of lumbar vertebrae just a little to the left side of the midline. As the artery crosses in front of convexity of lumbar vertebrae, its pulsation can be felt at the level of umbilicus, especially in slim persons.

Extent

Beginning: Abdominal aorta begins as continuation of descending thoracic aorta while passing through the **aortic opening** of the diaphragm which is bounded behind by lower border of body of twelfth thoracic (T$_{12}$) vertebra and in front by median arcuate ligament.

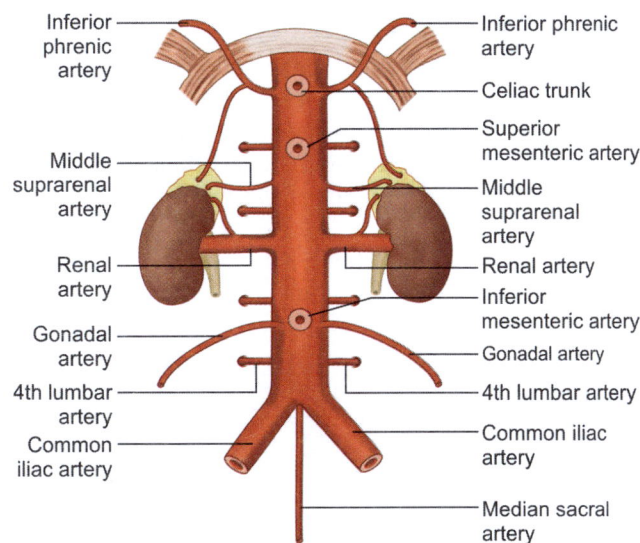

Fig. 27.4: Abdominal aorta with its branches.

End: Abdominal aorta ends at the level of body of **4th lumbar vertebera** to the left side of midline by dividing into right and left common iliac arteries.

Important Relations

Anteriorly

From above downwards
- Celiac and aortic plexuses of nerves

- Body of pancreas with splenic vein
- Left renal vein
- Third part of duodenum
- Coils of small intestine separated by parietal peritoneum.

Posteriorly
- Lumbar vertebrae with the intervening intervertebral disks
- Anterior longitudinal ligament
- Left lumbar veins.

To the Right
- Inferior vena cava
- Right sympathetic trunk
- Cisterna chyli
- Azygos vein
- Right crus of diaphragm.

To the Left
- Left sympathetic trunk
- Left crus of diaphragm.

Branches of Abdominal Aorta
Abdominal aorta gives rise to following sets of branches:
- **Ventral**—unpaired midline branches: Visceral branches
- **Lateral**—paired branches: Visceral branches
- **Dorsal**—paired branches: Parietal branches
- **Terminal**—paired branches: Parietal branches.

Ventral Branches of Abdominal Aorta
Ventral branches are midline unpaired 3 visceral branches, each one for abdominal part of foregut, midgut and hindgut. They are celiac trunk, superior mesenteric artery and inferior mesenteric artery.

(Celic trunk has been discussed in Chapter 25, superior and inferior mesenteric arteries in Chapter 26).

Lateral Branches of Abdominal Aorta
These are bilateral, arising from the sides of abdominal aorta.

Inferior phrenic artery
- It arises from beginning of abdominal aorta
- The artery runs upwards and laterally over the respective crus of the diaphragm medial to suprarenal gland
- The right artery passes behind inferior vena cava and the left passes behind abdominal part of esophagus
- Branches are—2 to 3 superior suprarenal branches and terminal phrenic branches.

Middle suprarenal artery
- It arises from the level of 1st lumbar vertebra

- The artery runs laterally and slightly upwards over the respective crus of diaphragm
- The artery enters the gland piercing the cortex, but not through hilum unlike the vein.

Renal artery
- Renal arteries are the largest lateral branch of abdominal aorta
- The artery arises at the level of L_2 vertebra
- The artery passes horizontally towards the hilum of kidney
- The right artery passes behind inferior vena cava and then right renal vein
- The left renal artery passes behind left renal vein
- Branches are—*inferior suprarenal* and *ureteric* arteries.

Gonadal (testicular or ovarian) artery
- This artery is narrower
- It arises from anterolateral aspect of abdominal aorta at the level of L_3 vertebra
- Initially the artery runs along the posterior abdominal wall downwards and laterally in front of psoas major muscle
- In case of male, testicular artery is included in the spermatic cord at the deep inguinal ring. It passes through the inguinal canal. At the upper pole of testis the artery divides into multiple branches. These branches supply testis and epididymis.
- In case of female, the ovarian artery reaches the true pelvis to enter between two layers of suspensory ligament of ovary and finally the mesovarium to supply the ovary. One descending branch anastomoses with the uterine artery. Ovarian artery also gives branches to the uterine tube.

Dorsal Branches of Abdominal Aorta
- *Paired branches*: Lumbar arteries
- *Unpaired branch*: Median sacral artery.

Lumbar arteries
- Lumbar arteries represent the segmental arteries of lumbar region
- Upper four lumbar arteries arises from the level of respective lumbar vertebrae
- The arteries cross the anterolateral aspect of the respective lumbar vertebra and then pass deep to the corresponding psoas arches
- Arteries of right side passes behind inferior vena cava
- Upper most pair of arteries pass deep to the crus of diaphragm
- The arteries pass deep to psoas major and quadratus lumborum. Only the 4th lumbar artery passes in front of quadratus lumborum. Dorsal branches of lumbar arteries pass backwards to supply muscle and skin of the back. Continuation of the lumbar arteries supplies muscles of the body wall.

Fifth lumbar artery
- It shows variation in origin
- It may be represented by lumbar branch of iliolumbar artery, or it may arise from median sacral artery.

Medial sacral artery
It arises from the dorsal aspect of terminal end of abdominal aorta. It runs along the midline of pelvic surface of sacrum accompanied by the median sacral vein on the right side. It supplies the structures of posterior pelvic wall.

Terminal Branches of Abdominal Aorta

Common iliac arteries

Abdominal aorta bifurcates into right and left common iliac arteries in front of body of 4th lumbar vertebra to the left side of midline. Each of the common iliac artery divides into external and internal iliac arteries in front of sacroiliac joint. Bifurcation of common iliac artery is an important landmark because it is crossed by:
- *Ureter*
- *Lower end of root of the mesentery* on the right side and *upper end of root of the pelvic mesocolon* on the left side.

Important relations
- Right common iliac artery crosses in front of beginning of inferior vena cava and right common iliac vein.
- Left common iliac artery is shorter. It is lateral to left common iliac vein and is crossed by the inferior mesenteric vessels.

LA 27.6 **Describe the inferior vena cava.**

INFERIOR VENA CAVA (FIG. 27.5)

Introduction
- Inferior vena cava in the longest and widest venous trunk of the body.
- It drains blood from the part of the body below diaphragm except the gut with related structures like gallbladder, pancreas and spleen.
- It ascends in front of lumbar vertebrae in the posterior abdominal wall.
- It enters the thorax piercing central tendon of diaphragm to open in right atrium of heart.

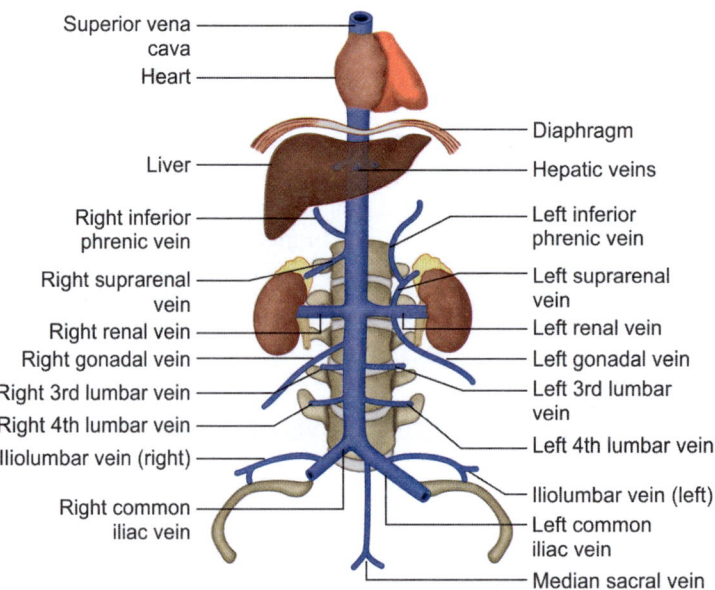

Fig. 27.5: Inferior vena cava with its tributaries.

Formation

Inferior vena cava is formed by union of right and left common iliac veins in front of the body of 5th lumbar vertebra to the right side of midline.

Termination

Inferior vena cava opens in lower and posterior part of right atrium of heart at the level of right 6th sternocostal junction.

Course and Important Relations

For easy understanding of course end relations, the vein is divided into segments, as follows.

Segment 1: This part runs upwards from the level of formation in front of lower lumbar vertebrae and to the right side of abdominal aorta. Anteriorly this part is covered by loops of small intestine.

Segment 2: It covered anteriorly by 3rd part of duodenum, head of pancreas and 1st part of duodenum from below upwards. Posteriorly, it is related to the upper lumbar vertebrae with the lumbar part of azygos vein and the cisterna chyli.

Segment 3: This part is above 1st part of duodenum where it forms posterior boundary of the epiploic foramen. So, in front of epiploic foramen it is related to the right free margin of lesser omentum.

Segment 4: This part runs upwards along the groove for inferior vena cava on posterior surface of liver. This segment of vena cava is fixed to the liver through the connection of hepatic veins.

Segments 5: Passing through the vena caval opening of the central tendon of the diaphragm at the level of lower border of body of 8th thoracic vertebra, this segment is a short thoracic part. It finally pierces fibrous pericardium of heart to open into lower and posterior part of the right atrium of heart at the level of right 6th sternocostal junction.

Anterior wall of vena caval orifice in right atrium is guarded by a semilunar endothelial fold called valve of inferior vena cava.

Tributaries

Following two points are to be noted first, before the tributaries of inferior vena cava are studied.
1. Tributaries of inferior vena cava almost correspond to the branches of abdominal aorta, except the ventral midline splanchnic branches, as the corresponding veins drain into portal vein.
2. Some of the veins of right side only drain into inferior vena cava directly.

Tributaries of formation: *Common iliac veins* of both sides, formed by union of external and internal iliac veins, join in front of the body 5th lumbar vertebra, to the right side of midline.
- Common iliac vein receives *iliolumbar vein* of respective side.
- Left common iliac vein receives *median sacral vein*.

Lumbar veins

Out of 4 lumbar veins, **3rd and 4th lumbar veins** of both sides drain into the inferior vena cava. *1st and 2nd lumbar veins* drain into the *azygos vein* in right side and the *hemiazygos vein* in left side.

Renal veins

Renal veins of both sides drain into the inferior vena cava from the kidney at the level of body of 2nd lumbar vertebra.

Below and above the renal veins, following **veins of two sides show variations in termination.**

Below renal vein:
- **Right gonadal (testicular or ovarian) vein** drains into *inferior vena cava*
- **Left vein** drains into *left renal vein.*

Above renal vein:
- **Right suprarenal vein** drains into **inferior vena cava**.
- **Left vein** descends downwards and medially to open into **left renal vein**.
  It is important to note here that though suprarenal arteries are three, superior, middle and inferior, the vein is single in each side.
- **Right inferior phrenic vein** opens into **inferior vena cava.**
- **The left vein** drains into **left suprarenal vein**.

Hepatic veins (last tributaries)

Hepatic veins drain the liver. These veins are primarily divided into two groups—upper and lower.
- **Upper hepatic veins** are most **constant**. They are **three in number**—right, middle and left. These veins come out from posterior surface of liver opposite the site of groove for inferior vena cava. These short and stout veins open into inferior vena cava immediately.
- **Lower hepatic veins** are **inconstant**. They are narrow small channels. Coming out from the back of **right lobe** and **caudate lobe**, they drain into the inferior vena cava.

> **Important Note**
>
> *Relations of inferior vena cava and abdominal aorta with their tributaries and branches:*
> - It is important to note that branches of abdominal aorta and the tributaries of inferior vena cava *always cross behind the two great vessels.*
> - Inferior vena cava lies to the right side of abdominal aorta. So, to drain into the vena cava, left-sided tributaries pass behind abdominal aorta. Again right-sided lateral and dorsolateral branches of abdominal aorta cross behind inferior vena cava.

LA 27.7 Describe the lumbar plexus of nerves.

LUMBAR PLEXUS OF NERVES (FIG. 27.6)

Introduction

It is the plexus of nerves which is formed mainly by the fibers of anterior primary rami or ventral rami of lumbar spinal nerves.

Nerves from this plexus are distributed mainly to the ventral aspect of lower limb and also to the lower part of abdominal wall.

Formation

Lumbar plexus is formed by:
- Ventral rami of **1st, 2nd and 3rd lumbar nerves**.
- **Upper division** of ventral ramus of **4th lumbar nerve**
- A small branch from subcostal (T_{12}) nerve.

Situation

The plexus is situated within the posterior part of psoas major muscle.

Stages of Formation
1. A small branch from subcostal nerve joins the root of 1st lumbar nerve
2. 4th lumbar nerve divides into upper and lower divisions. Upper division is for lumbar plexus. Lower division joins with whole of ventral root of 5th lumbar nerve to form *lumbosacral trunk*. This nerve trunk crosses ala of sacrum of pelvic brim and enters pelvic cavity to take part in formation of sacral plexus.
3. 2nd, 3rd and upper division of 4th lumbar nerves divide into ventral and dorsal branches.

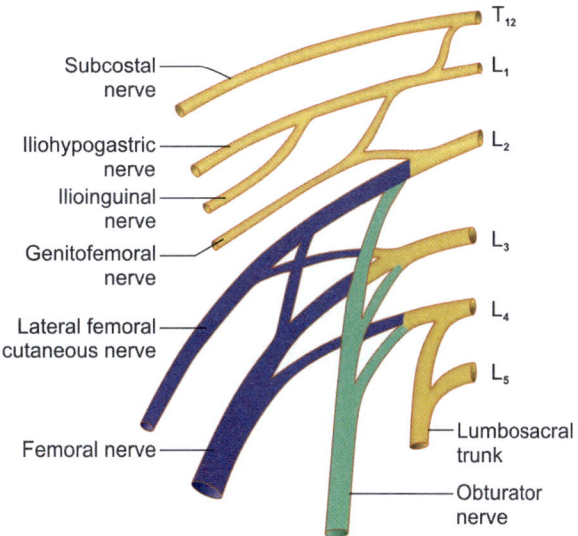

Fig. 27.6: Lumbar plexus.

Nerves Arising from the Plexus
- Branches from undivided ventral root of 1st and 2nd lumbar nerves join to form the **genitofemoral nerve**. The nerve runs initially in front of the psoas major muscle and finally lie in front of the external iliac artery. At the level of deep inguinal ring it divides into genital and femoral branches. **Genital branch** enters the inguinal canal through deep ring. It supplies cremaster muscle in male and sensory branches to labium majora in females. **Femoral branch** lying in lateral arterial compartment of femoral sheath supplies small areas of skin of front of thigh just below the groin.
- 1st lumbar nerve, after giving the twig for genitofemoral nerve, runs along posterior abdominal wall and gives out a *collateral branch*. The main nerve continues as **iliohypogastric nerve**. The collateral branch is known as **ilioinguinal nerve**. Iliohypogastric nerve, and ilioinguinal nerve below and parallel to the former enter the plane between transversus abdominis and internal oblique. Along this plane both the nerves approach towards anterolateral wall of abdomen. Both supply lower part of abdominal wall.
- The roots of 2nd, 3rd and 4th lumbar nerves divide into ventral and dorsal divisions.
- Branches from the dorsal division of 2nd and 3rd lumbar nerves unite to form **lateral femoral cutaneous nerve**. From posterior abdominal wall the nerve reaches the iliac fossa beneath the iliac fascia. Medial to anterior superior iliac spine the nerve finally passes deep to inguinal ligament to reach the lateral part of front of thigh and supplies the skin of that area.
- *Dorsal branches* of 2nd, 3rd and 4th lumbar nerves unite to form the **femoral nerve**. It appears lateral to the psoas major and approaches the groove between iliacus and psoas major muscles. Along this groove, the femoral nerve runs downwards deep to inguinal ligament and reaches front of thigh lateral to femoral sheath. It gives both motor and sensory branches to the front of thigh.
- *Ventral branches* of 2nd, 3rd and 4th lumbar nerves unite to form the **obturator nerve**. This nerve appears medial to psoas major muscle and runs downwards, lateral to lumbosacral trunk. Running along lateral wall of pelvis, the obturator nerve passes through obturator canal to reach the medial side of thigh. It is the nerve for adductor muscles of hip joint in the medial compartment of thigh.
- In some cases, branches from the ventral division of 3rd and 4th lumbar nerves form **accessory obturator nerve**. If present, it does not enter the pelvis, but crosses iliopubic eminence to reach the thigh.

Emerging Nerves Related to Psoas Major (Fig. 27.7)

In Front of Psoas Major
Genitofemoral nerve, emerging through anterior surface of the muscle runs downwards and slightly laterally.

Lateral to Psoas Major
Running laterally along posterior abdominal wall, from above downwards the nerves are:
- *Iliohypogastric nerve*
- *Ilioinguinal nerve*
- *Lateral femoral cutaneous nerve*
- *Femoral nerve.*

Medial to Psoas Major
- *Obturator nerve*
- *Accessory obturator nerve*, if present.
Medial to these nerves, lies the lumbosacral trunk.

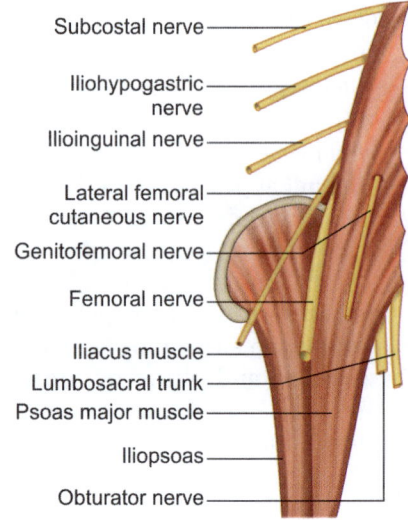

Fig. 27.7: Nerves of lumbar plexus related to psoas major.

LA 27.8 Describe briefly the autonomic nervous system in the posterior abdominal wall.

AUTONOMIC NERVOUS SYSTEM IN POSTERIOR ABDOMINAL WALL (FIG. 27.8)

Autonomic nerves of posterior abdominal wall are composed of both sympathetic and parasympathetic components.

Sympathetic
- **Greater** and **lesser splanchnic nerves**: Their preganglionic fibers are distributed through *celiac and aorticorenal ganglion*.
- **Lumbar part of sympathetic chain.**

Parasympathetic
- **Vagus nerve (Xth cranial nerve)**: Fibers are distributed through posterior gastric nerve containing fibers of vagus nerve of both sides.
- **Pelvic splanchnic nerves**: Fibers of these nerves originate from the neurons of intermediate area of S_2, S_3 and S_4 segments of spinal cord and come out through corresponding sacral nerves.

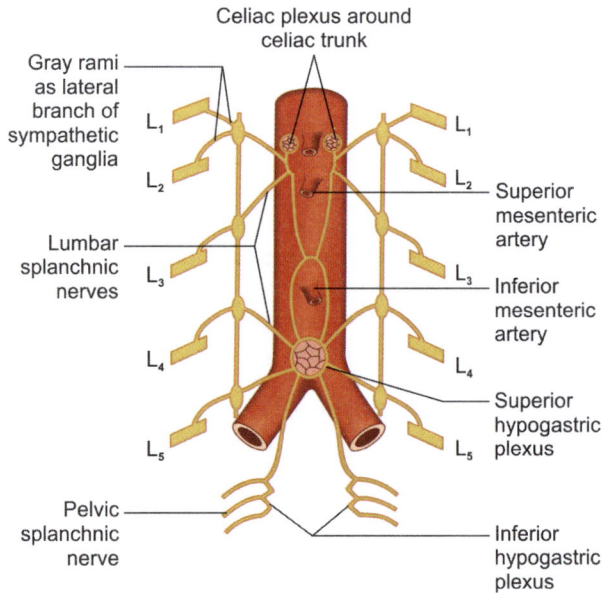

Fig. 27.8: Autonomic nerves of posterior abdominal wall.

Target Organs
- Smooth muscles of the abdominal and pelvic viscera—by parasympathetic nerves
- Mucous glands of gastrointestinal tract—by parasympathetic nerves
- Sphincters of viscera—by sympathetic nerves
- Blood vessels of viscera—by vasoconstrictor fibers of sympathetic nerves
- Blood vessels, sweat glands and arrectores pili muscle of the body wall of abdomen—by sympathetic nerves.

Distributions
It is important to note that the parasympathetic fibers for viscera join with the sympathetic fibers in ganglia and plexuses situated in relation to abdominal aorta and its main branches. Thereafter, both the autonomic nerve fibers follow the blood vessels supplying a particular viscera.

Celiac Ganglion (Fig. 27.8)
Celiac ganglion is the largest autonomic ganglion of the body belonging to sympathetic system. It is two in number situated on either side of the origin of celiac trunk from abdominal aorta. Each of the ganglia is irregular in outline and divided into two parts.
1. **Larger upper part:** It receives preganglionic sympathetic fibers as *greater splanchnic nerve* (T_5 - T_9)
2. **Smaller lower part:** It is named aortic-renal ganglion and it receives preganglionic sympathetic fibers as *lesser splanchnic nerve.*

Postganglionic fibers of sympathetic system arise from the coeliac ganglia and primarily form celiac plexus.

Celiac Plexus (Fig. 27.8)
Celiac plexus is a network of autonomic nerves situated adjacent to celiac ganglia, around the origin of celiac trunk and superior mesenteric artery in front of abdominal aorta.

Celiac plexus is made up of following fibers:
- *Postganglionic sympathetic fibers* from celiac ganglia
- Some of the *preganglionic sympathetic fibers* reach celiac plexus directly from greater and lesser splanchnic nerves.
- *Preganglionic parasympathetic fibers* from the vagus (Xth cranial) nerve. These fibers of vagus nerve reach celiac plexus via posterior gastric nerve which contain vagal fibers of both sides. It is to be noted here that vagal fibers relay in the parasympathetic ganglia related close to or in the wall of viscera.

Branches from Celiac Plexus
Branches of celiac plexus contain postganglionic sympathetic and preganglionic parasympathetic (vagal) fibers. They travel along the following routes:
1. Along the branches of unpaired ventral splanchnic branches of abdominal aorta, i.e. celiac trunk and superior mesenteric artery (not inferior mesenteric artery).
2. Along the paired lateral splanchnic branches of abdominal aorta, i.e. inferior phrenic, middle suprarenal, renal and gonadal arteries.

To reach the target point, these branches from the celiac plexus also run along the corresponding artery in the form of plexus which are named as per the name of the arteries as follows:
- **Left gastric plexus** passes to the stomach
- **Splenic plexus** supplies vasomotor branches to the spleen and its smooth muscles, if present in human spleen

- **Hepatic plexus** gives branches to liver, gallbladder and biliary tract
- **Superior mesenteric plexus** gives branches which are distributed to all parts of midgut along the arterial branches
- **Phrenic plexus** run along the inferior phrenic artery and its suprarenal branches to the *suprarenal gland*. These are *preganglionic fibers*
- **Suprarenal plexus** carries *preganglionic fibers* to *reach suprarenal medulla*. The cells of suprarenal medulla are considered to be modified postganglionic sympathetic neurons
- **Renal plexus** supplying the kidney and abdominal part of ureter is formed by nerves of following sources:
  - Celiac plexus
  - Aorticorenal ganglion
  - Least splanchnic nerve
  - Medial or splanchnic branch of 1st lumbar sympathetic ganglion
- **Gonadal plexus:**
  - *Testicular plexus* supplies testis, epididymis and vas deferens
  - *Ovarian plexus* supplies ovary and uterine tube.

Aortic Plexus (Intermesenteric Plexus) (Fig. 27.9)

This plexus of nerves is situated in front of abdominal aorta in between origin of superior mesenteric and inferior mesenteric arteries. *The plexus is formed by:*
- Branches from coeliac plexus
- Medial or splanchnic branches of 1st and 2nd lumbar sympathetic ganglia
- Branches from superior hypogastric plexus situated below the bifurcation of abdominal aorta.

Branches

Branches of intermesenteric plexus go to:
- Testicular plexus
- Superior hypogastric plexus.

Lumbar Part of Sympathetic Chain (Fig. 27.9)

This part of sympathetic chain is situated in posterior abdominal wall on either side of bodies of lumbar vertebrae. The chain presents four sympathetic ganglion (instead of five) as 1st and 2nd lumbar ganglion fuse to form one. Upper end of the chain is continued from thoracic chain which enters abdomen deep to the medial arcuate ligament. Below, it passes medial to psoas major muscle to be continuous as sacral part of sympathetic chain in the pelvis.

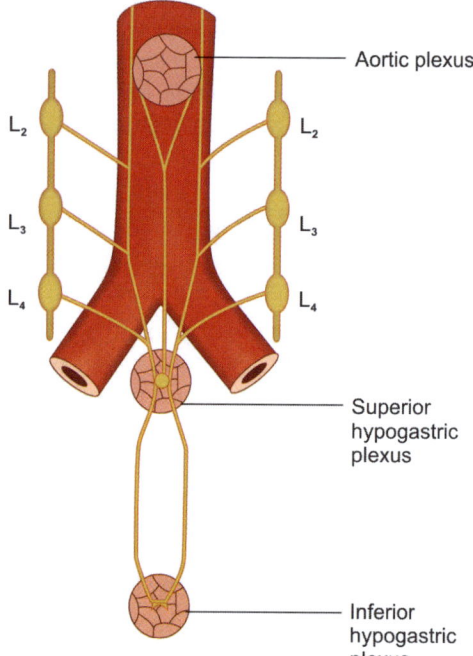

Fig. 27.9: Interrelation of aortic plexus with hypogastric plexuses.

It is important to note here that, as because the sympathetic center extends only up to L_1/L_2 segments of spinal cord, preganglionic white rami communicantes only pass via 1st and 2nd lumbar nerves to reach the 1st lumbar sympathetic ganglion **(Fig. 27.9)**.

Branches

Lateral branches

These are short postganglionic branches from 4 sympathetic ganglia which join 5 lumbar spinal nerves. These are nothing but gray rami communicantes. Gray rami from 1st lumbar ganglion join both 1st and 2nd lumbar nerves. These postganglionic sympathetic fibers supply following structures of abdominal part of body wall through lumbar somatic nerves.
- Smooth muscles of wall of blood vessels
- Sweat glands of skin
- Arrectores pili of skin.

Medial branches

These are splanchnic branches. The splanchnic branches are four in number arising from four lumbar sympathetic ganglia having following destination.
- Upper two join the celiac and intermesenteric (aortic) plexuses
- Lower two join the superior hypogastric plexus.

Short Notes: Celiac plexus

Chapter 28

Thoracoabdominal Diaphragm

LA 28.1 Discuss briefly the thoracoabdominal diaphragm. Write a note on its action and clinical anatomy.

THORACOABDOMINAL DIAPHRAGM

Introduction

Thoracoabdominal diaphragm or the diaphragm is a dome-shaped or curved musculo-aponeurotic sheet which separates the thoracic from the abdominal cavity (**Fig. 28.1**).

Its convex upper surface faces the thorax and concave lower surface is directed toward the abdominal cavity.

The central part of the diaphragm is aponeurotic or fibrous which is known as **central tendon**. Right and left domes are muscular and known as **cupolae**.

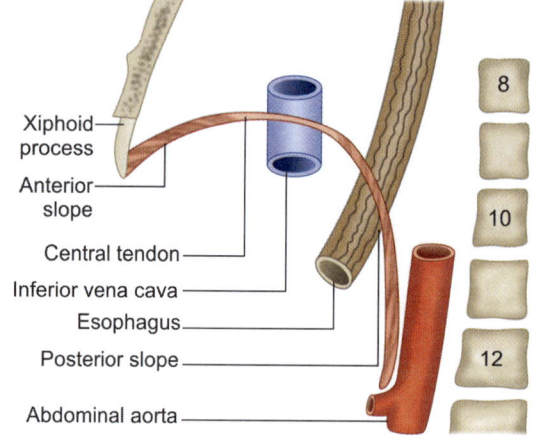

Fig. 28.1: Thoracoabdominal diaphragm in sagittal section.

Level of Cupolae

- In normal individual right cupola is at one rib higher level than the left.
- Level of cupola varies with the difference in body build. Cupola will be a higher in the short fat people than the tall thin people.
- In case of forced expiration, right cupola lies normally at the level of fourth costal cartilage, so left will be at the level of fifth.
- In case of deep inspiration right cupola descends at the level of tip of sixth costal cartilage.
- The persons with habit of overventilation of lung, as occurs in case of emphysema, the cupolae will show marked depression.

All these variations of level of cupolae are evident through a plain radiograph.

Attachments and Components

Peripheral fleshy or muscular attachment of the diaphragm is known as origin. It arises from highly oblique circumference of thoracic outlet. This attachments are low posteriorly and at the higher level anteriorly (**Fig. 28.1**).

From the periphery, the muscle fibers of diaphragm converge **centrally** in an **aponeurotic part** which is considered as **insertion**. This central part of diaphragm is known as **central tendon**.

Circumferential Attachment (Origin) (Fig. 28.2)

The muscle arises from three sources:
1. Anterior: Sternal
2. Lateral: Costal
3. Posterior: Vertebral (lumbar).

Anterior sternal origin

This component arises from two fleshy slips from back of xiphoid process. Occasionally these slips of origin may be absent (**Fig. 28.2**).

Lateral costal origin

From anterior to posterior, the costal slips of origin covers the circumferential outline of thoracic outlet. These slips arise from inner surface of **lower six (7th to 12th) costal cartilages** and adjacent areas of **corresponding ribs** (**Fig. 28.2**). These slips of origin of diaphragm interdigitate with the fibers of transversus abdominis.

Posterior vertebral (lumbar) origin

Origin of posterior slips of fibers of diaphragm is from following three sources *from lateral to medial*.
1. From lateral lumbocostal arch
2. From medial lumbocostal arch
3. From anterolateral aspect of bodies of upper 2-3 lumbar vertebrae and intervertebral disks.

Lateral lumbocostal arch (lateral vertebral origin)

Lateral lumbocostal arch or **lateral arcuate ligament** is a thickened band of fascia which represents condensed upper end of anterior layer of thoracolumbar fascia over upper end of quadratus lumborum. It is attached medially to the anterior surface of transverse process of

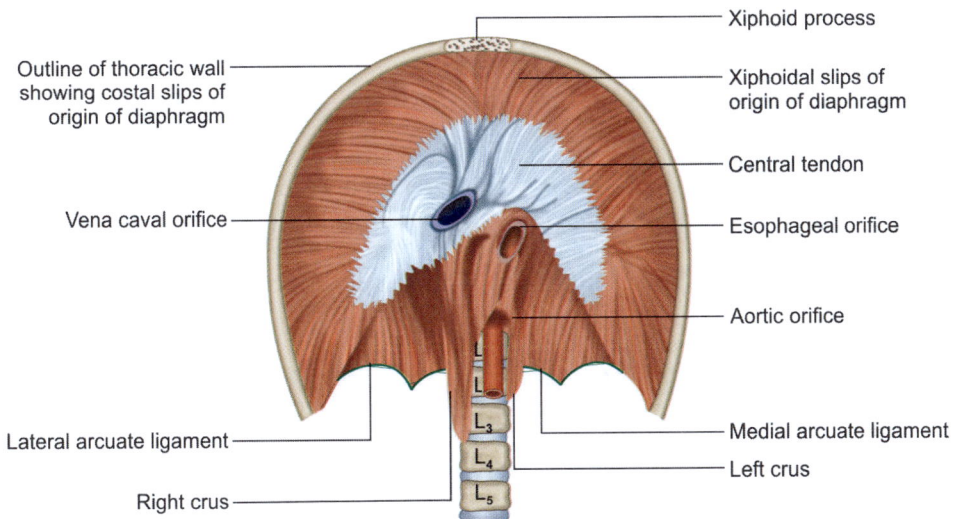

Fig. 28.2: Thoracoabdominal diaphragm viewed from abdominal surface to show its attachments and major openings.

first lumbar vertebra and laterally to the middle of lower border of twelfth rib. From this band of fascia diaphragmatic muscular slips originate to arch forwards and upwards (**Fig. 28.2**).

Medial lumbocostal arch (medial vertebral origin)

Medial lumbocostal arch is also known as **medial arcuate ligament**. It is the condensed upper end of psoas fascia or psoas sheath which covers anterior surface of psoas major muscle. This thickened band of fascia is attached medially to the side of the intervertebral disk between twelfth thoracic and first lumbar vertebrae and adjacent areas of bodies of these two vertebrae. Laterally the medial arcuate ligament is attached to anterior surface of transverse process of first lumbar vertebra. Fibers of diaphragm take origin from this band and arch upwards and forwards (**Fig. 28.2**).

Crura of diaphragm (median vertebral origin)

On either side of midline the anterolateral aspects of bodies of upper three lumbar vertebrae and the interposed intervertebral disks give origin to tendinous slips of origin of the diaphragm. These are known as crura of diaphragm *(singular—crus)* (**Fig. 28.2**). **Right crus** is **longer** and **broader** than the left. It arises from anterolateral aspect of bodies of **upper three lumbar vertebrae** and intervertebral disks. **Left crus, shorter** and **narrower**, arises from **upper two lumbar vertebrae** and the intervening disk. Medial tendinous fibers of two crura converge towards the midline and meet at the level of lower border of body of twelfth thoracic vertebra to form **median arcuate ligament**. Behind this ligament pass *aorta, cistern chyli* and *azygos vein*.

Lateral fibers of the crura diverge outwards, upwards and forwards to take part in formation of posterior part of the dome of diaphragm.

Specialized Fibers of Right Crus:

- Fibers from medial part of right crus run upwards and to the left, cross the midline and form a loop around lower end of the esophagus to form an elliptical opening called **esophageal orifice of diaphragm**.
- Some of the fibers of right crus run downward along posterior abdominal wall behind the parietal peritoneum. These fibers are contained within double fold of peritoneum and called **ligament of Treitz** which extends up to duodenojejunal flexure. This slip of voluntary muscle is known as **suspensory muscle of duodenum**. These striated muscular slips extend up to connective tissue around celiac plexus to duodenojejunal flexure. *As per recent concept, fibers of suspensory muscle of duodenum arise from left crus.*

Central Tendon (Insertion) of Diaphragm

All the muscular slips of diaphragm, from its circumferential attachment (origin) converge centrally into a central thin but strong aponeurosis. It is called **central tendon of diaphragm**. Central tendon is not exactly centrally located. It is more close to anterior xiphoidal aspect of thoracic outlet, so posterior muscular fibers are longer. Superiorly central tendon is related to **fibrous pericardium** with which it blends. It is trifoliate in appearance. The middle leaf is more anterior and its outline looks like an equilateral triangle with apex directed forwards. Right and left folia are tongue shaped and directed backwards and laterally. The left one is narrower.

Relations of Diaphragm

Superior Surface (Fig. 28.3)

Superior surface of central tendinous part is related to **pericardium** of heart with which it is blended. This area is comparatively flat and known as **cardiac plateau**. It extends more to the left side than the right.

One either side of cardiac plateau, right dome or cupola rises at a higher level than the left. **Diaphragmatic part of parietal pleura** separates superior surface of dome of diaphragm from the base of lung of the corresponding side.

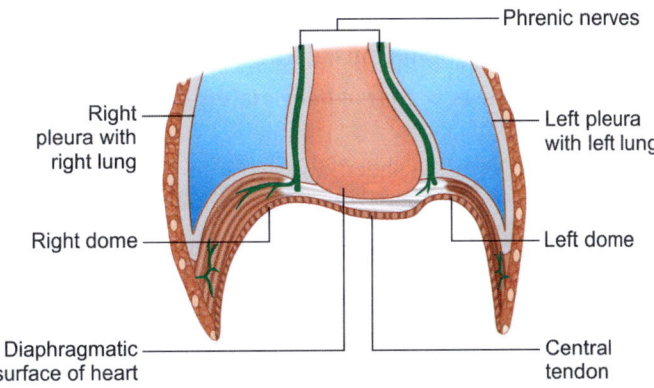

Fig. 28.3: Domes of the diaphragm on coronal section with its superior relations.

Inferior Surface

On the **right side**, inferior surface is more accurately adjusted with **right lobe of liver**. In addition, it is also related to **right kidney** and **right suprarenal gland**.

Inferior surface of diaphragm, on the **left side**, is related to **left lobe of liver, fundus of stomach, spleen, left kidney** and **left suprarenal gland**.

Apertures (Openings) of the Diaphragm

There are number of structures which pass from thorax to abdomen or in reverse direction through some apertures or openings. Aorta, esophagus and inferior vena cava pass through the major openings. Many other structures pass through smaller or minor openings.

Major Openings (Figs. 28.1 and 28.2)

Aortic opening

Aortic opening is the lowest and most posterior among the three major openings. It is situated at the level of lower border of body of **twelfth thoracic vertebra**. The aortic opening is bounded anteriorly by fibrotendinous median arcuate ligament which is formed by convergence of medial fibers of two crura of the diaphragm. Its posterior boundary is osseous as formed by lower border of body of twelfth thoracic vertebra. Structures passing through the opening are descending thoracic aorta continued as abdominal aorta, cisterna chyli continued upwards as thoracic duct and azygos vein.

Esophageal opening

Esophageal opening is located at the level of lower border of body of **tenth thoracic vertebra**. It is above, in front and to the left side of aortic opening in the left dome of the diaphragm. The opening is elliptical in outline with its long axis disposed obliquely. Esophageal orifice is formed by fibers of right crus of diaphragm which encircles or loops around the lower end of esophagus. The opening transmits **esophagus, gastric nerves, esophageal branches/tributaries of left gastric vessels** with some lymph vessels.

Phrenoesophageal ligament: *A band of elastic fibers* extends from undersurface of diaphragm to submucosal layer of esophagus penetrating its muscular wall. It is called phrenoesophageal ligament. It connects the esophagus to the diaphragm. The ligament possesses following functions.
- It permits some freedom of movement of esophagus during swallowing and respiration.
- It prevents upward displacement of esophagus during rise of intra-abdominal pressure.

Vena caval opening

Vena caval opening is the highest in level among three major openings of diaphragm. It is located at the level of lower border of body **eighth thoracic vertebra**. It is quadrilateral in outline and lies at the junction of central and right folia of central tendon of the diaphragm. So the margin of the opening is aponeurotic. It transmits **inferior vena cava** with some branches of **right phrenic nerve**. Margin of the vena caval opening is adherent to the outer adventitial coat of the venous trunk.

Minor Openings

Most of the minor openings are either gaps between adjacent slips of origin of the diaphragm or gaps between its peripheral outline and body wall. They are as follows:
- **Foramen of Morgagni**: This is a small gap between the **xiphoid** and **seventh costal slips** of origin of the diaphragm. This is triangular in outline and normally bridged by a layer of areolar tissue. Structures passing through it are **superior epigastric vessels** and some *lymph vessels* from abdominal wall and superior surface of liver. When the gap in this foramen is prominent, it is called **space of Larrey**. This deficiency may predispose occurrence of **retrosternal hernia**.
- **Lateral to foramen of Morgagni**, there is a gap between **seventh** and **eighth costal slips** of origin of the diaphragm. It transmits the **musculophrenic vessels**.
- **Gaps between adjacent remaining costal slips** of origin of diaphragm transmit corresponding **intercostal vessels and nerves**.
- **Gap behind lateral arcuate ligament** transmits **subcostal vessels** *and* **nerves**
- **Gap behind medial arcuate ligament** transmits **sympathetic trunk** and **lowest (least) splanchnic nerve.**
- **Small apertures of the crus** of the diaphragm transmit **greater** *and* **lesser splanchnic nerves**.
- **Foramen of Bochdalek** is a rare congenital deficiency of **posterolateral aspect** of the diaphragm which results due to failure of fusion between two embryological components of the diaphragm. When present, it may lead to herniation of abdominal content into thoracic cavity.
- **Multiple small apertures in central tendon** give passage to number of **minute veins**.

Vascular Supply of the Diaphragm

Arteries

The arteries of the diaphragm form a *branching and anastomosing pattern* both on superior and inferior surfaces.

Arteries of superior surface

- *Pericardiophrenic* and *musculophrenic arteries* which are branches of internal thoracic artery.
- *Superior phrenic arteries*: These are multiple branches from descending thoracic aorta.

Arteries of inferior surface

Inferior phrenic arteries: These are lateral set of branches arising from abdominal aorta. These arteries may arise from the celiac trunk.

Veins

Veins draining from superior surface

- *Pericardiophrenic and musculophrenic veins* which drain into internal thoracic vein.
- *Superior phrenic vein* is present on the right side and drains into inferior vena cava close to its termination.

- *Posterior phrenic veins* are multiple veins draining from posterosuperior part of the diaphragm and open into the azygos and hemiazygos vein.

Veins draining from inferior surface

Inferior phrenic veins are bilateral. Right inferior phrenic vein drains into inferior vena cava. Left-sided vein drains into the left suprarenal vein. Left vein is occasionally doubled. In such case, second one drains into inferior vena cava.

LYMPHATIC DRAINAGE

Lymph vessels draining the diaphragm form plexuses on both abdominal and thoracic surfaces. Lymphatic plexus is dense on abdominal surface which facilitates absorption of peritoneal fluid and other substances (drugs) injected through intraperitoneal route.

Primarily, lymph vessels from the plexus of inferior (abdominal) surface drain into **diaphragmatic, phrenic** and **superior lumbar lymph nodes**. As supposed to drain in centrepetal direction, lymph vessels from these abdominal lymph nodes, via the plexuses on thoracic surface drain into **anterior and posterior diaphragmatic lymph nodes**. Finally lymph vessels from these nodes terminate in **parasternal** and **posterior mediastinal lymph nodes**.

Innervation

The diaphragm receives its nerve supply from following two sources.
1. Phrenic nerve
2. Lower five intercostal nerves and subcostal nerve.

Phrenic Nerve

It arises in the neck, the original site of development of diaphragm. The nerve arises by union of fibers from roots of 3rd, 4th and 5th cervical nerves. But main contribution comes from 4th cervical nerve. Phrenic nerve, being the mixed nerve is the only motor nerve for the diaphragm and its sensory component caries sensory fibers from peripheral part of the diaphragm. While reaching the superior surface of diaphragm the phrenic nerve divides into sternal, anterolateral and posterior branches. Sensory fibers of phrenic nerve supply the central part of the diaphragm.

Lower Five Intercostal Nerves and Subcostal Nerve

These nerves supply sensory fibers for peripheral part of the diaphragm.

Referred Pain

In case of irritation of sensory fibers of phrenic nerve supplying the diaphragm, diaphragmatic pain is referred at the tip of the shoulder. It occurs when there is inflammation of diaphragmatic pleura due to lung/pleural diseases, or inflammation of diaphragmatic peritoneum due to disease of upper abdominal viscera, especially the gallbladder.

Variations in Position of Diaphragm

Height of diaphragm varies in level according to different position of body as follows.
- **In supine position**, abdominal viscera push the diaphragm superiorly, so it lies at a higher level. The height of the diaphragm is also raised during the phase of expiration due to elastic recoil of lung tissue.

- **In sitting position**, muscles of anterior abdominal wall are relaxed, capacity of abdominal cavity is increased. So height of the diaphragm is pushed down. It facilitates inhalation of air during inspiration in patients suffering from dyspnea.
- **But in standing position**, muscles of anterior abdominal wall contract which leads to rise of intra-abdominal pressure. Height of the diaphragm is raised upwards.
- **In right or left lateral position** on bed, hemidiaphragm of the corresponding side is raised at a higher level because of greater push of viscera on that side.
- **In Trendelenburg position**, which is the supine position of body with head end lowered down, required in some radiological or clinical investigations, the diaphragm is raised at its **highest level**.

Action of Diaphragm

Contraction of diaphragm in different physiological activities is known as **'descent of diaphragm'**. But during contraction, peripheral attachment of *diaphragm (origin) in ribs and cartilages remain fixed, the domes of the diaphragm only descend.*

So, the domes with the central tendon becomes flattened. It pushes the abdominal viscera downwards and increases the volume of thoracic cavity decreasing the intrathoracic pressure. **It results in intake of air in tracheobronchial tree in phase of inspiration**.

Compression of abdominal viscera squeezes venous blood from the organs more centrally. **It helps in venous return**, as more amount of blood is forced superiorly through inferior vena cava to the heart. The same factor also **facilitates return of lymph** through the thoracic duct.

The diaphragm is the **muscle of various expulsive acts**. During micturition, defecation and parturition, and also in case sneezing, coughing, vomiting, laughing, the act is preceded by deep inspiration. This brings out following two changes.
1. Deep inspiration leads to contraction and fixation of diaphragm.
2. Closure of glottis and larynx with a closed volume of inspired air further fixes the diaphragm which leads to rise of intraabdominal pressure.

The diaphragm **assists in weight lifting**. During this act, a person takes a deep breath and holds it which causes fixation of diaphragm. Raised intraabdominal pressure results in contraction of anterior abdominal wall muscles which prevents flexion of vertebral column. This helps postvertebral muscles in lifting of heavy weight.

Clinical Anatomy

Paralysis of Diaphragm

A single dome of the diaphragm may be paralyzed with eventual atrophy due to injury causing crushing or sectioning of the phrenic nerve in the neck. It causes paralysis of corresponding half of diaphragm except in persons who have accessory phrenic nerve. Radiological investigation confirms *permanent elevation of hemidiaphragm* with paradoxical movement. In this case, during inspiration, instead of descending, affected hemidiaphragm is forced upwards by increased intra-abdominal pressure which is the effect of marked descent of opposite unparalyzed hemidiaphragm.

Referred Pain from the Diaphragm

Sensory innervations from the diaphragm except the peripheral marginal part comes from sensory fibers of phrenic nerve which is formed by fibers of ventral rami of C3, C4 and C5 nerves. Somatic nerve fibers from same spinal cord segments supply skin over the tip of shoulder. So, in case of any disease causing irritation to diaphragmatic pleura or diaphragmatic peritoneum, irritation of sensory fibers of phrenic nerve causes perception of referred pain at the tip of shoulder.

Hiccups

Hiccups (hiccoughs) are involuntary, repeated, spasmodic contractions of diaphragm. It causes sudden inhalations which are rapidly interrupted by spasmodic closure of rima glottidis of larynx. It regulates the inflow of air and produces a characteristic sound. Spasmodic contractions of the diaphragm is due to irritation of fibers of phrenic nerve due to different local or central causes.

Diaphragmatic Herniae

Congenital diaphragmatic hernia (posterolateral hernia)

Posterolateral hernia is one of the very rare varieties of congenital diaphragmatic hernia which occurs as *1 in 1,200 births.* It results in herniation of abdominal contents into thoracic cavity. It is due to the defect or deficiency in different embryological components for development of diaphragm.

Existing gap leads to:
- Continuation of pleuroperitoneal canal
- Free communication between thoracic and abdominal cavities.

The deficiency through which posterolateral hernia takes place is known as **foramen of Bochdalek.**

Effect

It is usually an unilateral defect and common in left side due to early closure of right pleuroperitoneal membrane. *Herniation of abdominal content* leads to *inhibition of development of lung* which show hypoplasia.

Retrosternal hernia

In fully formed normal diaphragm, there is a small gap between xiphoidal and seventh costal slips of origin of the diaphragm. It is traversed by superior epigastric artery and usually bridged by a small amount of areolar tissue. The gap is known as **foramen of Morgagni.**

Rarely, there may be herniation through this retrosternal gap. It is less likely to be present in neonate. It later age, it may lead to retrosternal discomfort.

Retrosternal hernia is **commoner in right side** because pericardial attachment with central tendon of diaphragm is more extensive on the left side.

Herniation into thoracic cavity occurs between pericardial and pleural cavity. Sometimes pericardial sac may be invaginated by the hernia.

Congenital paraesophageal (rolling) hernia

Incidence of this type of hernia is because of a defect in the diaphragm, to the right and anterior to the esophagus at the site of esophageal hiatus.

Hernial sac of peritoneum is present into which *anterior wall of stomach rolls upwards* anteriorly and to the right of esophagus.

But the patient *does not suffer from regurgitation of stomach content* as because cardiac orifice so also cardiac notch of stomach are not altered from its normal position.

Cause

There is difference in opinion about the origin of the hernia as follows:
- Existence of a peritoneal recess in posterior mediastinum of thorax which facilitates upward rolling of stomach wall.
- Loss of clasping action of fibers of esophageal hiatus formed by right crus of the diaphragm.

Effect

It is a rare variety of hernia, which, if occurs, may cause compressive effect by the herniated mass on esophagus against vertebral column.

Acquired diaphragmatic hernia (sliding hernia)

It is the **most common variety of internal hernia** which occurs in middle aged persons due to weakness and/or deficiency of musculature of esophageal hiatus.

It is called **sliding hernia** because the cardiac end and part of fundus of stomach slides upwards. Particularly, it occurs in lying down position and forward and downward bending position of the body.

Effect

The patient suffers from regurgitation of stomach content because:
- Position of cardiac end and cardiac notch of stomach is displaced upwards.
- Loss of clasping action of fibers of right crus forming esophageal hiatus of the diaphragm.

Short notes: Lateral and medial lumbocostal arches; Crus of diaphragm

Short answers: Major and minor openings of the diaphragm; Actions of diaphragm; Anatomical concept of the diaphragmatic hernia

Chapter 29

Kidney and Suprarenal Gland

LA 29.1 Describe the kidney under following headings:
Surface features; Anatomical position and side determination (only for viva voce and practical); Relations; Coverings; Gross macroscopic structure; Arterial supply with vascular segments; Venous drainage and lymphatics; Nerve supply; Clinical anatomy.

KIDNEY

Introduction

- Kidneys are a pair of excretory organ placed in posterior abdominal wall. This organ is concerned with *excretion of waste product* of metabolism and *removal of excess amount of salts and water* from the blood in the form of urine.
- In living body kidneys are smooth, glistening and reddish brown in appearance.
- *Synonyms* of kidney are **renes** and **nephros.**
- Kidneys are oval in appearance with concavo-convex outline. Its long axis is vertical. Convex margin is lateral and medial margin is concave in the middle presenting the **hilum**.

Situation (Fig. 29.1)

Kidneys are situated:
- In posterior abdominal wall
- Behind parietal peritoneum
- Mostly in the lumbar region, on either side of the vertebral column, with extension into epigastric, umbilical and respective hypochondriac regions
- With long axis directed downwards and laterally along the long axis of psoas major muscle.

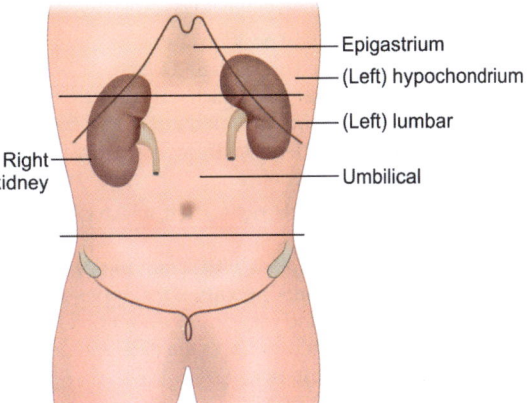

Fig. 29.1: Position of kidney in relation to areas of abdomen.

Parameters

Average weight of kidney is 150 g
Dimensions:
- Length   =   12 cm
- Breadth   =   6 cm
- Thickness =   3 cm

Surface Features (Figs. 29.2A and B)

Kidneys present 2 poles, 2 surfaces and 2 margins.

Anterior surface, very often, presents irregularity which explains that kidney is developmentally lobulated in origin.

Lateral margin is convex. But medial margin is concavo-convex with concavity or notching in the middle called hilum. Hilum is the gateway transmitting three major structures, renal vein, renal artery and pelvis of the ureter which is the proximal dilated end of ureter commencing from kidney.

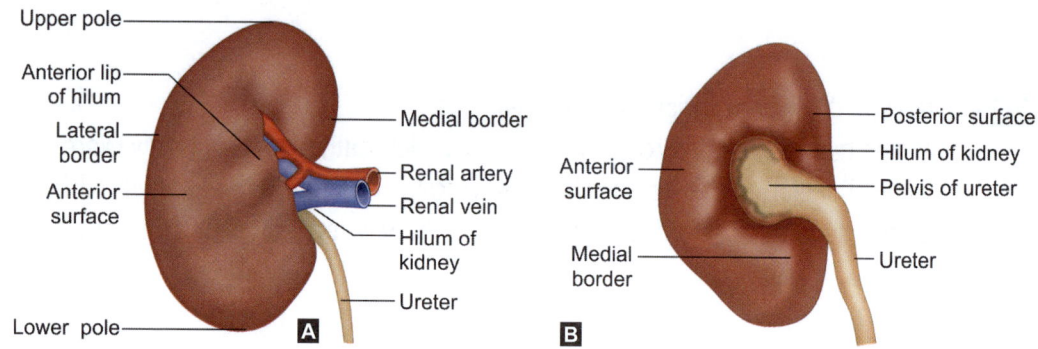

Figs. 29.2A and B: Surface features of right kidney. (A) Anterior view; (B) Medial view (renal vessels removed).

Anatomical Position and Side Determination

If single kidney is supplied with no structures at the hilum:
- **Differentiation of upper and lower pole**: Distance between upper pole and hilum is more than the distance of lower pole from hilum
- **Difference between lateral and medial border**: Hilum of the kidney bounded by anterior and posterior lips is present in the middle of medial border.
- **Difference between anterior and posterior surface:** From the anterior surface, hilum is visible more clearly because anterior lip of hilum is less projected medially than the posterior lip.

So, points for anatomical position and side determination are as follows:
- Upper pole, directed upwards and *slightly medially*, is known by its more distance from the hilum, in comparison to lower pole which is therefore directed downwards and *slightly laterally*.
- Hilum of the kidney, at the middle of medial border is directed medially.
- Anterior surface is identified by more clear visibility of hilum from this surface, as anterior lip of hilum is less projected than posterior.

Finally side of the hand, right or left, which is closer to the convex lateral border will determine the side of the organ.

If single kidney is supplied with structures at the hilum:
- In addition to the above points, if the upper end of the ureter is allowed to hang freely, for normal kink of the ureter, it will be found very close to lower pole.
- Anterior and posterior surfaces are differentiated by relationship of structure at the hilum, which are as follows from anterior to posterior.
  - Renal vein
  - Renal artery
  - Pelvis of ureter

If both the kidneys are supplied with renal vessels connected to segments of abdominal aorta and inferior vena cava:

In addition to the above points, kidneys of right and left side will be differentiated by inter-relationship of abdominal aorta and inferior vena cava as follows:
- Abdominal aorta is towards the left kidney, so right renal artery is longer than the left.
- Inferior vena cava is towards the right kidney, so left renal vein is longer than right.

Vertebral Level of Kidney
- Roughly, kidneys are situated at the level of bodies of L_1 to L_3 vertebrae.
- Due to pressure exerted by larger right lobe of liver, right kidney is at a slight lower level. **Transpyloric plane** cuts the **upper end of right hilum** and **lower end of left hilum**.

Relations of Kidney

Posterior Relations

Posterior relations of both the kidneys are common, as the posterior surfaces are in contact with the structures of posterior abdominal wall on either side of midline. These structures are muscles, vessels, nerves and fascia **(Fig. 29.3)**.

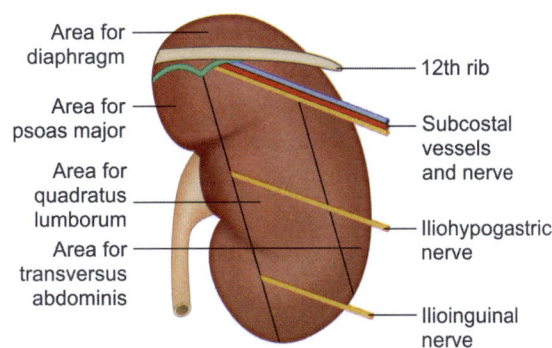

Fig. 29.3: Posterior relations of kidney (right).

Muscles:
- Diaphragm—in upper part
- Psoas major
- Quadratus lumborum
- Transversus abdominis—from medial to lateral.

Vessels and nerves:

From above downwards:
- Subcostal vein, subcostal artery and subcostal nerve
- Iliohypogastric nerve
- Ilioinguinal nerve.

Fascia:

Psoas fascia medially and anterior layer of lumbar fascia laterally intervene between posterior surface of kidney and muscles with neurovascular bundles.

Anterior Relations

Anterior relations of both the kidneys are different. If posterior surface of the organ is called **parietal surface**, anterior surface can be called **visceral surface** as it is related to different viscera as clarified in **Figure 29.4.**

Right Kidney (Fig. 29.4)
- Right suprarenal gland—nonperitoneal
- Second part of duodenum—nonperitoneal
- Right lobe of liver—peritoneal—separated by *hepatorenal pouch of Morison*
- Jejunum—peritoneal
- Right colic flexure—non-peritoneal.

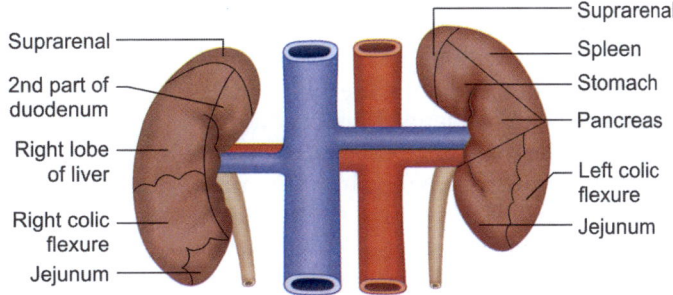

Fig. 29.4: Anterior relations of both kidneys.

Left Kidney (Fig. 29.4)

- Left suprarenal gland—nonperitoneal
- Stomach—peritoneal (*lesser sac*)
- Spleen—peritoneal
- Body of pancreas—nonperitoneal
- Jejunum—peritoneal
- Right colic flexure—nonperitoneal.

Coverings of Kidney (Figs. 29.5 and 29.6)

The kidney is invested by four layers of coverings of different types of connective tissue. From inside outwards the coverings are as follows:

1. **Capsule (fibrous capsule):** This is a thin layer of delicate *collagen fibers* with some *elastic fibers*. In healthy kidney, it can be stripped off the surface of kidney. In renal diseases, it becomes adherent. The capsule, covering all around enters the hilum to line the wall of the space of hilum called **renal sinus**.

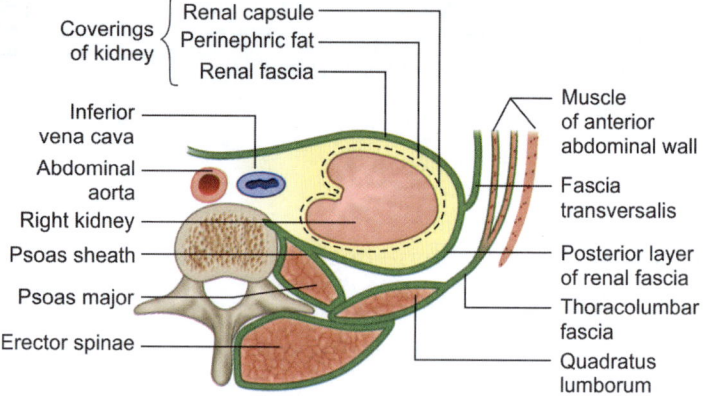

Fig. 29.5: Coverings of kidney.

2. **Perinephric fat (fatty capsule):** It is a *thin layer of fat* which covers the capsule all around, prominent at the margins and fills up the space of renal sinus.
   Perinephric fat plays an important role to retain the kidney in position. In case of severe loss of weight due to wasting disease, loss of perinephric fat will cause **nephroptosis** or *'floating kidney'.*

3. **Renal fascia (fascial capsule):** It is also known as **fascia of Gerota**.
   Renal fascia is the condensation of *fibroareolar tissue* around perinephric fat and thus prevents extension of perinephric abscess outside the kidney.
   At upper pole of kidney, the fascia forms common sleeve for suprarenal gland along with kidney. But a septum horizontally separates the two organs in two compartments. Moreover at the upper pole (end) of suprarenal, the fascia covering the suprarenal gland, fuses with diaphragmatic fascia. That is why during nephrectomy operation, the suprarenal gland remains well secured in position and it has no chance of displacement or accidental removal with the kidney.

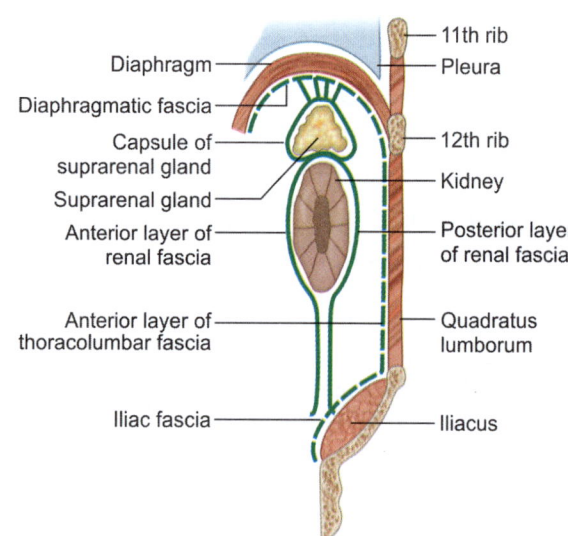

Fig. 29.6: Vertical disposition of renal fascia (sagittal section).

Below, anterior and posterior layers of renal fascia remain separate beyond lower pole of the kidney and blend with iliac fascia. In case of nephroptosis, kidney may drop down through this plane, but may be prevented by support of renal vessels from above. But there is chance of kinking of ureter leading to obstruction in urinary flow.

Medially, anterior layer of fascia blends with adventitia coat of renal vessels with abdominal aorta and inferior vena cava to become continuous with the renal fascia of opposite side. Posterior layer blends with psoas fascia.

Laterally, beyond margin of kidney, renal fascia becomes continuous with fascia transversalis.

4. **Paranephric fat:** It is a quantity of *extraperitoneal (retroperitoneal) fat* mainly on posterolateral aspect of lower part of kidney which acts as a packing material for support of kidney.

   True ad false capsule of kidney: *Original fibrous capsule* inside perinephric fat and fascial capsule outside (*renal fascia of Gerota*) are often termed as true and false capsule of kidney respectively.

Gross Macroscopic Structure of Kidney (Fig. 29.7)

Gross structure of kidney is ideally visible in naked eye through its coronal section. Coronal section primarily divides interior of kidney into three parts, **outer cortex, inner medulla** and space at the hilum called **renal sinus**.

In coronal section medulla presents about 10 pale triangular structures with their apices directed towards renal sinus. These are called **renal pyramids**. On the apex of each pyramid 2–3 openings are found called **renal papillae**.

Outer cortex is reddish brown in color and is divided into outer circumferential **cortical arches** and a part intervening between adjacent pyramids called **renal columns**.

Excretory units of kidney merges with conducting part which developmentally come from two sources. Through the renal papillae of pyramids open final order duct of structural unit of kidney called **duct of Bellini**. These ducts open in 7 to 13 small cup shaped structures called **minor calyces** (Kalyx means flower cup). These in turn open in 2–3 **major calyces** *(sing-calyx)* which unite at renal sinus to form upper proximal funnel-shaped **pelvis of ureter**.

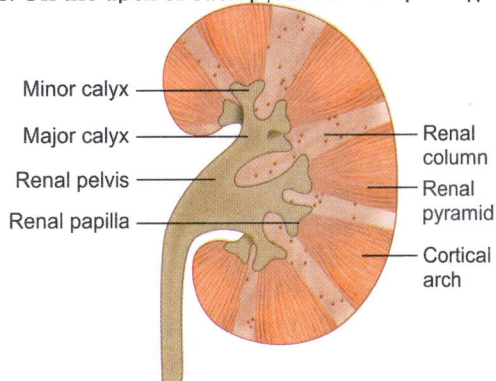

Fig. 29.7: Macroscopic features of kidney in coronal section.

(For integrated knowledge, a reader is advised to read a standard histology book with easier presentation for microscopic structures)

Arterial Supply and Vascular Segments of Kidney

Kidneys are supplied by renal arteries of corresponding side. Renal arteries arise at right angle as direct branch from abdominal aorta and they present wide caliber. For this reason, rate of blood flow through renal arteries is 1 liter per minute.

Usually for one kidney there is single renal artery which enters through the hilum. The artery divides into branches to supply five separate components of kidney which are called **vascular segments** named as follows **(Figs. 29.8A to C)**.

1. Apical
2. Upper ⎫
3. Middle ⎬ Anterior
4. Lower ⎭
5. Posterior

Renal artery initially divides into **anterior** and **posterior divisions**. Posterior division dividing into further branches supply posterior segment. Anterior division initially divides into upper and lower branches. **Upper branch** further subdivides to supply **apical** *and* **upper segments**. Middle and lower segments are supplied by divisions of **lower branch**.

Arteries of adjacent segments do not possess collateral circulation.

Accessory (aberrant) renal artery: This is an additional renal artery arising from abdominal aorta. Usually it arises from a lower level and enters the kidney close to lower pole. The artery may enter the kidney through hilum or at a higher level. Existence of accessory renal artery explains lobulated origin of kidney and it represents one of the multiple fetal lateral splanchnic arteries helping in ascent of kidney.

Accessory renal artery is not accompanied by corresponding vein.

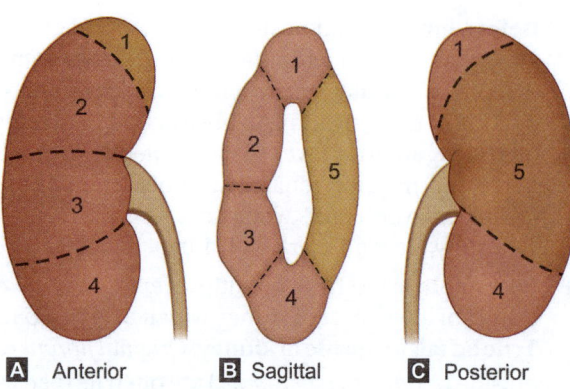

Figs. 29.8A to C: Vascular segments of (right) kidney. (1) Apical; (2) Upper; (3) Middle; (4) Lower; (5) Posterior.

Ramification of Segmental Arteries (Fig. 29.9)

Segmental arteries, being the example of end arteries, divide into **lobar arteries**. A lobar artery, reaching the level of apex of pyramid, divides into **interlobar arteries** which pass peripherally between adjacent pyramids. Interlobar artery, reaching beyond the level of base of pyramid, bifurcate in an arched fashion which run along opposite direction through the cortical arch, over the base of pyramid. These are called **arcuate arteries**. Branches from arcuate artery radiate towards the surface of cortex. These are called **interlobular arteries**. **Arterioles** from interlobular arteries extend to the **glomerulus**, which are tuft of capillaries. These glomeruli invaginate the blind end of microanatomical tubular unit of kidney called **renal tubule**.

Veins are formed in reverse order.

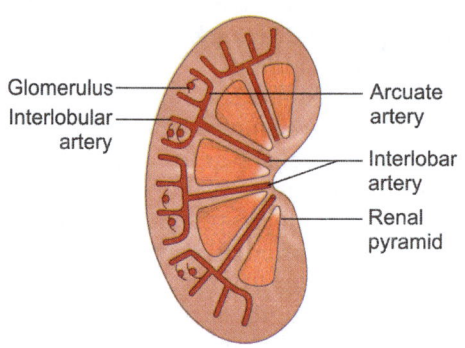

Fig. 29.9: Arterial ramification of kidney.

Venous Drainage

Veins draining the kidneys are renal veins. Tributaries of renal vein are **interlobar veins**. They unite at renal sinus. Renal vein formed at renal sinus comes out horizontally to drain into inferior vena cava.

Difference of the left renal vein from the right:
- As inferior vena cava into the right side of midline, the left renal vein is longer than the right
- Outside the hilum, the left renal vein receives following two important veins:
  a. Left suprarenal vein
  b. Left gonadal vein.

  On the right side, both these veins drain directly into the inferior vena cava.

Lymphatic Drainage

Lymph vessels from the kidney follow the course of veins. Final vessels run along the direction of renal vein, but drain into **para-aortic group** of lymph nodes lying adjacent to abdominal aorta at the level of origin of renal artery.

Nerve Supply

Kidney receives its innervations through sympathetic as well as parasympathetic components of autonomic nervous system. The nerves reach the organ through **renal plexus from celiac plexus**. **Parasympathetic** fibers come from the **vagus nerve**. **Sympathetic** fibers come from the centers situated at T_{12} **and** L_1 **segments** of spinal cord. The fibers come via thoracic (least) splanchnic nerve and lumbar (L_1) splanchnic nerves. **Vasomotor** fibers are carried via sympathetic. Pain fibers stimulated due to irritation of renal pelvis or calyces are carried through both sympathetic as well as parasympathetic. The pain known as **renal colic**. Due to transmission of pain fibers through sympathetic nerve (T_{12}, L_1), referred pain is felt from loin of the back (T_{12}) to groin with inguinal region (L_1). Nausea and vomiting in renal colic explains the vagal innervations.

Clinical Anatomy

Some Congenital Anomalies of Kidney
Anomalies in number
- In living individual, incidentally or accidentally absence of one kidney is detected. It is known as **agenesis**.
- In one side, there may be **duplication** of kidney. Additional one may remain separate or fused.

Anomalies in position
- Failure in complete ascent, may show the position of kidney anywhere **between pelvic and lumbar region**
- Both the kidneys may ascend in the **same side**, where they may lie one above the other or in the same level
- Both the kidneys may lie on reverse side due to faulty ascent, when both ureters may cross each other.

Anomalies in shape
- **Lobulated kidney**: In fetal life, the kidney develops by fusion of multiple lobulations. This lobulated condition may persist after birth.
- **Horse-shoe kidney**: Usually the lower poles (sometimes upper) of two kidneys may be fused through a connecting part known as isthmus lying in front of great vessels of abdomen. Isthmus is crossed in front by inferior mesenteric artery which prevents further ascent of horse-shoe kidney.
- **Pancake kidney**: Two kidneys may fuse to form one mass.

Failure of Communication between Excretory and Collecting Part

Metanephrogenic cap forms the excretory part and terminal end of ureteric bud forms the collecting part. If establishment of communication between these two fails, formation of multiple cysts inside the kidney occurs leading to a condition known as **congenital polycystic kidney**.

Stability and Mobility of Kidney

Perinephric fat and renal fascia helps to retain kidney in position, though in normal individual, kidney descends maximum up to 5 cm during full inspiration. In case of wasting diseases, when there is severe loss of weight, loss of perinephric and paranephric fat will cause **nephroptosis** or **'floating kidney'**.

Renal Pain

Pain fibers travelling through both sympathetic and parasympathetic get stimulated in case of irritation of renal pelvis or calyces by calculus (stone) or spasm of ureteric musculature. It is called **renal colic**. **Referred pain** is felt along the skin belts of loin (T_{12}) to groin (L_1) receiving same segmental somatic nerve supply.

Renal pain due to any disease ranging from pyelonephritis to renal calculus can be detected by the **tenderness of renal angle** between lateral border of erector spinae and twelfth rib.

Renal Injury

Kidney is well protected by muscles and fascia of posterior abdominal wall, and lower two ribs of thoracic cage. In spite of this fact range of renal injury varies from mild bruise on surface to complete laceration of the organ. As 25% of share of blood supply passes through kidney, patient may pass through the stage of shock due to severe blood loss in renal injury.

Common Renal Diseases

These are nephritis, pyelonephritis, renal stones (calculi), tuberculosis and sometimes renal tumors. Metastasis of malignant renal tumor occurs along the route of renal vein.

Protection of Costodiaphragmatic Recess in Renal Surgery

Lower end of costodiaphragmatic recess of pleura is related to upper part of posterior surface of kidney intervened by posterior slope of the diaphragm. The surgeons must take care of it while performing renal surgery.

Anatomical Concept of Kidney Transplantation

Following anatomical steps are adopted during transplantation of kidney:
- *Iliac fossa* is approached retroperitoneally through incision above the inguinal ligament
- Iliacus muscle is exposed
- Kidney to be transplanted is positioned on iliacus for vascular anastomosis
- **End to end anastomosis** is made between **renal artery** and **internal iliac artery**
- Renal vein is anastomosed with external iliac vein.

Following anastomosed with internal iliac artery, blood supply of the viscera on that side is still maintained through communication with branches of internal iliac artery of other side.

> *Special attention for theory*: Surface features with relations; Coverings; Vascular segments; Macroscopic structures; Clinical anatomy.

LA 29.2 Describe the Suprarenal gland under following headings:
Surface features; Anatomical position and side determination (only for Viva voce and practical); Relations; Coverings; Vascular supply; Lymphatics; Nerve supply; Basic structure; Clinical anatomy.

SUPRARENAL GLAND

Introduction

Suprarenal glands are a pair of endocrine glands situated in posterior abdominal wall in contact with anterosuperior aspect of upper pole of respective kidney. These are also known as *adrenal glands*.

The glands are asymmetrical in shape. **Right gland** is *triangular* or *pyramidal* in shape with the base related to anterosuperior aspect of upper pole of right kidney. **Left gland** is *semilunar (concavo-convex)* in shape with concave side related to medial aspect of left kidney extending from upper pole to hilum **(Fig. 29.10)**.

> **Anatomical Position and Side Determination**
> Single suprarenal vein for each of the glands *comes out through hilum*.
> Hilum with emerging suprarenal vein in on *anterior surface* of *right suprarenal gland*. The vein is directed *upwards and medially*. In case of left gland the hilum is *close to lower pole* and the vein is directed downwards and medially.
> So for anatomical position and side determination, following points are to be remembered **(Figs. 29.11A and B)**.
> - Right suprarenal gland is pyramidal with the base directed downwards. Its vein emerges from anterior aspect and directed upwards and medially.
> - Left suprarenal gland is semilunar in outline with concave side directed laterally. Its vein emerges from anterior surface close to lower pole and directed downwards and medially.

- **Size:** In average, dimensions of the gland are as follows:
  - Height = 5 cm
  - Breadth = 3 cm
  - Thickness = 1 cm
- **Weight:** 5 g

Inner medulla is one tenth of outer cortex of the gland.

Comparison with Size of the Kidney

- **At birth:** Suprarenal gland is **one-third (1/3)** of the size of kidney
- **In adult:** It is **one-thirtieth (1/30)** of the size of kidney.

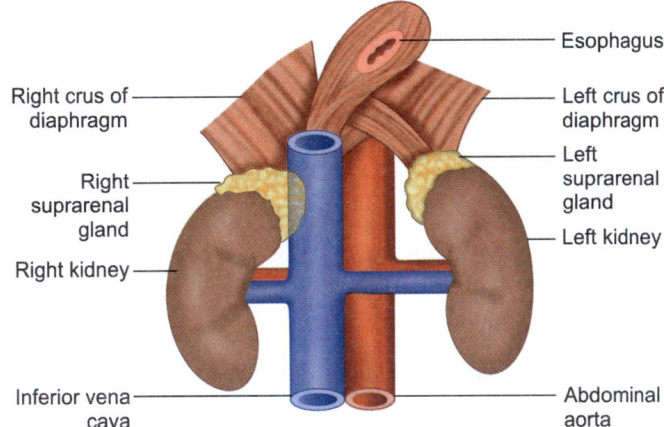

Fig. 29.10: Suprarenal glands with related structures.

Coverings of Suprarenal Gland (Fig. 29.12)

From within outwards:
- The suprarenal gland is covered by **layer of areolar tissue** all around
- **Continuation of renal fascia:** At the upper pole of the kidney, renal fascia splits to enclose suprarenal gland, which finally meet at the upper pole of gland to blend with diaphragmatic fascia.

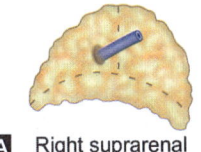
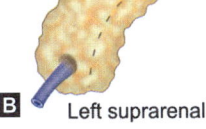

A Right suprarenal B Left suprarenal

Figs. 29.11A and B: Points for anatomical position of suprarenal gland. (A) Right suprarenal vein emeging from anterior surface is directed upwards and medially; (B) Left suprarenal vein emerging from anterior surface is directed downwards and medially.

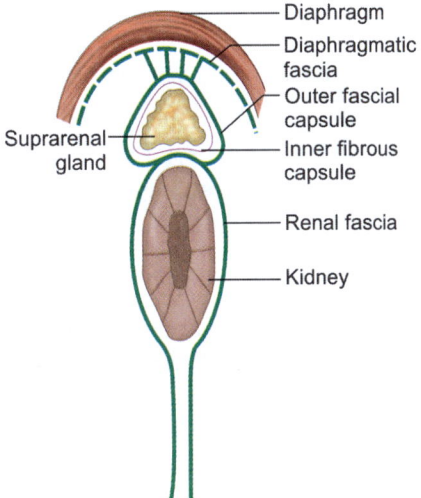

Fig. 29.12: Capsules (coverings) of suprarenal gland.

Surface Features (Comparison between Two Glands)

Anterior Surface (Fig. 29.13)

- **Right gland**: A vertical ridge divides anterior surface into lateral and medial half. Right suprarenal vein comes out through the hilum on this ridge, directed *upwards and medially*.
    - **Lateral half** = related to bare area of liver
    - **Medial half** = related to inferior vena cava
- **Left gland**: Anterior surface is divided into upper and lower half
    - **Upper half** = related to stomach
    - **Lower half** = related to pancreas

Left suprarenal vein, coming out through the hilum on anterior surface close to lower pole, is inclined *downwards and medially*.

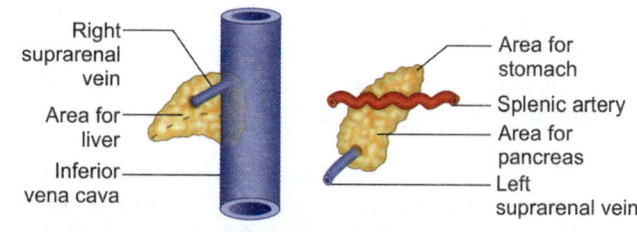

Fig. 29.13: Anterior relations of both suprarenal glands.

Posterior Surface (Fig. 29.14)

- **Right gland:**
    - **Lower part** = adjacent to base, is related to upper pole of right kidney
    - **Upper part** = related to right crus of diaphragm
- **Left gland:**
    - **Lateral part** = related to upper pole left kidney
    - **Medial part** = related to left crus of diaphragm.

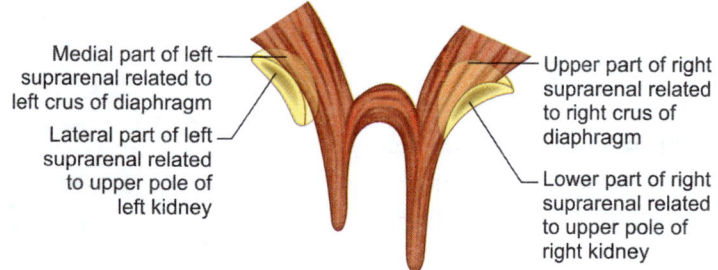

Fig. 29.14: Suprarenal glands seen from behind for posterior relations.

Peritoneal Relation of Suprarenal Gland

Suprarenal gland is a retroperitoneal organ. So **posterior surface** of both the glands are completely **nonperitoneal**. **Anterior surface** having different relations are **also nonperitoneal except upper half of left suprarenal gland**. This area, being related to stomach, is covered by peritoneum of lesser sac.

Arterial Supply (Fig. 29.15)

In fetal life suprarenal gland used to be proportionately larger. That is why it receives blood through multiple sources of arteries. These are superior, middle and inferior suprarenal arteries. These arteries, in embryonic period, represent the lateral splanchnic branches of abdominal aorta. Superior suprarenal artery used to give inferior phrenic branch, which, after birth, ultimately becomes direct branch of abdominal aorta. So, the superior suprarenal artery now becomes its branch. As kidney grows more and suprarenal undergoes to a stage of regression, finally renal artery, as a direct lateral branch of abdominal aorta, gives out inferior suprarenal artery.

All the suprarenal arteries enter the gland by piercing the anterior surface, but not through the hilum which transmits the single suprarenal vein.

Venous Drainage (Fig. 29.16)

Each suprarenal gland is drained by a single suprarenal vein which comes out through hilum. **Right vein** is *directed upwards and medially*, and drains into **inferior vena cava**. **Left vein** is *directed downwards and medially*, and drains into **left renal vein**.

Lymphatic Drainage

Lymph vessels from suprarenal gland, as usual, follow the course of its vein. The vessels drain into **para-aortic group** of lymph nodes which are retroperitoneal in posterior abdominal wall.

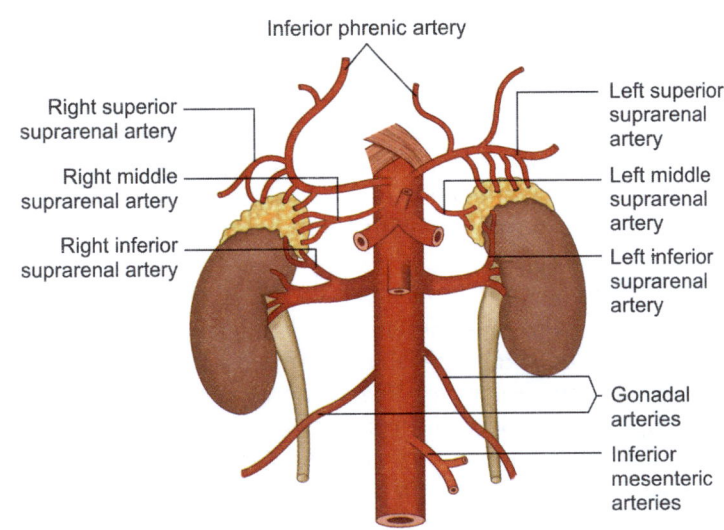

Fig. 29.15: Arterial supply of suprarenal gland.

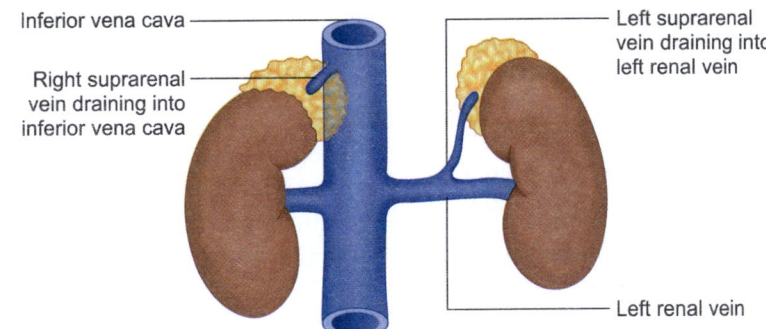

Fig. 29.16: Suprarenal veins.

Nerve Supply

Sympathetic vasomotor fibers for the gland are derived from greater and lesser splanchnic nerves. These fibers reach the gland **through celiac plexus**. These are **postganglionic fibers**.

In addition **preganglionic fibers** from the same source **enter the medulla** of the gland. The medulla is made up of cells belonging to chromaffin system. The cells behave as postganglionic neurons which receive preganglionic sympathetic fibers.

Basic Structure

Suprarenal gland is made up of larger *outer cortex* and *inner medulla* which is one tenth of cortex.

Cortex is developed from mesoderm of celomic epithelium. It is proportionately larger in fetal life being responsible for bigger size of the gland. **Suprarenal medulla** is developed from **neural crest cells**, so *ectodermal in origin*. Cells of medulla are as good as *postganglionic sympathetic neurons* and belong to *chromaffin system*.

Suprarenal cortex is made up of following three layers of cell groups from outside inwards.
1. **Zona glomerulosa**: Cells are present in cluster or clump. These cells liberate *mineralocorticoids* which *regulate water and electrolyte balance* of body.

2. **Zona fasciculata**: Cells are present in columns. These cells liberate *glucocorticoids* which maintain *carbohydrate balance* and *immune mechanism*.
3. **Zona reticularis**: Cells are present in the form of reticulum (network) and liberate sex hormones.

Suprarenal medulla is composed of cells which are **modified postganglionic sympathetic neurons**. These cells belong to the *chromaffin system* and are named **pheochromocytes**. Preganglionic sympathetic fibers end in these cells, stimulation of which release **epinephrine (adrenaline)** and **norepinephrine (noradrenaline)**.

Clinical Anatomy

- **Pheochromocytoma** is the tumor of suprarenal medulla. It is characterized by excessive secretion of adrenaline and noradrenaline. The disease is manifested by *hypertension, excessive sweating, palpitation* and *headache* with *pallor of skin*.
- **Hypoplasia** or **tuberculosis** of cortex causes insufficiency in secretion of cortical hormones. The clinical condition is known as **Addison's disease** which is characterized by *hypotension, muscular weakness, anemia* and *pigmentation of skin*. The disease is finally complicated by *circulatory and renal failure*.
- **Tumors of suprarenal cortex** are characterized by excessive secretion of cortical hormones. It is known as **Cushing's syndrome**.

> *Special attention for theory*: Relations with coverings; Vascular supply

SA 29.3 Write a brief note on chromaffin system.

CHROMAFFIN SYSTEM

Chromaffin system is made up of various groups of cells, all of which possess the common characteristics, that is the **affinity for staining with certain salts of chromic acid**. That is why these cells are called **chromaffin cells**.

These chromaffin cells *develop from neural crest cells*.
The cells secrete adrenaline and noradrenaline.

Types of Chromaffin Cells

1. **Suprarenal medulla:** These cells are incorporated inside the suprarenal cortex and receive preganglionic sympathetic nerve endings.
2. **Paraganglia:** In younger age these cells are present in the form of small rounded bodies of clusters of cells related to sympathetic ganglia. In adult they are microscopic in appearance.
3. **Para-aortic bodies**: These bilateral masses of chromaffin cells, 1 cm in size, are located in either side of abdominal aorta *at the level of origin of inferior mesenteric artery*. It gets atrophied by 14 years of life.
4. **Coccygeal body (glomus coccygeum):** It is a round body with 2 cm diameter situated in front of coccyx in close relation to terminal end of median sacral artery and the ganglion impar.
5. **Scattered chromaffin cells:** Small masses of chromaffin cells are found to be scattered in relation to *splanchnic nerves, autonomic plexus* and some organs like *heart, liver, kidney, ureter, prostate, spermatic cord* and *epididymis*.

Chapter 30

Pelvis

LA 30.1 Discuss the bony pelvis in reference to the following headings:
Anatomical position; False pelvis and true pelvis; Pelvic inlet; Pelvic outlet; Pelvic cavity; Pelvic parameters; Sex difference of pelvis; Types of female pelvis.
(For viva voce and practical examination)

BONY PELVIS

Orientation (Anatomical Position) of Bony Pelvis

At the outset, it is important for a student, to understand the exact orientation of the pelvis in relation to the position of trunk *in erect posture*.

The front of the **pubic symphysis** and the **anterior superior iliac spines** *of both sides* **should lie in same coronal plane** passing from side to side. Automatically, the pelvic surface of the sacrum will be directed downwards and forwards and, the pelvic surface of the symphysis pubis will face backwards and upwards.

FALSE PELVIS (FIG. 30.1)

False pelvis is so called because it is not truly the part of pelvis. Rather it lies in the lower part of abdominal cavity. It is bounded behind by the **lower lumbar vertebrae** and posterolaterally by the **iliac fossa** of hip bone and the **iliacus** muscle.

False pelvis supports the abdominal contents. After 3rd month of pregnancy, it supports the gravid uterus.

False pelvis is of less clinical significance.

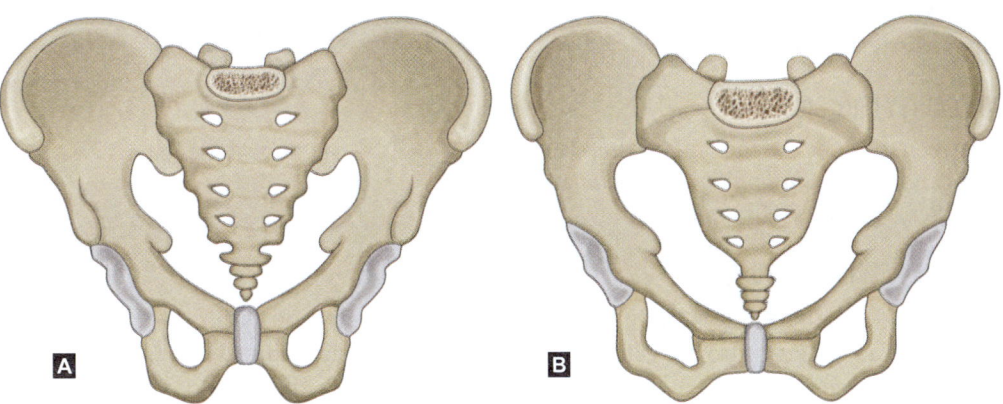

Figs. 30.1A and B: Pelvis: (A) Male pelvis; (B) Female pelvis.

TRUE PELVIS (FIG. 30.1)

True pelvis is the actual hollow of the basin. It presents superior and inferior apertures, called pelvic inlet and pelvic outlet respectively. Through the pelvic inlet, the pelvic cavity communicates above with the false pelvis of lower abdomen. Pelvic outlet presents following two basic characteristics.
1. It is bridged by a musculofibrous diaphragm (pelvic diaphragm), called pelvic floor, which slopes downwards and medially towards the midline from both sides.
2. In midline, it is traversed by the anorectal junction and the urethra behind and in front respectively. In addition, in females, the vagina traverses in between the two.

PELVIC INLET (PELVIC BRIM) (FIG. 30.1)

Pelvic inlet or pelvic brim is the line of demarcation between the false pelvis and true pelvis. The plane of the inlet is directed downwards and forwards making an angle of 60° with the horizontal plane.

Boundary of the pelvic brim is formed by the following on either side of midline.
- **Posteriorly**:
  - Sacral promontory—sacrum component
  - Ala of sacrum—sacrum component
- **Laterally**: Arcuate line of the ilium
- **Anteriorly**:
  - Pectineal line of the pubis
  - Pubic crest.

PELVIC OUTLET (FIG. 30.2)

Pelvic outlet is diamond or rhomboid shaped. It is bounded *from before backwards* as follows.
- **Anteriorly**: Inferior margin of pubic symphysis
- **Anterolaterally**: Conjoint rami of ischium and pubis.

The above two form together the pubic arch
- **Laterally**: Ischial tuberosity
- **Posterolaterally**: Sacrotuberous ligament
- **Posteriorly**: Coccyx.

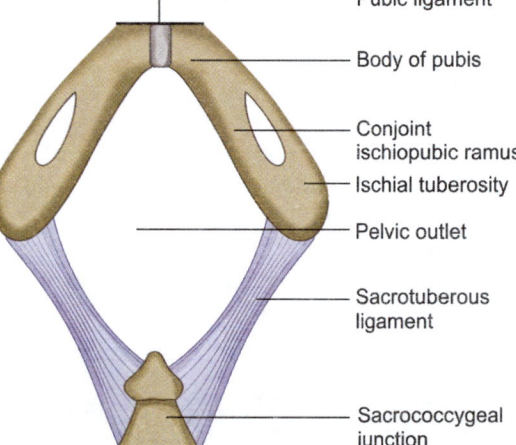

Fig. 30.2: Pelvic outlet.

PELVIC CAVITY (FIG. 30.3)

It is between the inlet and the outlet. It is a short curved canal with a *shallow anterior wall* and *deeper lateral and posterior walls*.

AXIS OF THE PELVIS (FIG. 30.3)

It is a curved imaginary line joining the central points of anteroposterior diameters of all the geometrical planes starting from the inlet up to the outlet. This line of the axis is clinically important because the curved course of the axis is taken by the fetal head as it descends through the pelvis during childbirth.

PELVIC PARAMETERS

Diagonal Conjugate (Fig. 30.3)

It is the distance between the midpoint of the sacral promontory and the lower border of *anterior surface* of pubic symphysis. It is normally about 5 inches (12–13 cm). If it is less in females, normal delivery of baby may be affected.

Interspinous Diameter

It is the distance between two ischial spines.

Pubic Arch

It is the angulation between two conjoint ischiopubic rami.

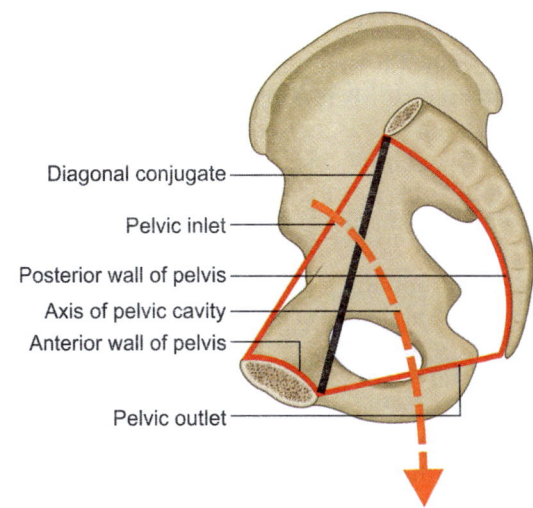

Fig. 30.3: Different pelvic lines.

SEX DIFFERENCES OF PELVIS

Bony Built

In females, the bones of pelvis with the head of femur are more slender and lighter. The articular surfaces and the acetabulum are smaller.

Pubic Arch (Subpubic Angle) (Fig. 30.4A)

In males, the angle is acute and pointed like a *Gothic arch*. In females, the angle is wide like a *Roman arch*.

Pelvic Brim (Pelvic Inlet) (Fig. 30.4B)

- In males, the outline of the brim is indented at the sacral promontory and the brim is widest towards the back (heart-shaped).
- In females, the brim is transversely oval and is widest in front.

Pelvic Outlet (Fig. 30.4C)

- In males, the rhomboid outlet is narrower or compressed from side to side.
- In females, the transverse measurement is wider.

Pelvic Cavity (Fig. 30.4D)

- In males, the pelvic cavity narrows down below, being *funnel-shaped*.
- In females, the cavity is more or less equally wide above and below and it is somewhat *barrel-shaped*.

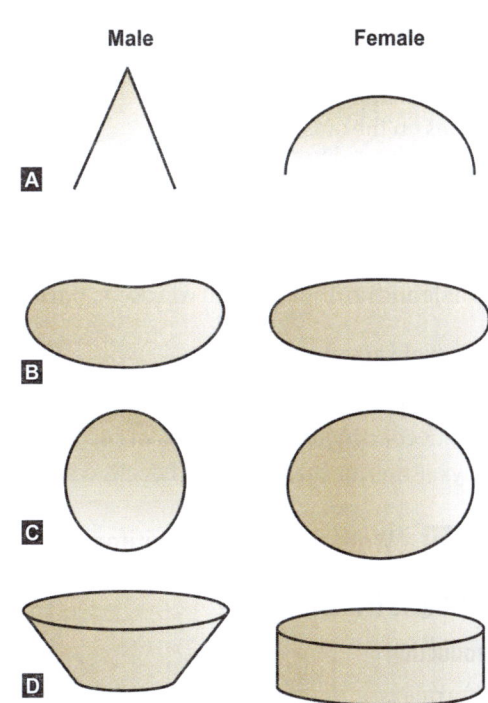

Figs. 30.4A to D: Sex difference of pelvis: (A) Pubic arch (subpubic angle); (B) Pelvic inlet; (C) Pelvic outlet; (D) Pelvic cavity.

TYPES OF FEMALE PELVIS (FIGS. 30.5A TO D)

(Caldwell and Moloy classification – 1933)

- **Gynecoid**: It is the typical female pelvis as described above **(Fig. 30.5A)**
- **Android**: It is the male type funnel-shaped pelvis **(Fig. 30.5B)**
- **Anthropoid**: It is long, narrow and oval shaped **(Fig. 30.5C)**
- **Platypelloid**: It is the rare variety. The pelvis is wide and flattened at the brim. The sacral promontory is pushed forwards **(Fig. 30.5D)**.

CLINICAL ANATOMY

Fracture of False Pelvis

Incidence of fracture of false pelvis is occasional due to direct trauma. Displacement of the upper part of ilium is very rare because of attachment of the iliacus muscle on the inside and the gluteal muscles on the outside.

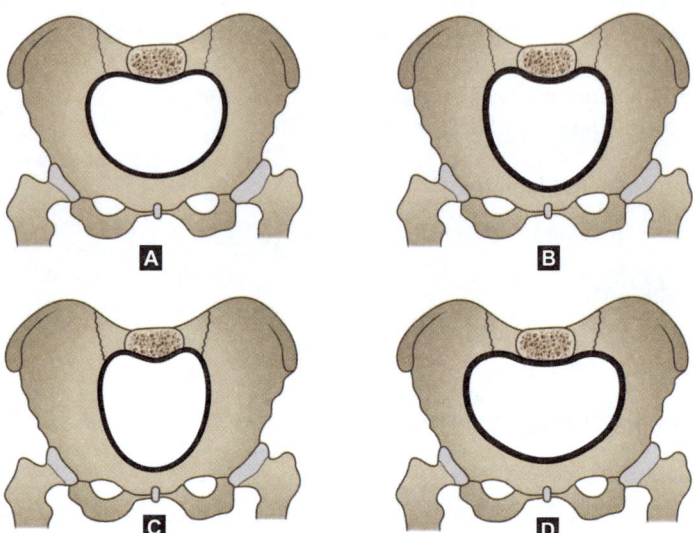

Figs. 30.5A to D: Types of female pelvis: (A) Gynecoid; (B) Android; (C) Anthropoid; (D) Platypelloid.

Fracture of True Pelvis

It breaks the ring of pelvis formed by pubic rami, ischium, acetabulum, ilium, sacrum joined by the strong ligaments of sacroiliac joint and symphysis joint. If the ring breaks at one point, the fracture will be stable and no displacement will occur. But the displacement will occur, if the ring breaks at two points.

Fracture of Sacrum and Coccyx

Fracture of lateral mass of sacrum may occur as a part of fracture of pelvis. Fracture of coccyx is rare. But **coccydynia**, dislocation of coccyx is common and is usually caused by direct trauma to the coccyx. Anterior surface of the coccyx can be palpated through per rectal examination.

SN 30.2 Write short notes on piriformis.

PIRIFORMIS (FIG. 30.6)

Introduction

Piriformis is a triangular muscle with broad origin end and narrower insertion end. It lies in front of posterior pelvic wall on either side of the midline.

Origin

Piriformis takes origin from the pelvic surface of **middle three pieces of sacrum** through three digitations. The digitations clasp the lateral aspect of the corresponding ventral sacral foramina.

Insertion

The fibers converge downwards and laterally and pass through the greater sciatic foramen to reach the gluteal region under cover of gluteus maximus. The muscle ends in a rounded tendon to be inserted into the **tip of greater trochanter of femur**.

Nerve Supply

Piriformis is supplied by ventral rami of **S_1 and S_2 nerves**.

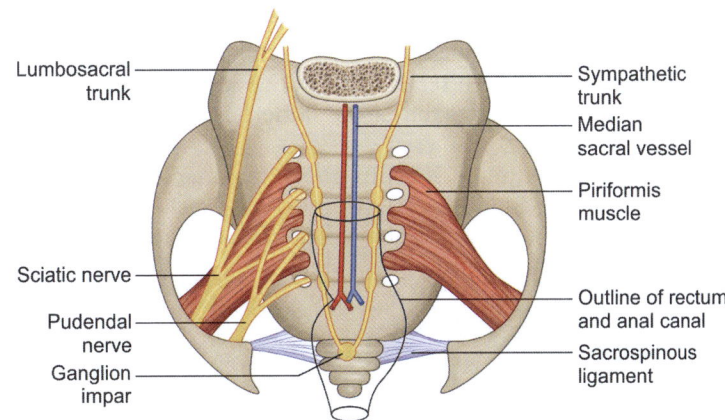

Fig. 30.6: Structures on posterior wall of pelvis.

Actions

- Piriformis is lateral rotator of hip joint in extended position of thigh. The same muscle acts a medial rotator when the thigh is flexed.
- Along with other short muscles around the hip, it stabilizes the hip joint.

SN 30.3 Write a short note on obturator internus.

OBTURATOR INTERNUS (FIG. 30.7)

Introduction

Obturator internus is a fan-shaped muscle which covers most of the lateral wall of the pelvis. Lower part of the muscle extends below the level of pelvic floor and forms the lateral wall of ischiorectal fossa.

Origin

The muscle shows following sources of origin:
- Pelvic surface of **obturator membrane**
- Pelvic surface of the margin of the **obturator foramen** except the region of obturator sulcus.
- **Pelvic surface of the ilium** in between the obturator foramen and the greater sciatic notch.

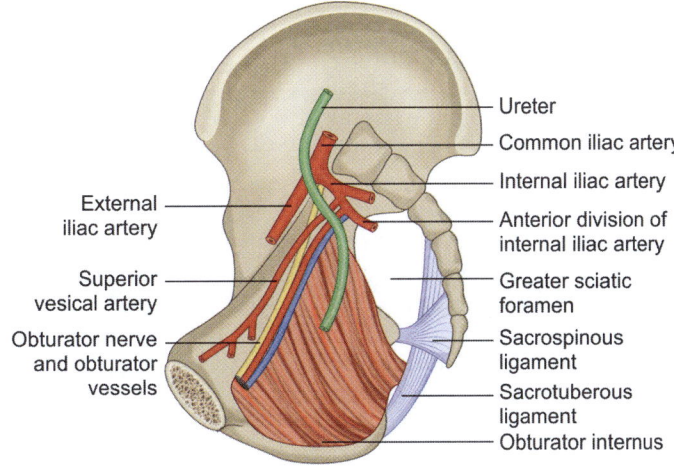

Fig. 30.7: Lateral wall of pelvis (right side).

Insertion

The muscle fibers converge backwards to form a tendon near the anterior margin of lesser sciatic foramen. The tendon makes sharply a lateral bend to leave the lesser pelvis through the lesser sciatic foramen and is inserted into the medial aspect of greater trochanter of femur.

Important Relations (Fig. 30.7)

Obturator internus is covered by a fascia called **obturator fascia**.

A thickened arched fascial band extends anteroposteriorly over the obturator fascia from pelvic surface of body of pubis to the ischial spine. It is called **arcus tendinous**. It gives origin to the levator ani of pelvic floor.

Part of the obturator internus above the attachment of pelvic floor is related to **obliterated umbilical artery** and **obturator nerve** and **vessels** from above downwards. Posterior part of the muscle is related to **internal iliac vessels** and **pelvic part of ureter**.

Part of the obturator internus below the pelvic floor forms **lateral wall of ischiorectal fossa** of perineum.

Nerve Supply

Obturator internus is supplied by the **nerve to obturator internus (L_5, S_1, S_2)** arising from the sacral plexus.

Actions

Obturator internus is **lateral rotator** of the hip joint **in extended position** of lower limb. The same muscle is **abductor** of hip **in flexed position** of thigh.

LA 30.4 **Describe the pelvic diaphragm under the following headings: Evolution; Composition; Attachment; Relations; Vascular and nerve supply; Actions; Clinical anatomy**

PELVIC DIAPHRAGM

Introduction

Pelvic diaphragm is a gutter-like musculotendinous shelf supporting from both the lateral walls of true pelvis towards the midline.

It forms the floor of pelvic cavity and thus separates the pelvic cavity from the perineum including ischiorectal fossa **(Fig. 30.8)**.

The diaphragm is formed by a pair of muscular sheet called **levator ani**.

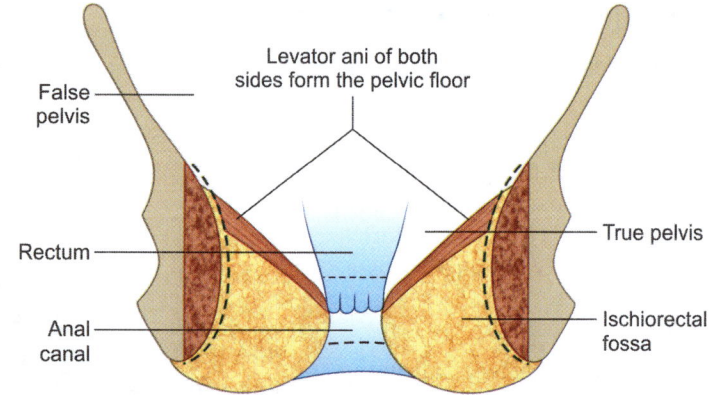

Fig. 30.8: Pelvis floor on coronal section.

Both the upper and lower surfaces of the muscular shelf are covered by **superior and inferior fasciae of pelvic diaphragm**.

Apart from the arched tendinous band over the fascia covering obturator internus on lateral wall of true pelvis, the pelvic diaphragm is also attached to the pelvic surfaces of body of pubis in front and ischial spine as well as the coccyx behind in such a manner, as if a funnel is suspended from these attachments.

Evolution

In case of quadrupedal animals, abdominopelvic viscera are mainly supported by their ventral body wall. Movements of their tail, supported by a number of caudal vertebrae, used to be controlled by following three muscles **(Fig. 30.9)**.

1. **Ischiococcygeus** : For dorsal flexion
2. **Iliococcygeus** : For lateral flexion
3. **Pubococcygeus** : For ventral flexion

Before the achievement of erect posture in primates, when the animals are habituated with sitting position, the following two changes take place.
1. **Changes in the caudal vertebrae**: Caudal part of vertebral column changes to be ventrally curved. The caudal vertebrae gets reduced in number which gives an indication for gradual loss of tail.
2. **Changes in three components of tail muscles**: Three flexor muscles of tail, gradually losing their separate identity, are approximated close to each other to form a composite muscle.

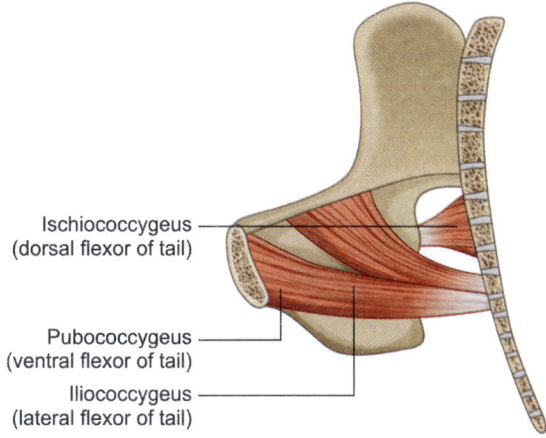

Fig. 30.9: Three flexor muscles of the tail of quadruped animals form morphological components of pelvic floor in bipedal human.

This composite muscle made up of ischiococcygeus, iliococcygeus and pubococcygeus will block the outlet of pelvis to form the pelvic floor. This composite muscle will be named as levator ani, as two muscles of both sides slopes downwards and medially towards the midline to hold the anorectal junction, along with urethra and, the vagina (in females).

Downward Sagging of Origin Levator Ani following Achievement of Erect Posture

With the achievement of erect posture, thrust of abdominopelvic viscera exerts downward pressure on pelvic floor formed by levator ani. This downward pressure pushed down the original origin of three components of levator ani from the level of pelvic brim to a curved line on the obturator fascia extending from pelvic surfaces of body of pubis to ischial spine. This curved line of thickened fascia on obturator internus is known as **arcus tendinous.**

Components of Levator Ani

Levator ani muscle is primarily divided into three morphological components attached to the three different components of hip bone forming pelvic wall. These are:
1. Ischiococcygeus
2. Iliococcygeus
3. Pubococcygeus.

Though these three components present three names, but they do not posses separate entity because:
- They are not distinguishable from one another
- In many cases, they perform jointly same physiological function.

Pubococcygeus muscle is further divided into different names as per their relations and attachments to different viscera. These are namely:
- Pubovesicalis
- Puboprostaticus (in male)
- Pubovaginalis (in female)
- Puborectalis and puboanalis.

These muscular components are also known together as **puboperinealis.**

Attachments of Levator Ani

Attachments of ischiococcygeus, iliococcygeus and pubococcygeus are as follows **(Fig. 30.10)**.

Ischiococcygeus

Ischiococcygeus forms posterosuperior part of levator ani and it is a **triangular musculotendinous sheet**.

By its apex the muscle takes origin from pelvic surface of tip of **ischial spine**. Its base is inserted into **lateral margin of coccyx** and **last piece of sacrum**.

Variations

- Ischiococcygeus is **partly muscular** and **partly tendinous**. Sometimes it is more tendinous than muscular
- This muscular part lies superior to the plane of sacrospinous ligament which is similarly triangular in shape
  Sacrospinous ligament is considered as **degenerated fibrotendinous part of ischiococcygeus muscle.**
- Sometimes ischiococcygeus is **absent**.

Iliococcygeus

This component of levator ani, connected to ilium of hip bone, takes **origin** from inner surface of **ischial spine** and **posterior half of arcus tendinous**.

Insertion of iliococcygeus shows typical characteristics as follows:
- Fibers are **inserted** to the **tip of coccyx** to **lower end of sacrum**
- Some fibers become fibrotendinous and show interlacement in the midline to form a strong band extending between tip of coccyx and back of anal canal. It is called **anococcygeal raphe**. Anococcygeal raphe lies on the superior aspect of a fibroelastic band containing some muscular fibers, called **anococcygeal ligament** which is coextensive with the raphe.

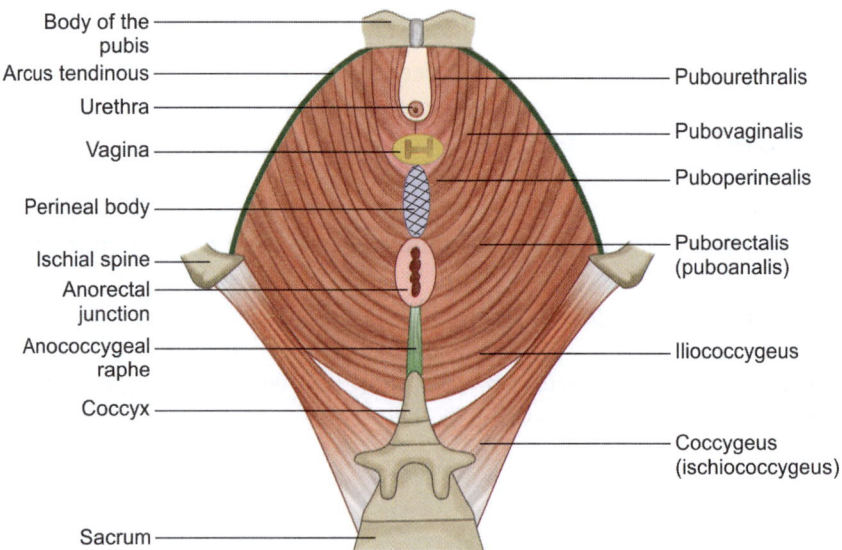

Fig. 30.10: Components of pelvic diaphragm.

Pubococcygeus

Pubococcygeus component of levator ani extends more horizontally backwards than downwards.

Most medial fibers of the muscle, from both sides, clasp the pelvic viscera which, from before backwards, are urethra, vagina (in females) and anorectal junction. For this reason, Pubococcygeus is also named as **pubovisceralis**.

Pubococcygeus takes **origin** from pelvic surface of body of **pubis** and **anterior part of arcus tendinous**.

Insertion of this component of levator ani shows visceral attachments and are subdivided into following parts.

- **Pubourethralis**: These are medialmost fibers of pubococcygeus. The fibers run backwards, below neck of urinary bladder on either side of upper end of urethra.
  Fibers of pubourethralis encircle this part of urethra, where it pierces the pelvic diaphragm. In case of males the fibers of pubourethralis blend on inferolateral aspect of prostate gland to form **puboprostaticus or levator prostatae**.
- **Pubovaginalis**: Behind the pubourethralis, fibers of pubococcygeus form a sling around posterior aspect of vagina to form pubovaginalis. Some of the fibers encircle to form **sphincter vaginae**.
- **Puboperinealis**: In both sexes, the muscle fibers of both sides show interlacement and blend at the **central tendon of perineum** or **perineal body**. The perineal body remains fixed in position in central midline position of perineum, as it is tied by various muscles of perineum from different sides along with the fibers of puboperinealis.
- **Puborectalis (puboanalis)**: Puborectalis part of pubococcygeus presents following components.
  - **Puborectal sling**: The fibers arising from body of pubis wind round anorectal junction from both sides. Pull of these muscle fibers forming anorectal sling maintains **anorectal flexure** or **perineal flexure** of anorectal junction.
  - **Puborectalis (puboanalis) conjoint tendon**: The fibers blend with longitudinal muscle coat fibers of rectum and descend as conjoint fibrotendinous band in the wall of anal canal from where the fibers form multiple septae to the perineum.

Relations of Pelvic Diaphragm (Fig. 30.11)
- **Superior surface**: *From below upwards,* superior surface is related to:
  - **Superior fascia of pelvic diaphragm (Fig. 30.11)**
  - Visceral layer of **pelvic fascia**

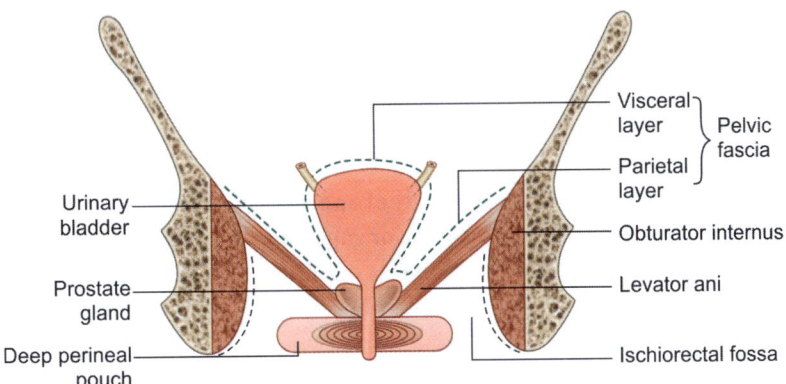

Fig. 30.11: Pelvic fascia with relation of pelvic diaphragm.

- Areolar tissue related to **urinary bladder, prostate, uterus, vagina** and **lower rectum**
- **Peritoneum**
- **Inferior surface**: This surface is covered by **inferior fascia of pelvic diaphragm** and it forms superomedial boundary of ischiorectal fossa.
- **Anteromedial border**: Anteromedial borders of levator ani of both sides are opposed to each other in the midline, but separated by a **narrow gap** for the passage of urethra, vagina and anal canal **(Fig. 30.10)**.
- **Posterolateral border**: This border of pelvic diaphragm is separated from coccyx by a narrow gap which is bridged by a layer of **areolar tissue.**

Vascular Supply of Pelvic Diaphragm

Pelvic diaphragm is supplied by all the arteries of the vicinity. But inferior gluteal, inferior vesical and pudendal arteries have main contributions.

Innervations of Pelvic Diaphragm

All the three components of levator ani are supplied by the nerve fibers arising from second, third and fourth sacral segments of spinal cord, but through different routes. Pubococcygeus is supplied by the fibers of *second and third sacral segments* via *pudendal nerve*. Iliococcygeus and ischiococcygeus components are supplied by direct branches of *sacral plexus,* fibers of which are derived from *third and fourth sacral segments.*

Actions of Pelvic Diaphragm

Evolution of pelvic diaphragm is an asset in bipedal animals including man, because with the achievement of erect posture, pelvic diaphragm prevents sagging down of abdominopelvic viscera. So fundamental action of pelvic diaphragm is **to support or hold the pelvic organs** in position.

Contraction of pelvic diaphragm **counteracts the raised intraabdominal pressure** which exerts a downward thrust. This function is evident during various physiological conditions like coughing, sneezing, laughing or in case of weight lifting.

Pelvic diaphragm can be considered as a muscle which **indirectly facilitates inspiratory phase of quiet breathing**. During inspiration, central tendon of thoracoabdominal diaphragm descends due to contraction of peripheral muscular slips. For this reason, intraabdominal pressure is raised which is adjusted by tone of pelvic diaphragm.

Pubococcygeus muscle of pelvic diaphragm acts as **compressor of the pelvic organs** traversing through, namely urethra, vagina and anal canal. Puborectalis part of this muscle, through the formation of conjoint puborectalis fascial band, assists external anal sphincter to **maintain the rectal continence**.

Puborectal sling **maintain forward convexity of anorectal flexure** and thus not only maintains anorectal continence, but also reduces the anterior gap of ano-urogenital hiatus.

Selective relaxation of one of the components of pubococcygeus **with increased tonicity of the remainder of muscle** units helps in various physiological acts like **micturition, parturition** and **defecation**.

Funnel-shaped and gutter-like architectures of the pelvic diaphragm **assists directing anteroposterior position of fetal head** in case of normal vaginal childbirth.

Clinical Anatomy

Injury to the Pelvic Diaphragm

Levator ani of pelvic diaphragm, pelvic fascia and the perineal body may be injured during childbirth. Pubococcygeus, the most important part of the levator ani is usually torn. It encircles the urethra, vagina and anal canal. Tear in the levator ani resulting from its stretching during childbirth may alter the position of bladder neck with urethra. This will cause dribbling of urine due to rise of intraabdominal pressure during coughing, sneezing, and laughing.

Spread of Infection through Hiatus of Schwalbe

Anterior and posterior ends of the arcus tendinous are attached to the pelvic surface of pubis and ischial spine respectively. Intermediate part is free from the obturator fascia to create a gap called hiatus of Schwalbe. This gap establishes a communication between the pelvic cavity and the perineum above and below the pelvic diaphragm respectively. Infection can spread from one part to the other through this gap in either of the two directions.

LA 30.5 Discuss briefly the internal iliac artery.

INTERNAL ILIAC ARTERY

Introduction

Internal iliac artery is the smaller of the two terminal divisions of common iliac artery. It is also shorter in length being 4 cm long. But it gives many branches for:
- **Most of the pelvic organs**
- **Part of the wall of pelvis including iliac fossa**
- **Perineum**
- **Gluteal region**

In fetal life, the artery is very prominent because it used to transmit the blood through the umbilical artery. After birth, proximal part of the umbilical artery persists as superior vesical artery. Distal part of the umbilical artery gets obliterated to form the medial umbilical ligament.

Origin

Internal iliac artery begins as bifurcation of common iliac artery in front of **upper end of the sacroiliac joint.**

Course and Important Relations

The artery runs **downwards** and **backwards** to reach the upper margin of greater sciatic notch where it divides into anterior and posterior division.

The trunk of the artery is very short and lies in front of **sacroiliac joint and lumbosacral trunk.** Anteriorly, it is crossed by the **ureter.**

Branches of Posterior Division (Fig. 30.12)

Posterior division gives following three branches which are **parietal**.
1. **Iliolumbar artery** runs upward in front of sacroiliac joint and lumbosacral trunk. Reaching deep to psoas major muscle it divides into iliac and lumbar branches.
   Iliac branch supplies iliacus muscle and gives a nutrient branch to the iliac fossa. It ends by a branch taking part in anastomosis at anterosuperior iliac spine.

Lumbar branch represents the 5th lumbar artery and supplies muscles of posterior abdominal wall after giving a spinal branch.
2. **Lateral sacral arteries** are usually two in number. These arteries run downwards and medially. Their branches enter through the pelvic sacral foramina to supply the structures of sacral canal. Their dorsal branches supply structure on back of sacrum emerging through the dorsal sacral foramina.
3. **Superior gluteal artery** runs backwards and leaves the pelvis through the greater sciatic foramen above the piriformis along with the superior gluteal nerve. It is distributed to the muscles of gluteal region.

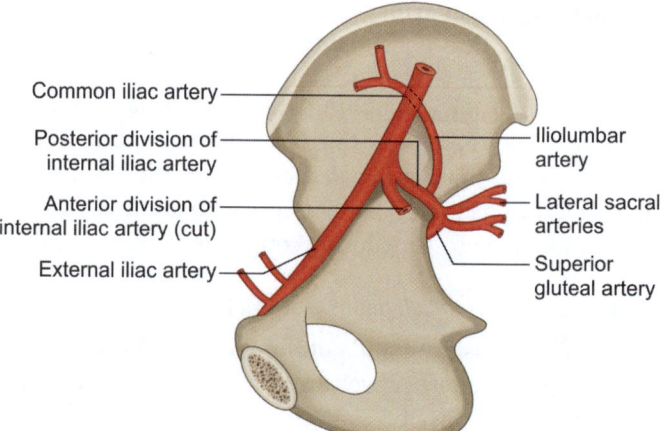

Fig. 30.12: Branches of posterior division of internal iliac artery.

Branches of Anterior Division (Fig. 30.13)

Branches of anterior division of internal iliac artery are **mostly visceral**. The branches are to be followed and remembered better if they are discussed in order from the level of pelvic brim downwards and backwards **(Fig. 30.13)**.

- **Superior vesical artery** is the persistent proximal part of the umbilical artery of fetal life. It runs downwards, forwards and medially below and parallel to the pelvic brim. The artery sends multiple short branches to the upper part of urinary bladder. One branch supplies vas deferens. Distal degenerated part of the artery is continued upwards forwards and medially in the lower part of anterior abdominal wall as **obliterated umbilical artery**.

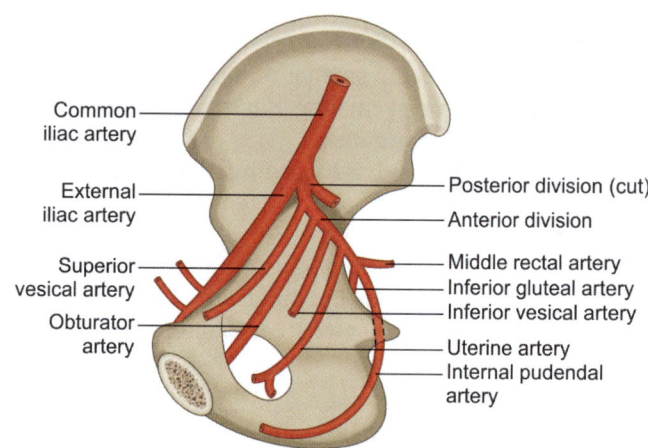

Fig. 30.13: Branches of anterior division of internal iliac artery.

- **Obturator artery** runs downwards forwards and medially over the obturator fascia and finally leaves the pelvis through the **obturator canal** with the obturator nerve and obturator vein above and below it respectively. Before it enters the thigh, it gives following branches in the pelvis.
    - **Iliac branch**: To iliac fossa
    - **Vesical branch**: It may replace the inferior vesical artery
    - **Pubic branch**: To anastomose with the pubic branch of inferior epigastric artery
- **Uterine artery** runs initially downwards, forwards and medially over the pelvic floor where it crosses the ureter. Finally, the artery changes its direction to pass upwards and laterally to pass in between the double fold of peritoneum attached to the lateral margin of uterus called **broad ligament**.

- **Inferior vesical artery** runs forwards and medially towards the base of urinary bladder. In addition to the branch to the terminal part of ureter, in case of male it supplies branches to the prostate, seminal vesicle and terminal part of vas deferens. In female, inferior vesical artery is present as **vaginal artery**.
- **Middle rectal artery** is a small branch. It may arise in common with the inferior vesical artery. It passes medially to supply the wall of rectum.
- **Inferior gluteal artery** is the **largest branch** of the internal iliac artery and is considered to be its continuation. It leaves the pelvis through the lower compartment of greater sciatic foramen to reach the gluteal region.
- **Internal pudendal artery** is the main artery of the perineum. It leaves the pelvis passing through the greater sciatic foramen. Crossing over the dorsal surface of ischial spine it enters the perineum passing through the lesser sciatic foramen.

SA 30.6 Discuss briefly the sacral plexus.
(For viva voce and practical)

SACRAL PLEXUS (FIG. 30.14)

Introduction
Sacral plexus gives rise to the nerves which are distributed to the back of lower limb with sole of foot and to the perineum.

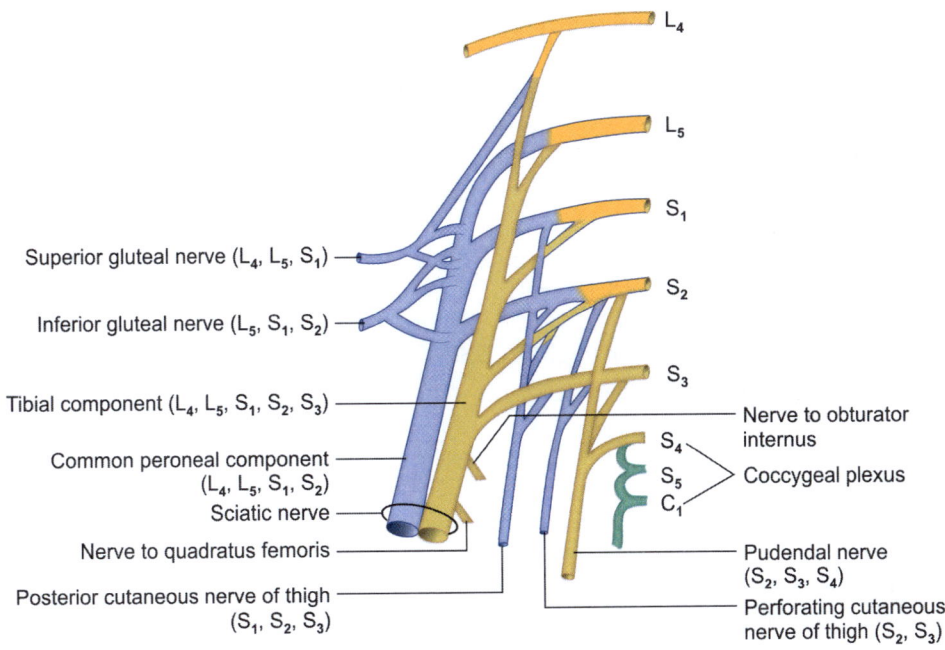

Fig. 30.14: Sacral plexus.

Situation
Sacral plexus is situated within the true pelvis in front of pelvic surface of sacrum.

Formation

Sacral plexus is formed by:
- Lumbosacral trunk (L_4 and L_5)
- Ventral rami of S_1, S_2 and S_3 nerves
- Part of the S_4 nerve.

Important Relations

- Lumbosacral trunk (L_4, L_5) and S_1 nerves are separated by **superior gluteal vessels.**
- S_1 and S_2 nerves are separated by **inferior gluteal vessels.**
- S_2, S_3 and S_4 nerves lie in front of the **piriformis** muscle under cover of **pelvic fascia**
- Plexus formation occurs in front of the piriformis.

Preplexus Connections and Branches

- Sacral nerves receive postganglionic sympathetic fibers via **gray rami communicantes.**
- Parasympathetic fibers come out from the S_2, S_3 and S_4 nerves to form the **pelvic splanchnic nerve.**
- **Muscular branches:**
  - **Piriformis:** S_2, S_3 S_4 nerves
  - **Levator ani:** S_4 nerve
  - **Sphincter ani externus:** Perineal branch of 4th sacral nerve.

Branches

- **Branches from both dorsal and ventral divisions**
  - **Sciatic nerve**
    - Dorsal divisions of L_4, L_5 S_1, S_2 nerves (common peroneal component)
    - Ventral divisions of L_4, L_5 S_1, S_2, S_3 nerves (tibial component)
  - **Posterior cutaneous nerve of thigh**
    - Dorsal divisions of S_1, S_2 nerves
    - Ventral divisions of S_2, S_3 nerves
- **Branches from dorsal divisions**
  - Superior gluteal nerve (L_4, L_5, S_1)
  - Inferior gluteal nerve (L_5, S_1, S_2)
  - Perforating cutaneous nerve of thigh (S_2, S_3)
- **Branches from ventral divisions**
  - Nerve to quadratus femoris (L_4, L_5, S_1)
  - Nerve to obturator internus (L_5, S_1, S_2)
  - Pudendal nerve (S_2, S_3, S_4).

Coccygeal Plexus

It is a small plexus of nerves formed by union of:
- Descending branch of S_4 nerve
- S_5 nerve
- Coccygeal nerve.

The three nerves join in front of coccygeus muscle and form the plexus. **Anococcygeal nerves** arise from the plexus. They pierce the sacrotuberous ligament and supply the skin in the region of coccyx and perianal region.

SA 30.7 Discuss briefly the autonomic nerves of the pelvis.

AUTONOMIC NERVES OF THE PELVIS

Autonomic nerves for the pelvic viscera, both sympathetic as well as parasympathetic, are distributed through the *inferior hypogastric plexus*. Sympathetic fibers for the plexus are derived from the *pelvic part of the sympathetic trunk*. Source of the parasympathetic fibers are the *pelvic splanchnic nerves*.

Pelvic Part of Sympathetic Trunk (Fig. 30.6)

As continuation of the lumbar part, pelvic part of sympathetic trunk enters the pelvis crossing over the ala of sacrum of respective side. It runs downwards and medially over the body of sacrum medial to the pelvic sacral foramina, on either side of the midline. The chain presents **four sacral ganglia**. Both the chains meet in front of the coccyx to form the small **ganglion impar**.

Branches from the sacral sympathetic ganglion are:
- **Gray rami communicantes** to all the sacral nerves and the coccygeal nerve
- **Branches to the inferior hypogastric plexus** from the upper ganglia
- **Branches to rectum** directly from the lower ganglia.

Pelvic Splanchnic Nerve

Pelvic splanchnic nerve is the **sacral outflow of parasympathetic nervous system**. It is formed by the fibers arising from **ventral rami of S_2, S_3, S_4 nerves**. These are called **nervi erigentes**.

Fibers of pelvic splanchnic nerves are distributed as follows:
1. Most of the fibers take part in the formation of **inferior hypogastric plexus**, through which parasympathetic fibers are distributed to the pelvic organs along with the sympathetic.
2. Some fibers ascend to the **superior hypogastric plexus** and then to the **inferior mesenteric plexus**
3. Some fibers ascend to supply **directly** to the part of **colon developed from the hindgut.**

Inferior Hypogastric Plexus

It is a combined plexus of nerves derived from both sympathetic as well as parasympathetic systems. As stated above, sympathetic fibers are derived from the **pelvic part of the sympathetic trunk.** Parasympathetic fibers reach the plexus through the **pelvic splanchnic nerves.**

Situation

Inferior hypogastric plexus divided into right and left halves is situated in the plane of extraperitoneal connective tissue in front of rectum, behind the base of urinary bladder and prostate in male and uterus with upper end of vaginal in female.

Formation

The plexus is formed by:
- Splanchnic branches from **upper sacral sympathetic ganglia**

- Pelvic splanchnic nerves
- Hypogastric nerve **from superior hypogastric plexus.**

Branches

Branches from the inferior hypogastric plexus containing both sympathetic as well as parasympathetic fibers are **carried along the visceral branches of internal iliac artery.** These are:
- **Rectal plexus**
- **Vesical plexus**
- **Prostatic plexus**
- **Uterovaginal plexus.**

Chapter 31

Pelvic Part of the Large Gut

LA 31.1 Discuss briefly the rectum under the following headings: Anatomical position (for viva voce and practical); Gross anatomy and relations; Blood supply, nerve supply and lymphatic drainage; Clinical anatomy.

RECTUM

Anatomical Position

The specimen of rectum is usually provided with the anal canal continued from its lower end. *Lower end of anal canal* is identified through its *skin lining*.

Anterior and posterior surfaces along with its upper and lower ends will also be identified by the following points:
- *Upper two-thirds* of the *anterior surface* of the rectum is *smooth* and *shining* as covered by *peritoneum*.
- Lower one-third of anterior surface as well as the whole of the posterior surface is rough and raw, as not covered by peritoneum.

How to Hold the Viscera

Rough and raw posterior surface of the rectum is to be held longitudinally on the palm of the left hand which is made curved in vertical direction and the wrist is to be extended.

Let the skin lined anal canal hang freely below the tips of the fingers.

Then, with the fingers of the right hand distal end of the anal canal is to be bent backwards to show the forward convexity of the anorectal flexure.

Introduction

The term **rectum** is derived from the Latin word *'rectus'* which means straight. Rectum, the distal part of the large gut is *straight in monkeys*. Human rectum is adapted to the concavity of the sacrum. Though it is a part of large gut, the rectum is **devoid of three cardinal features**, namely, taenia coli, haustrations and appendices epiploicae.

Extent

Beginning: Rectum begins at the **rectosigmoid junction** as continuation of sigmoid colon at the upper border of body of **3rd sacral vertebra**.

Termination: Rectum ends at **anorectal junction** which is 2–3 cm below and in front of the tip of coccyx.

Anorectal junction presents a forward convexity called **anorectal flexure** caused by the **puborectal sling** formed by the **puborectalis** fibers of levator ani muscle.

Length: 12 cm

Curvatures (Figs. 31.1A and B)

- **Anteroposterior curvature**: It is the forward concavity adjusted with the forward concavity of the pelvic surface of the sacrum **(Fig. 31.1A)**.
- **Lateral curvatures**: These are three lateral convexities at the upper, middle and lower third of rectum. Upper and lower thirds show convexity to the right and middle third shows convexity to the left **(Fig. 31.1B)**.

Lower end of the rectum shows dilatation called **ampulla** of rectum.

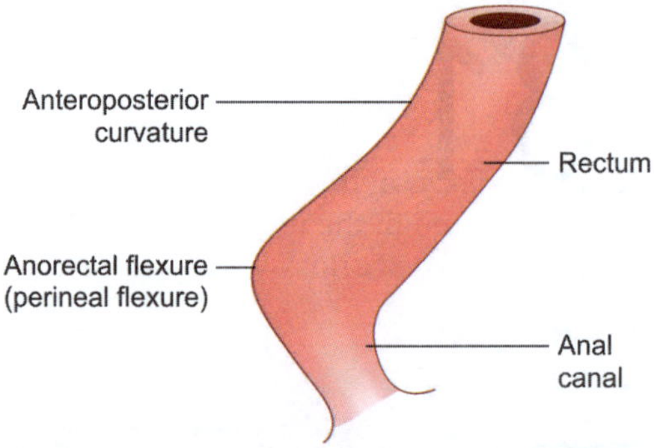

Fig. 31.1A: Anteroposterior curvature of rectum (lateral view).

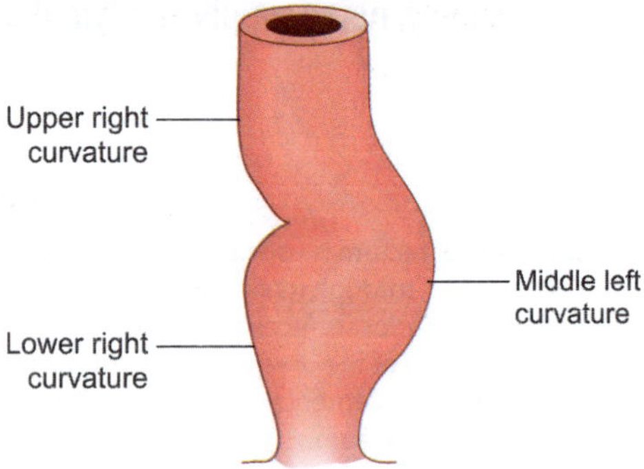

Rectal Fascia

Sigmoid mesocolon stops at the rectosigmoid junction and the rectum does not have its mesentery. However, the surgeons refer to *the connective tissue and the fat around the rectum as* **mesorectum**. The visceral fascia surrounding the mesorectum is known as **mesorectal fascia** which is grooved posteriorly in the midline to lodge the branches of superior rectal artery and tributaries of superior rectal vein with lymph nodes.

Fig. 31.1B: Lateral curvatures of rectum (anterior view).

Peritoneal Relations (Fig. 31.2)

Upper one-third of the rectum is covered by peritoneum in front as well as on the sides.

Middle one-third is covered by peritoneum only in front.

Lower one-third is completely nonperitoneal.

From the junction of upper two-thirds and lower one-third of the front of rectum, the peritoneum is reflected forwards to form **rectovesical pouch** in male and **rectovaginal pouch** in female.

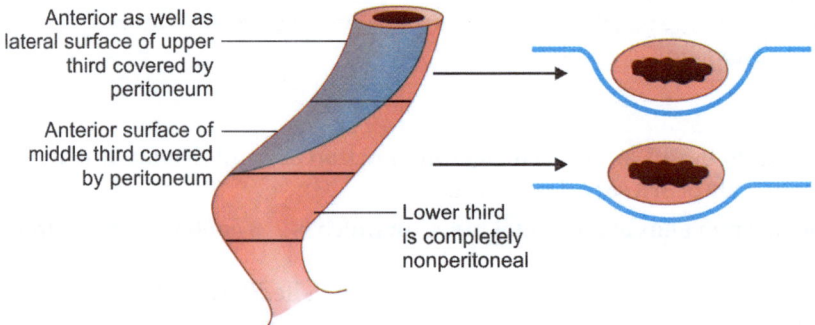

Fig. 31.2: Peritoneal relation of rectum.

Relations

Anterior

In male

Upper two-thirds of the rectum, covered by peritoneum, is related to sigmoid colon and coils of ileum contained in the rectovesical pouch. *Lower third,* devoid of peritoneum, is related to the posterior surface of urinary bladder, prostate, seminal vesicles and terminal end of vas deferens.

In female

Upper two-thirds of the rectum, covered by peritoneum, is related to sigmoid colon and coils of ileum contained in the rectovaginal pouch. *Lower third,* devoid of peritoneum, is related to posterior surface of vagina.

Anterior surface of lower one-third of rectum is separated from the pelvic viscera by the **rectovesical fascia (of Denonvillier)** and the **rectovaginal septum** in male and female respectively. These fascial septa act as line of barrier.

Posterior

Concavity of the **pelvic surface of sacrum** is separated from the posterior surface of rectum by the following structures from the midline to the lateral side.
- Median sacral vessels
- Bifurcation of superior rectal artery with corresponding vein, in the mesorectal fascia
- Pelvic part of the sympathetic trunk
- Piriformis, coccygeus and levator ani muscles
- Sacral plexus of nerves.

Special Features of the Wall

Muscular coat of rectum shows special characteristics in its outer longitudinal layer. The taenia coli of sigmoid colon come together at the rectosigmoid junction and the longitudinal muscle fibers from a broadband on both the anterior and posterior surfaces of the rectum. In addition, some muscle fibers from the puborectal sling blend with the longitudinal fibers of anorectal junction to form the **puborectalis.**

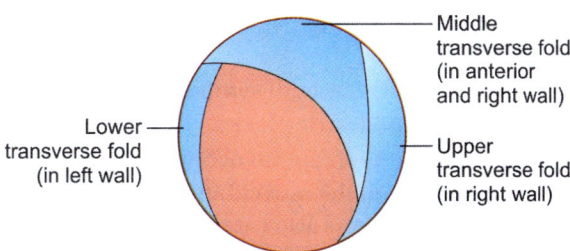

Fig. 31.3: Horizontal mucous folds of rectum (superior view).

Mucous membrane of the rectum, together with the circular muscle layer, form two or three **semicircular permanent folds** called the **transverse folds of rectum (Fig. 31.3).** Usual positions of these folds are as follows:
- **Upper fold:** It is at the upper end of rectum. It covers the **right wall**.
- **Middle fold**: It is **most constant**, at the level of the **ampulla**. It is on the **anterior** and **right walls**.
- **Lower fold:** It is occasionally present, a little below the ampulla. It is in the **left wall**.

Blood Supply

Arteries

Rectum is supplied by all the superior, middle and inferior rectal arteries.

Superior rectal artery is the direct continuation of the inferior mesenteric artery at the level of pelvic brim and the **chief artery supplying the rectal mucosa**. It descends along the root of pelvic mesocolon and divides into right and left branches which pass through the muscular coat to supply the mucosal lining. Right and left divisions anastomose with each other and also with the middle and inferior rectal arteries.

Middle rectal artery is a small branch of internal iliac artery and is mainly distributed to the muscular layer.

Inferior rectal artery arises from the internal pudendal artery in the perineum. It supplies rectum through anastomosis with the superior rectal and middle rectal arteries.

Veins

Veins draining the rectum correspond to the arteries. The **superior rectal vein** continued as inferior mesenteric vein is the tributary of the **portal venous system**. The **middle** and **inferior rectal veins** drain into the internal iliac vein, the inferior, via the internal pudendal vein. The communication among the three rectal veins in anorectal wall is one of the important portal-systemic anastomosis.

Lymphatic Drainage

Lymph vessels from the **upper part** of rectum follow the superior rectal vein and drain into **pararectal lymph nodes** and finally to the inferior mesenteric group of **preaortic lymph nodes**.

Lymph vessels from the **lower part** of rectum follow the middle rectal vein and drain into the **internal iliac lymph nodes**.

Nerve Supply

Rectum is supplied by both **sympathetic (L_1, L_2)** and **parasympathetic (S_2, S_3, S_4)** nerves through the **inferior hypogastric plexus**.

Sympathetic fibers are **vasoconstrictor** and **motor for the internal sphincter**. Parasympathetic fibers are **motor to the musculature** of the rectum.

Sympathetic fibers also carry sensory fibers which are **sensitive only to stretch**.

Clinical Anatomy

Digital Examination or Per Rectum (PR) Examination

In this type of clinical examination, finger is introduced through the anorectal region to feel any pathology inside anal canal and lower rectum or the surrounding viscera, e.g. urinary bladder, prostate, seminal vesicle, uterus, and ovary.

Prolapse of Rectum

Partial or complete prolapse of rectum through the anus is relatively common clinical condition. In **partial prolapse**, rectal mucosa with submucosa protrude for a short distance outside the anus. In case of **complete prolapse**, whole thickness of the rectal wall bulges outwards through the anus. Usual causes of partial or complete prolapse are damage of the pelvic floor muscles after childbirth or poor muscle tone in elderly persons.

Cancer of Rectum

Cancer (carcinoma) of rectum is a common variety of malignant disease. The disease remains confined in the wall of the rectum for a considerable period of time. Spread of the cancer initially occurs through the lymphatics. Later on, metastasis through the venous channel involves the liver through portal venous system.

LA 31.2 **Describe the anal canal under the following headings:**
Gross anatomy; Lining (interior); Musculature; Blood supply; Lymphatic drainage; Innervation; Clinical anatomy.

ANAL CANAL

Introduction

Anal canal is the short terminal part of large gut being devoid of its all the three cardinal features which are teniae coli, sacculations or haustrations and appendices epiploicae.

Position (Fig. 31.4)

Anal canal is the part of large gut which is situated
- Below the pelvic floor
- In the central part of anal triangle of perineum, being related to ischiorectal fossa on either side

Length = 3.8 cm (38 mm)

Extent

Proximal End

It is the junction with lower end of rectum, called *anorectal junction*.

Anorectal junction is a little below and 2–3 cm in front of tip of coccyx.

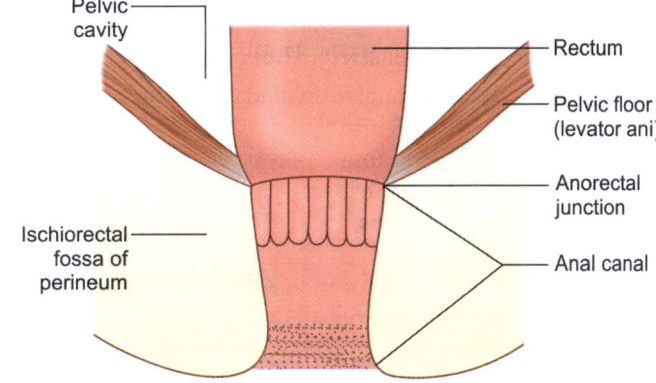

Fig. 31.4: Outline of anal canal on coronal section.

It presents a forward convexity called **anorectal flexure** or **perineal flexure**. The flexure or curvature is caused by pull of the muscular loop derived from pubococcygeus component of levator ani. The muscle fibers from both sides forming the loop around anorectal junction is known as **anorectal sling (Fig. 31.5)**.

Distal End

Distal end is known as **anus** which is 4 cm below the tip of coccyx.

Anal verge is the lowermost part of anal canal with cuticular lining. It is defined as '*sharp turn*' area where stratified squamous epithelium of lower anal canal becomes continuous with skin of perineum. The lining of anal verge is pigmented. Tonicity of external anal

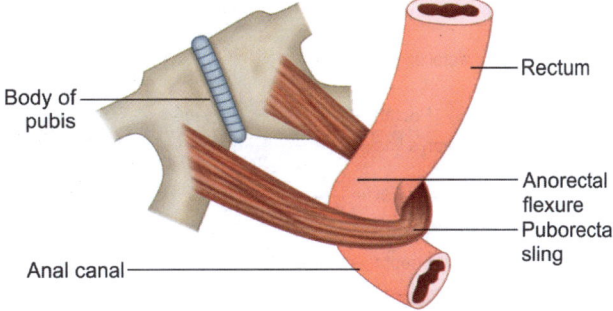

Fig. 31.5: Anorectal flexure maintained by puborectal sling.

sphincter at the level of anal verge keeps it in collapsed condition for which it presents number of folds and exists in the form of an anteroposterior slit between two buttocks.

From the proximal to distal ends, anal canal is directed *downwards and backwards*.

Relations

All around, the anal canal is encircled by *fibromuscular supporting tissue* and *neuronal network*. Beside this, relations of anal canal are as follows.

Anteriorly

In males: **Perineal body, membranous urethra** and **bulb of penis**.
In females: **Perineal body** and **posterior wall of lower end of vagina**.

Posteriorly

Anococcygeal ligament *and* **tip of coccyx**

Anococcygeal ligament connect posterior aspect of anal canal to the tip of coccyx. It is a midline *fibroelastic structure* which may contain *some skeletal muscle fibers*.

Above and parallel to this anococcygeal ligament, similarly extends in the midline the **anococcygeal raphe** having similar extent for the 'levator ani plate'. It is the plane of pubococcygeus component of levator ani muscle.

Lining (Interior) of Anal Canal (Fig. 31.6)

Mucosal lining of anal canal is divided into following three zones:
- Upper zone   = 15 mm
- Midline zone = 15 mm
- Lower zone   = 8 mm

Upper Zone

Upper 15 mm zone of anal canal is lined by **columnar epithelium** similar to that of rectum. It contains both secretory as well as absorptive cells. The submucosa of this zone contains numerous tubular glands opening through crypts and possesses following characteristics.

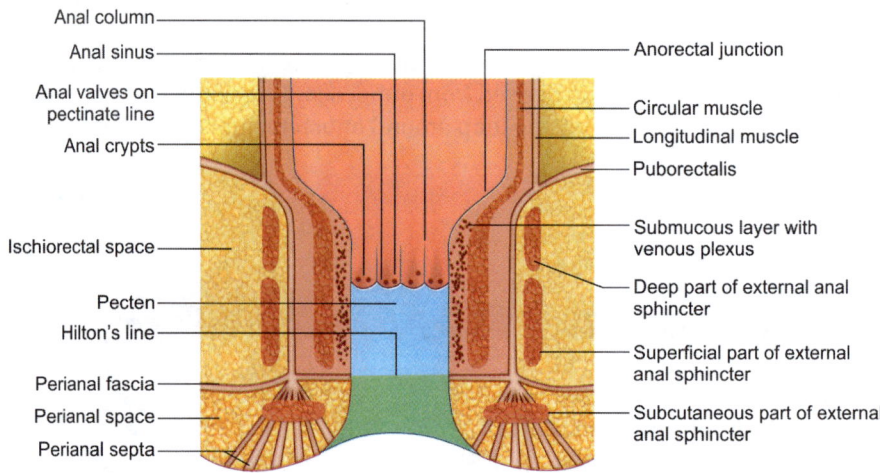

Fig. 31.6: Coronal section of anal canal to show its mucosal lining and musculature.

- The layer is more mobile
- It is relatively expansile or distendable
- It presents abundant arterial and venous plexuses

Mucosal lining of upper 15 mm zone presents following characteristics.
- There are 6 to 10 parallel vertical folds called **anal columns** which are more prominent in children, but less defined in normal adult individuals. Beneath the prominence of anal columns lie the terminal radicals of superior rectal artery and vein. The anal columns are most prominent in left lateral (3 O'clock), right anterior (7 O'clock) and right posterior (11 O'clock) position of wall of anal canal. Opposite these zones subepithelial connective tissue is expanded to form **anal cushions**.
- Lower end of anal columns unite to form crescentic or semilunar folds called **anal valves**. Small depressions above the curve of anal valves are known as **anal sinuses**. Anal sinuses present openings of **anal glands**, openings of which are called **anal crypts**. Cystic prolongations of anal glands may extend through internal anal sphincter, and even may pass through external anal sphincter. These prolongations are of surgical importance, as they predispose pathogenesis of **anal fistula**.
- The wavy line at the level of anal valves and anal sinuses is known as **pectinate line** or **dentate line**.

Anatomical and clinical importance of pectinate (dentate) line
- Embryologically, it represents the line of junction between **endodermal** and **ectodermal** components of anal canal lying above and below respectively.
- Thereby, it acts as **watershed line** between **visceral component** *above* and **somatic component** *below*.
- **Veins above the line** drain through superior rectal vein, so inferior mesenteric vein of **portal venous system**. **Veins below the line** drain via inferior rectal vein of **systemic venous system**.
- Lymph vessels above the line drain into inferior mesenteric group of **preaortic lymph nodes,** whereas those below the line end in **internal iliac group** of lymph nodes.
- **Internal hemorrhoids** due to engorgement of superior rectal venous radicles develop **above the dentate line.**
- Mucous membrane above the line is supplied by **autonomic nerves** and thereby insensitive to injurious sensory stimuli. But cuticular lining below is supplied by **somatic nerves**, i.e. inferior rectal branch of pudendal nerve and therefore sensitive to pain.
- *Anal papillae* are irregular folds, often found at the level of dentate line. These folds project from *free margin of anal valves* and represent torn (ruptured) margin of fetal anal membrane.

Middle Zone
- It is the part of inner lining of anal canal measuring **second 15 mm**. This area is called **pectin**.
- This area is smooth and lined by **nonkeratinized stratified squamous epithelium.**
- This area **lacks sebaceous** and **sweat glands** and **hair follicles**.
- This area of lining being **ectodermal** in origin, is supplied by numerous **somatic nerve endings.**
- This area is bounded below by an annular groove, called **intersphincteric groove**. The groove is at the level of lower border of internal anal sphincter. It is called intersphincteric groove because, the groove is between lower borders of internal anal sphincter and superficial part of external anal sphincter above, and subcutaneous part of external anal sphincter below.
- The groove, being paler in look, is named as **white line of Hilton**.
- The groove is formed because of **attachment** of inner most bands of **conjoint tendon of puborectalis** (see below).

Lower Zone
- It is the **lowermost 8 mm** of lining of anal canal *below the level of intersphincteric groove.*
- It is lined by hair *bearing* **keratinized stratified squamous epithelium.**
- It presents **sebaceous** *and* **sweat glands**
- It is **continuous with perianal skin**
- Subcutaneous plane of this area contains *abundance of connective tissue* and *venous plexus*. The venous plexus, called **external rectal venous plexus**, attributes to bluish coloration of the zone
- External rectal venous plexus is the **site for formation of external piles** or **external hemorrhoids.**

Anal Transition Zone
- Anal transition zone (ATZ) is the area of transition between mucosal zone lined by column epithelium and pectin lined by stratified squamous epithelium
- It is variable in height and does not correspond to pectinate line or dentate line
- This area extends upwards in the mucosal zone showing **islands of stratified squamous epithelium**
- *Function of ATZ:* Submucosa of anal transition zone is **highly sensitive** as it is **richly supplied by sensory nerves.** Due to relaxation of upper anal canal, when rectal content comes in contact in anal transition zone, it is recognized due to stimulation of nerve endings including thermoreceptors.

Musculature of Anal Canal
Anal canal, being part of gut as a continuation of rectum is lined by inner circular and outer longitudinal layers of smooth or visceral muscles. Peripherally, it is encircled by an additional layer of skeletal muscle fibers in a circular fashion. So, anal canal presents three layers of muscle fibers. Each of these three layers of muscle fibers possesses special characteristics. From inside outwards, they are as follows:
- Inner circular fibers which are condensed to form **internal anal sphincter**. This is visceral or smooth muscle.
- Intermediate longitudinal layer which blends with the fibers of pubococcygeus component of levator ani to form **conjoint longitudinal coat of puborectalis**. This layer is admixture of smooth muscle of anorectal wall and striated muscle of levator ani.
- Outer layer of circular muscle fibers which forms **external anal sphincter**. It is made up of striated or voluntary muscle and made up of *deep, superficial* and *subcutaneous parts.*

Internal Anal Sphincter
- Internal anal sphincter is *the thickened downward extension of inner circular muscle coat of rectum* beyond anorectal junction.
- It *extends up to upper two zones of anal canal* or up to the level of Hilton's line.
- The sphincter is made up of *smooth (involuntary) muscle* so under control of *autonomic nerves.*
- The lower part of sphincter is *traversed by conjoint fibromuscular band of puborectalis.*
- *Nerve supply*: The sphincter is supplied by both sympathetic as well as parasympathetic nerves through *inferior hypogastric plexus*. Sympathetic fibers are derived from *two lumbar spinal segments (L_1, L_2)*. Parasympathetic fibers are derived from *pelvic splanchnic nerves (S_2, S_3, S_4)*. Sympathetic fibers maintain tonicity of sphincter whereas parasympathetic fibers cause its relaxation. Sensory impulse is carried through both the components.

External Anal Sphincter (Figs. 31.6 and 31.7)
- External anal sphincter is a tube-like striated muscular complex in the wall of anal canal which forms an additional layer of muscle in this lowest part of the gut.

- This is composed of type I slowly contracting muscle fibers which are suitable for prolonged contraction.
- External anal sphincter is divided into following three parts:
  1. Deep part
  2. Superficial part
  3. Subcutaneous part

  Although these three components show different features in attachment, they are considered as a **single muscular unit**.

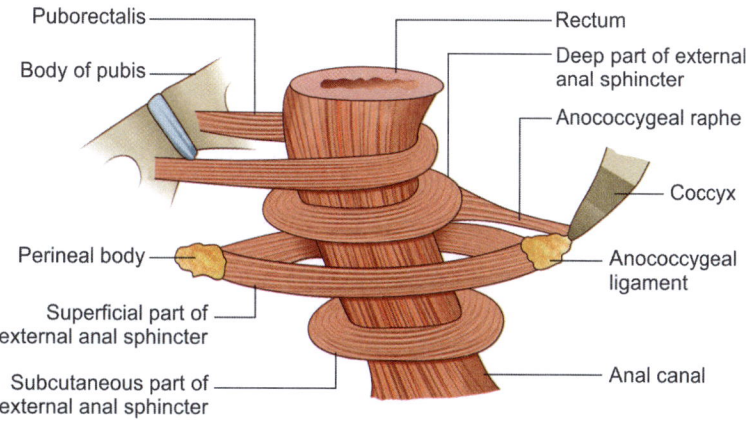

Fig. 31.7: Parts of external anal sphincter.

- Length and thickness of external anal sphincter varies between male and female.
  - **Deep part** of external anal sphincter form upper third of the muscle. Above it blends with fibers of puborectalis. Anteriorly some of the fibers decussate with *superficial transverse perineal muscle* and posteriorly some fibers are attached to **anococcygeal raphe** which is a **condensed band of fibrous tissue** of *'levator ani plate'* attached to the tip of coccyx. Deep part of external anal sphincter lies opposite the level of upper half of internal sphincter.
  - **Superficial part** of the external sphincter extends below up to lower border of internal anal sphincter. This is the component of muscle which shows attachment both in front as well as behind. **Anteriorly,** the fibers are **attached to central tendon of perineum or perineal body. Behind** the fibers are attached to a fibromuscular band extending from anal canal to tip of coccyx. It is called **anococcygeal ligament.** It is made up of **elastic fibers** along with **the muscle fibers** which are derived from the superficial part of external sphincter. The ligament is different from anococcygeal raphe which is devoid of muscle fibers and lies at a higher level as stated above.
  - **Subcutaneous part** lies below the level of internal anal sphincter and surrounds the lower part anal canal below white line of Hilton. Is has no bony attachment and encircle lower end of anal canal in the form of a flat band of 15 mm diameter. Fibrous bands as a continuation of conjoint tendon of puborectalis traverse the subcutaneous part to be attached to deep surface of perianal skin **(Fig. 31.6).**

Nerve supply of external sphincter

The external anal sphincter is mainly supplied by *inferior rectal nerve* which is a branch of pudendal nerve (S_2, S_3, S_4).

Ventral rami of same S_2, S_3 and S_4 nerves may give direct branches.

Conjoint Longitudinal Coat (Fig. 31.6)

- The longitudinal layer is situated between the internal and external sphincter of anal canal.
- It is called conjoint longitudinal coat because it is formed as downwards continuation of following two muscular elements.
  1. **Longitudinal smooth muscle fibers of rectum** continued beyond anorectal junction.
  2. **Innermost striated muscle fibers of puborectalis** which is named **puboanalis**.

- The longitudinal muscle layer formed by the visceral smooth muscle and the striated muscle fibers of puboanalis extend up to the level just above the lower margin of internal anal sphincter. Then the layer becomes completely *fibroelastic* and divides into number of septa which divide into following groups.
    1. *Lateral*: It is called **perianal septum** or **perianal fascia** which passes peripherally to cut off a subcutaneous part of main ischiorectal space called **perianal space** lying beneath perianal skin.
    2. *Central*: **Multiple fibroelastic bands** traverse through subcutaneous part of external anal sphincter to be attached to deep surface of perianal skin.
    3. *Medial*: These bands pass medially below the lower margin of internal anal sphincter and **attached to inner lining of anal canal forming the prominence of intersphincteric groove at the level of white line of Hilton.**

Blood Supply of Anal Canal

Artery
- Terminal branches of **superior rectal artery**
- Branches of **inferior rectal artery**
- A minor share by branches of **median sacral artery.**

Vein
- **Superior rectal vein**: Peripheral tributaries of superior rectal vein drain the *mucosa of upper anal canal*, the *internal anal sphincter* and *conjoint longitudinal muscle coat*.
- **Inferior rectal vein**: Tributaries of this vein drain the *lining of lower anal canal and the external anal sphincter.*

Lymphatic Drainage of Anal Canal

Lymph vessels from the anal canal follow two different directions like veins.
1. Lymph vessels from mucosal lining of **upper anal canal, internal sphincter** and **conjoint longitudinal muscle coat** run initially through *submucosal and intermural lymphatic plexus of rectum*. From there, the vessels pass via **mesorectal lymph nodes** to inferior mesenteric group of **preaortic lymph nodes**.
2. Lymphatics from lining of **lower anal canal** *and* **external anal sphincter** *form perianal lymphatic plexus*. Vessels from this plexus drain into **internal iliac group of lymph nodes** following the course of inferior rectal vein.
3. Besides lymph vessels from lining of lower anal canal, **below line of Hilton**, drain into **medial group of superficial inguinal lymph nodes**.

Innervation of Anal Canal

Anal canal, the lowest part of gut, is composed of the different embryological sources. Lining above the dentate or pectinate line is endodermal and that below the line is ectodermal in origin. Again internal anal sphincter and conjoint longitudinal muscle coat are made up of smooth (visceral) muscle fibers, whereas external anal sphincter is made up of striated (somatic) muscle fibers. That is why, anal canal is supplied by both *autonomic and somatic nerves.*

Autonomic innervations: **Sympathetic fibers** originate from *upper two lumbar segments* (L_1, L_2). Passing through corresponding sympathetic ganglia, fibers descend to sacral (S_1, S_2) sympathetic ganglia and come out as **sacral splanchnic nerves** to join *inferior hypogastric plexus.*

Parasympathetic fibers, coming from **pelvic splanchnic nerves** (S_2, S_3, S_4) also join *inferior hypogastric plexus.*

Sensory impulse from lining of upper anal canal, which is **rich in thermoreceptors** is carried by sympathetic fibers. Motor fibers of sympathetic causes spasm of lower rectal muscle by contraction of conjoint longitudinal muscle coat and internal sphincter of anal canal. Parasympathetic fibers cause relaxation of internal anal sphincter.

Somatic innervations: Somatic nerves for anal canal are derived from *second, third and fourth sacral spinal nerves via* **inferior rectal branch of pudendal nerve**. These fibers are:
- **Sensory to lower anal mucosa** below dentate or pectinate line, which is rich in *nociceptors* and *pressure receptors*.
- **Sensory branches to perianal skin**
- **Motor branches to external anal sphincter.**

Clinical Anatomy

Hemorrhoids (Piles)

Hemorrhoids or piles are surgical conditions which are characterized by prolapse of anorectal mucosa along with dilated veins of submucosa. Submucous coat of this area presents anastomosis between radicles of superior rectal vein of portal system and middle and inferior rectal veins of systemic system. Various clinical conditions leading to rise of portal venous pressure as a result of portal obstruction cause dilatation or engorgement of veins of anorectal submucosa which is one of the sites of portacaval anastomosis. Veins of this site of communication are dilated as they do not possess valves.

Internal hemorrhoids

Anal columns in upper and canal are filled by radicles of superior rectal veins and arteries. These are embedded in subepithelial connective tissue. This tissue with arteriovenous radicles is more prominent in left lateral (3 O'clock), right posterior (7 O'clock) and right anterior (11 O'clock) position of anal canal. Protrusion of radicles of superior rectal veins and arteries along with submucosa and mucosa opposite the abovementioned three landmarks are known as internal hemorrhoids. Internal hemorrhoids are categorized into following three degrees.
- *First degree*: Confined within the lumen of anal canal.
- *Second degree*: Hemorrhoids confined within anal canal, but comes out during defecation and get reduced after the act of defecation.
- *Third degree*: Herniation of hemorrhoids permanently outside anal canal.

External hemorrhoids

External hemorrhoids are developed from varicosities of tributaries of inferior rectal vein as they run laterally from lower anal canal close to anal margin. They are covered by skin or mucous membrane of lower end of anal canal. They are supplied by inferior rectal nerve, the nerve of somatic nervous system. That is why external hemorrhoids are sensitive to pain, temperature, touch and pressure, so tend to be painful.

Anal Fissure

At the level of pectinate or dentate line, lower end of anal columns are interconnected by **anal valves**. In case of chronic constipation, these anal valves are often torn. Prolongation of ulcers at the level of torn anal valves leads to formation of **anal fissure**. The fissure develops most commonly in the posterior median line and less commonly in anterior median line. This is because of lack of support of the inner wall by superficial part of external anal sphincter in the midline. Because the superficial part of external sphincter does not encircle the anal canal, but it sweeps alongside the lateral walls.

The anal fissure at the level of anal valve is painful because inferior aspect of the valve so also the fissure with cuticular lining is innervated by inferior rectal (somatic) nerve. The pain results in reflex spasm of external anal sphincter aggravating the condition.

Perianal Abscess

Anal crypts at the floor (bottom) of anal sinuses are the opening of anal glands. Infection can spread from the crypts to the cystic prolongation of the glands to the *intersphincteric space*. This may lead to abscess formation in perianal region. The abscess may be superficial below the level of perianal fascia beneath the perianal skin. It is called **subcutaneous perianal abscess**. If it is deep to perianal fascia, it will form **ischiorectal abscess**. Ischiorectal abscess may extend through retroanal recess to the ischiorectal fossa of other side forming **horseshoe-shaped abscess**. Ischiorectal abscess may be complicated by its spread through *hiatus of Schwalbe* to the pelvic cavity by the side of rectum to form **pelvirectal abscess**.

Anal Fistula

Anal fistula results from inadequate management or negligence in case of perianal abscess. The fistula opens in one side at the lumen of anal canal or lower rectum, and on the other side on the surface of perianal skin. If the track opens on one of the either side, it is called **sinus**. **Low anal fistula** is commoner which is *below the level of anorectal ring*. **High anal fistula** communicates with lower rectum.

Chapter 32

Urinary Bladder and Ureter

LA 32.1 Describe the urinary bladder under the following headings:
Anatomical position (only for viva voce and practical); Introduction; Situation, capacity and features; Peritoneal and visceral relations; Ligaments; Interior with trigone; Musculature; Vascular supply; Lymphatic drainage; Nerve supply; Clinical anatomy.

URINARY BLADDER

Anatomical Position

Following features of the urinary bladder (male or female) are to be identified fitst.
- **Surfaces:** Urinary bladder is tetrahedral having four surfaces as follows:
  - One superior surface: Widest, *smooth* and *glistening* as *covered by peritoneum*.
  - Two inferolateral surfaces: Intermediate in surface area
  - One posterior surfaces: Narrowest
- **Apex:** It is at the narrower end of the superior surface where this surface meets with the two inferolateral surfaces.
- **Base:** It is the smaller triangular posterior surface with it apex directed downwards to meet with the two inferolateral surfaces. This is known as the neck of the bladder.
- **Terminal end of the two ureters:** Connected to the superolateral angles of the base.

How to Hold the Viscera

Two inferolateral surfaces are to be held in contact with palms of two hands of respective side with the ulnar borders of the hand apposed.
 While holding the apex of the bladder is to be directed forwards with base facing backwards.
 Terminal ends of the ureters may be gripped through the tips of the thumb and index fingers of the corresponding hand.

If the specimen is male bladder: Before gripping the ureters, they are to be hooked by the terminal end of the vas deferens of respective side. The seminal vesicles lie lateral to the vas on either side.

Introduction
- Urinary bladder is a temporary reservoir of urine.
- It possesses thick muscular wall with remarkable power of expansibility.
- Its shape, size, position and relations vary with the amount of urine collected within and position of adjacent viscera.

Situation

In case of adults, empty urinary bladder is situated within lesser pelvis lying behind the pubis and below the pelvic brim.

When the bladder gets distended superior surface expands upwards and is rounded up above the level of pelvic brim behind lower part of anterior abdominal wall. The bladder as a whole becomes ovoid in outline and peritoneum reflected from its superior surface to the lower part of anterior abdominal wall is stripped off at a higher level from lower part of body wall (**Fig. 32.1A**).

In newborn, urinary bladder is not at all a pelvic organ, but it is situated above the level of pubic symphysis (**Fig. 32.1B**). When the child grows 6 years old, neck or lower end of bladder comes down at the level of upper border of pubic symphysis. At the age of puberty the urinary bladder reaches to its pelvic position.

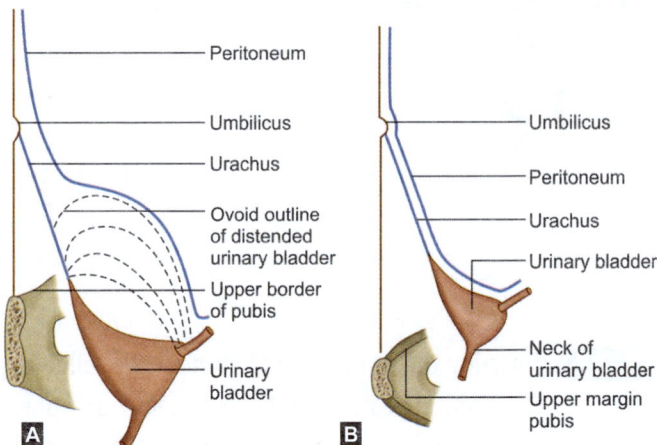

Figs. 32.1A and B: Position of urinary bladder in relation to pelvic inlet. (A) Adult; (B) Newborn.

Capacity

In case of adults, maximum amount of urine which can be stored in urinary bladder is 500 mL. The awareness for distension of the organ is felt due to stimulation of stretch receptors in its wall.

Features

Urinary bladder, when empty, is wedge shaped or more correctly to say, **tetrahedral in outline** with following features (**Fig. 32.2**).
- **Apex**: Apex is the tapering or pointed *anterior end* of the organ which is directed forward and slightly upwards towards superior margin of pubic symphysis. Form the apex, median umbilical ligament or urachus extends upwards to the umbilicus. It is the remnant of distal narrow part of allantois.

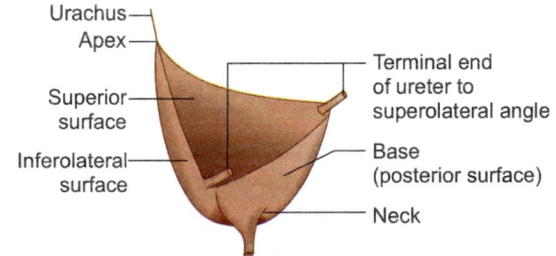

Fig. 32.2: Surface features of urinary bladder.

- **Base**: It is the posterior surface of bladder lying opposite the apex. It is directed backwards and slightly downwards. It is triangular in outline with slight convexity. Because of the bulging, base is also known as **fundus**.
- Angles of triangular base are as follows:
- **Two superolateral angles** present termination of ureter
- **Inferior angle** presents the commencement of urethra
- **Superior surface** is triangular when the bladder is empty. When distended, it becomes rounded
- **Two inferolateral surfaces** face downwards and laterally. These surfaces face to the pelvic surface of levator ani of corresponding half
- **Neck** of urinary bladder is the lower end from where starts the urethra.

Peritoneal Relations

Peritoneal lining of urinary bladder slightly varies in males and females.

In Males (Fig. 32.3A)

Peritoneum covering superior surface of urinary bladder is reflected on different sides as follows:

- **Anteriorly:** Beyond apex of the bladder peritoneum is reflected on posterior surface of infraumbilical part of anterior abdominal wall as parietal peritoneum.
- **Posteriorly:** From superior surface of male bladder, first peritoneum *covers uppermost part of posterior surface or base and upper end of seminal vesicle* from where, it is reflected on to the junction of upper two-thirds and lower one-third of anterior surface of rectum forming **rectovesical pouch**. Rectovesical pouch is the most dependent part of peritoneal cavity in male in both supine as well as erect posture. It is 7.5 cm deep to the level of anus. Its downward extension in fetal life up to the level of perineal body or apex of prostate, gets obliterated later on and called **rectovesical fascia of Denonvillier** which forms a primary line of barrier between rectum and anal canal behind and, urinary bladder with male reproductive organs in front.
- **Laterally:** Form superior surface, peritoneum is reflected towards lateral pelvic wall to form **paravesical fossa**.

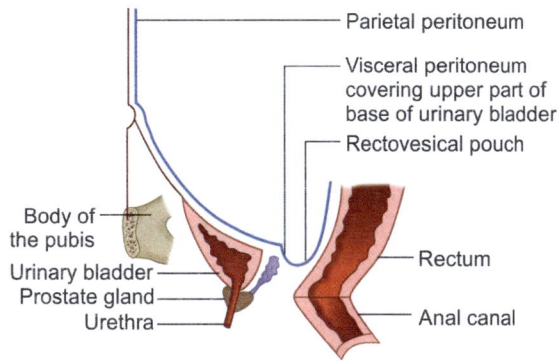

Fig. 32.3A: Peritoneal relation of male urinary bladder.

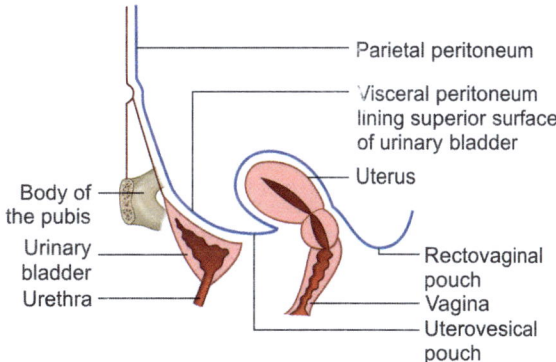

Fig. 32.3B: Peritoneal relation of female urinary bladder.

In Females (Fig. 32.3B)

Like male bladder, peritoneum covers the superior surface. *Its reflection anteriorly and laterally is similar as in males.*

Psteriorly its reflection is different as follows.

From superior surface of urinary bladder peritoneum is reflected at the junction of body and cervix of uterus to form **uterovesical pouch**. So unlike male bladder, upper part of posterior surface is not covered by peritoneum.

Visceral Relations

Superior Surface

Superior surface of urinary bladder is triangular in outline and bounded laterally by lateral borders extending from apex to base. Its posterior border separates the surface from base. In male, whole of superior surface (with uppermost part of base) is covered by peritoneum **(Fig. 32.4A).** In female, peritoneum covers the surface except its posteriormost part **(Fig. 32.4B).** In both the cases the surface is related to sigmoid colon and terminal coils of ileum.

Inferolateral Surfaces

Inferolateral surfaces (right and left) are related to pelvic fascia by which they are separated from slopes of levator ani. Anterior part of the surface is separated from lower part of pelvic surface of body of pubis by **retropubic space of Retzius** containing retropubic pad of fat. The surface is also related to **puboprostatic ligaments** in male and **pubovesical ligament** in female.

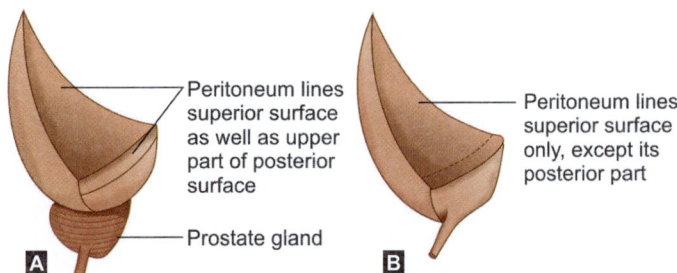

Figs. 32.4A and B: Peritoneal relation of male (A) and female (B) urinary bladder.

Base or posterior surface of urinary bladder facing posteroinferiorly present different relations in male and female. In females it is related to anterior wall of vagina. In case of males, base of urinary bladder is separated from anterior surface of rectum by seminal vesicle and vas deferens of both sides and fascia of Denonvillier (**Fig. 32.5**).

Apex is the anterior end of urinary bladder. From the apex extends **urachus** or **median umbilical ligament** upwards to umbilicus along the midline of posterior surface of infraumbilical part of anterior abdominal wall. It raises a fold of peritoneum named as **median umbilical fold**.

Neck of bladder is the lowermost end of the organ and it corresponds to beginning of urethra at the level of internal urethral orifice. It is the part of bladder which is *constant in position* independent of varying position of the organ itself and rectum.

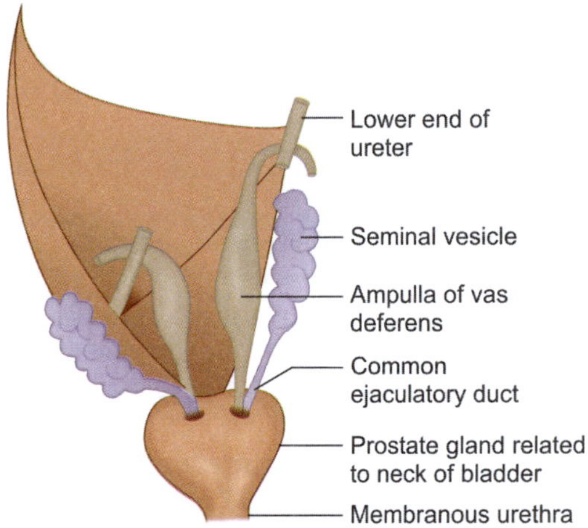

Ligaments of Bladder

True (Nonperitoneal) Ligaments

These are either *condensation of pelvic fascia* extending from bladder to wall of pelvis or *embryological remnants*.

Fig. 32.5: Structures related to the base and neck of male bladder.

- **Median umbilical ligament (urachus):** It is a cord-like structure extending from apex of urinary bladder to umbilicus passing through the plane of extraperitoneal tissue of infraumbilical part of anterior abdominal wall. It is the fibrosed remnant of distal narrow part of allantois.
- **Pubovesical ligament:** These are bilateral condensation of pelvic fascia extending from the lower margin of pubis to the neck of urinary bladder. These bands are *fibromuscular* in nature as it contains some fibers of detrusor muscle continued from bladder neck. In case of males, fibers of pubovesical ligament are prolonged at a lower level and blend with anterior surface of prostate to form puboprostatic ligament.
- **Posterior vesical ligaments:** These are actually condensations of connective tissue around neurovascular bundle with venous tributaries from vesical venous plexus which extends from posterolateral aspect of base of bladder to the ventral aspect of sacrum.

False (Peritoneal Ligaments) (Fig. 32.6)

False ligaments are folds of peritoneum raised from urinary bladder to the body of wall. These are as follows:
- **Median umbilical fold**: This is a midline fold of peritoneum extending from apex of urinary bladder to umbilicus. This peritoneal fold lies along the line of urachus which is called *median umbilical ligament*.

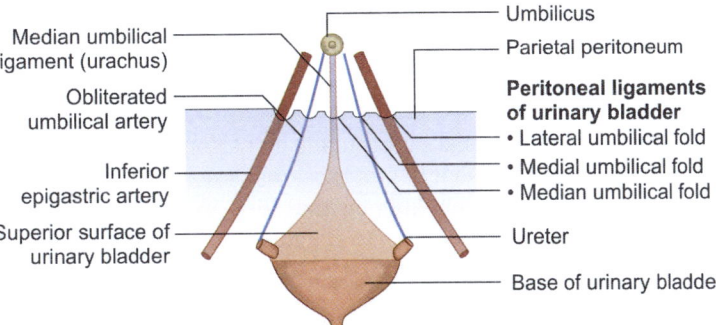

Fig. 32.6: Infraumbilical part of anterior abdominal wall viewed from behind with urinary bladder to show its ligaments.

- **Medial umbilical fold**: It is the bilateral fold of peritoneum extending along the line of **obliterated umbilical artery**. This degenerated part of artery is continued from superior vesical artery extending from the level of urinary bladder to umbilicus.
- **Lateral umbilical fold** is the bilateral fold of peritoneum extending upwards and medially along the line of inferior epigastric artery.

Interior of Urinary Bladder

Interior of urinary bladder is lined by mucous membrane. Except the area opposite the base of bladder, vesical mucous membrane is connected loosely to the subjacent muscular wall. That is why, mucosal surface presents prominent folds or rugosity when the bladder is empty. The folds disappear when the walls are stretched due to distension of organ.

The mucous surface is smooth in a triangular area on the inner surface of base of urinary bladder which is known as trigone of urinary bladder.

Trigone of Urinary Bladder (Fig. 32.7)

Trigone of urinary bladder is a small, smooth triangular area of mucous membrane at the level of lower part of base of the organ. The area is smooth because the mucous membrane is adherent to deeper muscular coat. The apex of the trigone is directed downwards and forwards at the level of internal urethral orifice. It is the site of commencement of urethra. Superolateral angles are the sites of opening of ureter. The ureteric orifices are guarded by mucosal folds called **ureteric**

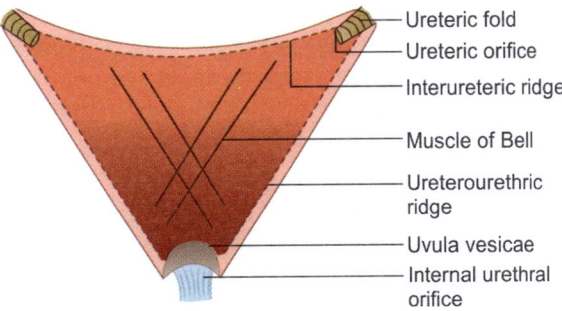

Fig. 32.7: Trigone of urinary bladder.

folds. In empty bladder distance between two ureteric folds is 2.5 cm. In distended condition of bladder the gap increases up to 5 cm. The base of trigone is formed by **interureteric ridge** on the mucosal surface which is formed due to continuation of longitudinal muscle fibers of one ureter to another. Sides of the trigone is formed by **ureterourethric ridge** deep to which longitudinal muscle fibers of ureter extend from ureteric orifice to internal urethral orifice. Beneath the mucosal lining of trigone, some detrusor muscle fibers of bladder present decussation or interlacement which are known as **muscles of Bell**. In case of trigone of male bladder, posterosuperior to inferior angle, an elevation called **uvula vesicae** is caused by median lobe of prostate.

Musculature of Urinary Bladder

Musculature of urinary bladder is made up of smooth muscles which are arranged in *three layers of interlacing bundles* present in cris-cross fashion. This is known as **detrusor muscle**. Characteristic feature of detrusor muscle fibers is that they are larger muscle fibers extending from one wall to another. Some of the fibers are arranged anteroposteriorly along the long axis of bladder passing from superior wall to inferolateral wall across the base. Again some fibers pass along the line at right angle to anteroposterior axis, from superior wall to inferolateral walls of both sides.

Musculature of Bladder Neck

Musculature of bladder neck is distinct from detrusor muscle of bladder wall structurally as well as functionally. That is why it is considered as separate functional unit which is again different in male and female.

Its function is disturbed following bladder neck surgery, particularly following the operation of transurethral resection of prostate (TURP).

Vascular Supply

Arteries

The urinary bladder is principally supplied by superior and inferior vesical arteries which are branches of anterior division of internal iliac artery.

Superior vesical artery: It supplies mainly the posterosuperior part of urinary bladder including the fundus or basal part. The artery gives *multiple branches*. One of the branches supplies vas deferens and is carried along the vas to anastomose with testicular artery. Superior vesical artery represents *proximal patent portion of fetal umbilical artery*. Distal part extends beyond urinary bladder up to umbilicus. It is named as *obliterated umbilical artery*. Superior vesical artery also supplies terminal part of ureter.

Inferior vesical artery: It arises often along with middle rectal artery from anterior division of internal iliac artery. This artery supplies *anteroinferior part of bladder including apex and neck, prostate, seminal vesicle and terminal part of ureter*. It may also supply branches to *vas deferens*.

For urinary bladder, vesical arteries are supplemented by **obturator and inferior gluteal arteries**. In females additional branches come from **uterine and vaginal artery**.

Veins

Veins draining urinary bladder follow the route which is different from arteries. Veins draining out the wall form a plexus on *inferolateral surface and base* known as **vesical venous plexus**. Adjacent to bladder neck, the plexus of veins joins with *prostatic venous plexus*. Finally the veins pass backwards from posterolateral aspect of base *along the route of lateral ligament* of bladder to terminate in the *internal iliac vein*.

Lymphatic Drainage

Lymph vessels draining urinary bladder starts from the plexuses which are arranged in following three planes from within outwards.
1. Mucosal
2. Intermuscular
3. Subserosal

Lymph vessels arising from these plexuses are arranged in the *three sets:*
1. Lymph vessels from **base with trigone** pass superolaterally to **external iliac lymph nodes**.
2. Lymph vessels from **superior surface** converge backwards towards posterolateral angle and pass superolaterally to drain in **external iliac lymph nodes**. From superior surface some vessels drain into **internal iliac** and **common iliac nodes**.
3. Lymph vessels from **inferolateral surface** pass in following two directions:
   a. Some merge with vessels of superior surface
   b. Some vessels pass upwards and forwards to **obturator group** of lymph nodes on obturator fascia.

Nerve Supply

Both parasympathetic and sympathetic components of autonomic nerve for the urinary bladder are distributed through **vesical plexus** embedded in relation to wall of the viscera. Vesical plexus is the part of **pelvic visceral plexus** related close to rectum, internal genitalia and urinary bladder. Nerves of vesical plexus come from **inferior hypogastric plexus** within true pelvis.

Sources of Nerves

- Parasympathetic fibers come from **pelvic splanchnic nerves** formed by the fibers of second, third and fourth sacral segments of spinal cord
- Sympathetic fibers reach the inferior hypogastric plexus from **lower two thoracic and first and second lumbar segments** ($T_{11} - L_2$) of spinal cord.

  Both the parasympathetic as well as sympathetic components contain **motor and sensory fibers**.

  In reference to the nerve supply of urinary bladder, parasympathetic component is known as **nerve of evacuation** and sympathetic as **nerve of filling**.

  When the urinary bladder gets distended, due to stimulation of stretch receptors in the bladder wall, impulse is carried through afferent component of pelvic splanchinc nerves. It results in awareness for fullness of bladder. Efferent component of pelvic splanchinc nerves is motor to detrusor muscle and inhibitory to internal urethral sphincter. So stimulation of this fibers causes evacuation of bladder.

  Sympathetic fibers ($T_{11} - L_2$) for urinary bladder passing through inferior hypogastric plexus and then through vesical plexus contain both afferent as well as efferent components. Physiological pain sensation due to overdistension of urinary bladder or pathological pain (due to calculus or malignancy) are carried through afferent component of sympathetic nerves. Sympathetic efferent fibers stimulates internal urethral sphincter with relaxation of detrusor, so closes the bladder neck.

Micturition

Act of micturition is a **reflex action under voluntary control** in the toilet-trained individual. The process is **under control of higher centers in the brain**.

As soon as the urinary bladder is distended with 300 mL of urine or more, **stretch receptors** in the wall of the bladder are stimulated. Impulse is carried through **afferent component of pelvic splanchnic nerves (S_2, S_3, S_4)** to second, third and fourth sacral segments of spinal cord, thereafter **through dorsal column** of spinal cord **to sensory area of cerebral cortex**. This transmission of impulse gives rise to sense of awareness for fullness of bladder. Parasympathetic **efferent impulse** pass out through second, third and fourth sacral segments of spinal cord and then pass through preganglionic parasympathetic **efferent fibers of pelvic splanchnic nerves** and finally through **inferior hypogastric plexus to the bladder wall**. Here they synapse with postganglionic neurons. Postganglionic fibers, when stimulated, detrusor muscles contract and smooth muscles of sphincter vesicae (internal urethral sphincter) relax. External urethral sphincter (sphincter urethrae) which is a voluntary muscle, also undergoes relaxation due to impulse carried through pudendal nerve (S_2, S_3 and S_4). Thereby as urine is voided from bladder and reach in urethra, **additional afferent impulse** pass **from urethra** to spinal cord **to reinforce the reflex action**.

But this act of micturition is under voluntary control under the influence of cerebral cortex. It means that, simply awareness for micturition as a result of functioning of stretch reflex is not followed by voiding of urine anytime anywhere. Until the time and place for micturition is favorable, the **act is inhibited by descending fibers** passing through **corticospinal tract** from cerebral cortex **to second, third and fourth sacral segments** of spinal cord. Act of micturition is **voluntarily controlled** by contraction of sphincter urethrae (external urethral sphincter). This is further assisted by contraction (stimulation) of sphincter vesicae (internal urethral sphincter) and relaxation (inhibition) of detrusor.

In case of infants, up to age 2–3 years, voluntary control on micturition is not established. Up to this age emptying of bladder is totally dependent upon activity of stretch reflex pathway.

Clinical Anatomy

Congenital Anomalies of Urachus (Figs. 32.8A to C)

Urachus, extending from apex of urinary bladder to umbilicus and representing the distal narrow portion of allantoic diverticulum, normally gets transformed into decanalized round fibrous cord called median umbilical ligament. Developmental defect may give rise to following conditions:

- **Patent urachus**: Urachus persists as a canalized duct extending from apex of the bladder to ubilicus. In case of newborns when umbilical cord is cut off, urine discharges through umbilicus. This condition is usually associated with outflow disorder of urinary bladder.

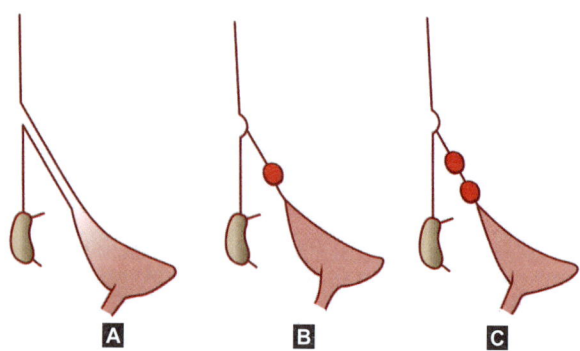

Figs. 32.8A to C: Congenital anomalies of urachus: (A) Patent urachus; (B) Urachal cyst; (C) Lacunae of Lushka.

- **Urachal cyst**: Urachus, while undergoing fibrotic change, may present existence of a small cavity which gradually enlarges into cystic form. It is called urachal cyst. It is usually situated in the midline below umbilicus. Sometimes it is lateral to the midline.
- **Lacunae of Lushka**: These are small multiple cavities in the line of urechus. These remain unnoticed throughout life.

Urinary Retention and Bladder Distension

This condition is called **bladder outflow obstruction**. It is commoner in males. In adult males it occurs as a result of obstruction to the urethra due to benign or malignant **enlargement of prostate** or **stricture of urethra**. Acute retention may also occur in **acute urethritis** or **acute prostatitis**. In females, though rare, acute retention may occur due to inflammation surrounding urethra following herpes.

Normal adult bladder has a capacity of about 500 mL. In case of urinary obstruction, when the urinary bladder remains distended up to limit of 1000 to 1200 mL. It will not cause any permanent damage to bladder wall. Distended bladder is drained through a catheter.

Suprapubic Cystostomy

When the urinary bladder gets distended, it is enlarged and become ovoid in shape to extend up to the level of umbilicus, being interposed in the plane between anterior abdominal wall and parietal

peritoneum. Suprapubic cystostomy is a surgical intervention in which cavity of the urinary bladder distended with water is approached for the following indication through extraperitoneal plane.
- For introduction of in-dwelling catheter for temporary or standby relief of bladder outflow obstruction
- For removal of urinary calculus, foreign bodies or small tumors
- For enucleation of prostate gland through suprapubic route for the management of benign hypertrophy of prostate.

Cystoscopy
It is the procedure of surgical examination, by which mucosa of urinary bladder, two ureteric orifices, internal urethral orifice with uvula vesicae are visualized through a tubular instrument inserted per urethra, called **cystoscope**. After bladder distended with fluid, an *illuminated tubular instrument*, fitted with the *lens*, is introduced into bladder through the urethra.

Cystocele
Cystocele is the herniation of part of urinary bladder occurring through vagina in females. It occurs following difficult childbirth which may cause perineal tear or injury to the pelvic floor.

Bladder Injuries
Urinary bladder may rupture intraperitoneally or extraperitoneally.
- **Intraperitoneal rupture** occurs in cases of *abdominal injury* in distended condition of urinary bladder. It *injures the superior surface* of bladder covered by peritoneum. This surgical condition is more complicated as it *soils the peritoneal cavity* with urine.
- **Extraperitoneal rupture** affecting inferolateral surface occurs in case of fracture of pelvis, when the bony fragments pierce the bladder wall.

Disrupted Motor Function of Urinary Bladder
Disordered act of micturition following **spinal cord injury** is characterized by following types of **neurogenic bladder.**

Atonic bladder
In normal condition, an individual can suspend the act of micturition by voluntary contraction of external urethral sphincter along with maintenance of detrusor muscle tone even with awareness of fullness of bladder. In case of spinal shock, awareness of fullness of bladder is lost with loss of voluntary contraction of external sphincter which becomes relaxed, but internal sphincter is tightly closed. So this condition of atonic bladder with overdistension, tightly closed internal sphincter and relaxed external sphincter causes overflow of urine.

When the period of spinal shock is over, dysfunction of urinary bladder may be one of the following two types depending upon the level of lesion.

Automatic bladder
This type of bladder dysfunction is observed if the lesion of spinal cord above the level of S_2, S_3 and S_4 segments. Following changes are observed.
- External urethra sphincter is relaxed
- When the bladder is distended, impulse from stretch receptor is carried to S_2, S_3 and S_4 segments by afferent fibers of pelvic splanchnic nerves. Stimulation of motor neuronal roots of same segments through interneurons completes the activity of local segmental reflex arc to lead to contraction of detrusor with relaxation of internal sphincter which results emptying of bladder.

So, through activity of local reflex pathway, bladder once distended, becomes empty automatically. That is why it is called automatic bladder.

Autonomous bladder

This type of urinary dysfunction occurs **when spinal injury causes lesion in sacral segments (namely S_2, S_3 and S_4) of spinal cord**. In this case, bladder is deprived of both supraspinal voluntary control as well as local reflex control. The bladder wall becomes flaccid and urine gets accumulated more and more with overdistension of the organ. As the sphincters are ineffective, overdistension of bladder is characterized by continuous dribbling.

SA 32.2 Write a brief note on the pelvic part of the ureter.

PELVIC PART OF URETER (FIG. 32.9)

Pelvic part of ureter begins as continuation of its abdominal part at the level of pelvic brim in front of sacroiliac joint. In the pelvis, the ureter lies in extraperitoneal areolar tissue. First, it runs **downwards and laterally** on the lateral wall of true pelvis **along the anterior border of greater sciatic notch**. Then, at the level of **ischial spine** it runs **forwards and medially** into the adipose tissue **above the levator ani** to reach the **superolateral angle of base of urinary bladder**.

In males, the pelvic ureter is **hooked by the vas deferens** near the superolateral angle of urinary bladder. Then it traverses obliquely the muscular wall of urinary bladder to open into the ipsilateral trigonal angle. Its terminal part is surrounded by the tributaries of vesical veins.

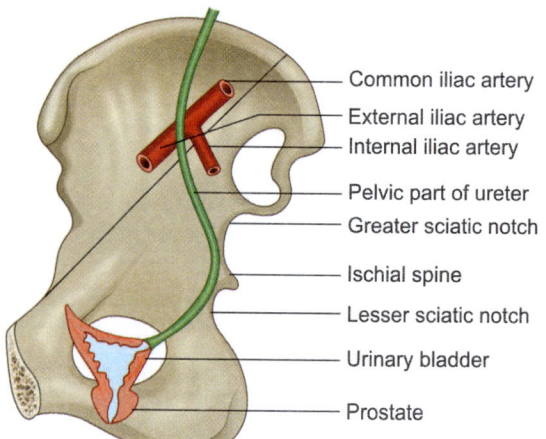

Fig. 32.9: Pelvic part of the ureter.

In females, anteromedial part of the course of pelvic ureter, while running above the levator ani, is related to the **uterine artery, uterine cervix** and **lateral fornices of vagina**. This part of ureter lies in the extraperitoneal connective tissue related to the inferomedial part of the **broad ligament**, bilayered peritoneal fold connecting the lateral margin of uterus to the lateral pelvic wall. Here, the ureter is crossed by the uterine artery 2 cm lateral to the uterine cervix. Then, the ureter inclines medially to reach the superolateral angle of the base of urinary bladder.

Chapter 33

Organs of Male Reproductive System

LA 33.1 Discuss briefly the prostate gland under the following headings:
Gross anatomy; Capsules and ligaments; Lobes; Relations; Interior (prostatic urethra); Vascular supply and lymphatic drainage; Nerve supply; Microstructure; Age changes; Zonal anatomy; Clinical anatomy.

PROSTATE GLAND

Introduction

Prostate is an organ of male reproductive system. It is a fibromusculoglandular organ having following ratio of three structural elements.
1. Fibrous tissue (25%)—mainly collagen fibers
2. Muscular tissue (25%)—mainly smooth muscles with some skeletal muscle fibers
3. Glandular tissue (50%)—exocrine glands
   Prostate is firm in consistency with the glandular element embedded in fibromuscular stroma.

Position of Prostate (Fig. 33.1)

- Prostate, looking like a chestnut, is pyramidal in shape with the base directed upwards and apex downwards.
- It rest below the neck of urinary bladder from which demarcated by a circular sulcus lodging plexus of veins.
- Beyond a small segment of urethra, from neck of bladder, called *preprostatic urethra*, prostate encircle proximalmost 3 cm of urethra, named p*rostatic urethra.*
- Below, the apex of prostate rests on urogenital diaphragm bounded by *superior and inferior fascia of urogenital diaphragm* outlining d*eep perineal pouch* which contains membranous part of urethra encircled by external urethral sphincter.

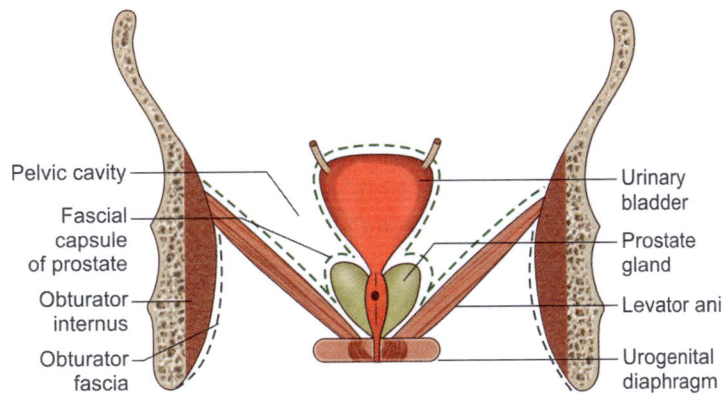

Fig. 33.1: Position and relations of prostate (coronal section view).

- Prostate is situated behind pubic arch with lower end of pelvic surface of body of pubis and in front of lower part of rectum.

Dimensions

- Transverse measurement = 4 cm
- Vertical measurement = 3 cm
- Anteroposterior measurement = 2 cm

Note: *Following structures in the body possess transverse measurement (breadth) more than vertical measurement (length)*
- *Pituitary gland*
- *Isthmus of thyroid gland*
- *Celiac trunk*
- *Cecum*
- *Prostate*

Weight

- In **young adults**, prostate weighs about **8 g**.
- But **after first five decades** of life, prostate usually enlarges as a result of **benign hypertrophy of prostate (BHP)** with increase in weight up to **40 g**.
- But sometimes weight may increase as much as **150 g**.

Functions

- Prostate, being a gland of male reproductive system, liberates a thin milky fluid which *increases the bulk of seminal fluid* at the time of ejaculation.
- Smooth muscles of the organ squeezes the secretion into prostatic urethra.
- Prostatic secretion contains **citric acid and acid phosphatase**. The **secretion is alkaline** in nature and neutralizes acid media of vagina.

Features of the Gland (Figs. 33.2 and 33.3)

Base of the pyramidal prostate is directed upwards and on it rests the *neck of urinary bladder*, separated by a *circular groove* containing *plexus of veins*.

Apex is directed downwards supported by *urogenital diaphragm*, two fascial layers of which, superior and inferior, outline *deep perineal pouch*. Through the pouch, membranous part of urethra passes vertically, encircled by external urethral sphincter made up of voluntary muscles.

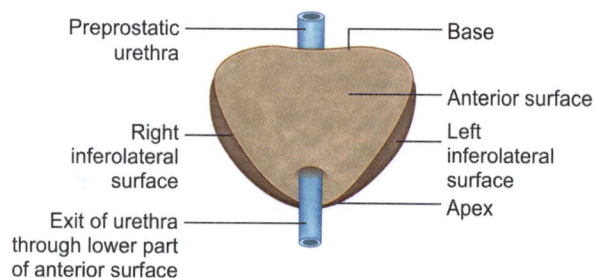

Fig. 33.2: Anterior view of prostate gland.

Beside the base (upper surface), prostate presents following surfaces:
- **Anterior surface**
- **Posterior surface**
- **Two (right and left) inferolateral surfaces.**

Proximal 3 cm of urethra, called **prostatic urethra** passes through the gland vertically to become continuous below with membranous urethra.

Prostatic *urethra traverses through the gland more close to anterior surface than posterior*. It comes out below not through the apex, but piercing lower part of anterior surface close to the apex.

Actually, prostatic urethra passes vertically between the anterior and middle third of gland (Fig. 33.3).

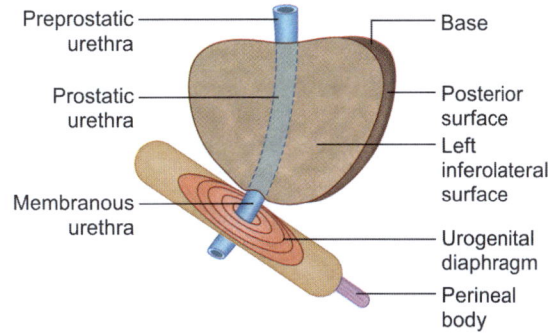

Fig. 33.3: Lateral view of prostate gland.

Capsules and Ligaments (Fig. 33.4)

Previously, the prostate was considered to have two capsules which used to be ideally termed as **inner and outer capsules**. Inner capsule, called *true capsule*, was considered to be the condensation of fibroconnective tissue on the surface of gland. But as per newer concept, in healthy normal prostate gland, till the age of onset of BPH, i.e. 50 years, there is no existence of inner capsule. It is only following BPH when proliferated glandular element pushes peripherally the connective tissue which is thus condensed to form **inner fibrous capsule** of the gland.

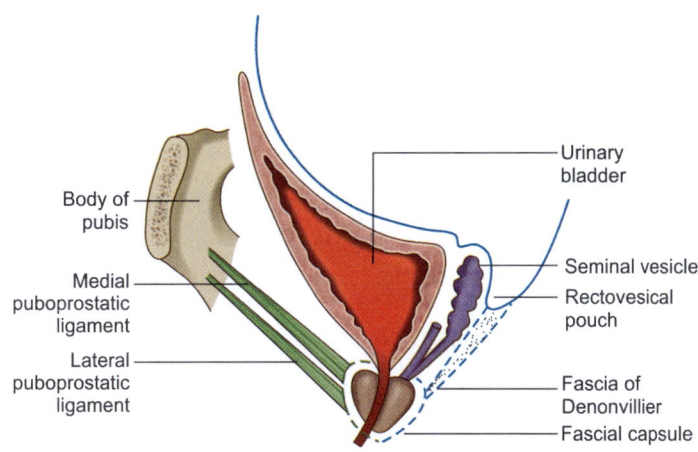

Fig. 33.4: Fascial capsule and ligaments of prostate.

The original capsule outside, formed by visceral layer of pelvic fascia, thereby called **fascial capsule** of prostate, **exists throughout the life as per modern concept**.

Structural characteristics of anterior and posterior parts of fascial capsule: Anteriorly, two pairs of bilateral fibrous bands extend from pelvic surface of body of pubis to anterior aspect of the capsule of prostate called:
1. **Medial puboprostatic ligament**: Attached more close to base of prostate.
2. **Lateral puboprostatic ligament**: Attached more close to apex of prostate.

Fascial capsule over posterior surface of prostate is condensed and named as **rectovesical fascia of Denonvilliers**. It is so called because it is prolonged upwards up to bottom of rectovesical pouch in between base of bladder and rectum. In fetal life rectovesical pouch used to extend up to perineal body. Subsequently lowermost part of the pouch obliterates with fusion of anterior and posterior layers. A potential space exists between the two layers. Anterior of the two layers is firmly attached to posterior aspect of prostate to form its fascial capsule. Posterior layer is loosely attached to visceral layer of pelvic fascia (Waldayer's fascia) of rectum. Bilaminar fascia of Denonvillier extends therefore from bottom of rectovesical pouch to perineal body.

In case of perineal prostatectomy operation, a surgeon must have anatomical knowledge of **space of Denonvilliers** which is a potential space between the two layers of fascia. As surgeon approaches through this plane, injury or damage to the rectum can be avoided.

Prostatic Venous Plexus in Relation to Capsule

Following benign hypertrophy of prostate (BHP), as inner fibrous capsule is defined by condensation of fibroconnective tissue of the gland on its surface, prostatic venous plexus is well secured in the plane between two capsules. It gives an advantage for enucleation of gland in prostatectomy operation, leaving the venous plexus secured and undisturbed between inner and outer capsules.

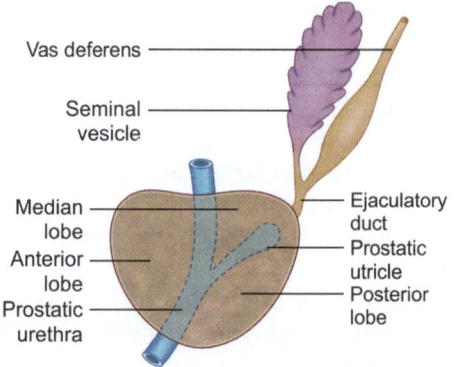

Fig. 33.5: Lobes of prostate in normal adult (lateral view).

In case of prostate of normal healthy young adult and also till the stage of BHP, prostatic venous plexus lies beneath the fascial capsule. Anterior part is known as **dorsal venous plexus**. It receives **deep dorsal vein of penis** lying in front of fascial capsule of prostate.

Neurovascular bundle is embedded bilaterally on the posterolateral aspect of fascial capsule. It contains *autonomic nerve* fibers, carried from inferior hypogastric plexus, which supply *prostate, urethra, seminal vesicle with ejaculatory duct* and moreover the *erectile tissue of penis*. Following radical prostatectomy for management of carcinoma of prostate, the patient may develop impotency as postoperative complication due to injury of these autonomic nerve fibers.

Lobes of Prostate

Earlier, the prostate gland was thought to be divided into five anatomical lobes as follows.

1. Anterior lobe
2. Posterior lobe
3. Median lobe
4. Right lateral lobe
5. Left lateral lobe

But nowadays, it is recognized that the five lobes can only be distinguished in fetal life **prior to 20 weeks'** of gestation. Beyond that period, the lobes are only three which are mentioned below (Fig. 33.5):

1. **Median lobe**: It is the upper and posterior part of the gland behind the upper part of the prostatic urethra and, above and in front of the **prostatic utricle** which opens in posterior wall of prostatic urethra and represents the caudal most part of the **paramesonephric duct** in male. It is the **wedge-shaped part** of the gland bounded posterolaterally by the intraprostatic part of common ejaculatory ducts.

   Median lobe of prostate is placed below the neck of urinary bladder in relation to the short segment of **preprostatic urethra**. Median lobe contains adequate glandular tissue. These are **subtrigonal** and **subcervical mucous glands** which are quite distinct from main prostatic glands. These glands are clinically important because mild degree of enlargement of these glands may even lead to obstruction to the urinary outflow **(outflow obstruction)**.

   Median lobe of prostate forms a crescentic elevation on the mucosal surface of posterosuperior margin of the internal urethral orifice. It is called **uvula vesicae**.

2. **Anterior lobe** is the part of the gland in front of the prostatic urethra. It is made up of only the fibromuscular stroma with little or no glandular tissue. So, the benign hypertrophy of the prostate gland is very rare to occur in this part of the gland.

3. **Posterior lobe** is behind the prostatic urethra and below the median lobe. Primary carcinoma starts from this lobe.

In normal adult prostate, both the anterior and posterior lobes merge with each other laterally.

In case of **benign hypertrophy of prostate (BHP),** as the prostatic anatomy is distorted, clinicians consider the prostate to be made up of **five lobes** with prominence of **additional two lateral lobes.**

Relations of Prostate (Figs. 33.1 and 33.4)

- **Base** of the prostate, directed upwards, is related to *neck of urinary bladder*. Junction of these two organs is related to a *venous plexus*.
- **Apex**, directed downwards, rests on *urogenital diaphragm* bounded by its *superior and inferior fascial layer* in between which lies *external urethral sphincter*.
- **Anterior surface** is related to *pubic arch* and lower part of *symphysis pubis* from which the gland is separated by *retropubic pad of fat* which contains *deep dorsal vein of penis*.
  - The space is traversed by *medial and lateral puboprostatic ligaments*.
  - Lower end of anterior surface, close to the apex, presents the *exit of prostatic urethra* which is continuous below with membranous part of urethra.
- **Posterior surface**, covered by specialized part of fascial capsule, *fascia of Denonvillier*, is related to lower *ampullary part of rectum*.
- **Inferolateral surfaces** are related to the gutter, on either side of midline, formed by *pelvic diaphragm*. *Levator ani muscle* of both sides, covered by its fascia forms the pelvic diaphragm.

Interior of Prostate (Fig. 33.6)

Prostate gland is vertically traversed from above downwards by **prostatic part of urethra** as a continuation of short segment of **preprostatic urethra** at the neck of urinary bladder.

Prostatic urethra, continued below as membranous urethra, is 3 cm long and fusiform in outline as viewed in coronal section **(Fig. 33.6)**. Posterior wall of prostatic urethra presents following specialized features:

- **Urethral crest**: It is a narrow vertical midline ridge.
- **Colliculus seminalis**: It is a small round bulge at the middle of urethral crest.

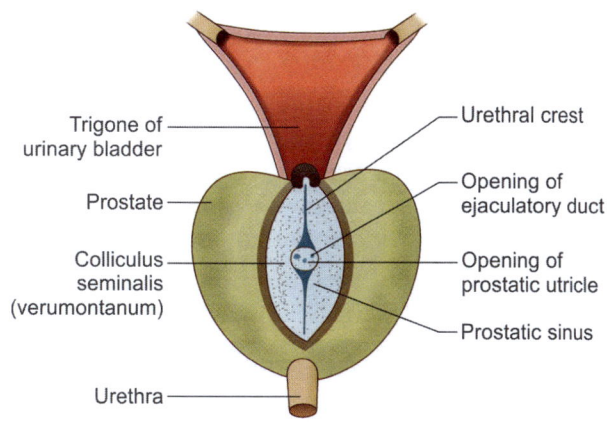

Fig. 33.6: Interior of prostate (features of posterior wall).

- Center of colliculus seminalis presents an opening of a tiny blind sac, called **prostatic utricle** which is directed upwards and backward along the midline of prostatic tissue, thus cutting off the median (middle) lobe from posterior lobe of the gland **(Fig. 33.5)**. Prostatic utricle embryologically represents the persistent fused lowermost end of both **paramesonephric ducts** in male.
- **Openings of common ejaculatory ducts** are present on colliculus seminalis on either side of opening of prostatic utricle. Before opening on prostatic urethra, ejaculatory ducts pass

downwards, forwards and medially through prostatic tissue, demarcating posterolaterally the median lobe from anterior and posterior lobes.
- **Prostatic sinus:** This is a narrow depression on either side of urethral crest on posterior wall of prostatic urethra. Ducts of the prostatic glandular follicles open here.

Vascular Supply and Lymphatic Drainage

Arteries Supplying the Prostate
- Inferior vesical artery
- Middle rectal artery and
- Internal pudendal artery

Branches from these arteries perforate the prostatic fascia along **posterolateral line from vesicoprostatic junction towards the apex of gland**. This line is important **guide for the neurovascular plane** in case of radical prostatectomy.

Veins from the prostate open into the venous plexus **(retropubic venous plexus)** behind arcuate pubic ligament and lower part of pubic symphysis. This plexus also receives **deep dorsal vein of penis** and communicates posteriorly through **vesical venous plexus** with **internal iliac vein**.

Lymphatic Drainage

Lymph vessels from prostate join with vesical lymph vessels and pass along two different routes.
1. *Anterolateral:* End in *internal iliac group* of lymph nodes.
2. *Posterior:* Drain in *external iliac nodes*.

Nerve Supply

Abundant autonomic nerve supply for the prostate is derived from **inferior hypogastric plexus**. Production as well as discharge of prostatic secretion are facilitated by both sympathetic and parasympathetic fibers.

A **periprostatic nerve plexus** is embedded in fascial capsule of prostate. These nerve fibers form a definable **neurovascular bundle** closely applied to the posterolateral part of fascial capsule, but easily separable. Nerve fibers from this bundle, apart from supplying prostate, ejaculatory duct, seminal vesicle, urethra, also supply erectile tissue of penis. During radical prostatectomy operation in carcinoma of prostate, these nerves need to be carefully preserved to avoid impotency as a postoperative complication.

Somatic nerve fibers through **pudendal nerve** supply **external urethral sphincter**. In case of radical prostatectomy operation, while neck of bladder and membranous urethra are sutured together, injury to these nerve fibers are avoided.

MICROSTRUCTURE (FIG. 33.7)

About 50% of the prostate gland is made up of **glandular element** and the remaining part constitutes the **fibromuscular stroma**. The glandular element is present in the form of **numerous follicles**. The follicles open in elongated canals which join together to form **15–20 main ducts**. Adjacent follicles, separated by fibromuscular stroma are separated by **connective tissue septa**. The stroma contains **smooth muscles fibers**.

Epithelium lining the follicles are **predominantly simple columnar**. It may be **pseudostratified**. The lining epithelium characteristically shows **infoldings** towards the lumen. Prostatic ducts are lined by **bilayered low columnar cells**. Some colloid material, called **amyloid bodies (corpora amylacea)** are often found within the follicles.

Prostatic secretion contains **acid phosphatase, amylase, prostate specific antigen (PSA), fibrinolysin** and **zinc**.

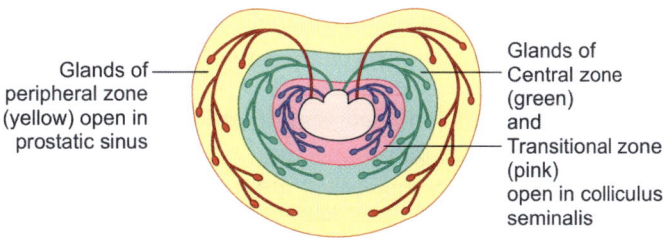

Fig. 33.7: Submucosal glands of different zones of prostate.

Neuroendocrine cells are present in the follicular epithelial lining. But their exact functions are not known. The number of these cells gets reduced after middle age.

Position of the glands are **submucosal.** They are broadly to **two types** arranged in *two zones* (Fig. 33.7):
1. **Glands of wider peripheral zone present long branched duct** which open in **prostatic sinus**.
2. **Glands of narrower central** and **transitional zones** possess **shorter ducts** which open in **colliculus seminalis** and also in **prostatic sinus**.

Some **small mucous glands** from **preprostatic urethra** open in **anterior wall** of the prostatic urethra. Though these glands are smaller, they may be enlarged in benign hypertrophy of prostate (BHP). It will cause enlargement of the median lobe of prostate which presses the internal urethral orifice from its posterior aspect (uvula vesicae).

Age Changes in Prostate

- **Before birth**: **Maternal estrogen** causes **squamous metaplasia of the ducts**
- **At birth:**
  - **Fibromuscular stroma** becomes proportionately the **larger component**
  - **Glandular element** is represented by **simple duct system**
- **At puberty (14–18 years):**
  - Size of the **glandular component** gets **doubled**
  - **Development of follicles** passes through the **maturation phase**
- **At the age of 17–18 years**
  - Initial **multilayered glandular epithelium is transformed into pseudostratified epithelium** with variety of following types of cells:
    ◊ Basal cells
    ◊ Exocrine secretory cells
    ◊ Mucous secreting cells
    ◊ Neuroendocrine cells
  - **Exocrine products are:**
    ◊ *Acid phosphatase*
    ◊ *Amylase*
    ◊ *Prostate specific antigen (PSA)*
    ◊ *B. microseminoprotein*
    ◊ *Zinc*
  - Stroma is condensed and proportionally reduced
- During third decades
  Follicles show infolding due to irregular multiplication of glandular epithelium.

- **Up to 45–50 years:**
  During this period, prostate passes through the **stage of involution** which shows following changes:
  - Follicular infoldings get abolished
  - Outlines of the follicles become more regular
  - Amyloid bodies increase in number
- **After 50 years:**
  The change is characterized by **benign hypertrophy of prostate (BHP)** with following features:
  - In an average, the size may increase up to **40 g**
  - **Glandular component is hypertrophied**, specially the **median lobe** part
  - **Fibroconnective tissue** component becomes **condensed** and pushed to the periphery to form the **inner fibrous capsule**.
- Instead of BHP, in some cases, the prostate may pass through the stage of **senile atrophy**.

Zonal Anatomy (Fig. 33.8)

From anatomical point of view, glandular element of prostate is divided into following three distinct zones:
1. Transitional zone = 5% by volume
2. Central zone = 25% by volume
3. Peripheral zone = 70% by volume.

Fibromuscular stroma (nonglandular tissue) fills up the gap between the right and left halves of peripheral zone in front of prostatic urethra.

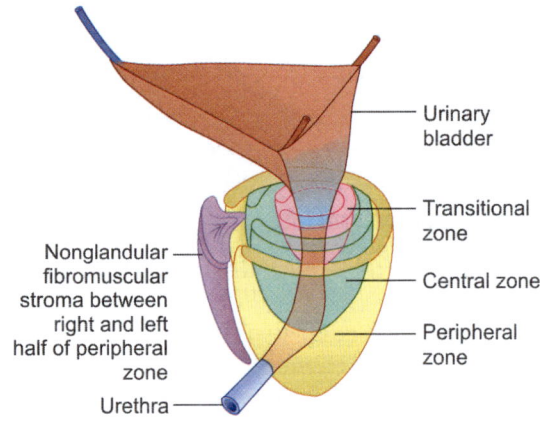

Fig. 33.8: Zones of the prostate.

- **Transitional zone** *encircles the distal part of preprostatic urethra and is positioned just proximal to apex of central zone.* Simple *mucus secreting glands* are situated in the tissue *around preprostatic urethra.* These glands are histologically not like the typical glands of prostate. Structurally they are *identical to glands of female urethra*. Transitional zone is so called because, it is situated between mucus secreting preprostatic glandular zone and main bulk of typical prostatic glands of other zones.
- **Central zone** *surrounds the ejaculatory ducts*, but lies *on the posterior aspect of preprostatic urethra*. It is conical in shape with the apex directed distally at the level of colliculus seminalis.
- **Peripheral zone** is the largest and encloses the posterior as well as both lateral aspect of preprostatic urethra and, transitional as well as central zone in a clasping manner. Anterior to urethra, two halves of peripheral zone are bridged by nonglandular fibromuscular stroma.

Clinical Anatomy

Clinical Examination of Prostate

Prostate gland is examined clinically for its pathology by digital examination per rectum **(PR examination).** Examiner's gloved index finger introduced per rectum palpates posterior surface of prostate **for its apparent size in enlargement, consistency** and **fixing to surrounding structures**.

Benign Hypertrophy of Prostate

Benign hypertrophy of prostate (BHP) is common in elderly men around the age of 50 years. The cause is possibly the imbalance in hormonal control of the gland. Enlargement of median lobe which corresponds to transitional zone of prostate with abundance of glandular element, is responsible for clinical manifestation of BHP. Median lobe enlarges upwards and encroaches towards posterior aspect of neck of bladder making the uvula vesicae more prominent, thus causing difficulty in micturition. Enlargement of median as well as lateral lobes as a whole will cause elongation and distortion of the prostatic urethra which results in narrow urinary stream. Further, leakage of urine in the prostatic urethra, through narrowed internal urethral orifice leads to *frequent and intense reflex desire for micturition* which explains the frequency. Due to enlargement of uvula vesicae at the bladder neck, a pouch of stagnant urine *(residual urine)* is formed within the bladder behind internal urethral orifice. The residual urine leads to *recurrent urinary tract infection*.

Prostate—its Normal Functioning and Disease

Normal secretory activity of glandular component of prostate in under influence of androgen and estrogen circulating in bloodstream. Prostatic secretion which adds to the bulk of seminal fluid contains an *enzyme* in large amount called **acid phosphatase**. In clinical condition, as in *carcinoma of prostate*, follicular cells fail to liberate this enzyme. So, the *serum acid phosphatase* level increases.

Normally, a small amount of protein is synthesized by follicular epithelial cells of prostate. For this **prostate specific antigen (PSA)** are found in blood. In case of diseases like cancer of prostate PSA level rises.

Carcinoma of Prostate

When the median lobe is the site for benign hypertrophy of the prostate, the lateral lobes, forming the peripheral zone are the sites for origin of carcinoma of prostate. Per rectal digital examination reveals hard and irregular surface of prostate.

Metastasis

Dissemination of cancer cells of prostate occurs through venous channels. Prostatic venous plexus joins with vesical venous plexus at the neck of bladder. The plexus also receives deep dorsal vein of penis. Veins from the plexus drain into internal iliac vein. Vertebral venous plexus also communicates with internal iliac vein through veins coming out through ventral sacral foramina. These veins are devoid of valves, so through venous channel, metastasis may occur in vertebral bodies.

Prostatectomy

As per recent concept, there is existence of only one fascial capsule of prostate derived from pelvic fascia. In case of benign hypertrophy of prostate fibrous tissue element of the gland becomes condensed to form another inner capsule keeping the venous plexus and neurovascular bundle outside it. This gives an advantage for enucleation of prostate gland, leaving behind both the capsules with neurovascular plexus. This kind of prostatectomy can be done through **transvesical route**. Other approaches for prostatectomy are as follows:
- **Retropubic route**: The gland is approached through capsule.
- **Perineal route**: Through the plane of fascia of Denonvillier
- **Transurethral route**: The operation is named *transurethral resection* (TUR).

SA 33.2 Describe the vas deferens with a note on clinical anatomy.

VAS DEFERENS

Introduction

Vas deferens or ductus deferens is a narrow thick-walled tubular structure derived from the mesonephric duct in male.

Function

- It is for transport of sperm from the epididymis to the urethra
- Recently, it is considered to have absorptive and secretory function.
- Extent:
  - **Beginning**: Vas deferens starts as continuation of tail of epididymis at the level of lower pole of testis within scrotal sac.
  - **Termination:** Distal end of vas deferens joins with the duct of seminal vesicle near the base of prostate within the true pelvis to form the **ejaculatory duct**. Finally through the ejaculatory duct, it opens in the posterior wall of the prostate urethra.
- **Length**: 45 cm (18 inches).
- **Caliber:** Lumen of the vas deferens is narrow with a thick, muscular wall for which it is felt like a cord.

Course and Relations (Fig. 33.9)

- **In the scrotum**: Vas deferens ascends along the posterior border of testis, medial to the epididymis. It joins with the other components of the spermatic cord at the level of upper pole of the testis.
- **In the inguinal canal**: As the most important constituent of the spermatic cord, it passes upwards, backwards and laterally through the inguinal canal from superficial inguinal ring to deep inguinal ring.
- **In the false pelvis**: Beyond the deep inguinal ring, the vas deferens hooks round the inferior epigastric artery to pass medially crossing the external iliac artery.

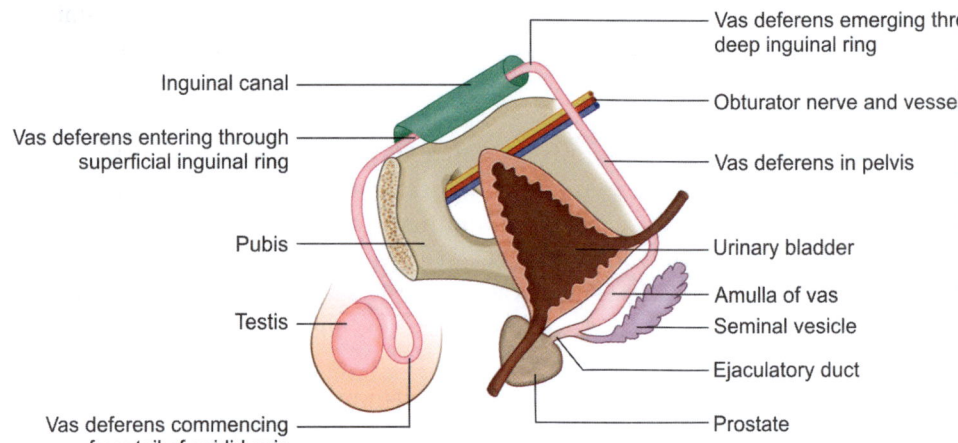

Fig. 33.9: Course and relations of vas deferens.

- **In the true pelvis**: It descends along the lateral pelvic wall crossing the obliterated umbilical artery and the obturator nerve and vessels and run for a short distance over the levator ani.
- **At the base of bladder**: Reaching the superolateral angle of the urinary bladder, the vas deferens kinks around the terminal end of ureter and change its direction again to pass downwards and medially behind the base of urinary bladder. It approaches the base of prostate lying medial to the seminal vesicle. This terminal end of the vas in relation to the bladder base is dilated and slightly tortuous to be called the **ampulla of vas deferens**.
- **As ejaculatory duct**: While passing downwards and medially in relation to the base of urinary bladder, the vas is joined from the lateral side by the duct of seminal vesicle to form the ejaculatory duct.

The ejaculatory ducts of both sides pierce the base of the prostate just behind the neck of urinary bladder and pass downwards forwards and medially forming the lateral boundary of the median lobe of prostate.

Finally, both the ducts open on the surface of colliculus seminalis on either side of the opening of prostate utricle.

Arterial Supply

- **Artery to the vas deferens** usually arises from the **superior vesical** and **inferior vesical arteries**
- It may be supplied by branches from the **testicular artery**, while in inguinal region
- Additional branch may arise from the **middle rectal artery**, while in the pelvis.

Venous Drainage

- Veins from the vas deferens drain into the **internal iliac vein** through **vesical venous plexus**
- Veins from lower proximal end of the vas drain into the **pampiniform plexus**.

Nerve Supply

Vas deferens receives the supply of rich postganglionic **sympathetic** nerves from the **pelvic plexus**.

Clinical Anatomy

Vasectomy is simple surgical operation adopted for sterilization in males. In this operation a short segment of vas within the scrotum is excised. The cut ends are ligated. It will stop the sperms to be added in seminal fluid. The sperms, continued to be produced, are degenerated and absorbed in the epididymis.

SA 33.3 Write a brief note on layers of scrotum with blood supply, nerve supply and clinical anatomy.

SCROTUM

Introduction

Scrotum is a Latin word meaning 'bag'. Scrotum is a sac of skin formed as an autpouching of lower part of anterior abdominal wall. It is posteroinferior to the penis. The sac is divided into two halves. Each half contains testis, epididymis and lower part of the spermatic cord.

Surface Features (Fig. 33.10)

Right and left halves of the scrotum is divided by a median ridge or raphe. The raphe is continued forwards to the midline of undersurface of penis. Posteriorly, it is continued along the midline of perineum up to the anus.

Skin of the scrotum is darker in color and presents corrugations (rugosity) on the surface, due to presence of the subcutaneous muscle called '*dartos*'.

The left half of the scrotum usually hangs slightly at a lower level due to a little more length of the left spermatic cord.

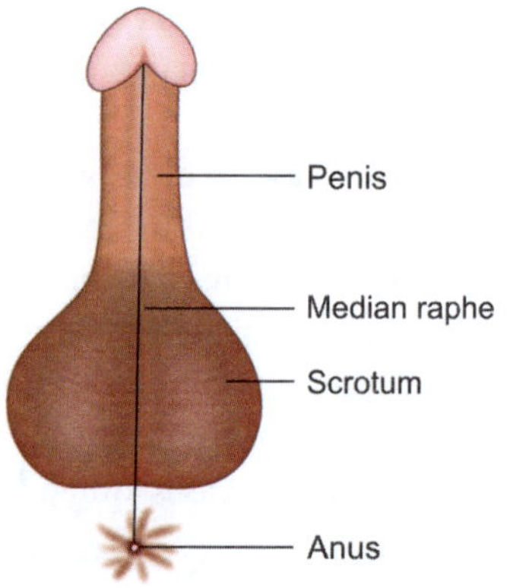

Layers of Scrotum (Fig. 33.11)

It has already been mentioned that scrotum is the outpouching from the lower part of anterior abdominal wall.

So the layers of the wall of scrotum correspond more or less to the layers of anterior abdominal wall. The layers of scrotum are as follows from outside inwards:

- **Skin** is thin and pigmented, hair bearing, devoid of fat and rich in sebaceous and sweat glands.
- **Dartos muscle** is a layer of **smooth muscle** representing the layer of superficial fascia of anterior abdominal wall. It is continuous with:
  - Fascia of Scarpa of anterior abdominal wall
  - Colles' fascia of perineum
  - Superficial fascia (dartos fascia) of penis.

  Layer of dartos muscle maintains optimum temperature within the scrotal sac to facilitate spermatogenesis in the testis.
- **External spermatic fascia** is continuation of the aponeurosis of external oblique.
- **Cremasteric muscle and fascia** is continuation of the internal oblique muscle.
  Transversus abdominis muscle is not continued in the scrotum.
- **Internal spermatic fascia** is continued from the fascia transversalis of anterior abdominal wall.
  Layer 3, 4 and 5 are prolonged in the scrotum beyond the spermatic cord.

Fig. 33.10: Scrotum with penis viewed from ventral aspect.

Blood Supply

Arteries supplying the scrotum are:
- Superficial external pudendal artery—branch of femoral artery
- Deep external pudendal arery—branch of femoral artery

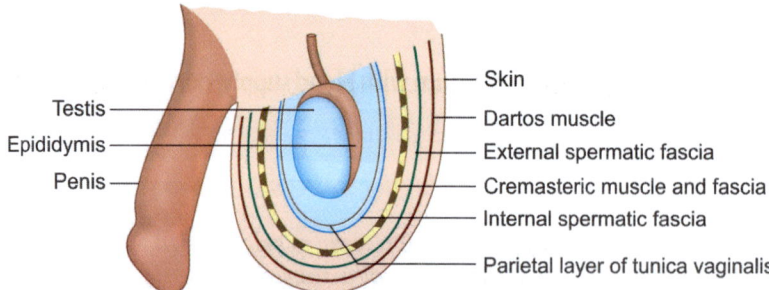

Fig. 33.11: Layers of the scrotum.

- Scrotal branch of internal pudendal artery
- Cremasteric branch of inferior epigastric artery.

Veins of the scrotum correspond to the arteries.

Lymphatic drainage: To superficial inguinal lymph nodes.

Nerve Supply

Sensory Nerves

- **Anterior one third:** Ilioinguinal nerve and genital branch of genitofemoral nerve.
- **Posterior two thirds:** Posterior scrotal branch of perineal nerve and perineal branch of posterior cutaneous nerve of thigh.

Motor Nerve

Dartos, being the involuntary (smooth) muscle, is supplied by the sympathetic nerves carried through the genital branch of genitofemoral nerve.

Clinical Anatomy

- **Scrotal edema** is characterized by swelling of scrotal skin and subcutaneous tissue following any infection in scrotum and surrounding area. This is due to the dependent position of the scrotum and laxity of its skin.
- **Sebaceous cysts** of scrotum are very often detected clinically due to abundance of sebaceous glands in its skin.
- **Scrotal swelling** is the clinical condition which is most commonly due to **complete inguinal hernia** or **vaginal hydrocele**. Swelling in case of vaginal hydrocele is due to accumulation of fluid with the peritoneal sac (tunica vaginalis) of the testis lying within the scrotum.
- **Elephantiasis of scrotum** is the clinical condition characterized by huge swelling of skin and subcutaneous tissue due to fungal infection or allergic reaction.

> **LA 33.4** Discuss briefly the testis under the following headings:
> Introduction with surface features; Anatomical position and side determination (for Viva voce and practical only); Coverings; Structure; Vascular supply, lymphatic drainage and nerve supply; Descent of testis; Clinical anatomy.

TESTIS

Introduction

Testis is the male gonad homologous to the ovary in female. It lies within the corresponding half of the scrotal sac and is suspended by the spermatic cord.

Function

- Testis produces spermatozoa
- It liberates the hormone, testosterone responsible for growth and maintenance of secondary sexual characteristics in male.

Gross Surface Features

Testis is ovoid in shape and flattened from side to side
It measures as follows:
- Vertically = 4 cm
- Anteroposteriorly = 3 cm
- Side to side = 2.5 cm

Ovoid testis presents **(Fig. 33.12)**:
- **2 poles**: Upper and lower
- **2 borders**: Anterior and posterior
- **2 surfaces**: Lateral and medial

Surface of the testis is smooth everywhere except the posterior border which is related to the spermatic cord. Smooth appearance is due to visceral layer of tunica vaginalis.

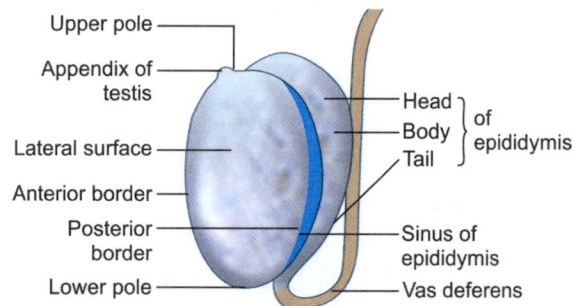

Fig. 33.12: Left testis with epididymis and vas deferens viewed from lateral side.

Anatomical Position and Side Determination

Specimen of testis is always found to be along with the epididymis and spermatic cord. Interrelation of these three structures are to be noted. Spermatic cord ascends along the posterior border of the testis which is masked. Epididymis, with its broader head end upward lies lateral to the spermatic cord.

A curved slit or narrow cleft, called the **sinus of epididymis** faces laterally. It is formed due to reflection of peritoneal lining, the visceral layer of tunica vaginalis, from the testis to the epididymis.

After confirmation of above-mentioned features, the following points are to be noted for anatomical position and side determination.
- **Upper pole** of the testis connected to the head of comma shaped epididymis is directed **upwards, forwards and laterally**
- **Anterior free border** faces forwards
- **Sinus of the epididymis** facing laterally will determine the side.

Coverings

From outside inwards, testis presents following three coverings:
1. Visceral layer of tunica vaginalis—serous layer of peritoneum.
2. Tunica albuginea—dense fibrous layer.
3. Tunica vasculosa—fine network of blood vessels embedded in reticular tissue.

Visceral layer of tunica vaginalis forms the outermost covering of the testis. Tunica vaginalis is a serous sac which represents the persistent distal part of the processus vaginalis. As this sac is invaginated by the testis from behind, the visceral layer of tunica vaginalis covers the testis all around except the posterior border which is closely related to the vas deferens medially and epididymis laterally in vertical disposition.

Tunica albuginea is the intermediate, thick fibrous coat of the testis. Along the posterior border of the testis this fibrous coat presents following characteristics:
- Along this line, tunica albuginea is not covered by tunica vaginalis
- Blood vessels and nerves of the testis traverse along this line
- An incomplete fibrous septum, called **mediastinum testis** enters the gland along this line vertically.

Tunica vasculosa is the innermost thin vascular layer of the testis. It is made up of network of finer blood vessels embedded in thin layer of fibroareolar tissue.

STRUCTURE OF THE TESTIS (FIG. 33.13)

The testis is made up of 200 to 300 tiny compartments called **lobules of the testis**. Each of the lobules are conical in outline with the narrow end directed backwards. Adjacent lobules are separated by fibrous septa which radiate from anterior border of the mediastinum testis to reach up to the deeper surface of tunica albuginea.

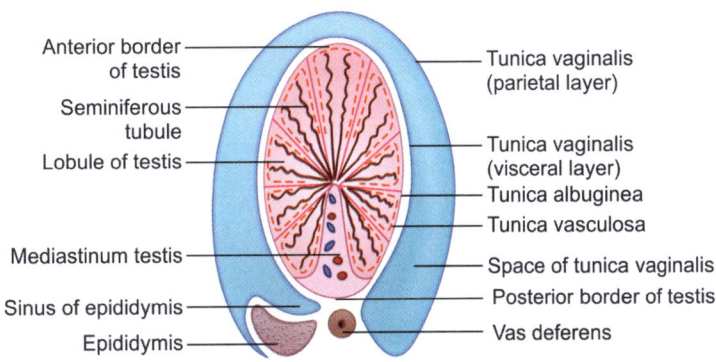

Fig. 33.13: Gross structure of testis on cross section (left).

Each of the lobules of the testis contains 2 to 3 narrow coiled **seminiferous tubules** with their blind peripheral end. The tubules measures *0.2 mm in diameter* and *60 cm in length*. Their walls are lined by multilayered *germinal cells* which produce spermatozoa. As the tubules proceed centrally they are changed into the straight tubules with the loss of the coils. The straight tubules form intercommunicating network of channels called **rete testis** in the mediastinum testis.

12 to 15 (even may be 30) **efferent ductules** emerge from the rete testis through the upper pole of testis. They join the duct of epididymis at its head end. Receiving the efferent ductules, the single duct of epididymis becomes hugely coiled on itself extending from the head end to the tail end. Finally it is continued as the vas deferens.

Within the lobules of testis, loose areolar tissue in between the tubules contains **interstitial cells of Leydig** which secrete *testosterone,* the male sex hormone.

ARTERIAL SUPPLY (FIG. 33.14)

As the testis starts developing in the intermediate cell mass of the dorsal body wall, it receives the testicular artery as a branch of abdominal aorta at the level of L_3 vertebra. Due to descent of the testis in the scrotum, the testicular artery becomes ultimately elongated along the posterior abdominal wall and inguinal canal. As the component of the spermatic cord, the artery reaches the posterior border of testis. It divides into multiple branches at the posterior border of the gland. **The short branches** pierce the posterior border. **The long branches** pierce tunica albuginea of both the lateral as well as medial surfaces and ramify as finer branches in the plane of tunica vasculosa.

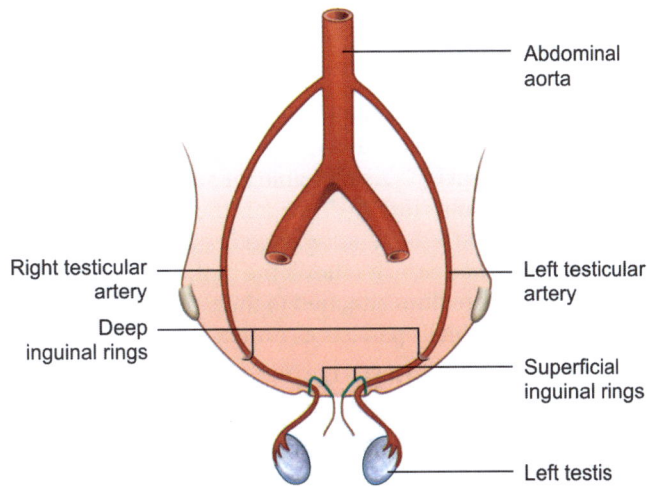

Fig. 33.14: Testicular arteries.

VENOUS DRAINAGE (FIG. 33.15)

Veins emerge along the posterior border of the testis. They form a network called **pampiniform plexus**. It is so called as it looks like a vine. The word pampiniform means 'Vine-like'. The veins of the plexus are arranged in 3 sets—anterior, middle and posterior. Anterior part is related to the testicular artery, intermediate part ascends along with the vas deferens and the posterior part is free. At the level of *superficial inguinal ring, four veins* are finally formed from the plexus. They form two veins along the inguinal canal up to the deep ring beyond which single testicular vein is formed. It runs upwards and medially along the posterior abdominal wall in relation to the testicular artery. The right testicular vein drains into the inferior vena cava whereas the left one ends in the left renal vein.

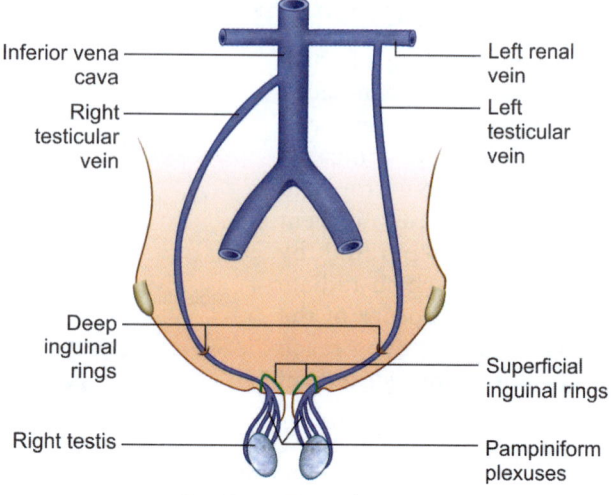

Fig. 33.15: Testicular veins.

LYMPHATIC DRAINAGE

Lymphatic vessels from the testis follow the route of testicular vessels and initially run as a component of spermatic cord. Finally they drain into preaortic and para-aortic group of lymph nodes below the level of 2nd lumbar vertebra.

NERVE SUPPLY

Testis is supplied by the sympathetic nerves coming from T_{10} segment of spinal cord. The fibers reach the organ through the renal and aortic plexuses. These are sensory and vasomotor in nature.

DESCENT OF TESTIS

Testis starts developing high up in the dorsal body wall at the level of T_{10} to T_{12} segment on the medial side of mesonephros. Finally, it needs to descend in the scrotum as the temperature within the abdominal cavity is not suitable for spermatogenesis.

Normal stimulus for the descent is the testosterone, the hormone liberated by the fetal testis. In late fetal life, it starts descending dragging its blood vessels, nerves and lymphatics, while descending behind the peritoneum, it follows the path of gubernaculum through the pelvis and inguinal canal. A slip of gubernaculum attached to the peritoneum, pulls its part as *processus vaginalis*. Distal part of processus vaginalis persists as tunica vaginalis which is invaginated by the testis from behind.

Gubernaculum of the testis is a mesodermal band extending from lower pole of testis to the bottom of scrotum. A slip from its proximal end is attached to the cephalic end of mesonephric duct. As the testis descends in the scrotum, proximal end of the mesonephric duct taken along with it, forms the epididymis.

Factors Promoting Descent

- Testosterone liberated by the fetal testis
- Differential growth of the body wall
- Intra-abdominal pressure and intra-abdominal temperature.

Gubernaculum is shortened as a consequence of the descent of testis to form the *scrotal ligament*. But t*he gubernaculum has no role in descent.*

Chronology of Descent (Fig. 33.16)

- Descent starts at 2nd month of fetal life
- Testis reaches iliac fossa by 3rd month
- It remains at the deep inguinal ring from 4th to 6th month
- It passes through the inguinal canal during 7th month
- It reaches the superficial inguinal ring during 8th month
- It enters the scrotum at 9th month.

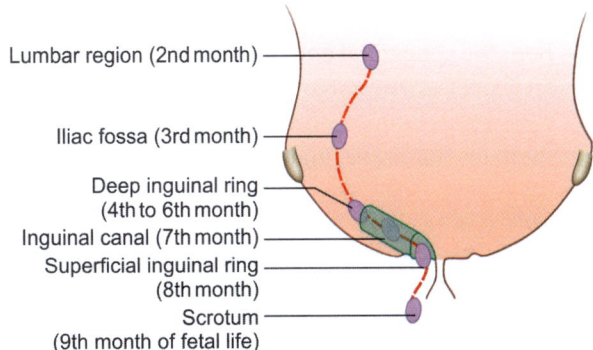

Fig. 33.16: Chronology of descent of testis in fetal life.

Clinical Anatomy

Congenital Anomalies

- **Monorchism** is the congenital absence of the testis in one side. If the testis is absent on both the sides, the condition is known as **anorchism.**
- **Cryptorchidism** explains the clinical condition of **undescended testis**. It occurs when the journey for the descent is incomplete. Then it may lie in lumbar, iliac and inguinal region. Even it may lie in upper scrotal region.
- **Ectopic testis** is a congenital anomaly in which case testis deviates from its usual path of descent and may be lodged in various abnormal positions as follows.
    - Interstitial: Superficial to the aponeurosis of external oblique in lower part of anterior abdominal wall.
    - In the proximal part of medial aspect of thigh.
    - Dorsal to the penis
    - In the perineum.

    Ectopic testis occurs when a part of the gubernaculum passes to an abnormal direction and the testis follows it.

Hydrocele

It is a clinical condition characterized by accumulation of fluid in some part of processus vaginalis. Normally, the proximal part of the processus vaginalis connected to the peritoneal cavity becomes obliterated just before birth and the distal part remains as tunica vaginalis related to the testis.

Types of the hydrocele are the following **(Figs. 33.17A to D):**

- **Vaginal hydrocele**: In this variety fluid accumulates in the normally existing cavity of tunica vaginalis. In this case the patient presents a *scrotal swelling*. This type is simply termed as hydrocele.

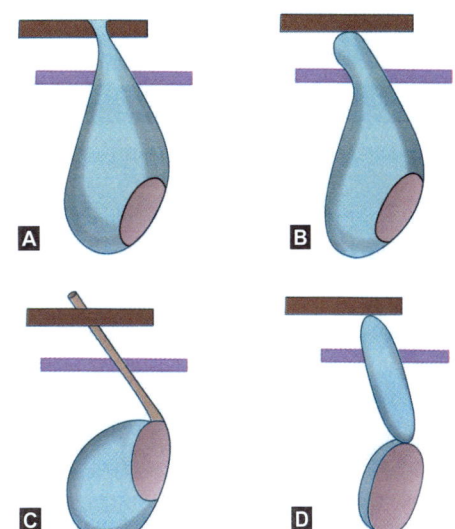

Figs. 33.17A to D: Types of hydrocele. (A) Congenital hydrocele; (B) Infantile hydrocele; (C) Vaginal hydrocele; (D) Hydrocele of the cord.

- **Congenital hydrocele**: This types of hydrocele occurs due to persistence of whole of the processus vaginalis. It is intermittent hydrocele due to existence of a tiny communication between the processus vaginalis and the peritoneal cavity.
- **Infantile hydrocele**: In this type, the processus vaginalis is occluded at the deep inguinal ring. Both the congenital and infantile hydrocele present *inguinoscrotal swelling*.
- **Hydrocele of the cord**: In this case, fluid accumulates in the proximal part of processus vaginalis which is disconnected from both the peritoneal cavity as well as the distal part of processus vaginalis (tunica vaginalis).

Vericocele

It is a condition in which veins of pampiniform plexus of the testis are dilated. It is a common disorder in young adult. It occurs mostly on the left side. This is because of the reason that left testicular vein drains into the left renal vein, in which the venous pressure is higher.

Torsion of Testis

In this disorder, testis is rotated around the spermatic cord within the scrotum. It is often associated with abnormally large sized tunica vaginalis. Torsion of the testis needs prompt management. Otherwise occlusion of the testicular artery may quickly lead to necrosis of the testis.

Malignant Tumor of the Testis

- Testicular tumors are of two main verities. *Seminoma* of testis is the carcinoma arising from seminiferous tubules. *Teratoma* arises from the totipotent cells of the organ.
- *Metastasis* (secondary spread) of the testicular malignancy occurs through lymphatics to the para-aortic lymph nodes at the level of L_2 vertebra.
- During later stage, when the malignancy spreads locally to the wall of the scrotum, then the superficial inguinal lymph nodes are involved.

Chapter 34

Organs of Female Reproductive System

LA 34.1 Describe the uterus under the following headings: Introduction with surface features; Parts; Angulated position; Peritoneal relations and visceral relations; Cavity; Ligaments; Supports; Vascular supply, lymphatic drainage and nerve supply; Age changes; Zonal anatomy; Clinical anatomy.

UTERUS

Introduction

Uterus is the *hollow, thick-walled, mobile muscular organ* of female reproductive system. It is also called *hysteria*.

Situation (Fig. 34.1)

In young adult nulliparous (till first pregnancy) women, uterus is situated within the true pelvis between urinary bladder in front and rectum behind. Lower end of uterus invaginates through upper end of anterior wall of vagina.

Function

Uterus is the *nidus, nest* or *house* for:
- *Reception*
- *Retention*
- *Nutrition* and
- *Growth of fertilized ovum up to the stage of fully matured fetus, till the birth of newborn.*

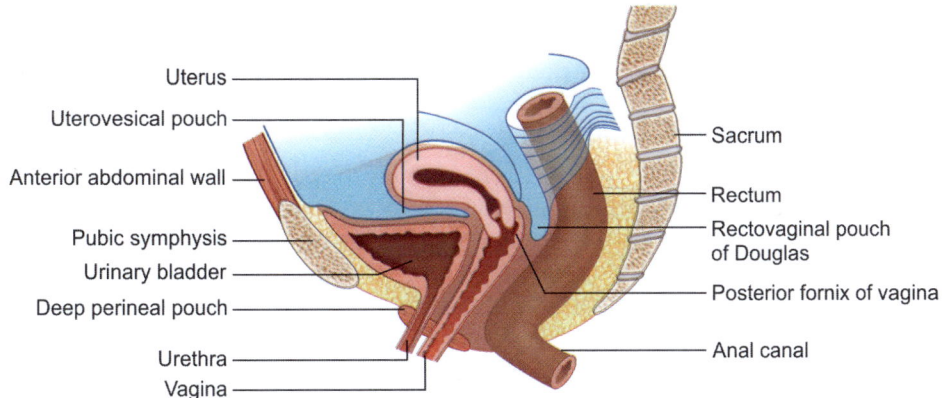

Fig. 34.1: Position and relations of uterus in sagittal section.

Shape and Size

Uterus of nulliparous young adult women is *pear-shaped* with following dimensions
- Vertical measurement (length)   =   7.5 cm
- Transverse measurement (breadth)   =   5 cm
- Anteroposterior measurement (thickness) =   2.5 cm

Muscle fibers of thick muscular wall (myometrium) *possess enormous power of elongation*, which is responsible for huge increase in size of the organ during the entire period of pregnancy.

Parts (Fig. 34.2)

From above downwards, uterus presents following parts.

- **Fundus:** It is the upper blind rounded end around which anterior and posterior surfaces of uterus are continuous with each other.
- **Body (corpus uteri):** It is the intermediate flattened part of uterus which is demarcated from the fundus by a transverse plane joining the medial ends of two uterine tubes opening into the cavity of uterus at its lateral angles. These lateral angles of the uterus are known as **cornu of uterus**.
- **Cervix:** It is the lowermost, narrower, fusiform part of uterus below the body. Junction between the body and the cervix presents a constriction over the surface known as **isthmus**. Invagination of lower half of cervix into uppermost part of anterior wall of vagina divides it into:
    - **Supravaginal part:** Part projected above vaginal canal
    - **Vaginal part:** Part invaginated within vaginal canal
  Uppermost invaginated end of vagina is known as *vaginal vault*.

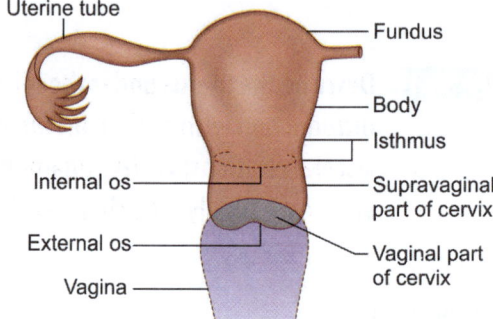

Fig. 34.2: Parts of uterus.

Pockets or recesses between the invaginated cervix and the vaginal vault on different aspects are known as anterior, posterior, right lateral and left lateral fornices **(Fig. 34.2)**.

As the cervix projects from the front of upper end of vagina, the posterior fornix is deeper than the anterior fornix.

At the level of isthmus, upper aperture of the cervix communicating with the cavity of body is known as **internal os**. Lower aperture of cervix opening into vaginal canal is known as **external os**.

In nulliparous women, external os is a circular aperture. But after parity or childbirth, it is a transverse slit guarded by anterior and posterior lips **(Fig. 34.6B)**.

Length of body and fundus (5 cm) is double the length of cervix (2.5 cm).

Angulated Position of Uterus (Figs. 34.3A and B)

Uterus of young adult nulliparous women is bent ventrally to rest on superior surface of empty or partly filled urinary bladder. In this position, long axis of cervix of uterus forms angle of 90°, open forwards, with the long axis of vagina. This angulation is known as **'anteversion' (Fig. 34.3A)**.

Again, uterus itself is bent forwards at its junction of body and cervix forming an obtuse angle of 125°. This angle between the long axis of body and that of cervix is known as **'anteflexion' (Fig. 34.3B)**.

Angle of anteversion is maintained by a ligament known as **'uterosacral ligament'** extending from the cervix uteri to the lateral aspects of lower part of sacrum. Angle of anteflexion is maintained

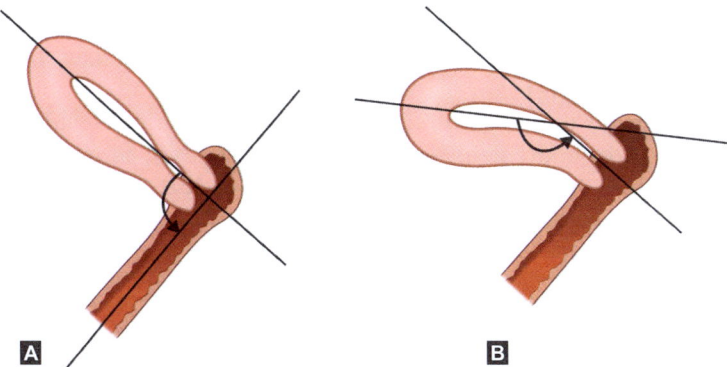

Figs. 34.3A and B: Angulations of uterus: (A) Anteversion; (B) Anteflexion.

by **tension of round ligament of uterus** having a line of pull downwards and forwards from its attachment at lateral cornu of uterus **(Fig. 34.4)**.

In 10 to 15% of cases, uterus presents a variable degree of backward tilt when its long axis is approximated towards the long axis of vagina. This condition is known as **retroversion** and **retroflexion (Fig. 34.5)**.

This position of the uterus predisposes sagging of uterus **(prolapse of uterus)** downward into vaginal canal. Incidence of prolapse is resisted by various factors maintaining the **supports of uterus**.

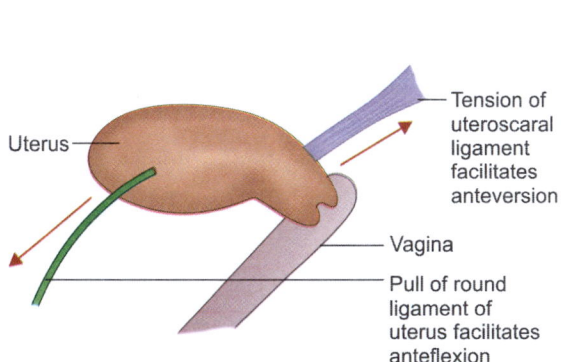

Fig. 34.4: Normal anteverted and anteflexed position of uterus.

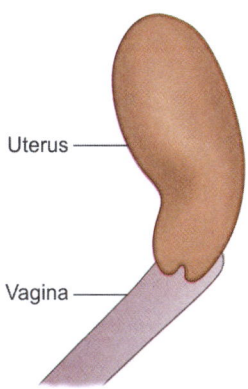

Fig. 34.5: Retroverted uterus.

Communication

Uterus being the hollow organ, communicates in two directions as follows:
1. **At lateral angles**: uterus communicates with medial end of **uterine tube**, which, at its lateral end, communicates with **peritoneal cavity**.
2. **At lower end**: Through external os, cavity of cervix uterus communicates with **vaginal canal** which opens through vaginal orifice to the exterior **(introitus)**.

Clinical Importance of Communication

Through cavity of uterus and canal of uterine tube and vagina, peritoneal cavity is open to the exterior. So, infection of peritoneal cavity (peritonitis) may occur more commonly in females than males.

Peritoneal Relations (Fig. 34.1)

Peritoneal cavity of the pelvic region is invaginated by uterus from below. This invagination is partial. So uterus is partially covered by peritoneum.

Fundus is covered by peritoneum all around its surface. Anteriorly, beyond fundus, peritoneum covers anterior surface of the body. At the junction of body and cervix, peritoneum is reflected on to the superior surface of urinary bladder to form *shallow* **uterovesical pouch**. Two sides of the pouch is bounded by a crescentic peritoneal fold called *uterovesical fold*.

Anterior surface of supravaginal part of cervix is therefore **nonperitoneal,** but its **posterior surface** is **peritoneal,** as peritoneum covering posterior surface of body continues over the supravaginal part of cervix. Further downwards, covering upper end of posterior surface (*posterior fornix*) of vagina, peritoneal membrane is reflected on to the junction of upper two-thirds and lower one-third of anterior surface rectum. *A deeper pouch of peritoneum* is thus formed between anterior surface of rectum and posterior fornix of vagina, which is called **rectovaginal pouch or pouch of Douglas**.

Pouch of Douglas is the *most dependent part of female peritoneal cavity* in erect position, and also along with *hepatorenal pouch of Morison* in supine position. So due to any pathological condition causing peritonitis, fluid starts accumulating in this pouch which can be felt through vaginal examination at the depth of 5 cm from the anus.

In fetal life, bottom of the pouch of Douglas used to be deeper in extent up to the level of perineal body. This lower part of the pouch obliterates by fusion of anterior and posterior lining of the pouch to form a septal barrier called **rectovaginal septum**.

Rectovaginal septum is *functioning as barrier* between rectum and anal canal behind and uterus and vagina in front *against the spread of infection*. Functionally, it is homologous to *rectovesical fascia of Denonvillier* in males.

Pouch of Douglas is bounded laterally by peritoneal fold called *rectovaginal fold*.

Pairs of **uterovesical fold** and **rectovaginal folds**, forming lateral boundaries of corresponding pouches act as **peritoneal** *or* **false ligaments of uterus**.

From the *lateral margins* of body (and posterior aspect of supravaginal portion of cervix), a double fold of peritoneum extends to the lateral wall of pelvis to form the **broad ligament of uterus** which are also peritoneal (false) ligaments of uterus.

So, it is clear that following areas of uterus are **nonperitoneal.**
- Anterior surface of supravaginal part of cervix below the level of uterovesical pouch.
- Whole of vaginal part cervix
- Lateral margins of the body, along the line of attachment of broad ligament.

Features with Relations (Fig. 34.1)

- **Fundus** is the upper round blind end of uterus above the level of openings of medial end of uterine tubes. Posterior wall of narrow slit-like cavity of fundus is the **site for implantation of fertilized ovum.**
- **Body of uterus**, in its empty condition, with empty urinary bladder and rectum in erect posture, presents **anteroinferior** and **posterosuperior surfaces**. In this *typical position of uterus*, anteroinferior surface rests on urinary bladder (superior surface) separated by uterovesical pouch. Posterosuperior surface is separated from anterior surface of rectum by rectovaginal pouch or pouch of Douglas. Fundus and posterosuperior surface of body are related to coils of ileum and distended sigmoid colon.

  Lateral borders of body are slightly convex and give attachments to double fold of peritoneum called **broad ligament of uterus** extending up to lateral pelvic wall.

- **Cervix of uterus (cervix uteri)**, the lower 2.5 cm of uterus is narrower and more cylindrical than body. It is wider in the middle than the ends. The cervix extends from internal os to external os, and is divided into **supravaginal part** and **vaginal part**. Upper third of cervix is called **isthmus**. Isthmus does not show any change during first month of pregnancy. But in second month, this part of cervix is '*taken up*' (incorporated) in the body for further changes during pregnancy. Isthmus portion of cervix is considered as **lower uterine segment** in reference to the body, the **upper uterine segment**.

Relations of Supravaginal Part of Cervix

- **Anteriorly**: Base of urinary bladder
- **Posteriorly**: Rectum, from which it is separated by pouch of Douglas containing coils of ileum and sigmoid colon.
- **Laterally**: Fibro fatty tissue below broad ligament, known as **parametrium**. 2.5 cm lateral to cervix, the ureter inclines *downwards forwards* and *medially* through parametrium from the level of ischial spine towards superolateral angle of urinary bladder. At this site, the ureter is crossed by uterine artery which enters the plane between the two layers of broad ligament. Lateral to cervix uteri, interrelationship between ureter and uterine artery is important because, during hysterectomy operation, ureter is to be identified and secured by the surgeon, while ligating the uterine artery.

Cavity of Uterus

- **Cavity of the body** of uterus extends from the wall of fundus to the level of internal os of cervix. In anteroposterior plane, the cavity is flat. It is triangular in outline with the base towards the fundus, in coronal section **(Fig. 34.6A)**. Superolateral angles of the cavity communicate with the uterine tubes.
- **Cavity of cervix** is known as **cervical canal**. It is narrower and fusiform in shape. Above, the cervical canal communicates with the cavity of body through *internal os*. Below it opens into vaginal canal through *external os*. In nulliparous women, external os is a circular aperture **(Fig. 34.6B)**. After birth it is a transverse slit guarded by *anterior* and *posterior* lips. Following childbirth, external os is also found to be a transverse aperture with prominent anterior and posterior lips **(Fig. 34.6B)**. Inner lining of cervical canal presents two longitudinal ridges, one each in anterior and posterior walls. The longitudinal ridges give rise to *oblique palmate folds* directed upwards and laterally like branches of a tree. That is why these are named **arbor vitae uteri (Fig. 34.6A)**. The oblique folds on opposing walls interdigitate to close the cervical canal.

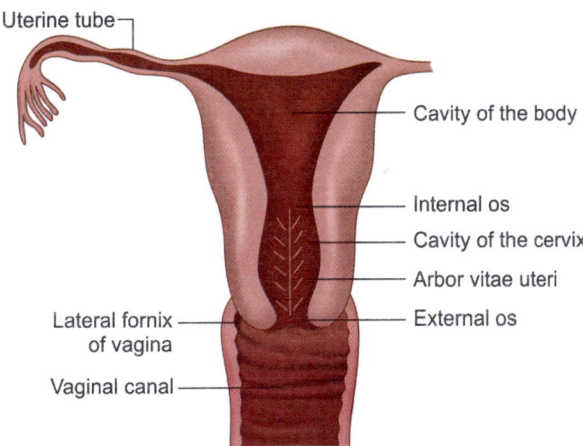

Fig. 34.6A: Cavity of uterus (with uterine tube and vagina) in coronal section.

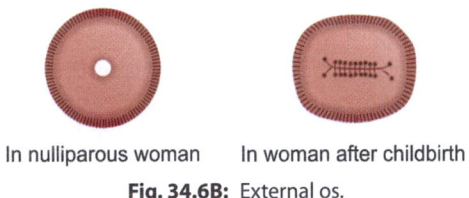

Fig. 34.6B: External os.

Ligaments of Uterus

Ligaments of uterus are broadly classified into following two groups.
1. True (nonperitoneal) ligaments
2. False (peritoneal) ligaments.

True (Nonperitoneal) Ligaments

True ligaments of uterus are either *embryological remnants* or *condensation of fibroconnective tissue* attached to the organ. Embedded into the fibroconnective tissue of the true ligaments, there may be *blood vessels*. True ligaments contain some *smooth muscles*.

True ligaments are:
1. Round ligament of uterus
2. Uterosacral (sacrocervical) ligament
3. Lateral cervical ligament (Mackenrodt's ligament)
4. Pubocervical ligament

Round ligament of uterus (Fig. 34.7)

Round ligament is a 10 cm long, narrow flattened band. Proximally, it is attached to the level of cornu of uterus, anteroinferior to medial end of uterine tube. The ligament, thereafter, is divided into two parts.
1. **Proximal part** passes laterally in between two layers of broad ligament to reach lateral wall of pelvis.
2. **Distal part**: At the site of origin of inferior epigastric artery, the ligament changes its direction to curve forwards from lateral pelvic wall and enter deep inguinal ring. While traversing the inguinal canal it presents following characteristics.

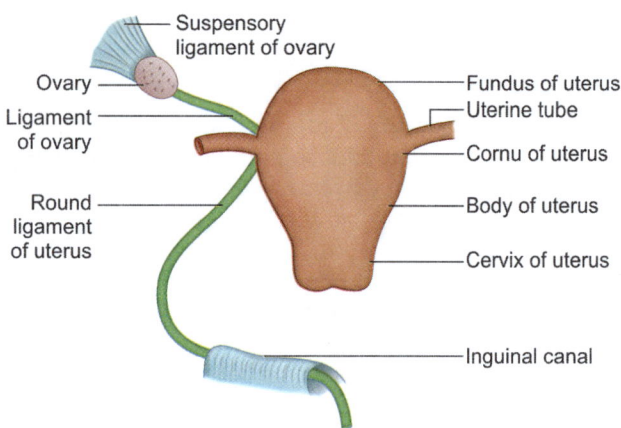

Fig. 34.7: True ligaments of uterus (embryological remnants).

   - The ligament is enclosed by the same coverings as those of spermatic cord in male, but comparatively thinner and gradually are lost on the surface of the ligament.
   - Some fibrous strands from the ligament are attached to the wall of the inguinal canal.
   - Finally the ligament comes out through superficial inguinal ring to be attached to the tissue of mons pubis at the upper end of labium majus.

Structural composition of round ligament

Round ligament of uterus is structurally **fibromuscular** in nature. Its **proximal end** consist of **smooth muscle fibers**. **Distally,** it is more **fibroelastic** in nature and while inside inguinal canal, it contains **skeletal muscle fibers**, representing **cremasteric muscle** fibers of male and thereby derived from loop of fibers of internal oblique muscle.

Morphology of round ligament

Round ligament of uterus is the remnant of distal part of **gubernaculum of ovary**. The proximal part is represented by the ligament of ovary, which extends from inferomedial pole of ovary to the cornu of uterus posteroinferior to the opening of uterine tube.

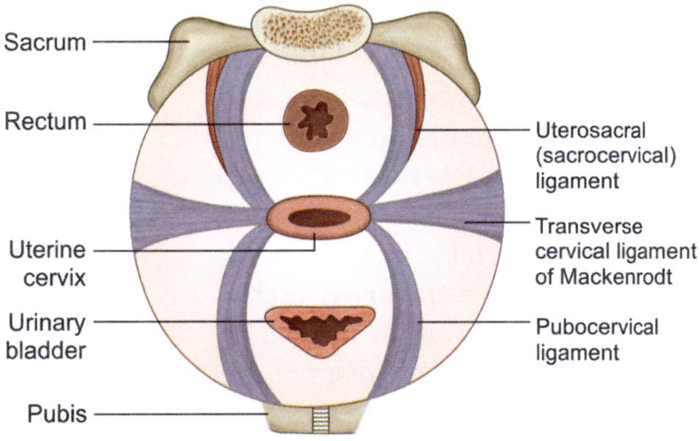

Uterosacral ligament (Fig. 34.8)

Clinically it is also named **sacrocevical ligament**. This is a **bilateral fibromuscular band** with the character of stretchability. Anteriorly, the ligaments are attached to the lateral aspect of cervix at the level of internal os.

The ligamentous bands clasp the rectal wall from both sides and pass backwards through the rectouterine peritoneal folds to be attached to the sides of *second and third pieces of sacrum*.

Fig. 34.8: True ligaments of uterus (condensations of pelvic fascia).

Transverse cervical ligament (Fig. 34.8)

Transverse cervical ligament is also known as **Mackenrodt's ligament** or **cardinal ligament**. The ligament is formed by condensation of pelvic fascia. This paired ligament extends from the side of the cervix uteri and the lateral fornix of the vagina to have extensive attachment to the lateral pelvic wall. The lower part of the ureter and the pelvic blood vessels traverse the transverse cervical ligament.

Pubocervical ligament (Fig. 34.8)

This is also the paired ligament which extends from the pelvic surface of the body of pubis to the anterior aspect the cervix uteri, clasping the sides of the urethra below the level of urinary bladder.

False (Peritoneal) Ligaments

Main peritoneal ligament (fold) of the uterus is the *broad ligament of uterus*. Besides this bilateral broad peritoneal fold, uterus is connected through pairs of *uterovesical* and *rectovaginal folds* in front and behind respectively.

- **Uterovesical folds** are simple paired curved peritoneal ridge forming the lateral outline of the uterovesical pouch, as the visceral peritoneum is reflected from the front of uterus to the urinary bladder.
- **Rectovaginal folds** are similar peritoneal folds forming the lateral boundary of the rectovaginal pouch of Douglas as the peritoneum is reflected from the front of rectum to the posterior fornix of vagina.

Broad ligament of uterus (Fig. 34.9)

Introduction

It is the bilateral double fold of peritoneum which extends from the lateral border of uterus to the lateral wall of the pelvis.

Disposition

In anteverted and anteflexed position of uterus, the plane of the broad ligament faces downwards and forwards or backwards and upwards.

Borders and surfaces

- **Medial border** is attached to the lateral border of uterus.
- **Lateral border** of both the layers falls on the lateral pelvic wall.
- **Superior border** is free where the anterior and posterior layers of the ligament are continuous with each other around the uterine tube.

- **Inferior border** of anterior layer extends up to the level of junction of body and cervix where it is reflected forwards. This border of the posterior layer extends up to the level of lateral fornix of vagina and then it is reflected backwards.
- **Surfaces** are **anteroinferior** and **posterosuperior** formed by the corresponding layers of the peritoneal fold.

Parts

- **Mesosalpinx:** It is the upper marginal part of the broad ligament adjacent to the uterine tube *(salpinx)*.

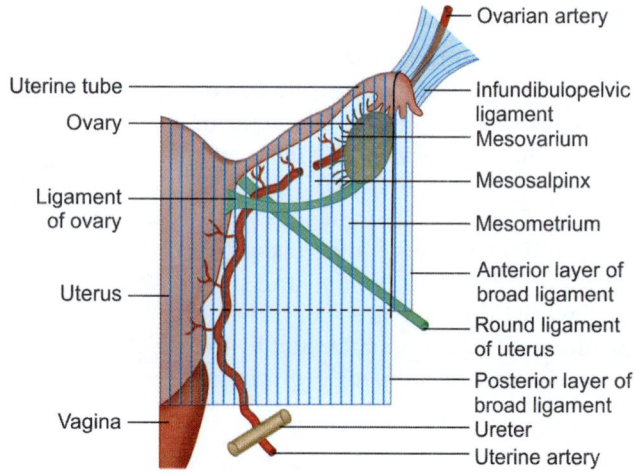

Fig. 34.9: Broad ligament of uterus (posterior view).

- **Mesometrium**: It is the main part of the ligament attached to the uterus.
- **Mesovarium**: It is the part which extends from the posterior layer of broad ligament to be attached to the ovary.
- **Infundibulopelvic ligament**: It is also known as the **suspensory ligament of ovary.** This part of the broad ligament extends from the lateral infundibular end of the uterine tube upwards and laterally to the wall of the *false pelvis*.

Contents

- **Uterine tube**: Along the upper free border of broad ligament
- **Two arteries**: *Uterine* and *ovarian arteries* with corresponding veins
- **Two ligaments**: *Round ligament of uterus* and *ligament of ovary*
- **Two embryological rudiments**: *Epoophoron with its duct (Gartner's duct)* and *paroophoron*
- **Usual components** of any mesentery (peritoneal fold): Lymph vessels with lymph nodes, autonomic plexus nerves and fibroconnective tissue.

Supports of Uterus

Uterus is a mobile muscular organ which possesses enormous power of increase in size during pregnancy and great variation in appearance during the reproductive period of life. For these age changes, the uterus has the tendency to sag downwards through the vaginal vault. This is prevented by various factors or mechanisms which are known as supports of uterus.

The supports are fundamentally of two types, primary and secondary.

Primary Supports

- Pelvic diaphragm
- Perineal body
- Urogenital diaphragm
- True (nonperitoneal) ligaments
- Relationship with other viscera.

Secondary Supports

These are peritoneal folds of uterus, mainly the broad ligament.

Primary supports play very important role to maintain the position of the uterus. *Broad ligaments* with other peritoneal folds of uterus, namely the *uterovesical folds* and *rectovaginal folds* have less significant role as supports of uterus.

Mode of functions of various primary supports are discussed below.

Pelvic diaphragm

Pelvic diaphragm, formed by levatores ani muscles, acts as the important support of uterus in different ways.
- Fundamentally, forming the pelvic floor, it **holds the uterus** along with other pelvic viscera in weight-bearing postures.
- In addition, muscular tone of the pelvic diaphragm, **resists downwards sagging** of uterus **whenever there is rise of intraabdominal pressure**.
- Part of the pubococcygeus is attached to the perineal body. Along with other perineal muscles attached, these fibers **fix the perineal body**.
- Part of the pubococcygeus **winds round the vaginal vault** from both sides to **form a sling** and the encircling fibers form **sphincter vaginae**. This arrangement supports the vaginal vault, so also the uterus.
- The component of pubococcygeus forming **puborectal sling** pulls all the pelvic viscera including the uterus in **upward and forward direction** along the oblique line.

Perineal body

Perineal body, also called the **central tendon of perineum**, is actually aggregation of fibromuscular tissue situated in the midline of the perineum just below the plane of pelvic floor. It gives attachment to the part of levator ani (pubococcygeus part) along with many other muscles of perineal pouches in a radiating fashion from all directions. Due to the fixed position, as tied from the different sides, the perineal body acts **as an anchor** and thereby **maintains the integrity of pelvic diaphragm**.

Urogenital diaphragm

It is a musculomembranous shelf bridging across the anterior pubic arch component of the pelvic outlet. Below the anterior part of pelvic diaphragm, the urogenital diaphragm acts as an additional support of the uterus.

True ligaments of uterus

The true (nonperitoneal) ligaments, which are condensations of pelvic fascia, tie the uterine cervix to the anterior, posterior and both the lateral walls of true pelvis. These ligaments, described in previous section, are following **(Fig. 34.8)**.
- **Anterior:** Pubocervical ligament
- **Posterior:** Uterosacral (sacrocervical) ligament
- **Lateral:** Transverse cervical ligament of Mackenrodt or cardinal ligament.

Combined role of uterosacral ligament and round ligament of uterus for uterine support:

Anteverted and anteflexed position of uterus in an important factor maintaining the support of the organ. This position of uterus prevents the sagging of uterus downwards through the vagina.

When there is rise of intraabdominal pressure, fundal end of the uterus will be pushed downwards and forwards towards the urinary bladder and pubic symphysis. This is facilitated by the tension of round ligament of uterus. Pull of the cervix upwards and backwards is maintained by the uterosacral ligament **(Fig. 34.4)**.

Arterial Supply (Fig. 34.10)

Uterus is supplied by:
1. Uterine artery—main source
2. Ovarian artery—additional source

Uterine artery, arising from anterior division of internal iliac artery, first runs medially towards the cervix. 2 cm lateral to the cervix, the artery crosses the ureter above the level of lateral formix of vagina. Next part of the uterine artery ascends with a tortuous course lateral to the uterus between two layers of broad ligament. Finally, it runs laterally towards the ovary and ends by anastomosing with the ovarian artery.

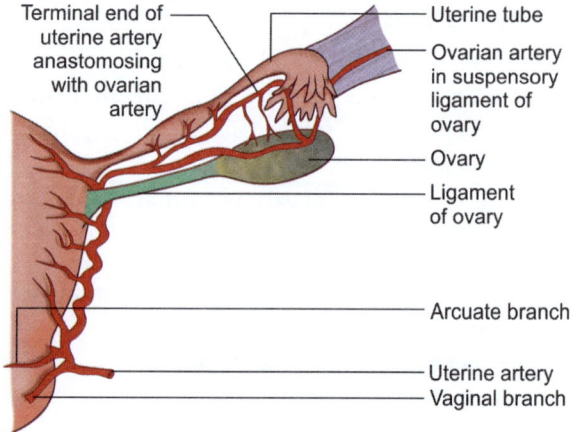

Fig. 34.10: Arteries supplying the uterus.

Branches

- **Near the cervix:**
  - *Cervical branches* encircle in front of and behind the cervix and anastomose with the corresponding arteries of opposite side.
  - *Vaginal branches*
  - *Ureteric branches*
- **Near the body: Arcuate branches** encircle the body of uterus and anastomose with the branches of the opposite side.
- **Near the uterine tube: Tubal** and **ovarian** branches supply corresponding structures.

Venous Drainage

Veins draining the uterus correspond to the arteries. They form a plexus along the lateral border of the uterus extending upwards up to the level of the uterine tube. This plexus drain through the **uterine** and **vaginal veins** to the internal iliac vein. Some veins from the upper end of the plexus drain into the **ovarian vein**.

Lymphatic Drainage (Fig. 34.11)

Lymph vessels draining the uterus initially form plexuses in three different planes of the wall of the uterus. These are **endometrial, myometrial** and **subserous plexuses**. These plexuses are connected through the vessels which are directed from within outwards. Finally, the lymph vessels come out to the sides of the uterus to drain into various groups of lymph nodes as follows.
- From the *fundus* and *upper part of the body*: Most of the lymph vessels follow the route of ovarian vessels to drain in **preaortic** and **paraaortic groups** of lymph nodes.
- From the area of *cornu of uterus*: The lymph vessels follow the *route of the round ligament of uterus* and drain into the **medial group of superficial inguinal lymph nodes**.

- From the *lower part of the body*: The vessels pass laterally *through the plane of broad ligament* to the lateral wall of pelvis to drain into the **external iliac group of nodes**.
- *From the cervix*: Lymph vessels follow the following three directions
    1. *Laterally:* To the **external iliac and obturator lymph nodes**
    2. *Posterolaterally:* To the **internal iliac nodes**
    3. *Posteriorly:* To the **presacral group of nodes**.

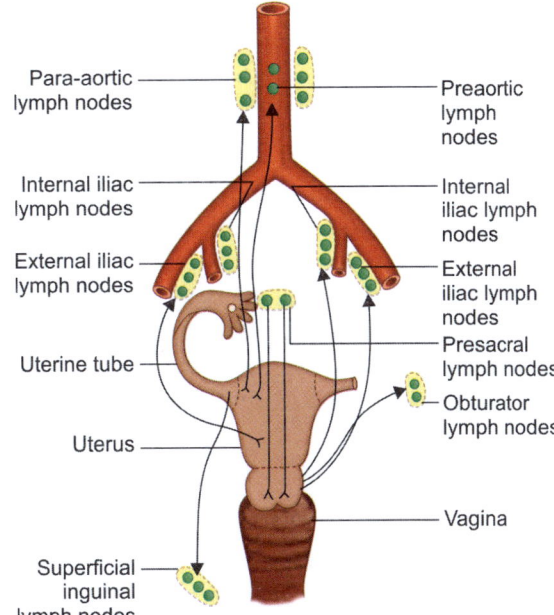

Fig. 34.11: Lymphatic drainage of uterus.

Nerve Supply

Both the sympathetic as well as parasympathetic fibers supply the uterus through the **inferior hypogastric plexus** and **ovarian plexus**.

Sympathetic fibers from T_{12} to L_2 spinal segments are for **uterine contraction** (of myometrium) and **vasoconstriction**. Parasympathetic fibers from the *pelvic splanchnic nerves* are **vasodilator** and **inhibitory to the myometrium.**

Pain fibers from the uterus follow the following two different courses.
1. Pain sensation **from the body** follows the **sympathetic route (T_{12} to L_2)**. So, the referred pain is felt in the **back, inguinal region** and upper part of **front of thigh**.
2. Pain **from the cervix** follow the **parasympathetic route (pelvic splanchnic nerves)**. Its referred pain is felt in **perineum, gluteal region** and the **back of thigh**.

Age Changes of the Uterus

In Fetal Life
- Fundus end of the uterus projects a little above the inlet of true pelvis.
- Cervix is larger than the body.

At Puberty
- Uterus enlarges proportionately in size
- It descends below the pelvic inlet
- Arbor vitae uteri appear in the cervical mucosa.

During Menstruation
- Uterus is slightly enlarged
- It becomes more vascular
- Lips of the external os become more prominent.

During Pregnancy
- Uterus becomes enormously enlarged due to hyperplasia of myometrium with huge elongation of individual muscle fibers
- With the advancement of pregnancy, the uterine wall becomes gradually thinner.

After Childbirth

Size of the uterus gradually returns towards the pre-pregnancy size. It is known as involution of uterus.

In Old Age

- Following menopause, the uterus becomes atrophic and smaller in size.
- The texture of the wall becomes condensed
- The internal os becomes obliterated
- The lips of the external os disappear.

Clinical Anatomy

Congenital anomalies of uterus may result due to abnormalities of fusion of distal parts of the paramesonephric duct. Common anomalies are **bicornuate uterus** or **septate uterus**. Septate uterus apparently looks normal, but its cavity is subdivided through a vertical septum, when both the paramesonephric ducts do not fuse. If only the upper part of the septum persists, it gives rise to the bicornuate uterus. Double uterus results from complete failure of fusion of distal ends of both the paramesonephric duct.

Retroverted position of uterus may be congenital or acquired in origin. In these cases, the uterus is deviated backwards more towards the line of the axis of the vagina. It may predispose the incidence of prolapse of uterus.

Prolapse of the uterus is the clinical condition characterized by sagging of the organ downwards through the vagina. It may occur due to weakness of the supports of uterus mostly after difficult or repeated childbirth. Incidence of the prolapse is also found after manopause due to atrophy of the pelvic fascia along with the pelvic organs.

Cesarean section is the operative procedure adopted to deliver the baby cutting open the lower abdominal and uterine walls, to avoid the obstructed or difficult normal vaginal delivery. This operation is so named as Julius Caesar, the great Roman emperor, was born through this method.

Hysterectomy is the name of operation for removal of the uterus. It is so called because, the Greek terminology of the uterus is *'hystera'*. This operation is indicated for various pathological conditions of uterus including carcinoma. During this operation, the ureter is accidentally ligated or injured as a serious complication, as it crosses 2 cm lateral to the cervix of the uterus.

Carcinoma of the cervix is the most common variety of the uterine malignancy. It is again the most common malignant disease in females. Metastasis of this cancer rapidly occurs through the lymphatic spread.

Fibromyoma (fibroid) of uterus is the benign tumor of the uterus. It is common in the body of the uterus.

LA 34.2 **Discuss briefly the uterine tube with a note on clinical anatomy.**

UTERINE (FALLOPIAN) TUBES

Introduction

Uterine tubes, also called fallopian tubes, are thin-walled narrow tortuous tubes which are connected to the lateral angle (cornua) of the uterus.

Functions

- During regular menstrual cycle, the uterine tube transports the ovum from the ovary to the cavity of uterus.
- Uterine tube provides the site for fertilization of ovum, after the spermatozoa reaches the tube through the vagina and uterus.

Situation

Uterine tube is situated in the upper free margin of the broad ligament of uterus.

Measurement

The tube is 10 cm long.

Extent

- **Medially,** the uterine tube opens into the lateral angle of the cavity of the uterus at the junction of fundus and body.
- **Laterally,** the tube opens into the peritoneal cavity and is in close relation to free medial surface of the ovary.

Parts of the Tube (Fig. 34.12)

From **medial to lateral**, the parts of the uterine tube are as follows.

- **Intramural** part is so called because, this short segment of the tube measuring 1cm traverses through the myometrium of the uterus. It opens through the **uterine ostium** at the lateral angle of the cavity of the uterus which indicates the level of junction between the fundus and body.
- **Isthmus** is so called because it is the **narrowest** part of the tube. It is **thick-walled** and **cord-like** due to abundance of muscle fibers in its wall.
- **Ampulla** is the *dilated, elongated* and *thin-walled* part of the uterine tube lateral to the isthmus. It is the usual **site for fertilization** of ovum. It may be more than the half of the length of whole tube, measuring 6 to 7 cm. The ampulla is directed upwards, laterally and slightly backwards to arch over the ovary.
- **Infundibulum** is the funnel-shaped lateral end of the uterine tube. It presents the opening at its end called **abdominal ostium** which opens into the peritoneal cavity. The margin of the ostium is surrounded by number of short finger like processes called **fimbriae** *(singular—fimbria)*. One fimbria is longer than the other and is attached to the tubal pole of the ovary. It is called **ovarian fimbria**.

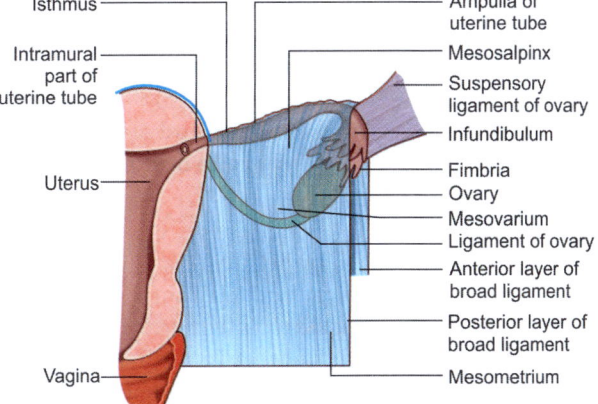

Fig. 34.12: Uterine tube and ovary with related structures viewed from behind.

Mesentery of the Tube (Fig. 34.13)

Uterine tube is contained in the upper free margin of the broad ligament. From the posterior layer of the broad ligament, the mesentery of the ovary, called *mesovarium* extends to the ovary. The uppermost part of the broad ligament extending from the uterine tube up to the level of mesovarium is called **mesosalpinx** which can be considered as the mesentery of the uterine tube. The mesosalpinx contains the **ligament of ovary** and the **round ligament of uterus** which are posteroinferior and anteroinferior to the uterine tube respectively.

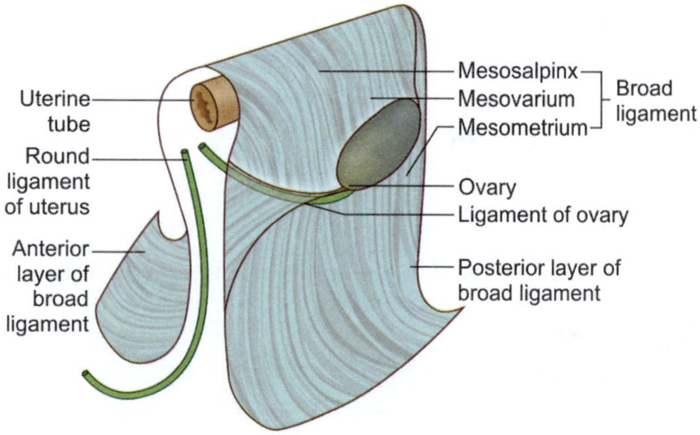

Fig. 34.13: Uterine tube (cut section) with related structures.

Blood Supply

- **Arteries** supplying uterine tube are derived from both the uterine and ovarian arteries. **Medial two-thirds** of the tube is supplied by the branches of the **uterine artery**. Branches of **ovarian artery** supply the **lateral one-third**.
- **Veins** from the uterine tube correspond to the arteries. They drain into the **uterine** and **ovarian veins**.

Lymphatic Drainage

- Lymph vessels from the **lateral one-third** of uterine tube follow the route of ovarian vessels and drain into the **paraaortic group** of lymph nodes
- Lymph vessels from **medial two-thirds** follow the course of uterine artery and drain into the **internal iliac group** of lymph nodes
- Lymph vessels from the **medial end** of the tube **(isthmus)** follow the round ligament of uterus and drain into the **medial group of superficial inguinal lymph nodes**.

Nerve Supply

Uterine tube is supplied by both sympathetic as well as parasympathetic nerves.
- **Sympathetic fibers** are derived from T_{10} to L_2 segments of spinal cord and these are distributed through the **hypogastric plexuses**. Sympathetic nerves supplying the uterine tube are **vasoconstrictor** and **sensory** in nature.
- **Parasympathetic fibers** reach the uterine tube through two different routes. **Medial half** of the tube is supplied by the **pelvic splanchnic nerves (S_2, S_3, S_4). Vagus nerve** supplies the **lateral half.** Parasympathetic fibers are **vasodilator** in function. They **inhibit peristalsis** of the tube which is mostly under hormonal control.

Clinical Anatomy

Uterine Tube, a Channel Predisposing Peritonitis

The uterine tube is a direct route of communication from the vulva to the peritoneal cavity in female through the vagina and uterine cavity. So, infection of the female genital tract, if not managed properly, may lead to **peritonitis**.

Salpingitis

Infection of the uterine tube, called salpingitis, is interrelated to the peritonitis, as either of the two condition may result from the another one. Salpingitis may result from **pelvic inflammatory disease.** It may lead to some serious complication like **pelvic abscess** and **general peritonitis.**

Sterility

Sterility in female may result, if there occurs **blockage in the lumen** of the uterine tube which **interferes with the transport of ovum** required for fertilization.

Ectopic Pregnancy

Implantation and **growth of fertilized ovum** may occur outside the uterine cavity in the **wall of the uterine tube**. As formation of decidua is not possible in the thin wall of the tube, **tubal abortion** is the consequence. **Rupture of the tube** with effusion of blood into the peritoneal cavity **(hemoperitoneum)** is a serious complication.

Tubal Ligation

Ligation and division of uterine tubes is the common procedure for obtaining birth control in case of women who already have children.

Hysterosalpingography

It is a radiological examination, through which patency of the cavity of uterus and the lumen of the uterine tube is visualized after injecting the radiopaque dye through vaginal route.

LA 34.3 **Describe the gross anatomy of the ovary with ligaments, vascular supply, lymphatic drainage, nerve supply and clinical anatomy.**

OVARIES

Introduction

Ovaries are female gonads concerned with production of female gametes called *oocyte* (mature ovum). These are homologous to the testes in male. Ovary also produces the hormones, *estrogen* and *progesterone*.

Gross Appearance

In adult nulliparous (nonpregnant) women, the ovaries are **oval almond shaped** structure of **grayish-pink** color.

Measurement

Length = 4 cm
Breadth = 2 cm
Thickness = 1 cm

Situation (Fig. 34.14)

- Ovary is **connected to the posterior layer of the broad ligament** of uterus through **mesovarium**.
- It is suspended from the lateral wall of **false pelvis** through the **suspensory ligament of ovary**.

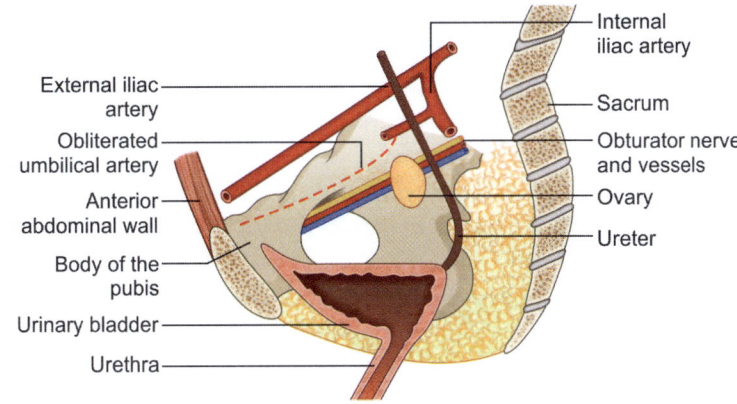

Fig. 34.14: Position and relations of ovary in lateral wall of pelvis.

- Ovary lies in close apposition to the area of the lateral wall of **true pelvis** called **ovarian fossa** which is a small peritoneal depression bounded as follows:
  - **Posteriorly:** Ureter and internal iliac vessels
  - **Anteriorly:** Obliterated umbilical artery
  - Floor of the fossa is related to the **obturator nerve** and **obturator vessels**.

External Features and Relations with Disposition (Figs. 34.12 to 34.14)

Ovary, being oval in outline like testis presents two poles, two surface and two borders:
- **Two poles** are tubal and uterine poles. **Tubal pole** is in close contact with the infundibular end of the uterine tube. It is directed upwards and laterally. **Uterine pole** is directed downwards and medially towards the body of the uterus **(Fig. 34.12)**.
- **Two surfaces** are lateral and medial. **Lateral surface** is opposed to the ovarian fossa **(Fig. 34.14)**. **Medial surface** is free and related to the fimbriated end of infundibulum of uterine tube. One longer fimbria is in contact with the medial surface of the ovary, called **ovarian fimbria.**
- **Two borders** are anterior and posterior. **Anterior border** is considered as the **mesenteric border**. It gives attachment to the **mesovarium** through which the ovary is connected to the posterior layer of broad ligament **(Fig. 34.13)**. Anterior border of ovary is the line of demarcation between simple squamous epithelium (mesothelium) of mesovarium and cubical germinal epithelium lining the surface of the ovary. It is called **white line of the ovary.** Posterior border of the ovary is the free **antemesenteric border**.

Ligaments of the Ovary (Fig. 34.12)

Nonperitoneal ligament is the ligament of ovary and peritoneal ligaments are mesovarium and suspensory ligament of ovary.
- **Ligament of ovary** is a band-like structure which extends from the **uterine pole of the ovary** to the posteroinferior aspect of the **lateral cornu of the uterus**. It is **contained in the broad ligament.** It represents the **proximal part of the gubernaculum of ovary**.
- **Mesovarium** is short double fold of peritoneum which extends from the posterior layer of broad ligament of uterus to the anterior border of ovary. Mesovarium is considered as the **mesentery of the ovary** through which pass the **ovarian vessels** with autonomic nerves of ovarian plexus.
- **Suspensory ligament of ovary** is truly the part of the broad ligament of uterus. It is so called and also considered as the peritoneal fold of the ovary because it suspends the ovary from the lateral wall of the false pelvis. It is also called the **infundibulopelvic ligament.** Through this peritoneal fold ovarian artery approaches the mesovarium.

Important Relations (Figs. 34.12 and 34.14)

Upper pole is directed *upwards and laterally*. It is called the **tubal pole** as it is related to the lateral infundibular end of the uterine tube. **Vermiform appendix** may be related to the right ovary, when it is pelvic in position. **Ovarian fimbria** is in contact with the upper pole which gives attachment to the suspensory ligament of ovary.

Lower pole is directed *downwards and medially* towards the uterus, so it is called the **uterine pole**. It is connected by the **ligament of ovary** to the lateral angle of uterus posteroinferior to the medial end of the uterine tube.

Lateral surface of the ovary is in opposition to the **ovarian fossa** of the lateral wall of the true pelvis. Floor of the fossa lodges the obturators nerve and obturator vessels separated by the parietal peritoneum.

Medial surface is relatively free but covered by the **infundibulum** of the uterine tube as the tube arches round the upper pole of the ovary. The surface is related to a small peritoneal recess called **ovarian bursa**.

Anterior border gives attachment to the **mesovarium** from the posterior layer of the broad ligament. It presents the **hilus** of the ovary transmitting ovarian vessels.

Posterior border is free and more *convex*. It is related to the curve of the lateral end of the **uterine tube**.

Arterial Supply

Ovarian artery is the chief source of arterial supply to the ovary. Though the ovary lies in the pelvis, ovarian artery is the lateral splanchnic branch of abdominal aorta as the fetal position of ovary is in dorsal abdominal wall before its descent. The artery reaches the ovary passing through the suspensory ligament and the mesovarium. After giving branches to the ovary, the artery is further continued between the layers of broad ligament and end by anastomosing with the uterine artery. Distal part of the artery also supplies branches to the uterus, uterine tube and ureter.

Uterine artery gives some additional branches to the ovary which also enter through the mesovarium.

Venous Drainage

Multiple small veins come out through the hilus of ovary and form a plexus around the ovarian artery called **pampiniform plexus**. From this plexus, single ovarian vein is formed at the level of the pelvic inlet. Ascending along the posterior abdominal wall, the **right ovarian vein** drains into the **inferior vena cava** and the **left vein** drains into the **left renal vein**.

Lymphatic Drainage

Lymph vessels from the ovary come out through the hilus along with the tributaries of ovarian vein. The vessels follow the course of the ovarian vein and drain into the **paraaortic group** of lymph nodes.

Nerve Supply

Both sympathetic as well as parasympathetic fibers pass to the ovary as **ovarian plexus** following the course of ovarian artery. The ovarian plexus is formed by the fibers coming from **aortic, renal** and **hypogastric plexuses**. Sympathetic fibers derived from T_{10} and T_{11} **spinal segments** are **sensory** and **vasoconstrictor** in function. Parasympathetic fibers derived from **pelvic splanchnic nerves** (S_2, S_3, S_4) are **vasodilator** in nature.

Gross Structure

Surface of the ovary is lined by *simple cubical epithelium* called **germinal epithelium** which represents the peritoneal lining and is continuous with the mesothelium of mesovarium.

Beneath the germinal epithelium, a thin layer of connective tissue is known as **tunica albuginea**.

Outer **cortex** of the ovary presents **ovarian follicles** which are found at various stages of development. Each of the follicles contains one female gemmate called **oocyte**. Every month one follicle shows maturation to shed out one oocyte. The fully mature ovarian follicle prior to the shedding of oocyte (mature ovum) is known as **Graafian follicle**. Discharge of the oocyte from the follicle is known as **ovulation**. Ovulation occurs at 14th day of the usual 28 days menstrual cycle. Following ovulation, the Graafian follicle is converted into **corpus luteum**. The cells of the wall of ovarian follicle liberates the hormone **estrogen**. Another hormone, **progesterone** is liberated by the cells of corpus luteum.

Medulla of the ovary is made up of **connective tissue stroma**. It is richly vascular containing blood vessels with nerve fibers and lymphatics.

Clinical Anatomy

Displacement of Ovary

Ovary is kept in position by the normal broad ligament and mesovarium. Following pregnancy and childbirth, the broad ligament may be lax. It may give rise to abnormal mobility of ovary resulting following conditions.
- **Prolapse of ovary** may occur in the pouch of Douglas. Then the ovary can be felt through vaginal examination.
- **Ovarian torsion** is an acute abdominal painful condition in which case the ovary is twisted due to abnormally long broad ligament components (mesovarium and suspensory ligament).

Ovarian Cysts
- **Small follicular cysts** are common and these originate from the unruptured Graafian follicles. They *rarely exceed 1.5 cm* in diameter.
- **Large ovarian cyst (luteal cyst)** with encysted fluid may be formed in the corpus luteum. The fluid is retained in the cyst as the corpus luteum fails to be fibrosed. Usually, it *does not exceed 3 cm in diameter*. Rarely, it becomes hugely enlarged to fill up the abdominopelvic cavity.

Ovarian Carcinoma

Carcinoma of ovary is not uncommon. Incidence is 15% among all the cancers.

Ovarian Dysgenesis

Ovaries are found to fail to develop in cases of Turner's syndrome.

Imperfect Descent of Ovary

Very rarely, the ovary may fail to descend into the pelvis or may be drawn downward along the route of the round ligament of uterus into the inguinal canal or even into the labium majus.

SA 34.4 How to hold the uterus (with its appendages) in anatomical position? (Only for viva voce and practical).

If only the specimen of uterus is provided:
- The rounded fundus of the uterus is to be directed upwards with the external os (ostium) of the cervix looking downwards.
- Anterior and posterior surfaces are to be differentiated as follows:
  Fundus and body are smooth and shining both in front and behind due to peritoneal lining. But only the upper part of the posterior surface of the cervix is smooth and shining as it is also covered by peritoneum. The lower part of posterior surface and the whole of the anterior surface of the cervix are raw in appearance as not covered by peritoneum.
- To represent the anteverted position of the uterus the long axis of the specimen is to be tilted upwards and forwards.

If the uterus is provided with the broad ligament, uterine tube and ovary:
- Posterior aspect of the broad ligament is identified by the attachment of the ovary which is connected to its posterior layer by mesovarium.
- The lateral wider infundibular end of the uterine tube is more close to the ovary.

Chapter 35

Perineum and Urethra

SN 35.1 Write a short note on perineal body.

PERINEAL BODY
Perineal body is the midline condensed fibrotendinous body located in the midline of perineum in front of anus. This strong fibrous nodular structure is called **central tendon of perineum** because many small muscles of perineum along with a part of levator ani attached to it radiate in different direction. Pull of these muscles in a radiating manner maintains the central fixed position of the perineal body in normal individual. Perineal body, through the radiating pull of these muscles, supports not only the structures of the perineum, but also the pelvic diaphragm for holding the pelvic viscera.

Muscles Attached to the Perineal Body
The following muscles are attached to the perineal body as they converge to this central point of the perineum from different directions.

Superficial Plane (Fig. 35.1A)
- **Anteriorly:** Bulbospongiosus
- **Laterally:** Superficial transverse perinei
- **Posteriorly:** Superficial part of external anal sphincter.

Intermediate Plane (Fig. 35.1B)
- **Anteriorly:** Sphincter urethrae
- **Lateral:** Deep transverse perinei.

Deep Plane (Fig. 35.1C)
Anteriorly: Part of pubococcygeus with sphincter vaginae.

Function
Perineal body is the important support for the pelvic organs including the uterus in female. As this central tendon is tied by various muscles radiating in different directions, increased tone of these muscles during rise of intraabdominal pressure fixes the perineal body.

Clinical Anatomy
Perineal tear is a complication which results in females following difficult childbirth. It leads to injury to the perineal muscles or the perineal body itself. In this condition, the tone (tension)

of the perineal body is lost. Effect will be prolapse of the uterus through the vaginal vault. Prolapse of urinary bladder or rectum may occur through anterior or posterior wall of vagina which are called *cystocele* or *rectocele* respectively.

SA 35.2 Write a brief note on ischiorectal fossa with clinical anatomy.

ISCHIORECTAL FOSSA (FIG. 35.2)

Introduction

Ischiorectal fossa, presently called *ischioanal fossa* is a wedge-shaped space situated on each side of anal canal below the pelvic diaphragm. It is often referred as *ischioanal space*.

The *base* of the wedge-shaped space is directed downwards towards the perineal skin. The *edge* is directed upwards.

Two ischioanal fossae are joined together behind the anal canal by a narrow connecting part giving a horseshoe-shaped appearance.

Dimensions

- Vertical: 5–6 cm
- Anteroposterior: 5 cm
- Transverse: 2.5 cm.

Boundaries

The wedge-shaped fossa presents following boundaries.
- **Base**: It is convex in outline and is formed by the perineal skin lateral to the anus.
- **Lateral wall**: it is vertical and is formed by:
  - Obturator internus muscle with its covering fascia
  - Medial surface of ischial tuberosity
- **Medial wall**: It inclines upwards and laterally and meets the lateral wall to form the edge of the fossa. It formed as follows.
  - *Lower part*: External anal sphincter around anal canal
  - *Upper part*: Inferior surface of levator ani
- **Edge (linear apex)**: It is formed by a condensed fascial line where obturator fascia meets with the anal fascia on undersurface of levator ani.

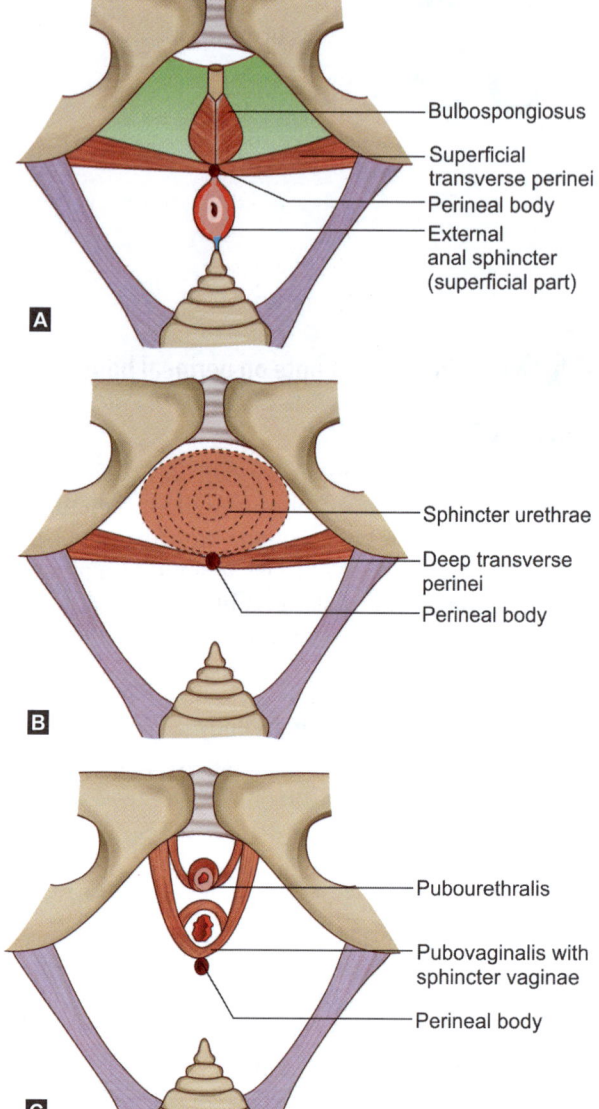

Figs. 35.1A to C: Muscles attached to the perineal body: (A) Superficial plane; (B) Intermediate plane; (C) Deep plane.

Anteroposterior Extent

Anteriorly, the fossa extends up to the perineal membrane.

Posteriorly, the fossa reaches up to the lower border of gluteus maximus and the sacrotuberous ligament.

Recesses

These are the narrow extensions of the ischioanal fossa which are as follows:
- **Anterior recess**: It extends forwards above the urogenital diaphragm in the urogenital triangle of perineum.
- **Posterior recess**: It is the narrow extension underneath the sacrotuberous ligament.

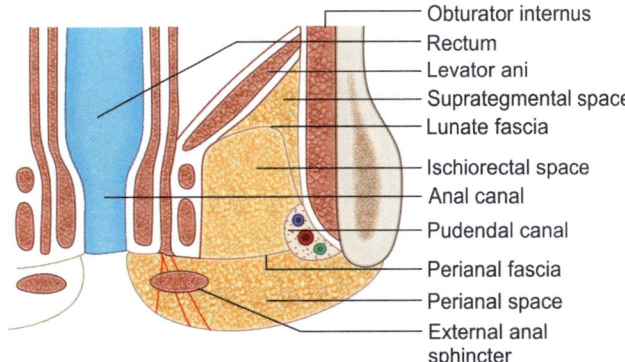

Fig. 35.2: Ischiorectal fossa through coronal section of perineum.

Intercommunication of Two Fossae

A narrow communicating part of the fossa lies behind the anal canal. It gives a horseshoe-shaped appearance of the two fossae together.

Clinical Importance of the Recess and Communication

These are the site for spread of infection from one fossa.

Subdivisions of the Fossa

A transverse fascial septum extends from the undersurface of conjoint puborectalis longitudinal muscle coat of rectum from medial to lateral direction. It is called **perianal fascia**. The fascia is attached medially to the level of Hilton's line of anal canal and laterally to the obturator fascia at the level of pudendal canal (*see* below). This horizontal septum of perianal fascia divides ischioanal fossa (ischiorectal fossa) into lower perianal space and upper ischiorectal space.

Perianal space is the shallow subcutaneous space beneath the subcutaneous part of the external anal sphincter. The fat in the perianal space is arranged in the form of small loculi separated by short fibrous septa. Infections of the perianal space are more painful because of unyielding nature of fat loculi and rich sensory nerve supply.

Ischiorectal space is larger and deep to perianal fascia. It is filled by larger loculi of fat separated by incomplete fibrous septa. It acts as a *'dead-space'* to allow distension of anal canal during defecation. Upper part of the ischorectal space is traversed by a curved fascia called *lunate fascia* which extends from lateral to medial wall of the fossa. It divides the ischiorectal space into the lower **tegmental space** and upper **suprategmental space (Fig. 35.2)**.

Suprategmental space may communicate with the pelvic cavity through a slit-like gap at the level of arcus tendineus along the line of attachment of levator ani from the obturator fascia. This linear communicating slit is known as **hiatus of Schwalbe (Fig. 35.3)**. If the hiatus is present, infection may spread from the pelvic cavity to the ischioanal space or in reverse direction.

PUDENDAL CANAL (FIG. 35.2)

Introduction

It is a narrow fascial canal on the lateral wall of ischioanal fossa. The canal is directed *forwards, upwards* and *slightly medially* over the fascia covering obturator internus on medial surface of the body of ischium.

Formation

Pudendal canal is formed by meeting of the following fasciae from different sides.
- **Laterally:** Obturator fascia
- **Medially:** Perianal fascia
- **Superiorly:** Lunate fascia

Contents

Pudendal nerve (S_2, S_3) and internal pudendal artery.

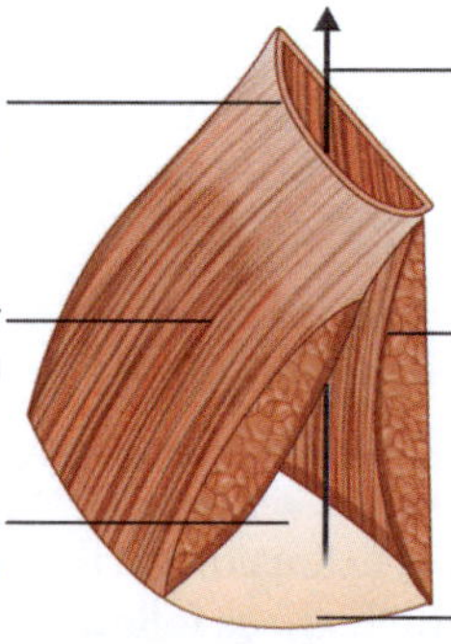

Fig. 35.3: Hiatus of Schwalbe.

Clinical Anatomy (Pudendal Neve Block)

It is a clinical procedure where the pudendal nerve is anesthetized ('blocked') by injecting local anesthetic drugs to abolish sensation in the perineum. The procedure is adopted during difficult and/or instrumental childbirth per vagina. Position of the block is located through digital examination per vagina by which position of the ischial spine is identified.

Contents of Ischioanal (Ischiorectal) Fossa (Fig. 35.4)

- Ischioanal (ischiorectal) pad of fat.
- Pudendal nerve and internal pudendal vessels in the pudendal canal lying in the lateral wall of the fossa. These are main nerve and vessels of the fossa.
- Inferior rectal nerve and vessels passing from lateral wall to medial wall of the ischioanal fossa.
- Posterior scrotal or labial nerve and vessels crossing the anterolateral angle of the anal triangle to reach the urogenital triangle.
- Perineal branch of fourth sacral (S_4) nerve—at posterior angle of the anal triangle.
- Perforating cutaneous nerve (S_2, S_3). It appears at ischioanal fossa piercing the sacrotuberous ligament.

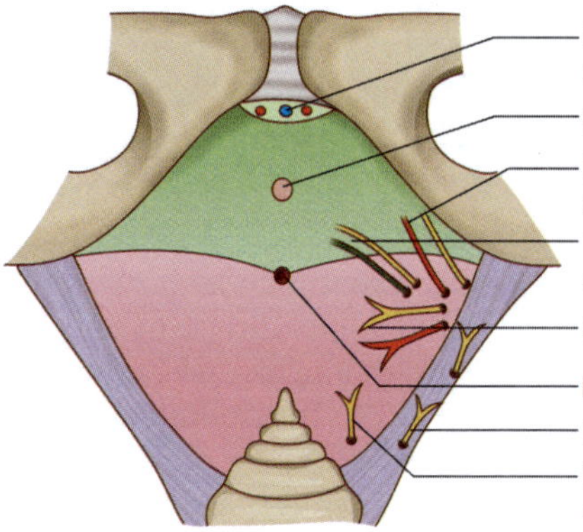

Fig. 35.4: Perineal vessels and nerves.

Clinical Anatomy

Ischiorectal Fossa Infection

Ischiorectal fossa (ischioanal fossa) is filled up with fat and it is poorly vascularized. As the fossa is close to the anal canal, chance of infection is very common. Apart from the anal mucosa, infection can spread from the perianal hair follicles or sweat gland. Rarely, perirectal abscess may burst through the levator ani to spread into the ischioanal fossa.

Ischiorectal abscess may spread into the opposite fossa through the communication behind the anal canal.

Anorectal Fistula or Anal Fistula

Sometimes ischiorectal abscess may burst internally on the surface of anorectal mucosa and externally on the surface of perianal skin. This will give rise to the formation of the track of anal fistula.

Hiatus of Schwalbe

It is a narrow linear or crescentic gap between the obturator fascia and the tendinous arch of origin of levator ani. It may lead to spread of abscess from ischiorectal fossa to the pelvic cavity or in reverse direction. This gap may also lead to herniation of pelvic organ (ileal loops). The condition is known as ischiorectal hernia.

SN 35.3 Write a short note on superficial perineal pouch.

SUPERFICIAL PERINEAL POUCH (FIGS. 35.5 AND 35.6)

Superficial perineal pouch or space is the *superficial or lower* of the two perineal spaces occupying the urogenital triangle.

Boundary

The pouch is bounded below by the membranous layer of the superficial fascia (fascia of Colles) and above by the perineal membrane.

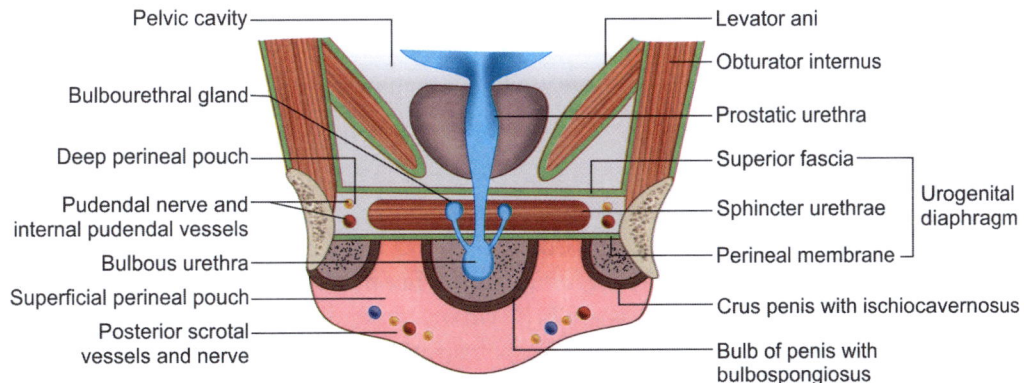

Fig. 35.5: Superficial and deep perineal pouches in male (coronal section).

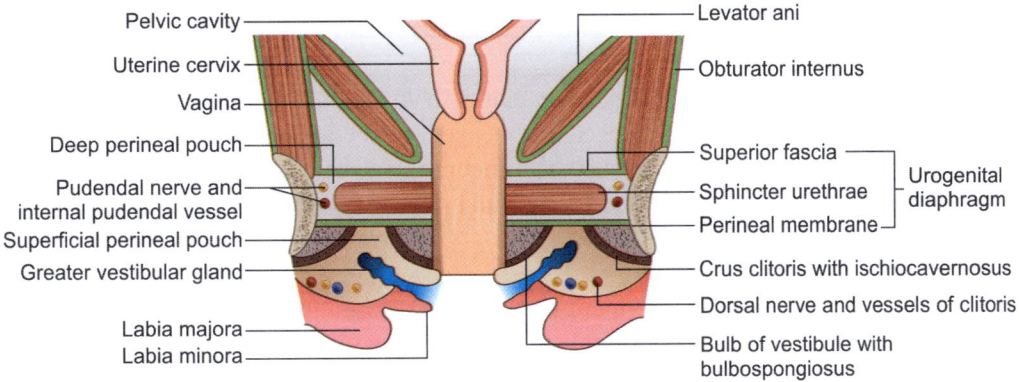

Fig. 35.6: Superficial and deep perineal pouches in female (coronal section).

Extent

Superficial perineal pouch extends laterally up to ischiopubic rami:
- *Posteriorly*, the pouch is closed along the line of posterior border of perineal membrane.
- *Anteriorly*, the pouch communicates freely with the potential space lying between the membranous layer of superficial fascia and the external oblique aponeurosis of abdominal wall.

Contents

In Male

- Two components of the root of penis, namely bilateral *crura of the penis* and *midline bulb of the penis*.
- Muscles of the crura and the bulb, called *ischiocavernosus* and *bulbospongiosus*.
  - *Ischiocavernosus* covers the crus of penis on each side. Its action is to compress the crus penis and helps in the process of erection of penis.
  - Bulbospongiosus muscle is bipennate in nature having two halves radiating from a midline raphe. It covers the bulb of penis with proximal part of corpus spongiosum. Its function is to compress the penile part of urethra to empty it for residual part of urine or semen.
- *Superficial transverse perinei muscle*: This bilateral muscle is transverse in disposition. It arises from the ischial tuberosity and is inserted into the perineal body. Its action is to fix the perineal body at the center of perineum.
- *Perineal branch of pudendal nerve* terminates in superficial perineal pouch sypplying the abovementioned muscles.
- *Perineal body*: It is a small mass of fibrotendinous tissue attached at the center of posterior margin of perineal membrane as well as the whole urogenital diaphragm. It functions as a *central tendon of perineum* for attachment of different muscles of perineum.

In Female

- Components of the root of the clitoris which are rudimentary as compared to the root of penis.
- *Crura of clitoris* are bilateral. Midline portion of the root is known as the *bulb of the vestibule* which is divided into right and left halves due to presence of the vagina in the midline.
- Muscles related to the root of clitoris are *ischiocavernosus* and *bulbospongiosus* like male. But the muscle are less prominent and the bulbospongiosus is divided into the right and left halves because of vagina.
- *Superficial transverse perinei muscle* are bilateral and transversely disposed. It is identical in structure and function to that of male.
- *Perineal branch of pudendal nerve*: It ends in superficial perineal pouch supplying the muscles of the pouch.
- *Perineal body*: Perineal body is *larger* than that of male and is more clinically important. It is *wedge-shaped* mass of fibrotendinous tissue between lower end of vagina and the anal canal. It gives attachment to various muscles of the perineum and also the fibers of levator ani. The later assists the perineal body in supporting the vaginal vault so also the uterus.

Clinical Anatomy

Traumatic rupture of urethra in the perineum may cause extravasation of urine from the superficial perineal pouch to the anterior abdominal wall between the planes of the fascia of Scarpa and external oblique muscle.

SN 35.4 Write a short note on deep perineal pouch.

DEEP PERINEAL POUCH (FIGS. 35.5 AND 35.6)

Deep perineal pouch is deep to the perineal membrane, but unlike the superficial pouch, it is a closed space all around. It is traversed by the membranous part of urethra and in addition, the vagina is female.

Boundary
- **Superficial:** Perineal membrane (inferior fascia of urogenital diaphragm)
- **Deep:** Superior fascia of urogenital diaphragm.

Extent
- *Laterally:* Both the superior as well as inferior fasciae of urogenital diaphragm are attached to the conjoint ischiopubic rami.
- *Anteriorly*: Both the layers meet at the transverse perineal ligament closing the pouch anteriorly.
- *Posteriorly*: Superior fascia fuses with the posterior border of the perineal membrane.

Contents

In Male
- *Membranous part of urethra*: It is 0.5 inch long traversing the deep pouch and lying between the two layers of fascial membrane. It is encircled by sphincter urethrae muscle. It is continuous above with the prostatic urethra and below with the penile urethra. It is not only the shortest but also the narrowest part of the urethra.
- *Sphincter urethrae muscle*: This muscle encircles the urethra in the deep perineal pouch. It arises from the pubic arch on both the sides. The fibers pass medially to surround the urethra. Sphincter urethrae is supplied by the perineal branch of pudendal nerve.
  Action: During the act of micturition, the muscle remains relaxed. It contracts to compress the membranous part of urethra, when the micturition process can be voluntarily stopped.
- *Bulbourethral glands*: These are paired small glands which lie beneath the sphincter urethrae muscle on either side of the membranous urethra. Their ducts pierce the perineal membrane to open into the penile part of urethra.
- *Deep transverse perinei muscle*: On either side, these muscles are transversely disposed posterior to the sphincter urethrae. They arise from the respective ischial ramus and pass medially to be inserted into the perineal body. These muscles are not significant clinically.
- *Internal pudendal artery*: Terminal part of the internal pudendal artery on each side enters the deep perineal pouch and passes forwards to give rise to the following branches.
  - Artery to the bulb of penis
  - Artery to the crus penis
  - Dorsal artery of penis
- *Dorsal nerve of penis*: It runs forwards through the deep perineal pouch and supplies the skin of penis.

In Female
Deep perineal pouch in female contains the structures as in male *except the bulbourethral glands*. In addition, like urethra, vagina also traverses the deep perineal pouch in female. So the contents are the following:
- Urethra

- Vagina
- Sphincter urethrae muscle
- Deep transversus perinei muscles
- Internal pudendal vessels
- Dorsal nerve of clitoris.

SN 35.5 **Write short note on urogenital diaphragm.**

UROGENITAL DIAPHRAGM

Introduction
It is a musculofascial septum bridging over the urogenital triangle of the perineum.

Extent
Urogenital diaphragm fills up the gap of the pubic arch. *Laterally,* the diaphragm extends up to the conjoint ischiopubic rami.

Urogenital diaphragm is made up of the fasciae and muscles of **deep perineal pouch**. So, *anteriorly* the diaphragm extends up to the transverse perineal ligament.

Posteriorly, the urogenital diaphragm extends up to the posterior margin of the perineal membrane.

Composition

Fascial Membranes

- *Superiorly:* **Superior fascia of urogenital diaphragm**
- *Inferiorly*: Inferior fascia of urogenital diaphragm which is called **perineal membrane**. **Central tendon of perineum or perineal body** connected at the middle of posterior border of perineal membrane is also considered as component.

Muscular Component

- Sphincter urethrae—encircling the urethra
- Two deep transverse perinei muscles.

Contents

- The urogenital diaphragm is traversed by a short segment of urethra being 0.5 inch long. It is called membranous part of urethra.
- Bulbourethral gland in male—two in number, right and left. They lie deep to sphincter urethrae.
- Internal pudendal vessels
- Dorsal nerve of penis or clitoris.

Functions

- Urogenital diaphragm, bridging across the anterior part of the pelvic outlet, mechanically supports the pelvic organs.
- Tonicity of the diaphragm containing the muscles resists the raised intraabdominal pressure during physiological and pathological condition, thus prevents sagging of the pelvic organs downwards.
- Sphincter urethrae contracts to close the urethral lumen at the end of the act of micturition.
- Some fibers of sphincter urethrae, encircle the vagina to form the sphincter vaginae, which supports the vaginal vault, so the uterus.

Clinical Anatomy

Integrity of the pelvic floor is maintained by the tonicity of the central tendon of the perineum (perineal body) through attachment of perineal muscles. In case of difficult childbirth in women, perineal tear with injury to the muscles of pelvic diaphragm interferes with the supports of uterus resulting uterine prolapse.

LA 35.6 Describe the male urethra.

MALE URETHRA

Introduction

Male urethra is a mucosa lined membranous conduit or channel for external discharge of urine and also seminal fluid.

Male urethra is 18–20 cm long as it passes through the penis for a length. It extends from *internal urethral orifice* at the neck of urinary bladder to the *external urethral orifice (meatus)* at the tip of glans penis. At its whole length, the male urethra presents two bends.

Parts of Male Urethra (Fig. 35.7)

Basically, male urethra presents two parts—posterior (proximal) and anterior (distal) urethrae.

- *Posterior urethra* is 4 cm long and lies *in the pelvis* where it is controlled by urogenital sphincter mechanism.
- *Anterior urethra* is 16cm long and lies *within perineum* proximally and *in the penis* distally, surrounded by the corpus spongiosum.

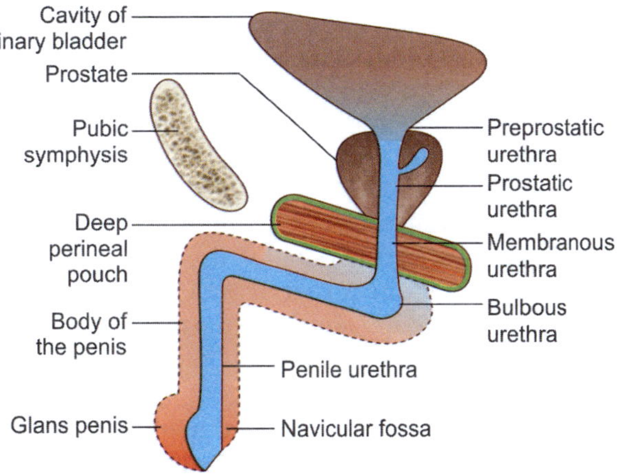

Posterior Urethra

Posterior urethra is subdivided into following components:
- Preprostatic urethra
- Prostatic urethra
- Membranous urethra

Fig. 35.7: Male urethra seen through sagittal section.

Anterior Urethra

Anterior urethra is subdivided into following components:
- *Bulbous or perineal urethra*: It is within the bulb of penis covered by bulbospongiosus
- *Penile urethra*: It is within the corpus spongiosum of penis.

Lumen of urethra

Urethral canal is a mere slit except during passage of the fluid. Outline of the lumen on cross-section of different regions shows following appearance.
- **Prostatic part:** Concavoconvex with wider transverse diameter and concavity backwards
- **Preprostatic and membranous parts:** Stellate

- **Bulbous and penile parts:** Transverse *slit*
- **External orifice:** Sagittal slit.

Preprostatic urethra (Fig. 35.8)

The preprostatic urethra is approximately 1cm in length. It extends from the neck of urinary bladder to the base of prostate. It is surrounded by small periurethral glands. These glands contribute to the formation of benign prostatic hypertrophy (BPH). Enlargement of these periurethral glands around preprostatic urethra gives rise to the symptoms of outflow obstruction in old age.

Prostatic urethra (Fig. 35.8)

It is the part of posterior urethra, 3-4 cm in length traversing the prostate. It passes through the substance of the gland more close to the anterior than the posterior surface.

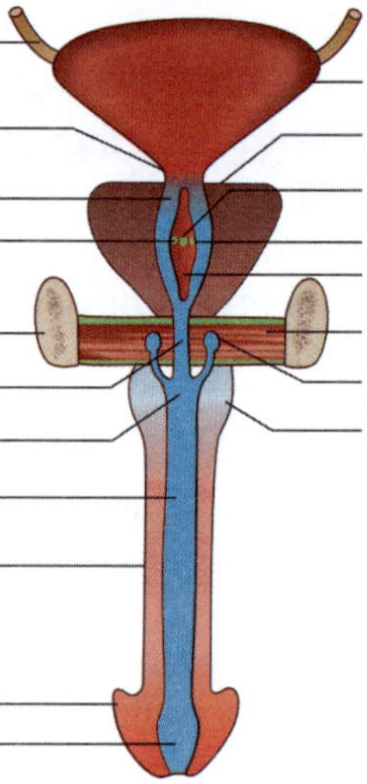

Extent

Prostatic urethra is continuous proximally with the preprostatic part and distally comes out from the prostate through the anterior surface close to the apex.

Features of the wall

Throughout most of its length, the posterior wall of prostatic urethra presents a midline ridge, called **urethral crest**. Projection of the urethral crest on the posterior wall gives a crescentic appearance of the lumen on transverse section.

Fig. 35.8: Coronal section through straightened male urethra with related structures.

On each side of the crest, a shallow depression on the posterior wall is known as **prostatic sinus.** Floor of the sinus shows openings of 15-20 *prostatic ducts*.

An elevation at the middle of the urethral crest is known as **verumontanum** or **seminal colliculus**.

Center of the verumontanum presents a slit-like orifice of **prostatic utricle**. Verumontanum is a surgical landmark for the level of urethral sphincter during transurethral resection of benign hypertrophy of the prostate. Small **opening of the ejaculatory duct** is present on either side of the opening of prostatic utricle.

Prostatic utricle is 6 mm long blind sac which extends upwards and backwards through the prostate gland behind its median lobe. The wall of the sac presents *fibrous* and *muscular* tissue with the inner lining of *mucous membrane*. The mucosal lining is pitted by the openings of number of small glands. The prostatic utricle develops from the *paramesonephric duct* or *urogenital sinus* and it is thought to be homologous with the vagina of the female. The more accepted view is that it is 'uterine homologue' and that is why it is called 'the utricle'.

Lowermost part of the prostatic urethra is immobile as this part is fixed by the puboprostatic ligaments.

Membranous urethra

Membranous part of urethra is so called because it lies in between two fascial membranes which are the superior and inferior fasciae of urogenital diaphragm. It is the *shortest* (2-2.5cm) and the *least dilatable* part of the urethra. With the exception of the external meatus, it is the *narrowest* segment of the urethra.

Extent

It descends downwards and forwards with slight ventral concavity from the *prostate to the bulb of penis*. It passes through the perineal membrane, 2.5 cm posteroinferior to the pubic symphysis.

Structure of the wall

The membranous urethra passes through the musculofascial layer of the *deep perineal pouch (urogenital diaphragm)*. Peripherally, the wall presents muscle fibers. Inner muscular layer is made up of relatively *thin layer of smooth muscles*. Peripherally, it presents prominent layer of *striated muscles* which form the **external urethral sphincter**. The luminal **epithelial layer** is separated from the muscular layer by a narrow **layer of fibroelastic connective tissue**.

Bulbourethral glands are covered by the sphincteric muscle fibers and their discharge is poured into the membranous urethra during sexual excitement.

Factors maintaining the urinary continence:
- Radial folds of urethral mucosa
- Submucosal connective tissue
- Intrinsic smooth muscles of urethra
- Striated muscle fibers of pubourethralis component of levator ani.

Anterior/spongiose/penile urethra

This part of male urethra lies within the spongy cavernous tissue of the penis.

Length

In the flaccid penis, it is 15 cm long.

Extent

It extends from the membranous urethra to the external urethral meatus on the glans penis.

Anterior urethra starts below the perineal membrane as the *bulbar urethra* within the bulb of penis covered by bulbospongiosus.

Curvatures

Anterior urethra presents two curves. First it turns forwards below the perineal membrane within the bulb of penis in the superficial perineal pouch. It is the widest part of the urethra. Next the urethra shows the second bend as its penile part.

Features

- The *bulbourethral glands* open into the bulbar urethra about 2.5 cm below the perineal membrane.
- Penile urethra is a narrow *transverse slit* when empty. The diameter is 6 mm during passage of urine.
- Terminal end at the glans shows a dilatation called *navicular fossa*
- The *external urethral meatus* is the *narrowest* site and is a *sagittal slit*, bounded on each side by a small labium.
- The urethral mucosa, particularly in bulbar and distal penile segment presents numerous small *orifices of mucous glands*.
- The mucosal surface also shows small pit-like recesses called *lacuna*. The large lacuna, called *lacuna magna* is situated on the roof of the navicular fossa.

Blood Supply

The urethral artery arises below the perineal membrane from the *internal pudendal artery* or *common penile artery*. The artery passes through the corpus spongiosus and supplies the urethra and also the erectile tissue. The urethra is also supplied by the *dorsal artery of the penis*.

Veins from the *posterior (proximal) urethra* drain into vesicoprostatic venous plexus, which ends in the internal iliac vein. *Anterior (distal) urethra* is drained by the *dorsal veins of penis* and *internal pudendal vein*.

Lymphatic Drainage

Lymph vessels from the *posterior urethra* mainly drain into the *internal iliac lymph nodes*. Lymphatics from the *anterior urethra* proceed to the following destinations.
- Mostly the vessels go to the *deep inguinal nodes*
- Some follow the inguinal canal and drain into the *external iliac group*
- Those from the glans penis go to the *superficial inguinal lymph nodes*.

Sphincters of the Urethra

Internal Urethral Sphincter

It is the smooth muscle sphincter called **sphincter vesicae** present at the level of urinary bladder neck in both the sexes.

In case of male, bladder neck at the commencement of urethra is completely surrounded by the distinct smooth muscle arranged circularly with its sympathetic innervation. The sphincter extends distally to surround the preprostatic urethra. These muscle fibers are distinct from the smooth muscle fibers extending from bladder neck to the prostate. These fibers in the bladder neck are known to form *internal sphincter mechanism*. It contributes to the *urinary continence*.

In the female, the bladder neck consists of morphologically independent smooth muscle forming the internal urethral sphincter.

External Urethral Sphincter

External urethral sphincter takes part in the formation of *urethral sphincter mechanism*. It is composed of both striated and smooth muscle fibers.

Striated component is formed by the fibers of sphincter urethrae of urogenital diaphragm. Upper circular element surrounds the urethra in female and the apex of the prostate in male. These fibers are lodged between the neck of bladder and the perineal membrane.

Lower fibers are different in nature in male and female. **In female**, these fibers extend laterally outside the urethra at the level of perineal membrane and are divided into two components. A part, known as **compressor urethrae** follows the pubic arch and is attached to the connective tissue. The other part, called **urethrovaginal sphincter**, extends downwards and backwards to surround the lateral sides of the vaginal wall. In male, later extension of the sphincter is not well developed. The sphincter of this level primarily encircles the membranous urethra forming a powerful constrictor.

Smooth muscle component is arranged between the striated component of the sphincter and the longitudinal muscle layer of the urethra. However, it is not well developed.

Nerve Supply

Probably, the *perineal branch of the pudendal nerve* supplies the sphincter in the perineum. As the urethral sphincter mechanism extends upwards through the urogenital hiatus, it receives nerve supply in the pelvic cavity from the *direct branches from sacral plexus* and the *pelvic splanchnic nerves*. All these nerves originate from the 2nd, 3rd and 4th sacral segments of spinal cord.

Clinical Anatomy

Urethral Infection

The most dependent part of urethra in male is the bulbar part. It is the most common site for inflammation and stricture formation.

In case of female, urethral infection may ascend upwards to the urinary bladder causing cystitis. This occurs due to short length of female urethra.

Rupture of Urethra

Severe trauma in perineum may lead to a complication like rupture of urethra. The common site of rupture is the bulbar part of urethra below the perineal membrane. Extravasation of urine occurs from the superficial perineal pouch to the scrotum and also anterior abdominal wall beneath the membranous layer of superficial fascia. If the membranous part of urethra is ruptured, urine outflows in the deep perineal pouch first. Then it may escape in the pelvis around the prostate and bladder or downwards into the superficial perineal pouch.

Urethral Catheterization in Male

During introduction of a catheter or other instrument through the male urethra, the following anatomical facts are to be remembered.
- External urethral meatus is the narrowest site of the urethra
- Within the glans, the urethra dilates to form navicular fossa
- A fold of mucous membrane projects towards the lumen of urethra, from the posterior end of navicular fossa
- Membranous part of urethra is the fixed and narrow part
- By holding the penis upward, S-shaped curve of the urethra is converted into J-shaped curve.

Chapter 36

Explanatory Notes (Clinical/Embryological/Morphological)

36.1 Umbilicus has both anatomical as well as clinical importance.

Anatomical Importance of Umbilicus

- The umbilicus represents the site of meeting of four folds (head fold, tail fold and two lateral folds) of the embryonic disk.
- The level of umbilicus is considered as the 'water shed line' of anterior abdominal wall. Superficial veins above the umbilicus drain upwards into the axillary vein and those below the umbilicus drain into the great saphenous vein. Lymph vessels above and below the umbilicus drain into the axillary and inguinal lymph nodes respectively.
- The belt of skin (*dermatome*) of anterior abdominal wall at the level of umbilicus is supplied by cutaneous nerves arising from the anterior ramus of the tenth thoracic (T_{10}) spinal nerve. Any pathological condition of viscera supplied by the autonomic fibers of same spinal cord segment (T_{10}) causes referred pain around umbilicus.

Clinical Significance of Umbilicus

- The umbilicus is the site of portocaval anastomosis. In case of the diseases due to portal venous obstruction, the superficial veins around the umbilicus become engorged and tortuous in a radiating fashion which is known as **Caput Medusa.** It is so called because the dilated veins look like the snakes radiating from the head of the Greek goddess Medusa.
- Due to the deficiency in closure of fetal umbilical ring, a newborn presents protrusion of abdominal organ like intestinal loop through the umbilicus. It becomes visible through the transparent layer of amniotic membrane. This condition is known as **exomphalos** or **omphalocele**.
- Due to weakness or deficiency of abdominal wall at the site of umbilicus, sometimes there is incidence of **congenital** or **acquired umbilical hernia**.
- In case of persistence of whole length of *vitellointestinal duct* extending from the midgut loop to the umbilicus, the communication may cause **leakage of intestinal content** through the umbilicus.
- When the *urachus*, representing the distal part of allantoic diverticulum, remains patent, **leakage of urine** occurs through umbilicus from urinary bladder.

36.2 In case of abdominal operations, paramedian incisions are preferred to midline incisions.

During exploration of abdominal cavity in surgical operations, abdominal wall is incised layer by layer. During these stages, first the skin, superficial fascia and anterior wall of the rectus sheath are

incised. Rectus abdominis muscle is retracted laterally to prevent undue stretching of the nerves which approach from the lateral aspect of the muscle. Posterior wall of the rectus sheath along with the succeeding layer of the abdominal wall up to the peritoneum are then incised in the similar fashion. Incision of these layers are preferred along the paramedian line instead of the midline incision because:
- Along the midline, the aponeurotic collagenous fibers show maximum lamellations and interlacement. During closure of the incision, these will give less chance of healing of the scar.
- Maximum avascularity of the fibers in the midline will cause more hindrance in repair.
- Fibers of the linea alba are thinnest, so weakest in the midline.
- Postoperative closure line of the paramedian incision opposite the line of the rectus abdominis will get additional support due to tonicity of the muscle.

36.3 Shutter mechanism of inguinal canal prevents occurrence of inguinal hernia in normal individual.

In normal healthy individual, protrusion of abdominal organs through the inguinal canal to cause the inguinal hernia is prevented by the following factors which results in shutter mechanism.
- **Obliquity of the canal:** The deep inguinal ring and the superficial inguinal ring are not in the same line anteroposteriorly as well as from side of two side. The deep ring is not only lateral to the superficial ring, but also it is at a higher level and in the deeper plane.
- **Flap valve mechanism:** Lowermost arched fibers of internal oblique and transversus abdominis extend from the lateral part of the anterior wall to the medial part of the posterior wall of the inguinal canal. During rise of intraabdominal pressure, contraction of these muscle fibers leads to apposition of anterior and posterior wall of the canal.
- **Ball valve mechanism:** The mechanism comes into action in case of males. During rise of intraabdominal pressure, loops of the fibers of cremaster muscle formed by the internal oblique pull up the ball of the testis to plug the superficial inguinal ring from below.
- **Slit valve mechanism:** Through this mechanism, the slit of the superficial inguinal ring is narrowed due to shrinkage of the intercrural fibers connecting the lateral and medial crura of the superficial ring as a result of contraction of external oblique.

36.4 Indirect inguinal hernia occurs more commonly in young adults, whereas direct inguinal hernia is common on old age groups.

- **Indirect inguinal hernia:** It protrudes through the deep inguinal ring to pass through the inguinal canal. In this clinical condition, persistence of whole of the processus vaginalis from the general peritoneal cavity acts as a predisposing factor. The patent processus vaginalis takes part in the formation of the hernial sac which is followed by tendency of protrusion of bowel loops since the childhood of the individual. So, the indirect inguinal hernia is found to occur in case of young adults.
- **Direct inguinal hernia:** It protrudes through the inguinal canal not through the deep ring, but pushing the posterior wall of the canal directly. In normal healthy individual, this is prevented by the tonicity of the conjoint tendon of the posterior wall formed by internal oblique and transversus abdominis. In old age due to loss of tonicity and elasticity of the muscles, the conjoint tendon becomes lax to give rise to the chance of occurrence of the direct inguinal hernia.

36.5 Direct inguinal hernia occurs through the triangle of Hesselbach, whereas the indirect inguinal hernia occurs lateral to it.

The triangle of Hesselbach in the anterior abdominal wall is bounded as follows:
- **Laterally:** Inferior epigastric artery
- **Medially:** Lateral border of rectus abdominis muscle
- **Inferiorly:** Medial half of the inguinal ligament forming the base of the triangle.

Deep inguinal ring is just lateral to the lower end of inferior epigastric artery which forms the lateral boundary of the triangle of Hesselbach. So, the indirect inguinal hernia occurring through the deep ring is lateral to the triangle.

As the direct inguinal hernia protrudes through the posterior wall of the canal, it is medial to the deep inguinal ring through the area of Hesselbach's triangle.

36.6 Hepatorenal pouch of Morison and rectovaginal pouch of Douglas are the most dependent part of the peritoneal cavity.

Hepatorenal pouch of Morison is the right posterior subphrenic space which is bounded as follows:
- **Anteriorly:** Inferior surface of the right lobe of liver below the level of inferior layer of coronary ligament.
- **Posteriorly:** Peritoneum covering anterior surface of right kidney
- **Superiorly:** Inferior layer of coronary ligament
- **Inferiorly:** The pouch is open to merge with the general cavity of greater sac of peritoneum.

In supine position the Morison's pouch is the deepest part of the peritoneal cavity of abdomen above the pelvic brim.

Rectovaginal pouch or pouch of Douglas is behind the uterus and upper end of the vagina, so it is present only in females. This pouch is the deepest part of the peritoneal cavity in females, both in spine as well as erect posture. The pouch is bounded as follows:
- **Posteriorly:** Anterior surface of upper two-thirds of the rectum.
- **Anteriorly:** Posterior surface of the uterus and posterior fornix of the vagina.
- **Laterally:** Right and left rectouterine folds
- **Inferiorly:** Reflection of peritoneum from the rectum to the uterus.
- **Superiorly:** The pouch communicates with the greater sac of peritoneum.

In spine position both the hepatorenal pouch of Morison as well as the rectovaginal pouch of Douglas are equally dependent part of the peritoneal cavity. So, if there is collection of ascitic fluid, blood or pus due to any pathological condition of abdominopelvic organ, it will be accumulated first in these two pouches. Fluid accumulated in the pouch of Douglas can be clinically confirmed even through per vaginal digital examination.

36.7 Strangulated intestinal loops protruded inside the lesser sac in case of internal hernia cannot be reduced by widening the outline of the epiploic foramen.

Epiploic foramen is the window or aditus to the lesser sac from the greater sac. In case of internal abdominal hernia, intestinal loops are squeezed through the epiploic foramen (foramen of Winslow) inside the narrow cavity of the lesser sac. This foramen in the site for the neck of the herniated sac. If the herniated loop gets further distended, it will be strangulated at the site of neck at epiploic foramen.

To release the strangulation, the epiploic foramen needs to be widened through incision on any of the margins which is not practically possible because all the four outlines of the foramen present vital structures as mentioned below.

- **Anteriorly:** Right free margin of lesser omentum containing the portal vein, hepatic artery and bile duct.
- **Posteriorly:** Inferior vena cava and right suprarenal gland.
- **Superiorly:** Caudate process of the caudate lobe of liver
- **Inferiorly:** First part of the duodenum and a segment of the hepatic artery.

The strangulated hernia is reduced by aspirating the contents of the distended intestinal loops with the help of aspirating needle.

36.8 The greater omentum of stomach is known as the policemen of abdomen.

The greater omentum of stomach is an elongated, free and thin double layered fold of peritoneum hanging freely from the greater curvature of stomach in front of the loops of small intestine. Initially, the two layers extend downwards (as 1st and 2nd layers) for some length and then turn upwards (as 3rd and 4th layers) to be attached to the transverse colon. As the abdominal cavity is packed with the bowel loops with other abdominal viscera, all the layers of the greater omentum are closely apposed. The thin omental layers containing adipose tissue and network of fine blood vessels are freely mobile.

If there is incidence of any inflammatory process in any viscera, e.g. in case of appendicitis, the disturbed inflamed area will be sealed by the tag of the greater omentum like the policeman rushing towards the disturbed area of a locality. That is why the greater omentum is called the policeman of the abdomen.

36.9 Gastric ulcers most commonly occur along the lesser curvature of stomach.

Gastric ulcers are found most commonly to occur along the mucosa of the lesser curvature of the stomach due to the following reasons.
- Oblique muscle fibers of the innermost layer of musculature of stomach falls a little short of the lesser curvature of stomach on both anterior as well as posterior walls of stomach. At the end of the third phase of deglutition, when the food bolus or the liquid reaches the stomach, it passes initially along the gastric canal, which is the part of the gastric cavity extending from cardiac orifice to pyloric orifice adjacent to the line of lesser curvature of stomach. So the hot, irritant or spicy liquid or food bolus comes first in contact with the mucosa of the gastric canal, to give rise to the formation of erosion so also the ulcer in this part of the gastric mucosa.
- More vascularity of any tissue facilitates quicker healing or repair of an ulcer. The blood vessels arising from the right and left gastric artery supply more directly the gastric wall with the lack of formation submucous vascular plexus. So due to less vascularity of the gastric mucosa along the lesser curvature of stomach, ulcers formed in this area have the less chance of healing.

36.10 A patient suffering from acute inflammation of gallbladder (acute cholecystitis) may present pain in the right shoulder and in the back and epigastrium.

These are the sites of referred pain on the different areas of the body as the pain fibers from the gallbladder are carried by the multiple routes of the nerves which are:
- Phrenic nerve (C_3, C_4, and C_5)
- Sympathetic nerves (T_7, T_8, and T_9)
- Parasympathetic nerve (vagus).

Localized pain in the right upper abdomen is due to irritation of the parietal peritoneum over the under surface of right dome of the diaphragm supplied by the right phrenic nerve.

Referred pain in the following areas is felt due to the reasons as stated below.
- **Pain in the right shoulder:** Among the C_3, C_4, and C_5 segments of spinal cord giving fibers to the phrenic nerve, C_3, and C_4 segments give fibers for the suprascapular nerve which supplies the skin over the tip of right shoulder.
- *Pain in the back:* This pain is felt over the inferior angle of the right scapula which is supplied by T_7, T_8 and T_9 spinal nerves. The same spinal nerves also carry sympathetic nerve fibers from the gallbladder.
- *Pain in the epigastrium*: This is due to the reason that the skin of the epigastric region of anterior abdominal wall is supplied by T_8 and T_9 nerves which also carry the sympathetic fibers from the gallbladder to the corresponding segments of spinal cord.

36.11 Calot's triangle is the clinically significant landmark for hepatobiliary surgery.

Calot's triangle is bounded by the following structures.
- **Superiorly:** Inferior surface of the liver
- **Medially:** Common hepatic duct
- **Inferolaterally:** Cystic duct

The triangle contains cystic lymph node, the cystic artery and the right hepatic artery. During gallbladder operation (cholecystectomy), the cystic artery is to be identified in this triangle for ligation as it lies behind the cystic lymph node.

During surgical operation when the Calot's triangle is exposed, the cystic lymph node is also to be identified. This lymph node is often found to be enlarged due to hidden pathological conditions of liver and gallbladder. The cystic lymph node is the first lymph gland to be enlarged in carcinoma of gallbladder. Once this node is found to be enlarged, the porta hepatis is also required to be examined.

36.12 Courvoisier's law differentiates extrinsic and intrinsic obstruction of the biliary tract.

As per the Courvoisier's law, the gallbladder is clinically noticed distended and palpable if the cause of obstruction of the biliary tract is extrinsic as found in case of carcinoma of head of pancreas which causes obstruction of the common bile duct. In case of intrinsic pathology of the biliary tract gallbladder is not distended to be clinically palpable. For example, in case of cholelithiasis (gallstone) causing obstruction of the neck of gallbladder, the wall may be thickened but the organ is usually contracted due to fibrosis of the wall. So it is not enlarged in size.

36.13 A patient of carcinoma of head of pancreas may present obstructive jaundice.

The infraduodenal part of common bile duct passes downwards and to the right along the groove on the posterior surface of the head of the pancreas. Occasionally, it may be embedded within the substance of the head of pancreas.

About 10 cm distal to the pyloric end of the stomach, the common bile duct opens on the posteromedial wall of the second part of the duodenum along with the pancreatic duct through the major duodenal papilla at the summit of the ampulla of Vater. Bile is discharged in the second part of duodenum for digestion of fat.

In case of carcinoma of head of pancreas, the common bile duct is obstructed by compression of the cancerous growth and by infiltration of the duct by cancer cells. It results in stagnation of bile with subsequent rise of bilirubin level in the blood that causes the jaundice. Increased level of the bile pigment will cause yellow coloration of the skin, mucous membrane and conjunctiva. This sign is known as jaundice which comes from the French word *jaune* meaning yellow.

36.14 Following splenectomy operation, a patient may develop diabetes mellitus.

In splenectomy operation, the following structures of the splenic pedicle are ligated and cut before the spleen is removed.
- Terminal branches of the splenic artery entering the hilum of spleen.
- Tributaries of the splenic vein coming out of the hilum
- Gastrosplenic ligament
- Lienorenal ligament

During ligature of the lienorenal ligament, care is to be taken to preserve the tail of pancreas which is contained in between the two layers of the ligament. If the tail of the pancreas is accidentally removed, the patient may develop following complications.
- Tail of the pancreas contains abundant beta cells of islets of Langerhans. Loss of these cells will lead to suppression of insulin liberation which will raise the blood glucose level resulting diabetes mellitus.
- Damaged pancreas due to accidental removal of its tail along with lienorenal ligament releases enzymes that start to digest the surrounding tissue with serious consequences.
- Activated pancreatic enzymes due to the damaged pancreatic tissue produce signs and symptoms of acute peritonitis.

36.15 In case of pathologically enlarged spleen (splenomegaly), if the organ is hugely enlarged, it grows towards the right iliac fossa.

The spleen is situated in the left hypochondrium under the left dome of the diaphragm. Its convex diaphragmatic surface lies opposite the left 9th, 10th and 11th ribs with the axis lying at the level of the 10th rib directed downwards, forwards and medially. Broader anterolateral end of the spleen is anteriorly obstructed by the phrenicocolic ligament which extends from the undersurface of the left dome of the diaphragm to the left colic flexure which is directly related to the anterior aspect of the lateral end of the spleen.

So, in pathological condition, when the spleen is enlarged, it will not be able to grow forwards directly due to the phrenicocolic ligament and directly downward due to the left colic flexure. Enlarged spleen proceeds *downwards, forwards* and *medially* along the line of direction of the 10th rib which corresponds to the direction of the long axis of the spleen. From the left hypochondrium this line extends to the diagonally opposite right iliac fossa up to which level the spleen may extend if it is hugely enlarged.

36.16 A newborn infant presents discharge of intestinal content through umbilicus.

Discharge of intestinal content through the umbilicus may be found in newborn infant due to presence of *Meckel's fistula*. In 2% of individuals only proximal part of the vitellointestinal duct persists after birth in the form of a small outpouching from the antemesenteric border of the ileum. It is called Meckel's diverticulum. It is 2 inches in length and is situated 2 feet proximal to the ileocecal junction. But in rare occasion whole of the vitellointestinal duct may persist and remain patent after birth connecting the summit of the 'U' shaped midgut loop with the umbilicus. In such case lumen of the small intestine establishes a communication to the exterior at the site of umbilicus through the patent vitellointestinal duct. It is called Meckel's fistula. After birth, as umbilical cord is cut, there occurs leakage of intestinal content through the umbilicus as the umbilical end of the whole vitellointestinal duct is cut open.

36.17 A patient suffering from acute appendicitis initially complains of pain around umbilicus but finally the pain is localized in the right iliac fossa.

Initially, the pain of acute appendicitis is *visceral pain* which is felt due to *distension* of the appendicular wall and *spasm* of the muscle. Afferent fibers carrying visceral pain pass through the sympathetic fibers to the superior mesenteric plexus. Then the fibers enter the 10th thoracic segment of spinal cord via the lesser splanchnic nerve. Pain is felt at this stage around the umbilicus because the dermatome (skin belt) at this level is supplied by 10th intercostal (thoracic spinal) nerve. This is the vague referred pain which is visceral in nature.

Later on, when the inflammatory process extends beyond the vermiform appendix and involves the parietal peritoneum of right iliac fossa, precise, severe and localized pain, somatic in nature, is felt in the right iliac fossa. It is clinically detected through maximum tenderness at McBurney's point which corresponds to the position of the base of appendix. The point is at the junction of right one-third and left two-thirds of the line joining the right anterior superior iliac spine and the umbilicus.

36.18 Sites of collateral portovenacaval anastomosis are of embryological, anatomical or clinical significance.

In case of obstruction of the normal portal venous blood flow through the liver to the inferior vena cava, portal venous blood is reshunted through the following sites of communication between the tributaries of portal and systemic veins. These anastomoses are called portosystemic anastomosis. It is also to be noted that engorgement of some of this collateral venous circulation may give rise to various clinical manifestations.

- **At umbilicus:** Paraumbilical veins will shunt portal venous blood from the left division of the portal vein to the veins radiating from the umbilicus at anterior abdominal wall. Engorged tortuous veins radiating around umbilicus are termed as Caput Medusa as these veins resemble the snakes radiating from the head of Greek goddess Medusa.
- **At the lower end of esophagus:** Esophageal tributaries of the left gastric vein (portal system) communicate with the esophageal tributaries of the inferior hemiazygos vein at the lower end of esophagus. Engorgement of these veins due to portal obstruction may cause their rupture. It will be manifested by vomiting of blood. Clinically, it is known as hematemesis.
- **At the anal canal:** Superior rectal vein of the portal system communicates with middle rectal and inferior rectal veins of the systemic system. Engorged and tortuous veins at this site leads to the development of *hemorrhoids or piles.*
- **At the bare area of liver:** Minute veins draining the liver (portal system) communicate with the veins draining the diaphragm (systemic system).
- **At the posterior abdominal wall:**
    - Veins draining the retroperitoneal parts of the gut, e.g. duodenum, ascending colon and descending colon (portal system) communicate with the veins of the posterior abdominal wall and the kidneys (systemic system). These communicating veins are called veins of Retzius.
    - Splenic vein of the portal system sometimes communicates with the renal vein of the systemic system.
- *Persistent ductus venosus*: Vary rarely the ductus venosus may be persistent after birth connecting the left division of portal vein (portal system) and the inferior vena cava (systemic system).

36.19 Cold abscess (caseous material) in patient of caries spine (tuberculosis) of thoracolumbar vertebrae may trickle down in the femoral region.

Tuberculosis of the vertebrae is known as caries spine. Prolonged untreated or complicated cases of this disease may lead to necrosis of the bony tissue forming *caseous material* which is semisolid in nature. The necrotic material is initially collected in the paravertebral region following the course of the spinal nerve. As this necrotic substance is noninflammatory but looks like pus, the clinical condition is known as cold abscess.

In the lumbar region the psoas major muscle is paravertebral in position and it is covered by a fascial envelop called *psoas sheath*. Medial border of the psoas sheath presents five crescentic gaps called psoas arches. In case of caries spine of thoracolumbar vertebra caseous pus of cold abscess are initially collected beneath the psoas sheath protruding through the psoas arches.

The psoas major muscle extends over the paravertebral region and iliac fossa to the femoral region to be inserted into the lesser trochanter of femur. The psoas sheath covering the anterior surface of the muscle also extends up to the femoral region. So the pus (caseous material) may trickle down up to the femoral region beneath the inguinal ligament.

36.20 Knowledge of Brodel's line is important for the surgeons while doing segmental resection of kidney.

Brodel's line runs along the lateral border of the kidney along which passes a coronal plane through the kidney which is least vascular. Kidney is divided into vascular segments which are supplied by independent divisions of renal artery. The vascular segments are as follows:
- Apical
- Upper
- Middle
- Lower
- Posterior

At the hilum of the kidney, the renal artery primarily divides into anterior and posterior divisions. Posterior division supplies the posterior segment of the kidney through multiple branches. Anterior division further divides into upper and lower branches. The upper branch divides to supply the apical and upper segments. The lower branch divides similarly to supply the middle and lower segments. Each of the final divisions of the renal artery is the example of an end artery which does not anastomose with each other. Brodel's line divides the kidney coronally into anterior and posterior halves. The anterior half is made up of apical, upper, middle and lower segment.

In case of *nephrolithotomy* operation for removal of renal stone, segmental resection of kidney is done to the remove stone through the least vascular plane which corresponds to the Brodel's line.

36.21 A patient suffering from an attack of renal colic, pain is felt to be radiating from loin to groin.

In general, the term renal colic is used in case of ureteric pain. A calculus (stone) in the ureter is characterized by severe agonizing pain. By mistake it is commonly termed as renal colic. Pain is felt due to distension or spasm of the muscular wall of the ureter by the impacted calculus. Pain fibers from the ureter traverse via T_{11} - L_2 sympathetic ganglia to the corresponding segments of spinal cord. As a result of impaction of the stone, obstruction in the ureter is gradually forced downwards as a result of propagative muscular spasm. That is why the pain is felt radiating from loin to groin, successive belts of skin. The pain is also felt over the genitalia and uppermost part of the front of the thigh supplied by genitofemoral nerve (L_1, L_2).

If the pain is of renal origin, due to infection, calculus or any other pathology, it is felt over the loin. Sympathetic fibers carrying pain sensation from kidney, passing through the aortico- renal ganglion and finally via the least splanchnic nerve (T_{12}) enter the 12th thoracic segment of spinal cord. That is why the renal pain is felt over the skin belt of loin supplied by the same segmental somatic nerve (T_{12}) which is the subcostal nerve.

36.22 A newborn baby presents leakage of urine through the umbilicus.

Leakage of urine through the umbilicus in a newborn baby is a congenital anomaly characterized by presence of patent urachus. The urachus, extending from the apex of the urinary bladder to the umbilicus, represents the distal narrow portion of the allantoic diverticulum. Normally, it is transformed into a decanalized round fibrous cord called median umbilical ligament. On rare occasion, the urachus persists as a canalized duct extending from the apex of the urinary bladder to the umbilicus. In case of newborn, when the umbilical cord is cut off, urine discharges through the umbilicus due to patency of the whole duct. This condition is usually associated with outflow disorder of the urinary bladder.

36.23 A patient of benign hypertrophy of prostate (BHP) may present following symptoms:
   a. Difficulty in micturition with narrow urinary stream
   b. Frequent desire for micturition
   c. Recurrent urinary tract infection

Benign hypertrophy of prostate (BHP) is common in elderly men around the age of 50 years. The cause is the imbalance in hormonal control of the gland. Enlargement of the *median lobe of the prostate* which corresponds to the transitional zone of prostate with abundance of glandular element, is responsible for clinical manifestation of BHP. The median lobe enlarges upwards and encroaches towards the posterior aspect of the neck of urinary bladder making the bulge of the uvula vesicae on the posterior aspect of the internal urethral orifice more prominent. This causes *difficulty in micturition.*

Enlargement of the median lobe as well as the lateral lobes as a whole will cause elongation and distortion of prostatic urethra which results in *narrow stream during micturition.*

Leakage of urine in prostatic urethra through the narrowed internal urethral orifice leads to *frequent and intense reflex urge (desire) for micturition,* which explains the frequency.

Due to enlargement of uvula vesicae at the bladder neck, a pouch of stagnant urine (*residual urine*) is formed within the bladder behind the internal urethral orifice. The residual urine leads to *recurrent urinary tract infection.*

36.24 A patient suffering from carcinoma of the prostate may develop metastasis (secondary deposit) in the vertebral bodies and even in skull.

When the median lobe is the site for benign hypertrophy of prostate, the *lateral lobes,* forming the peripheral zone, are the sites for origin of the carcinoma of prostate. In case of prostatic cancer per rectal (PR) digital examination reveals hard and irregular surface of the prostate when the finger is gently pressed forwards.

Anatomical knowledge of metastasis: Dissemination of cancer cells of prostate occurs *through the venous channels.* Prostatic venous plexus is mainly embedded in the posterior aspect of the fascial capsule. It also establishes communication superiorly at the neck of the urinary bladder.

The plexus also receives the deep dorsal vein of penis. Veins from the prostatic venous plexus drain posterolaterally into the internal iliac vein, which in turn communicates with the internal vertebral venous plexus via the veins passing through the ventral sacral foramina. Internal vertebral venous plexus receives basivertebral veins from the ventral bodies. So the route for the metastasis are as follows:
- Prostatic venous plexus
- Vesical venous plexus
- Internal iliac vein
- Ventral sacral veins
- Internal vertebral venous plexus
- Basivertebral veins
- Vertebral bodies.
- All these communicating veins are devoid of valves.
- The internal vertebral venous plexus communicates with the basilar venous plexus at the base of skull through the foramen magnum. So the cancer may spread up to cranium.

36.25 In prostatectomy operation, the gland is enucleated leaving behind the capsules.

As per recent concept, there is existence of only one fascial capsule of the prostate in normal healthy male derived from the pelvic fascia. In case of benign hypertrophy of the prostate the fibrous tissue element of the gland becomes condensed to form another inner capsule keeping the venous plexus with the neurovascular bundle outside it. Then the gland becomes enveloped by two capsules which are outer original fascial capsule and inner thick and condensed fibrous capsule formed by peripheral fibrous tissue of the gland itself. The prostatic venous plexus remains well secured in between the fascial and fibrous capsules. This gives rise to an advantage for removal of the gland leaving behind both the capsules with the intact venous plexus which will prevent postoperative bleeding. The operative procedure is known as *enucleation of prostate*. This is conventionally done through the *transvesical route* in which case the gland is approached through the cavity of urinary bladder. Other approaches of the prostatectomy are as follows:
- **Retropubic route:** The gland is approached through the capsule
- **Perineal route:** The gland is approached from its posterior aspect through the rectovesical fascia of Denonvillier.
- **Transurethral route:** The operation is known as transurethral resection of prostate (TURP).

36.26 Per vaginal digital examination is very significant for diagnosis of pelvic pathological conditions in females.

In female pelvic cavity, the vault of the vagina with its fornices is superiorly related to the uterus, uterine tube and ovary with the broad ligament. Anteriorly, lie the urinary bladder and urethra. The uterus with the vagina is posteriorly related to the rectum and anal canal. Visceral layer of pelvic peritoneum is reflected from the junction of upper two-thirds and lower one-third of anterior surface of rectum to form the rectovaginal pouch or pouch of Douglas. The bottom of the pouch is the most dependent part of peritoneal cavity in females and it is 5 cm deep to the level of anus.

Through per vaginal digital examination any pathology related to the structures of female pelvic cavity can be clinically detected as follows:
- Base and neck of the urinary bladder may be felt anteriorly

- Rectum and anal canal may be felt posteriorly
- If the finger is gently pushed upwards and forwards, the uterine cervix may be felt
- Any collection of free fluid in the pouch of Douglas may be felt digitally if the finger through the vaginal vault is pushed upwards and backwards.

36.27 Prolapse of the uterus may occur in elderly lady following repeated and difficult childbirth and/or after menopause.

Prolapse of the uterus is the clinical condition characterized by sagging of the organ downwards through the vagina. It may occur due to weakness of the support of the uterus mostly after difficult and/or repeated childbirth.

Primary supports of the uterus are the following that resist the sagging of the organ whenever there is rise of intraabdominal pressure.

- **Pelvic diaphragm:** The levator ani muscle of the pelvic floor grossly holds the pelvic organ through its tone. It also resists the downward pressure of the uterus through its contraction when there is rise of intraabdominal pressure due to physiological or pathological conditions.
- **Perineal body with urogenital diaphragm:** The perineal body is the central tendon of the perineum which is tied by many perineal muscles from different directions. The plane of perineal muscles forming urogenital diaphragm with its superior and inferior fascia acts as an additional support for the uterus.
- **Axis of anteversion and anteflexion:** This is maintained by anteroinferior pull of both uterine cornu by the round ligaments of uterus and posterosuperior pull of uterine cervix by the uterosacral ligaments.
- **True ligaments of the uterus:** These are pubocervical, uterosacral and lateral (transverse) cervical ligaments of the uterus which are formed by condensation of the pelvic fascia.

In case difficult or repeated childbirth, due to loss of tone of the muscle of pelvic floor and perineal tear, the support of the uterus becomes weaker. In addition after menopause, the true ligaments become lax due to atrophy of the pelvic fascia.

36.28 When compared to the testis, the ovary experiences incomplete journey of descent in intrauterine life.

The gonads (testis and ovary) develop in dorsal body wall inside the abdominal cavity in fetal life in intermediate cell mass. A band of mesenchymal tissue known as gubernaculum of testis or ovary extends from the caudal pole of the gonad to the pudendal region where the genitalia (scrotum or labium majus) is developed. In case of males, the testis follows the whole path of the gubernaculum to descend along the lumbar region, iliac fossa and inguinal canal to reach in the scrotum, where the temperature is suitable for spermatogenesis.

Normal stimulus for the descent is the testosterone, the hormone liberated by the fetal testis. Differential rate of growth of the body walls and growth of other viscera inside the abdominal cavity are considered to be the other factors responsible for the descent. However, dragging by or shrinkage of the gubernaculum does not have any role for the descent.

In case of females, the ovary also follow the same route of the descent following the line of its gubernaculum. But the gubernaculum of the ovary gets attached to the lateral cornu of the uterus in between. Thus the gubernaculum of the ovary is divided into following two parts.
1. *Proximal part:* From the ovary to the uterus—called ligament of ovary
2. *Distal part*: From the uterus to the labium majus—called round ligament of uterus.

As the ovary descends up to the level of pelvic cavity where it is connected to the uterus through the ligament of ovary, it fails to descend further along the route of the round ligament of uterus. So, it faces the incomplete journey for descent unlike the testis.

36.29 Undescended and maldescended testis are the types of ectopic testis.

The testis starts developing in the dorsal body wall at the level of T_{10} to T_{12} segment at the medial side of the mesonephros. Finally, it descends in the scrotum as the temperature within the abdominal cavity is not suitable for spermatogenesis.

During the normal descent, following the line of the gubernaculum (but not due to its pull), the testis passes along the posterior abdominal wall, iliac fossa, whole length of inguinal canal to reach the scrotum.

If the descent of the testis is arrested anywhere in its normal path, the condition is known as *cryptorchidism* (undescended testis). In that case, the testis may lie in lumbar, iliac region or in the inguinal canal up to the superficial inguinal ring.

Ectopic testis is a congenital anomaly in which case testis deviates from its usual path of descent and it may be lodged in various abnormal positions as follows:
- **Interstitial:** Superficial to the aponeurosis of external oblique in the lower part of anterior abdominal wall.
- In proximal part of the *medial aspect of the thigh*
- *Dorsal to the penis*
- In the *perineum*

Ectopic testis occurs when a slip of the gubernaculum passes to an abnormal direction and the testis follows it along with the processus vaginalis.

36.30 Rupture of bulbar or membranous urethra will cause extravasation of urine in the scrotum, penis and anterior abdominal wall.

Both the superficial and deep perineal pouches are situated in the urogenital triangle of the perineum and laterally bounded by the ischiopubic rami. The perineal membrane, which is also called inferior fascia of the urogenital diaphragm, separates the two pouches. The deep perineal pouch is bounded superiorly by the superior fascia of the urogenital diaphragm. The deep pouch is traversed by the membranous part of the urethra and it is a closed pouch, as its two fascial boundaries fuse with each other both in front as well as behind. The superficial perineal pouch is bounded superficially by the fascia of Colles which is the superficial fascia of the perineum. This fascial layer merges with the posterior border of perineal membrane. So the superficial pouch is closed posteriorly. The fascia of Colles is continuous anteriorly with the dartos muscle sheet of scrotum, fascia of penis and the deep membranous layer of superficial fascia of the infraumbilical part of anterior abdominal wall, which is known as fascia of Scarpa. The superficial perineal pouch contains the bulbar part of the urethra in the bulb of penis.

In case of rupture of membranous or bulbar part of urethra, extravasated urine accumulates first in the superficial perineal pouch. This is due to the reason that deep perineal pouch is closed on all sides. From the deep pouch urine will be extravasated in the superficial pouch through the apertures of the perineal membrane. The superficial pouch is open anteriorly beneath the fascia of Colles. So urine will be extravasated beneath the dartos of serotum and the fascia of penis making the genitalia swollen. Further, urine will be accumulated in the infraumbilical part of anterior abdominal wall beneath the plane of the fascia of Scarpa.

Index

Page numbers followed by *f* refer to figure.

A

Abdomen 367*f*
   horizontal disposition in 263
   infracolic compartment of 264*f*
   policemen of 469
Abdominal aorta 309, 347, 347*f*
   branches of 348
   dorsal branches of 349
   extent 347
   terminal branches of 350
Abdominal cavity, peritoneal membrane in 261
Abdominal content, herniation of 365
Abdominal ostium 447
Abdominal wall
   anterior 239, 411*f*, 477
   deficiency of 240
   muscles of posterior 343*f*
   part in posterior 345
   posterior 341, 342, 342*f*, 354, 354*f*, 472
   weakness of 240
Abdominis muscle 240
Abductor digiti minimi 189
Abductor hallucis 220
Abductor pollicis longus 60, 62, 63
   tendons of 96
Abscess
   cold 345, 473
   drainage of 90
   horseshoe-shaped 406
   ischiorectal 406, 456
   pelvic 448
   pelvirectal 406
   perianal 406
   subcutaneous perianal 406
Acetabular fossa 190
Acetabular labrum 191, 193, 232
Acetabular notch 190
Acetabulum 140
Acid phosphatase 418, 423, 425
Acromioclavicular dislocation 40
Acromioclavicular joint 35, 37, 38*f*
Acromioclavicular ligament 38
Acromiothoracic artery 15

Addison's disease 378
Adductor brevis 150
   action 150
   nerve supply 150
Adductor canal 142
   contents of 142, 143*f*
   location of 134*f*
   perforator 225
Adductor longus 135, 150
   action 150
   nerve supply 150
Adductor magnus 150
   hamstring part of 150, 160
   tendon of 141
Adhesive capsulitis 46
Adipose tissue 6
Adrenaline 378
Afferent vessels 18
Ampulla 447
   of Vater 278, 303
Amylase 423
Amyloid bodies 423
Anal canal 261, 341, 399, 472
   blood supply of 404
   coronal section of 400*f*
   innervation of 404
   lining of 400
   lymphatic drainage of 404
   musculature of 402
Anal columns 401
Anal crypts 401
Anal fissure 405
Anal fistula 401, 406
   high 406
   low 406
Anal glands 401
Anal sinuses 401
Anal sphincter
   external 402
      parts of 403*f*
   internal 402
Anal valves 401, 405
Anal verge 399
Anatomical snuff box 94, 98, 98*f*, 128
Anconeus muscle 33, 72
Anesthesia 123

Angular notch 270
Ankle
   dislocation of 214
   flexor retinaculum of 183, 183*f*
   injuries 214
   sprain 236
Ankle joint 209, 213, 236
   factors maintaining stability of 213
   in coronal plane 210*f*
   relations of 212
   right 211*f*
Ankle perforator
   lateral 227
   lower medial 227
   middle medial 227
   upper medial 227
Annular fibers 78
Annular ligament 71, 71*f*, 126
Annular pancreas 279, 310, 314
Anococcygeal ligament 386, 400, 403
Anococcygeal nerves 392
Anococcygeal raphae 386, 403
Anomalous arterial branch 305
Anorectal fistula or anal fistula 457
Anorectal flexure 387, 388, 395, 399, 399*f*
Anorectal junction 399
Anorectal sling 399
Antebrachial interosseous membrane 72
Antemesenteric border 281
Antigravity muscle, powerful 184
Antigravity venous return 224
Anus 399
Aorta, coarctation of 167
Aortic plexus 356, 356*f*
Aorticorenal ganglion 354
Ape-like deformity 125
Aponeurotic fibers 240
   specialization of 241
Appendices epiploicae 324
Appendicitis 286
   pain of 332
   perforation in 331
   visceral pain for 332

Appendicular orifice 327f, 328
Appendix
  base of 329
  body of 329
  mesentery of 329
  positions of 330
  tip of 329
  to infection, predisposition of 331
Arch of foot
  functions of 222
  lateral longitudinal 221f
  medial longitudinal 220, 221f
Arch support, structural mechanism of 220
Arcuate arteries 372
Arcuate ligament
  lateral 347, 359
  medial 345, 360
Arcuate popliteal ligament 200, 200f
Arcus tendinous 384, 385
  anterior part of 387
  posterior half of 386
Areola 7
  lymphatic drainage of 8f
Areolar tissue 388
  layer of 375
Arm
  anterior compartment of 26
  medial
    cutaneous nerve of 21
    intermuscular septum of 112
  median nerve in 109f
  posterior compartment of 32, 116
  radial nerve in 115f
  ulnar nerve in 112f
Arteria cauda pancreatica 313, 322
Arteria nervi 160
Arteria pancreatica magna 313, 322
Arteria princeps pollicis 84
Arteria radialis indicis 84
Arteria recta 282, 335
Arterial arcade 282, 335
Arterial pulsation 224
Arterial pulse 136
Arterial supply, sources of 304
Artery
  advantage for compression of 146
  appendicular 330f
  fifth perforating 163
  forming network, source of 56
  fourth perforating 163
  musculophrenic 362
  of Drummond, manginal 336f, 337
  pericardiophrenic 362
  superficial 84f
Arthritis, traumatic 104
Arthroscopy 209
Articular surface 190, 200, 210
  congruence of 193, 232

Articularis genu 142
Ascitis 266
Atonic bladder 415
Automatic bladder 415
Autonomic nerves 354f, 401, 402
Autonomic nervous system 354
Autonomous bladder 416
Axilla 123
  and arm 112
  and scapular region 11
  apex of 11
  base of 12
  boundaries 11
  contents of 11, 13
  fibrofatty tissue of 18
  injuries in 117
  nodular swelling in 120
  radial nerve injury at 123
  suspensory ligament of 3
Axillary artery 14, 15f
  branches of 6, 15
  continuation of 28
  extent 14
  part of 14-16, 20
Axillary fascia 4, 12
Axillary lymph nodes 7, 12, 16, 17f
  apical group of 8
Axillary lymphadenopathy 18
Axillary nerve 21, 105, 122
  branches 106
  causes of 106
  clinical anatomy 106
  clinical manifestations 106
  course of 105, 105f
  distribution of 106f
  injury to 47, 122
  origin 105
  relations 105
  remote effect of 123
Axillary sheath 14
Axillary tail of Spence 4, 120
Axillary vein 14, 15f
Azygos vein 351

B

Back of thigh
  arterial anastomosis in 162f
  arteries of 162
Baker's cyst 168, 209
Ball valve mechanism 252, 467
Baseball finger 98
Basivertebral veins 475
Beneath skin 30
Biceps brachii
  muscle 11, 26, 26f
  tendon of 31
Biceps femoris 161, 207
Bicipital aponeurosis 26
Bilaminar fascia of Denonvillier 419

Bile canaliculi 297
Bile duct 278, 302, 308
  exogenous obstruction of 305
  joins, end of 303
  sphincters of 303f
Bile salt cholesterol complex 304
Biliary apparatus 299
  arterial supply of 303
  components 300
  extrahepatic part of 299, 300, 300f, 301f
  intrahepatic part 299
Biliary colic 304
Biliary diverticulum 256
Biliary fistula, postoperative 305
Biliary tract 470
  lymphatic drainage of 304
  venous drainage of 304
  with gallbladder, nerve supply of 304
Bladder
  injuries 415
  outflow obstruction 414
  wall 413
Blind sac, ends in 81
Blood
  anticoagulant of 287
  vessels 24, 188
Body weight, distribution of 222
Bone
  fracture of 127
  long 119
Bony configuration 219f, 220, 221
Bony factor 231
Bony pelvis 379
  orientation of 379
Bowleg 234
Bow-stringing displacement 76
Brachial artery 14, 28, 28f, 30
  bifurcation of 31
  branches of 29, 55
  origin 28
  termination 28
Brachial plexus 18, 19
  branches from 20
  formation of 20f
  location of 20
  lower
    lesion of 121
    trunk of 122
  nerve of 14
  posterior cord of 105
  roots of 19
  upper lesion of 121
Brachialis muscle 27, 27f
Brachioradialis 59, 60
Breast 4, 5
  abscess 9, 120
  develops 120
  incidence of 9

arterial supply of 6f
blood supply of 6
carcinoma of 10, 120, 121
clinical anatomy of 7
deep relations 5
extent 4
fixation of 120
inferior crescent of 5
lobes of 5
lobules of 6
location of 4f
lying beneath deep fascia, part of 4
lymphatic drainage of 7, 8f
parenchyma of 8f
prognosis of cancer of 10
quadrants of 4f
relations of 4
skin 120
soft tissue architecture of 5, 5f
support of 6
to peritoneum, spread from 9
Brodel's line 473
Bucket handle type injury 208
Bulbar urethra, rupture of 477
Bulbospongiosus 458
Bulbourethral glands 459, 463
Bursa, small 97

C

C7 and C8 nerves, fibers of 61
Calcaneal artery, median 183
Caldwell and Moloy classification 382
Calf muscle 186
   deep veins of 227
   pump 226
Caliber of lumen 285
Calot's triangle 302, 302f, 322, 470
   clinical importance of 305
Canal of Guyon 76
Cancer
   cells, dissemination of 425
   primary origin of 299
Cancerous retraction 10
Capsular ligament 100, 216
Caput medusa 239, 239f, 341, 466
Cardiac notch 270
Cardiac orifice 268, 270
Cardiac plateau 360
Cardinal ligament 441
Caries spine 136
Carpal bones
   front of 75
   osteoarthritis of 111
Carpal tunnel syndrome 76, 111, 125
   effects of 111
Carpal tunnel, formation of 75
Carpometacarpal joint 102
   extension of 63

first 103f
movements of first 104f
Carries blood vessels 257
Cartilage
   cells, devoid of 192
   intra-articular 201
   medial semilunar 202
Caseous material 473
Caudal vertebrae, changes in 385
Caudate lobe 289, 295
Cecal artery, posterior 331
Cecal branches, anterior and posterior 328
Cecal diverticulum 324
Cecum 321, 324
   abnormal position of 328
   appendix 325f
   clinical anatomy 328
   interior of 327f
   morphology 324
   peritoneal relation of 326, 326f
   posterior relations 326
   relations of 326
   shape and size 325
   situation 324
   special features of 327
   types of 325
Celiac ganglion 354, 355
Celiac lymph nodes 290
Celiac nodes 298
Celiac plexus 299, 355, 377
   branches from 355
   renal plexus from 373
Celiac trunk 320, 321
   branches of 273
   distribution of 320f
Central tendon 358, 359
Central vein 297, 298
Cephalic vein 1
Cerebral cortex, sensory area of 413
Cervical
   canal 439
   lower deep 7
Cervicoaxillary canal 11, 12, 12f
Cervix 436
   carcinoma of 446
   cavity of 439
   supravaginal part of 438, 439
   uteri 439
Cholecystectomy 305
Cholecystitis 304
   acute 469
Cholelithiasis 304
Chromaffin cells 378
   types of 378
Chromaffin system 378
Chyme 275
Cisterna chyli 342
   variations of 342
Citric acid 418

Clavicle
   fracture of 119
   sternal end of 36
Clavicular head 1, 2
Clavicular notch 36
Clavipectoral fascia 3, 3f, 5, 11
Claw foot 223
Claw hand 22, 114, 124
Clergyman's knee 205, 235
Clitoris, crura of 458
Cloquet's lymph node 132, 137
Clubfoot 237
Coccygeal plexus 392
Coccyx
   lateral margin of 386
   upper part of 155
Colic artery
   left 336, 337
   middle 336
   right 336
      division of middle 308
   superior left 337
Colic flexure
   left 333
   right 278, 296, 332
Colic impression 317
Collagen fibers 215
   small bundles of 320
Collagenous disease 102
Collateral artery 57
Collateral ligament, medial 211f
Collateral portocaval anastomosis 340
Collateral portovenacaval anastomosis 472
Colle's fracture 102
Colliculus seminalis 421, 423
Colon
   ascending 261, 261f
   descending 261, 261f
Columnar epithelium 400
Common bile duct 300f
Common iliac
   arteries 350
   veins 351
Common palmar digital
   arteries 84
   branch 87
Communicating veins 223, 226
Communicating vessels 223
Compartment muscles, posterior 59
Compartments beneath retinaculum 96
Compressor urethra 464
Concavoconvex articular disk 36
Condylar joints, two 196
Congenital anomalies 314, 414
Congenital defect 229
Congenital deformity 237

Connective tissue
 septa 6, 422
 stroma 5, 6, 452
 trabeculae 319
Coracobrachialis muscle 11, 27, 27f, 108
Cord
 branches, lateral 21
 hydrocele of 433f, 434
Cornua 446
Coronal disposition 204
Coronary artery, disorder of 228
Coronary bypass surgery 228
Coronary ligament 202
 inferior layer of 289f
Corpora amylacea 423
Corpus luteum 451
Corpus uteri 436
Costodiaphragmatic recess, protection of 374
Courvoisier's law 305, 470
Coxa valga 196, 229
Coxa vara 196, 229
Cremasteric muscle 249, 428
 fibers 440
 loop of 250f
Cribriform fascia 133, 135
Critical point of Sudeck 338
Cruciate ligament 166, 202, 203, 234
Cruciform fibers 79
Crutch paralysis 123
Cryptorchidism 433
Cubital fossa 30, 30f, 48, 108
 anterior compartment of 26
 content of 31, 31f
 floor of 31f
 median nerve in 108f
 roof of 30f
Cuboid bone 180
Cupola 358
 level of 358
Cushing's syndrome 378
Cutaneous nerve 174, 174f
 of calf, lateral 166
Cystic artery 301, 303, 322
 superior division of 301
Cystic duct 300f, 302
Cystic lymph node 301
Cystocele 415, 454
Cystoscopy 415

D

Dartos muscle 428
Deep perineal
 nerve 174-177
 pouch 459, 460
Deep vein 223, 227
 thrombosis 223, 228
Deltoid ligament 211, 214, 220, 237

Deltoid muscle 23
 under cover of 24
Deltoid tuberosity 23
Deltopectoral groove 1, 1f
Dermal plexus 7
Dermatome 466
Detoxication 287
Detrusor muscle 412
Diabetes mellitus, develop 471
Diaphragm
 action of 364
 apertures of 361
 central tendon of 296, 360
 crura of 360
 descent of 364
 domes of 361f
 esophageal orifice of 360
 left dome of 296
 openings of 361
 paralysis of 364
 referred pain from 364
 relations of 360
 right dome of 295, 296
 vascular supply of 362
Diaphragmatic hernia
 acquired 366
 congenital 365
Diaphragmatic pleura 296
Digital arteries, branches of 90
Digital nerves 117
Digital pulp space 89, 89f, 93
 infection 128
Digital synovial sheath 82, 128
Dimple 120
Dislocation
 anterior 40
 posterior 40, 195
Distal articular surface 210
Disuse atrophy 114
Diverticulitis 286
Dorsal digital expansion 61, 96, 97, 97f, 173
Dorsal interossei muscles 85, 85f, 97, 114, 176
Dorsalis pedis artery 178, 186
Dorsiflexion and plantar flexion 213
Dorsum of hand, cutaneous nerves of 94, 94f
Drawer signs, anterior and posterior 234
Duct of Bellini 371
Duodenal cap 276
 deformed 276
Duodenal compression 279
Duodenal diverticula 279
Duodenal flexure, superior 276, 277
Duodenal papilla 278f
 major 278, 303, 313
 minor 278, 303, 313
Duodenal ulcer 276

Duodenojejunal flexure 280, 283
Duodenum 260, 274, 341
 anatomical position of 274
 anterior relation of 277f
 curvature of 275
 descending part of 277
 first part of 276, 296, 308
 functions 275
 interior of 278f
 length 275
 location of 275, 275f
 muscle of 279
 nomenclature 275
 of Zygosis 260f
 parts 275
 posterior relation 278f
 second part of 277, 296
 suspensory muscle of 279, 280f, 360
 with related structures 276f
Dupuytren's contracture 78, 127

E

Ectopic pancreas 314
Ectopic pregnancy 449
Ectopic testis 433, 477
 types of 477
Efferent ductules 431
Efferent vessels 18
Ejaculatory duct 426, 427, 462
 openings of common 421
Elastic fibers 279, 403
Elbow
 action on 28
 arterial anastomosis around 56f
 effusion of 70
 flexor of 60
 lesion at 114
 muscle acting on 58
 posterior dislocation of 70
Elbow joint 31, 49, 56, 67, 69f, 71
 arterial
  anastomosis around 56
  supply 69
 articular surfaces 67
 capsule of 33
 clinical anatomy 70
 fibrous capsule of 67, 68f
 lateral side of 34
 ligaments 68
 movements 70
 nerve supply 70
 radial collateral ligament of 69f
 relation of 69
 synovial membrane of 68
Endocrine component 287
Endoscopic retrograde cholangiopancreatography 279
Enterocytes 282
Enteroliths 331

Index

Enzyme, collagenase 127
Epicondylitis, lateral 70, 126
Epididymis, sinus of 430
Epigastric artery
    inferior 243, 253*f*
    superior 243
Epigastric hernia, cause 246
Epigastric region 275
Epigastric vessels
    inferior 264
    superior 362
Epigastrium
    pain in 470
    right 287
Epinephrine 378
Epiploic foramen 259, 263
Epithelial layer 463
Epithelium 422
    gastric body type 286
Erb's point 21
Erb-Duchenne palsy 22, 121
    deformity in 22, 121
Esophageal branches 361
Esophageal opening 361
Esophageal orifice 268
Esophageal varices 274
Esophagus 361
    abdominal part of 295
    lower end of 341, 472
Estrogen 449, 451
Exomphalos 240, 466
Extensor carpi
    radialis 62
        brevis 60
        longus 60
    ulnaris 62
        tendon of 62
Extensor digiti minimi 61
    tendon of 97
Extensor digitorum 60, 61, 97
    longus
        muscle 172, 172*f*, 176, 213
        tendon of 212
    tendon of 61
Extensor hallucis longus
    muscle 172, 172*f*, 176, 178, 213
    tendon of 175, 212
Extensor indicis 64
    tendon of 97
Extensor pollicis
    brevis 60, 63
    longus 63, 64, 94
        tendon of 64, 98
Extensor retinaculum 96
    functions of 96
    inferior 171, 176
    superior 171, 175
Extensor tendon apparatus 96
Extraperitoneal fatty tissue 250
Extraperitoneal rupture 415

F

Fabellofibular ligament 200
Falciform ligament 257, 263, 289, 293*f*, 296
    reflection of 293*f*
Falciform margin 133
Falciform process 155
Fallopian tubes 446
Falx inguinalis 250, 254
Fascia
    covering popliteus 161
    cruris 179
    deep 59, 62
        to deep 223
    lata 134, 135, 241
        infolding of 139
    of Denonvillier 421
    of Gerota 370
    system, superficial 5
    transversalis 250
Fascial capsule 370, 419, 419*f*
    posterior parts of 419
Fascial layer
    inferior 421
    superior 421
Fascial lining 93
Fascial septum 137
Fasciocutaneous branches 179
Fatty capsule 370
Femoral artery 135, 137, 143, 144, 144*f*, 153, 169
    aneurysm of 146
    branches of 144*f*, 145
    in adductor canal 145
    in femoral triangle 145
    lateral circumflex 146, 154
    medial circumflex 146, 154
    pulsation of 146
    superficial subcutaneous branches of 135
    termination 144
Femoral branch 353
Femoral canal 137
    contents of 137
    function of 137
Femoral condyles, tibial articular surface of 197*f*
Femoral cutaneous nerve
    lateral 353
    medial 224
Femoral fossa 137
Femoral hernia 133, 137, 138, 230
    bulge of 136
    clinical diagnosis of 230
    direction of 230
        bulge of 138
    protrudes inferolateral 138
    strangulated 230
Femoral intercondylar notch 206

Femoral neck, ossification of 229
Femoral nerve 135, 145, 146, 353
Femoral ring 137
    medial margin of 138
Femoral septum 137
Femoral sheath 136, 136*f*, 137, 145
    compartments 137
    medial compartment of 137
    shape and size 136
Femoral triangle 134
    boundaries 134
    content of 134, 135*f*
Femoral vein 136, 137, 143, 224, 227
Femoral vessels 135, 136
Femur
    and deficiency, shaft of 142
    articular surface of 196
    lateral condyle of 203
    lateral epicondyle of 200
    patellar articular surface of 197*f*
Fenestrated endothelial cells 297
Fetal life, testis in 433*f*
Fibers
    deep 140
        transverse 77
    direction of 95
    lowest 240, 241
    middle and upper 241
    nerve carry 53
    superficial 54, 140
    types of 78
Fibrinolysin 423
Fibrocartilage, covered by 36
Fibrocartilaginous facet 215
Fibroconnective tissue, condensation of 440
Fibroelastic bands, multiple 404
Fibroelastic connective tissue, layer of 463
Fibromuscular arch 70
Fibromuscular stroma 422, 423
Fibrous band 286
    diverticulum with 285*f*
Fibrous capsule 41, 41*f*, 100, 103, 191, 191*f*, 198, 210, 214, 370
    deficiency in 42
    distal attachment 68, 191
    inner 419
    original 371
    proximal attachment 68, 191
Fibrous flexor sheath, components of 78*f*
Fibrous pericardium 360
Fibrous septa 10
Fibrous tissue 89, 462
Fibula
    lateral malleolus of 210, 237
    malleolus of 212
    neck of 166
Fibular artery 185
    circumflex 185

Fibular collateral ligament 200
Fibular malleolus 214
Fibular nerve 166, 236
    common 166
    deep 174-177, 178f, 212
    superficial 174, 182
Fibular retinacula 181, 181f
Fibular retinaculum
    deep to inferior 180
    inferior 181
    superior 180, 181
Fibular trochlea 180
Fibular vein 236
Fibularis brevis
    muscle 174, 180, 180f, 186
    tendon of 179
Fibularis longus
    muscle 179, 186
        part of 177
    tendons of 181
Fibularis tertius
    muscle 172f, 173, 174, 213
    tendon of 175, 212
Fimbriae 447
Fingers
    abduction of 114
    dorsum of 61
    fibrous flexor sheath of 78
    pulp space of 128
First metacarpal bone, base of 63
Flap valve mechanism 251, 467
Flat foot 222, 237
    acquired 222
Flat tendon 150
Flexion deformity 78
Flexon digitorum superficialis 50f
Flexor carpi
    radialis 49
        origin 49
        tendon of 76
    ulnaris 51, 69
Flexor creases, posterior limit of 90
Flexor digiti minimi, superficial to 84
Flexor digitorum
    accessorius 186, 189
    brevis 188
    longus, tendon of 183, 186
    part of 52
    profundus 52
    superficialis 50
Flexor halluces
    brevis 188
    longus 220
        tendon of 183, 186
Flexor muscles 385f
Flexor pollicis longus 53
Flexor retinaculum 49, 50, 53, 75f, 76f, 81
Flexor tendon
    common 82f

    synovial sheath of 81, 81f, 81f
    with lumbricals 89
Follicles, development of 423
Follicular cysts, small 452
Food
    digestion of 268, 275
    reservoir of 268
Foot
    arch of 218, 220f
    causes eversion of 180
    dorsum of 171, 173f, 174f, 182
    eversion of 216
    extensor retinacula of 175, 175f
    factors maintaining arches of 220
    forcible eversion injury of 214
    inversion of 216
    off ground 206
    sole of 183
    transverse arch of 219f
    twisting of 223, 237
Foramen
    of Bochdalek 362, 365
    of Morgagni 362, 365
    of Winslow 259
Forearm
    anterior compartment of 48
    arteries of front of 56f
    back of 62, 116
    deep fascia of 50
    lateral cutaneous nerve of 107
    lower end of 89
    margins of lower end of 129
    medial cutaneous nerve of 21
    midprone position of 60
    muscles
        of front of 48
        of posterior compartment of 58, 59f
    nerves of front of 56f
    posterior compartment of 58, 63f, 65
    radial artery in 55
    space of Parona 89, 92, 93, 93f
    superficial flexors of 109
    ulnar nerve in 112f
Forefoot, tarsal bone of 209
Foregut, artery of 273, 320
Fovea capitis 43
    femoris 191
Frenulum
    left anterior 327
    right posterior 327
Froment's sign, positive 124
Frozen shoulder 46
Fundus 408

G

Gallbladder 277, 300, 300f, 301f, 314
    acute inflammation of 469
    fossa for 290, 296, 301

    neck of 301
    removal of 302
Gallstone 304
Gangrenous change 252
Gastric and epiploic branches 322
Gastric artery
    left 273, 321
    right 273, 322
    short 322
Gastric canal 272
Gastric carcinoma 274
Gastric impression 296, 317
Gastric mucosa 268
Gastric nerves 361
Gastric plexus, left 355
Gastric ulcers 469
Gastric veins
    esophageal tributaries of left 341
    left 273
    right 273
    short 273
Gastric vessels
    short 318
    tributaries of left 361
Gastroduodenal artery 321
    origin of 322
Gastroepiploic artery
    left 273, 322
    right 273, 322
Gastroepiploic lymph nodes, right 274
Gastroepiploic vein
    left 273
    right 273
Gastroesophageal junction 273
Gastrointestinal tract, longest compoment of 280
Gastrophrenic ligament 255, 256, 263, 270, 271
Genicular anastomosis 168
Genicular artery
    branch of inferior 168
    descending 143
    inferior 169
    middle 167
    superior 169
Genicular branch, descending 169
Genicular nerve 166
Genital branch 353
Genitalia swollen 477
Genitofemoral nerve 145, 353
    femoral branch of 135, 137, 145
Genu valgum 209, 233
Genu varum 209, 233, 234
Germinal epithelium 451
Gland
    largest 287
    left 375, 376
    right 375, 376
    suprarenal 367

Glandular element 422, 423
Glandular epithelium, multilayered 423
Glandular parenchyma 5
Glenohumeral joint 35, 40
  dislocation of 46
Glenohumeral ligament 43, 43f, 44
Glenoid fossa 41f
Glenoid labrum 41, 41f, 44, 125
Glisson's capsule 290
Glucagon 306
Glucocorticoids 378
Gluteal artery
  inferior 160, 162, 391
  superior 160, 162, 390
Gluteal branch curls 159
Gluteal lines, anterior and inferior 156
Gluteal nerve
  inferior 157, 159
  superior 156, 157, 159
Gluteal region 155
  arteries of 160
  nerve of 159
  right thigh with 161f
  skeletal background of 155f
Gluteal vessels
  inferior 157
  superior 157
Gluteus maximus muscle 134, 157, 159, 194
  structures undercover of 158f
Gluteus medius muscle 155, 156, 159, 194
  and minimus, paralysis of 156, 232
Gluteus minimus muscle 155, 156, 159, 194
Gonadal artery 349
Gonadal plexus 356
Graafian follicle 451
Gracilis muscle 149, 231
Great toe, medial side of 174
Greater omentum 256, 262f, 270, 271, 333
Greater sac, communication with 265
Greater trochanter, medial surface of 158
Gubernaculum 247
  of ovary, proximal part of 450
Gut
  facilitates motility of 257
  part of 273
Guyon's canal 87, 88
Gynecomastia 9

H

Hair follicles 401
Ham 160

Hamstring
  muscles 160
  nerve supply of 162
Hand 75
  deformity of 124
  dorsal spaces of 93, 94
  dorsum of 89, 117, 129
  extensor retinaculum of 95
  facial spaces of 89, 90f
  flattening of 111
  flexor retinaculum of 75
  interossei muscles of 85
  intrinsic muscles of 79
  movement of 74
  pain in 88
Head of femur
  artery of 194, 233
  ligament of 191, 193
  round ligament of 193
Head of pancreas, carcinoma of 279, 310, 314, 470
Heart, diaphragmatic surface of 296
Hematemesis 274, 341
Hemiazygos vein 351
Hemidiaphragm, permanent elevation of 364
Hemolymphoid organ 315
Hemoperitoneum 449
Hemorrhoids 341, 405, 472
Heparin 287
Hepatic artery 298
  common 321
  left 322
  right 322
Hepatic duct 300, 300f
  accessory 300, 305
  common 300, 300f, 305
Hepatic flexure 332
Hepatic group 274
Hepatic laminae 297, 339
Hepatic lobes 289
  physiological subdivision of 290
Hepatic lobules 297, 298
Hepatic nodes 298
Hepatic pedicle 290
Hepatic plexus 356
Hepatic segments, subdivisions of 291
Hepatic sinusoids 298
Hepatic veins 291, 298, 352
  lower 298, 352
  upper 298, 352
Hepatobiliary surgery 470
Hepatocytes 297
Hepatopancreatic ampulla 303
  of Vater 313
Hepatorenal pouch 266
  of Morison 259, 265, 294, 369, 468
Hernia 254
  complete 253

  diaphragmatic 365
  internal 366
  posterolateral 365
  pushes 254
  sliding 366
  strangulated 267
Herniation, facilitating factor for 284
Herring bone pattern 312
Hesselbach's triangle 254f
Hiatus of Schwalbe 389, 406, 455, 456f, 457
Hiccups 365
Hilton's line 402, 455
Hilum 316, 367
Hindgut, dorsal mesentery of 255
Hinge joint, modified 67, 196, 206
Hinge movement 196
Hip joint 147, 158, 159, 190, 191f, 195, 232
  abduct 156
  acquired dislocation of 195, 233
  adductor of 139
  anterior dislocation of 195
  articular surfaces of 190f
  bursae around 194
  congenital dislocation of 195, 232
  diseases of 196
  dislocation of 195
  ischiofemoral ligament of 192, 192f
  lateral rotator of 158
  ligaments of 191
  nerve supplying 194
  trunk at 194
Hormonal mechanism 252
Horn
  anterior 201, 202
  posterior 201, 202
Horseshoe kidney, stability and mobility of 373
Housemaid's bursa 204
Housemaid's knee 205, 208, 235
Humeral artery, circumflex 16
Humeral head 48
Humeroradial joint 67
Humeroulnar head 51
Humeroulnar joint 67
Humerus
  lateral epicondyle of 33, 56, 126
  medial epicondyle of 57
  nutrient artery for 29
  trochlea of 67
Hunter's canal 142
Hydrocele 433
  congenital 433f, 434
  infantile 433f, 434
  types of 433f
Hydrochloric acid 268
Hypochondrium
  left 287
  right 287

Hypogastric plexus 356f, 448
  inferior 393, 398, 402, 404, 413, 422, 445
  superior 393
Hypophysis cerebri 321
Hypoplasia 378
Hypothenar muscles 79, 80
  paralysis of 114
Hysterectomy 446
Hysterosalpingography 449

I

Ileal arteries 282
Ileal papilla 327
Ileocecal junction 281, 283
Ileocecal orifice 327, 327f
  landmark of 327
Ileocecal sphincter 327
Ileocecal tuberculosis 329
Ileocecal valve 327
  functions of 328
Ileocolic artery 328, 336
  inferior division of 331
  superior branch of 336
Ileocolic lymph nodes 331
Ileum 284
Iliac artery
  external 426
  internal 374, 389, 390f, 394
  superficial circumflex 145
Iliac branch 389
Iliac crest 345
  tubercle of 156
Iliac fossa 374, 379
  cecum in right 327f
  right 472
Iliac lymph nodes
  external 132, 413
  internal 398
Iliac spine, anterior inferior 140, 192
Iliac vein, internal 422, 427, 475
Iliac vessels, internal 384
Iliacus muscle 134, 343, 344, 379
Iliococcygeus 386
Iliofemoral ligament 191, 192f
Iliohypogastric nerve 353
Ilioinguinal nerve 135, 353
Iliolumbar artery 389
Iliolumbar vein 351
Iliopsoas fascia 326
Iliotibial tract 133, 134, 134f, 156
Ilium, pelvic surface of 383
Index finger 97
  radial side of 84
Infant's feet 222
Infection 284
Inferior vena cava 277, 289, 308, 350, 350f, 362, 451
  formation 351

groove for 295
  termination 351
  tributaries 351
Inflammatory retraction 10
Infracolic compartment
  horizontal disposition at 264
  spaces in 265
Infrapatellar bursae 205
Infrapatellar fat pad 203
Infraspinatus bursa 44
Infundibulopelvic ligament 442, 450
Infundibulum 447, 451
Inguinal canal 246, 246f, 247, 252, 426, 467
  boundaries of 250
  clinical anatomy of 252
  content of 249
    female 249
    male 248
  extent 246
  male 247f
  shutter mechanism of 251
  wall of 250, 251f
Inguinal fossa
  lateral 264
  medial 264
Inguinal hernia 138, 252
  clinical diagnosis of 230
  complete 429, 252
  contents of 252
  direct 253, 254, 254f, 467, 468
  incomplete 252
  indirect 253, 253f, 467, 468
  oblique 254
  obstructed 252
  protrusion of 138
  strangulated 252
Inguinal ligament 132, 137, 241, 246
Inguinal lymph nodes 131, 229, 230
  deep 132
  superficial 131, 131f, 135, 444, 448
Inguinal ring
  deep 246
  superficial 230, 241, 246, 254
Inguinoscrotal swelling 434
Insulin 306, 312
Intercarpal joints 66
Interclavicular ligament 37
Intercondylar spines 206, 235
Intercostal muscles 11
Intercostal nerves, lower five 243, 363
Intercostal spaces 11
Intercostobrachial nerve 12
Interlobar arteries 372
Interlobar stroma 6
Interlobar veins 372
Interlobular arteries 372
Interlobular stroma 6
Interlobular veins 298
Intermesenteric plexus 356

Intermetacarpal joints 66
Intermuscular septum
  lateral 116
  medial 27
Interosseous membrane 52, 53, 63, 66, 72, 72f, 170
  anterior surface 73
  attachments 72
  direction of fibers 72
  functions of 73
  part of 64
  posterior surface 73
  surfaces 73
Interosseous muscles 187
  dorsal interossei 188
  plantar interossei 187
Interosseous nerve 61
  anterior 53, 54, 109
  palsy, posterior 66
  posterior 60-62, 64-66, 116
Interosseous talocalcanean ligament 214
Interphalangeal joint, proximal 97
Intersegmental ties 220
Intersphincteric groove 401
Interstitial cells of Leydig 431
Intertubercular sulcus, lateral lip of 1
Interureteric ridge 411
Intestinal content, leakage of 240, 466
Intestinal loops, strangulated 468
Intestinal obstruction 286
Intestinal villi 281
Intestine, small 268, 314
Intraperitoneal rupture 415
Intrathoracic pressure, negative 224
Ischial spine 386
Ischial tuberosity
  upper lateral part of 160
  upper medial part of 161
Ischioanal fossa 454, 456
Ischioanal space 454
Ischiocavernosus 458
Ischiococcygeus 386
  muscle, part of 386
Ischiorectal fossa 454, 455f, 456
  anteroposterior extent 455
  clinical anatomy 456
  contents 456
    of ischioanal 456
  formation 456
  infection 456
  ischiorectal 456
  lateral wall of 384
  pudendal neve block 456
  recesses 455
  subdivisions of 455
Ischiorectal space 455
Islets of Langerhans 306, 312
Isthmus 436, 447
Ito cells 297

Index

J

Jaundice, obstructive 305, 310, 314, 470
Jejunal and ileal
  arteries 335
  branches 282
Jejunal arteries 282
Jejunum 284
  coils of 308
  length of 280
Jejunum and ileum 280, 284
  antemesenteric border of 282
  arterial supply of 282
  borders and surfaces 281
  extent of 280f
  layers 281
  mesenteric border 281
  mucosal surface 281
Joint
  axis of 71
  bursae around 44
  calcaneocuboid 216
  compound 196
  displacement of 37
  factors maintaining stability of 193
  fibrous capsule of 71
  interphalangeal 97
  ligaments of 43, 71
  locking of 207
  of right foot, ligaments of 215f
  posterolateral aspect of 200
  relations of 72, 193
  socket of 43
  unlocking of 206, 207

K

Keystone 220
Kidney 367
  anterior
    relations 369, 369f
    surface of right 296
  arterial
    ramification of 372f
    supply of 371
  clinical anatomy 373
  congenital anomalies of 373
  coverings of 370, 370f
  floating 370, 374
  horse-shoe 373
  left 370
  lobulated 373
  lymphatic drainage 373
  macroscopic features of 371f
  nerve supply 373
  pancake 373
  parameters 367
  position of 367f

posterior relations 369
relations of 369
right 361, 368f, 369
situation 367
size of 375
structure of 371
surface features 368
transplantation, anatomical concept of 374
true and false capsule of 371
vascular segments of 371, 372f
venous drainage 372
vertebral level of 369
Klumpke paralysis 22, 121, 122
Knee
  bursitis around 208
  deformities 209
  extension of 203
  genicular anastomosis around 168f
  level perforator 227
  perforator
    above 227
    below 225
  replacement 209
    arthroplasty 209
Knee joint 138, 142, 148, 163, 196, 201f, 202, 206, 235
  abnormal angulations of 233
  anterior part of capsule of 198f
  around 168
  bursae around 204
  collateral ligament of 151, 160, 167
  effusion of 209
  injuries 207
  locking of 206
  movements of 206
  partially flexed 206
  relations of 204
  right 201f
  unlocking muscle of 235
Knock knee 233
Krukenberg's tumor 9, 121
Kupfer cells 297

L

L_2 vertebra, body of 283
Lactiferous duct 5
Lacuna 463
  magna 463
  of Lushka 414, 414f
Lacunar ligament 137, 138, 230, 241, 251
Laparoscope 267
Large gut, pelvic part of 395
Large intestine 323
  cardinal features of 324
  components of 323, 323f

functions of 323
haustrations 324
sacculations 324
teniae coli 324
Left lobe 289
  ridge on 289f
  segments 291
Leg
  anterior compartment of 178
  anterolateral compartment of 171
  artery of anterior compartment of 174
  back of 183
Lesser omentum 256, 263, 270, 290
  hepatoduodenal part 294
  hepatogastric part 294
  parts of 294
Lesser sac, superior recess of 265, 295
Levator ani 384
  attachments of 386
  components of 385
  plate 403
Lieberkuhn, crypts of 282
Ligament
  accessory 35, 37
  and spleen, peritoneal relations of 317f
  bifurcate 215
  broad 390, 416
  calcaneofibular 212, 237
  coracoacromial 43
  coracoclavicular 35
  coracohumeral 2, 43
  costoclavicular 35, 37
  costocoracoid 3
  dorsal 103
  extra-articular 199
  false 441
  intra-articular 201, 202
  lateral 103, 211
  lienorenal 255, 256, 263, 312
  medial 211
  median arcuate 360
  morphology of round 440
  nonperitoneal 294
  of Treitz 279, 360
  reinforcing 200
  resection, precaution during 138
  superficial part of 199
  three strong 193, 232
Ligamentous sprains 207
Ligamentum mucosum 203
Ligamentum patellae 141, 200
Ligamentum teres femoris 193
Ligamentum teres hepatis 289, 294
  fissure for 290
Ligamentum venosum 289
  fissure for 289, 289f, 295

Limb
  lateral 215
  medial 215
Linea alba 241, 242
  clinical anatomy 242
  formation 242
  layers of fibers of 242
  supraumbilical part of 246
  weakness of 242
Lip
  lower 327
  upper 327
Lister's tubercle 64
Little finger
  base of terminal phalanx of 81
  flexion deformity of 127
  medial side of 84
Liver 9, 277, 287, 296f, 298
  anatomical position of 287, 288
  and stomach, anteroposterior relation of 258f
  architecture of 297, 297f
  arterial supply 298
  bare area of 293, 295, 341, 472
  biopsy 299
  blood supply of 298
  cells 292
  cirrhosis of 299, 340
  clinical anatomy of 298, 299
  coronary ligament 294
  falciform ligament 293
  false ligaments 293
  functions 287
  gross features 287
  hilum of 290
  inferior surfaces of 295f
  largest organ 287
  left
    lobe of 361
      superior border 288
      triangular ligament 294
  lesser omentum 294
  ligaments of 293
  ligamentum venosum 295
  lymphatic drainage of 298
  malignant disease of 299
  nerve supply of 298, 299
  nonperitoneal areas of 293
  peritoneal
    ligaments 293, 294
    relation of 292
  posterior
    border 288
    surfaces of 295f
  right
    inferior border 288
    triangular ligament 294
  segments of 291, 291f
  spaces around 265
  supports of 291

veins draining 298
venous drainage 298
visceral relations of 295
Lobar arteries 372
Lobe
  anterior 420
  large right 289
  of liver, right 361
  posterior 421
Lower limb 131, 176
  axis artery of 160
  joint of 190
  venous
    drainage of 223
    pump of 227
Lower trunk 299
Lumbar artery 349
Lumbar lymph nodes, superior 363
Lumbar plexus 353f
Lumbar somatic nerves 357
Lumbar veins 351
Lumbar vertebra 346f
  lower 379
  third 239
  upper 360
Lumbocostal arch, medial 345, 360
Lumbosacral trunk 389
Lumbrical branches 110
Lumbrical canals 83, 91, 94
Lumbrical muscles 79, 82, 83, 83f, 187
Lumen, blockage in 449
Lunate fascia 455
Lunate surface 190
Lurching gait 156, 232
Luteal cyst 452
Lymph node 7, 8, 8f, 290
  apical group of 18
  appendicular 331
  celiac group of 274
  cystic group of 301
  deltopectoral group of 1
  groups of 17, 444
  hepatic group of 274
  internal
    iliac group of 401
    thoracic group of 8
  left gastric group of 274
  pancreaticosplenic 274
  posterior
    diaphragmatic 363
    intercostal 9
    mediastinal 363
  pyloric group of 274
  supraclavicular group of 18
Lymph vessels 7, 8, 9, 362
  deep 299
  from breast, receive 7
  of breast, groups of 7
  superficial 298
Lymphadenitis 18

Lymphatic flow, direction of 17
Lymphatics draining skin, blockage of 10
Lymphocytes, manufactures 315
Lymphoid tissue 331

M

Mackenrodt's ligament 441
Macromastia 9
Male bladder, neck of 410f
Male urethra 461, 461f, 462f
  anterior 461
  blood supply 464
  clinical anatomy 465
  lymphatic drainage 464
  nerve supply 464
  parts of 461
  posterior 461
  sphincters of 464
Male urinary bladder, peritoneal relation of 409f
Malleolar artery
  anterior lateral 179
  anterior medial 179
Malleolar network, medial 179
Malleolar perforators, medial 225
Mallet finger 98
Mammography, advantage of 10
Manubrium 1
Masculophrenic vein 362
McBurney's point 329, 332
Meckel's cyst 285f, 286
Meckel's diverticulum 285, 285f, 314, 471
  blood supply 285
  clinical anatomy 286
  incidence 285
  inflammation of 286
  length 285
  location 285
  mucosa 286
Meckel's fistula 240, 285f, 286, 471
Medial malleolus, fracture of 214
Median nerve 31, 49, 108, 108f
  branches of 84, 109
  clinical anatomy 110
  distribution of 109f
  injury 125
  lateral root of 21
  lesion at wrist 111
  medial root of 21
  muscular branch of 86
  origin 108
  palm of hand 109, 110
  palmar
    cutaneous branch of 76
    digital branches of 95
  principle of distribution 108
Mediastinum testis 430
Medical meniscus 234

Medullary cavity 119
Membranous urethra, rupture of 477
Menisci tear, types of 208
Meniscofemoral ligaments 202
Meniscotibial joint 206
Menopause 476
Mesenteric arterial occlusion 284
Mesenteric artery 323
　inferior 336f, 337, 355
　superior 282, 335, 336f
Mesenteric lymph nodes 282, 284
Mesenteric plexus
　inferior 393
　superior 331, 356
Mesenteric vein, superior 313
Mesenteric venous thrombosis 284
Mesenteric vessels, superior 284, 310
Mesentery 280, 283, 285
　clinical anatomy 284
　contents of 284
　cyst 284
　functions 284
　intestinal border of 284
　morphology 283
　root of 283
　tumor 284
Mesoappendix 329, 330f
Mesoduodenum 260
Mesogastria
　dorsal 255
　subdivision
　　of dorsal 255
　　of ventral 255
Mesogastrium, dorsal 255
Mesorectal fascia 396
Mesorectum 396
Mesosalpinx 448
Mesotendon 81
Mesovarium 447, 450, 451
Metacarpal bone
　adjacent 60
　fourth 49
Metacarpal heads 78
Metacarpophalangeal joint 61, 83
Metal staples interlock 220
Metastasis 299
Metatarsal bone, second 180
Metatarsalgia 222, 237
Metatarsophalangeal joint, first 148
Micturition, difficulty in 474
Midcarpal joint, movements in 101
Middle finger
　right 97f
　tendons for 91
Midpalmar space 83, 90
Midtarsal joint 216, 216f
Milk ridge 9
Miromastia 9

Monk's hood 278
Motor branches 19
Motor fibers 413
Mucinous fluid 102
Mucoid degeneration 102
Mucous membrane 281, 397, 462
Mucous glands
　orifices of 463
　small 423
Mucous secreting
　cells 271
　glands 271
Murphy's sign 305
Muscle 65
　abductor
　　digiti minimi 80
　　pollicis brevis 80
　action of 28
　adductor
　　part of 151
　　pollicis 80
　belly ends 60
　compression of 227
　deep group of 52
　fibers 156, 403
　　direction of 152
　　nonstriated 279
　flat 245
　　quadrilateral 139
　flexor
　　digiti minimi 80
　　pollicis brevis 80
　name of 80
　nerve supply of 27
　of back, superficial 161f
　of Bell 412
　of perineum, small 453
　opponens digiti minimi 80
　opponens pollicis 80
　palmaris brevis 80
　part of 150
　producing
　　movements 70, 104, 216
　　plantar flexion 213
　short 193, 232
　tendon, relations of 179
　thenar 114
　tibialis
　　anterior 171, 171f, 213, 216, 220
　　posterior 216
　unlocking 235
　wasting of thenar 110
Muscular arteries 146
Muscular branches
　lower 167
　upper 167
Muscular tissue 462
Musculocutaneous nerve 21, 27, 107, 107f

N

Navicular fossa 463
Neck of femur, fracture of 195, 229, 233
Neck of fibula, fracture of 236
Neck with axilla, root of 12f
Nephrolithotomy 473
Nephroptosis 370
Nephros 367
Nerve 188
　around elbow, compression of 70
　bifurcation of 152
　circumflex 16, 105
　injury, disability for 123
　lumbar plexus of 352
Nervi erigentes 393
Neural crest cells 377
Neuralgic pain 222, 237
Neuroendocrine cells 423
Neurogenic bladder, types of 415
Neurovascular bundle 135, 420, 422
　structures of 165
Nipple
　and areola
　　lymph vessels from 8
　　skin of 7
　congenital retraction of 10
　except 7
　lymphatic drainage of 8f
　retraction of 120
　supernumerary 9
Nonarticular intercondylar notch 197
Noradrenaline 378
Norepinephrine 378
Nutrient artery 233
Nutrient branch supplies 186

O

Oblique abdominis muscle, external 240, 241f
Obturator artery 390
　abnormal 138, 231
Obturator fascia 384
Obturator foramen 151, 383
Obturator internus 158, 383
　insertion 383
　nerve to 157-159
　origin 383
　tendon of 157
Obturator membrane 151, 383
Obturator nerve 152, 353, 384
Olecranon, back of 70
Omental bursa 259, 263, 265
Omental tuberosity 307
Omphalocele 240, 466
Oocyte 449, 451
Osseofibrous tunnel 183
Ossification, membranous type of 119
Osteoarthritis 196, 209, 222

Osteophytes 196, 209
Osteoporosis 196
Ovarian artery 349, 451
Ovarian carcinoma 452
Ovarian cysts 452
Ovarian dysgenesis 452
Ovarian fimbria 447, 450
Ovarian follicles 451
Ovarian fossa 450
Ovarian plexus 445, 451
Ovarian torsion 452
Ovarian vein, right 451
Ovarian vessels 450
Ovary 449, 449f, 476
   arterial supply 451
   clinical anatomy 452
   descent of 248
   displacement of 452
   external features 450
   gross appearance 449
   gross structure 451
   gubernaculum of 440
   imperfect descent of 452
   ligament of 247, 448, 450, 476
   lymphatic drainage 451
   measurement 449
   medulla of 452
   mesentery of 450
   nerve supply 451
   prolapse of 452
   protruding, gubernaculum of 248f
   situation 449
   suspensory ligament of 442, 449, 450
   venous drainage 451
Ovulation 451
Ovum, mature 451
Oxyntic cells 271

P

Pain
   fibers 304, 445
   referred 153, 363, 374
   vague 332
Palm
   entry in 86
   median nerve in 110f
   midlevel of 81
   nerves of 84f
   of hand, lateral aspect of 125
   ulnar nerve in 87
Palmar aponeurosis 50, 76, 77, 77f, 89
   clinical anatomy 78
   functions 78
   planes of fibers 77
Palmar arch
   deep 88f
   superficial 84
Palmar cutaneous branch 86

Palmar digital
   artery 85
   branch 87
   nerves, two 87
Palmar division, medial 87
Palmar fascial
   septa 77
   space, medial 83
Palmar interosseous 85, 85f, 97
Palmar radiocarpal ligament 100
Palmar septum
   intermediate 91
   medial 77, 91
Palmar spaces, infection of 129
Palmar ulnocarpal ligament 100
Palmaris brevis 87
Palmaris longus 50, 76
   origin 50
   tendon of 76
Pampiniform plexus 427, 432, 451
Pancreas 306
   anatomical position 307
   arteries of 313f
   body of 310, 311f, 318
   ducts of 312, 312f
   endocrine part 306
   exocrine part 306
   functional components 306
   head of 308, 308f
   location 306, 306f
   lymphatic drainage of 313
   malignancy of 314
   measurement 307
   neck of 310, 310f
   parts of 307, 307f
   relations of 312f
   shape 306
   spleen and celiac trunk 306
   tail of 312, 314
   trauma of 314
   vascular supply 313
Pancreatic arteries 322
Pancreatic disease, diagnosis of 314
Pancreatic duct 278, 303f
   accessory 309, 313
Pancreatic enzymes 306
Pancreatic fibrocystic disease, congenital 314
Pancreatic impression 317
Pancreatic islets 306
Pancreatic veins 313
Pancreaticoduodenal artery
   inferior 278, 309, 313, 336
   superior 278, 309, 313, 322
Pancreaticoduodenal vein
   inferior 313
   superior 313
Pancreatitis 314
Para-cardiac nodes 298
Paracentesis abdominis 266

Paracolic gutter 264
Paraesophageal hernia, congenital 365
Paramesonephric duct 420, 421
Parametrium 439
Paranephric fat 371
Pararectal lymph nodes 398
Parasympathetic fibers 334, 373, 404, 445, 448
Paraumbilical veins 340
Paravertebral gutter 264
Parenchyma, lymph vessels from 8
Paresthesia 88
Parietal cells 271
Parietal pain 332
Parietal peritoneum 250
Parietal pleura, diaphragmatic part of 361
Parona's space 94
Parthe's disease 196
Partietal peritoneum 137
Patella 141
   articular surface of 197
   displacement of 141
   factors maintaining stability of 141
   femoral condylar articular surface for 197f
   lateral dislocation of 231
   lateral displacement of 231
Patellar articular area 197
Patellar ligament 141, 200, 201f, 204
Patellar plexus 147
   infrapatellar branch for 148
Patellar retinacula 141, 198f
Patellar tendon 200
Patent urachus 240f, 414, 414f
Patent vitellointestinal duct 240f
Peau d'orange appearance 10, 120
Pectinate ligament 241
Pectineal fascia 137, 139
Pectineus muscle 139
Pectoral fascia 2, 5
Pectoral muscles 2
   actions of 2
   nerve supply of 2
Pectoral nerve
   lateral 21
   medial 21
Pectoral region wraping, deep fascia of 2
Pectoralis muscle
   major 1, 1f, 2, 11, 14
   minor 1, 2, 2f, 3, 11, 15, 40f
Pelvic
   brim 380, 381
   colon 260
   fascia 387, 387f, 441f
   floor, morphological components of 385f

inflammatory disease 448
inlet 380
lines, different 381f
mesocolon 260, 262
outlet 380, 380f, 381
visceral plexus 413
Pelvic cavity 380, 381
　female 475
　peritoneum 262
　　in female 263f
　spaces in 266
Pelvic diaphragm 380, 384, 387f, 443, 476
　actions of 388
　components of 386f
　evolution 384
　inferior fasciae of 384
　injury to 389
　innervations of 388
　integrity of 443
　relations of 387
　superior fascia of 384, 387
　vascular supply of 388
Pelvic organs 388
　compressor of 388
Pelvic parameters 381
　diagonal conjugate 381
　interspinous diameter 381
Pelvic splanchnic nerve 354, 392, 393, 402, 404, 413, 445, 448
　fibers of 393
Pelvis 379, 379f
　autonomic nerves of 393
　axis of 380
　difference of 381, 381f
　false 379, 426
　female 379f
　floor 384f
　fracture
　　of false 382
　　of true 382
　lateral wall of 383f, 449f
　level of 264
　male 379f
　ring of 382
　true 380, 427, 450
　types of female 382, 382f
Penicillar arterioles 319
Penile artery, common 464
Penile urethra 461, 463
Penis 477
　deep dorsal vein of 420, 421, 422
　dorsal
　　artery of 464
　　nerve of 459
　　veins of 464
　erectile tissue of 420
Pepsin 268
Per rectum examination 398
Per vaginal digital examination 475

Perianal fascia 404, 455
Perianal septum 404
Perianal space 404, 455
Periarteriolar lymphatic sheath 319
Pericardium 360
Perineal body 387, 403, 443, 453, 458, 403, 460
　clinical anatomy 453
　function 453
　muscles attached to 453, 454f
　with urogenital diaphragm 476
Perineal flexure 387, 399
Perineal membrane 460
Perineal pouch, superficial 457, 457f
Perineal vessels and nerves 456f
Perinephric fat 370
Perineum, central tendon of 387, 403, 443, 453, 460
Peripheral heart 184, 226, 236
Periprostatic nerve plexus 422
Peritoneal cavity 259f, 261, 265
　complex 259
　　foregut making 257
　infection of 266
　lesser sac of 265
　vertical disposition of 261f
Peritoneal dialysis 257
Peritoneal ligaments 411, 441
Peritoneum 255, 264f
　clinical anatomy of 266
　functions of 257
　greater sac of 258
　lesser sac of 258, 262
　visceral layer of 281
Peritonitis 266, 448
　acute 314, 414
Peroneal artery 184, 185
Peroneal nerve 177, 182, 212, 236
Peroneal retinacula 181, 181f
Peroneal trochlea 180
Peroneal vein 236
Peroneus brevis 180, 180f
Peroneus tertius 173, 175, 213
Persistent ductus venosus 341, 472
Pes cavus 222
Pes planus 222, 237
Peyer's patch 281f, 282
Phalanx
　distal 61, 97
　middle 97
Pheochromocytoma 378
Pheochromocytes 378
Phrenic artery
　inferior 348
　superior 362
Phrenic nerve 363
Phrenic plexus 356
Phrenicocolic ligament 333
Phrenoesophageal ligament 361
Pierces clavipectoral fascia 15

Pierces supinator muscle 60
Piercing clavipectoral fascia, structures 3
Piercing retinaculum, structures 183
Piles 405, 472
Piriformis 158, 382
　actions 383
　insertion 383
　origin 382
Pisiform bone 95
Pituitary gland 321
Plantar aponeurosis 176
Plantar arch 189
Plantar artery 188
　lateral 185, 189
　medial 185, 188
Plantar calcaneonavicular ligament 215
Plantar calcaneocuboid ligament 216
Plantar flexors, chief 184
Plantar ligament
　long 216
　short 216
Plantar metatarsal arteries 189
Plantar nerves, medial and lateral 174
Plastic component 209
Plexus formation, stages of 19
Plica circularis 281f
Plica longitudinalis 278
Plicae circulares 278, 278f, 281
Polycystic kidney, congenital 373
Polythelia 9
Popliteal aneurysm 168
Popliteal artery 163, 209, 166
　ascending branch of 162
　branches of 167
　upper muscular branch of 163
　with branches 167f
Popliteal cyst 209
Popliteal fascia 164
Popliteal fossa 155, 163, 164f, 166, 178, 236
　apex of 164
　boundaries of 164
　contents of 164, 165f
　deeper structures of 168f
　floor of 164, 165f
　inferolaterally 164
　muscles of 165
　nerves of 166f
　neurovascular structures of 165
　roof of 164, 164f
　superolaterally 164
　superomedially 164
Popliteal ligament, oblique 161, 164, 201, 201f
Popliteal pulsation 167
Popliteal thrombosis 168
Popliteal vein 227
Popliteofibular ligament 200

Popliteus muscle 168f, 169
   actions 170
   additional head of 169
   fascia covering 169
   insertion 169
   nerve supply 170
   origin 169
   tendon of 199
Porta hepatis 289, 289f, 290, 292, 300
   level of 300
   peritoneal folds of 290
Portal hypertension 299, 314, 340
Portal lobule 297
Portal pressure 340
Portal triad 297
Portal vein 313, 323, 338
   clinical anatomy 340
   course with relations 339
   formation of 310, 338
   intrahepatic part 339
   significance of 338
   termination of 338, 339f
   tributaries of 339, 339f
Portal venous
   obstruction 299, 310
   system 398
   thrombosis 340
Portosystemic anastomosis 340f, 472
Positive anterior drawer sign 208, 234
Positive Froment's sign 114
Positive posterior drawer sign 208, 234
Postganglionic fibers 377
Postganglionic sympathetic
   fibers 355, 357
   neurons 378
Pott's fracture 237
   dislocation 214
Pouch of Douglas 263, 266, 438
Pouch of peritoneum 438
Preaortic lymph nodes 328, 398, 401
Preganglionic fibers 377
   parasympathetic 355
Prepatellar bursitis 208
Preprostatic urethra 417, 420, 421, 423, 462
Prepyloric vein 270
Prestyloid recess 100
Processus sacciformis 100
Processus vaginalis 253, 432
Profunda brachii artery 29, 34
   branches 34
   origin 34
   terminal branches 34
   termination 34
Profunda femoris artery 145, 153, 154f, 162
   branches of 154, 163
   course 154
   origin 154
   terminal end of 163

Progesterone 449, 451
Pronator quadratus 54, 54f
Pronator teres 48
   muscle, heads of 49
   origin 48
Pronators of forearm, paralysis of 110
Prostate 417f, 420, 425
   arteries supplying 422
   benign hypertrophy of 420, 421, 425, 474
   carcinoma of 425, 474
   enlargement of 414
   interior of 421f
   ligaments of 419f
   lobes of 420f
   median lobe of 474
   specific antigen 423, 425
   zones of 423f, 424f
Prostate gland 321, 417, 418f, 419f
   age changes in 423
   capsules and ligaments 419
   clinical anatomy 424
   features of 418
   functions 418
   interior of 421
   lobes of 420
   lymphatic drainage 422
   nerve supply 422
   position of 417
   relations of 421
   vascular supply 422
   zonal anatomy 424
Prostatectomy 425
   operation 475
Prostatic ducts 462
Prostatic hypertrophy, benign 462
Prostatic secretion 423
Prostatic sinus 422, 423, 462
Prostatic urethra 417, 419, 421, 462
   exit of 421
   traverses 419
Prostatic utricle 420, 421, 462
Prostatic venous plexus 412, 475
Proximal limb, deep layer of 176
Pseudocoxalgia 196
Pseudocyst 314
Pseudoganglion 66, 106
Psoas arches 473
Psoas major 135, 354
   emerging nerves related to 354
   lateral to 354
   medial to 354
   muscle 342-344
Psoas sheath 345, 473
   clinical anatomy of 345
Pubic arch 381, 381f
Pubic symphysis 144
Pubic tubercle 241, 253
   acts 230
   medial to 230
Puboanalis 387, 403

Pubocervical ligament 441
Pubococcygeus 387
Pubofemoral ligament 192, 192f
Puboperinealis 385, 387
Puboprostatic ligament 410
Puborectal sling 387, 399f
Puborectalis 387, 395
   conjoint tendon of 387, 401
   muscle fibers of 403
Pubourethralis 387
Pubovesical ligament 410
Pubovisceralis 387
Pudendal artery
   deep external 145
   internal 160, 391, 459, 464
   superficial external 145
Pudendal canal 455
Pudendal nerve 157, 159, 160, 422
   perineal branch of 458
Pudendal vein, internal 464
Pudendal vessels, internal 157
Pulmonary embolism 228
Pulp
   space 90
   white 319
Pyloric antrum 271
Pyloric canal 271
Pyloric constriction 270
Pyloric orifice 269, 270
Pyloric sphincter 272
Pyloroduodenal junction 276
Pyramidalis muscle 243, 243f, 244

Q

Q angle, increased 231
Quadrangular space 24f, 25
   boundaries 25
   communication 25
   location 25
   structures passing through 25
Quadrate ligament 71
Quadrate lobe 290, 296
Quadratus femoris 158
   nerve to 157-159
Quadratus lumborum muscle 344
Quadratus plantae 186, 189
Quadriceps femoris
   components of 140f
   muscle 140
   tendon of 141
Quadriceps tendon, anterior lamina of 140

R

Rabbit hole 237
Radial artery 28, 30, 55
   clinical anatomy 56
   muscular branches 56
   palmar carpal branch 56

recurrent 56
  superficial palmar branch of 56, 76
  termination 56
Radial bursa 81, 93
  extent 81
Radial collateral
  artery 29
  ligament 69, 100
Radial nerve 21, 31, 59, 60, 72, 115
  branch of 98
  causes of 117
  clinical anatomy 117
  course 115
  deep 60, 61, 65f, 117f
    branch of 60, 116
  divisions of 56
  entry from axilla to arm 115
  in axilla 115
  in back of arm 116
  injury, effect of 123
  muscular branches 115
  origin 115
  principles of distribution 115
  relations and distribution 115
  sensory branches 115
  superficial 65, 116, 117
    branch of 94
    terminal branch 117
Radial notch 71
Radiocarpal joint 99
Radiocarpal ligament, dorsal 100
Radioulnar joint 67
  acts on 64
  complex 73
  distal 66, 72f
  muscle acting on 58
  proximal 71, 71f
  superior 68, 71
Radioulnar syndesmosis, ligament of 72
Rectal artery
  inferior 398, 404
  middle 391, 398, 427
  superior 337, 398, 404
Rectal mucosa 398
Rectal vein
  inferior 404
  middle and inferior 398
  superior 398, 404
Rectocele 454
Rectosigmoid junction 395
Rectovaginal pouch 263, 266, 396, 438
Rectovaginal septum 397, 438
Rectovesical fascia 397, 419
Rectovesical pouch 266, 396
Retracted nipple 10
Rectum 261, 395
  anteroposterior curvature of 396f
  blood supply 398

  cancer of 399
  clinical anatomy 398
  curvatures 396
  lateral curvatures of 396f
  lymphatic drainage 398
  muscular coat of 397
  nerve supply 398
  peritoneal relation of 396, 396f
  prolapse of 398
  rectal fascia 396
  relations 397
  transverse folds of 397
Rectus abdominis muscle 243, 243f, 254
  actions 244
  insertion 243
  nerve supply 244
  origin 243
Rectus femoris
  muscle 140
  nerve to 147
Rectus sheath 244
  clinical anatomy 246
  formation of 245f
  walls 244
Red pulp 319
Reinforce reflex action 414
Renal artery 349, 374
  accessory 372
Renal colic 374
  attack of 473
Renal columns 371
Renal diseases, common 374
Renal fascia 370
  continuation of 375
  vertical disposition of 370f
Renal impression 317
Renal injury 374
Renal papillae 371
Renal plexus 356
Renal pyramids 371
Renal sinus 370, 371
Renal surgery 374
Renal tubule 372
Renal veins 351
Reproductive system
  organ of female 435
  organ of male 417
Rete testis 431
Retention band, superior 275, 280
Reticular cells, network of 320
Retinacular arteries 196, 233
Retinacular fibers 191, 233
Retinaculum
  accessory slips of 75
  structures attached to 76
Retropubic space of Retzius 410
Retropubic venous plexus 422
Retrosternal hernia 365
Rheumatoid arthritis 102, 104

Rhomboideus minor 20
Rickets 229
Rider's bone 150, 290
Right ankle joint, lateral ligament of 212f
Right foot, dorsal interossei of 188f
Right knee joint
  capsule, posterior aspect of 199f
  collateral ligaments of 199f
  cruciate ligaments of 203f
Right patella, femoral articular surface of 197f
Right popliteal fossa, content of 165f
Right shoulder, pain in 469, 470
Right triangular ligament, layers of 293
Ring finger
  flexion deformity of 127
  lateral half of 95
Road traffic accident 319
Root lesion 23
Rosenmuller's lymph node 137
Rotator cuff 42
  around shoulder joint 42f
  functions of 42
  injuries 46
  joint by 44

S

Sacciform recess 71
Sacral artery
  lateral 390
  medial 349
  median 404
Sacral ganglia, four 393
Sacral plexus 391, 391f
  branches 392
  formation 392
  preplexus connections 392
Sacral sympathetic ganglia, upper 393
Sacral vein, median 351
Sacroiliac joint 389
Sacroiliac ligament, posterior 155
Sacrospinous ligament 155, 159, 386
Sacrotuberous ligament 155
Sacrum, pelvic surface of 397
Salpingitis 448
Saphenous nerve 143, 148, 174, 175
Saphenous opening 132, 133f
  clinical anatomy 133
  formation 133
  margin 133
  situation 132
  size and shape 133
  structures at opening 133
Saphenous vein
  accessory 225
  great 131f, 175, 224, 224f, 228, 229, 236
  short 225, 225f

Sartorius
    muscle 138
    nerve to 147
Scaphoid, fracture of 102
Scapula 35
    coracoid process of 3
    depression of 2, 39f
    elevators of 39f
    glenoid fossa of 41
    infraglenoid tuberosity of 32
    movements of 39
    protractor of 40f
    retractor of 40f
    rotation of 39
    winging of 14, 122
    with ribs, muscles connecting 35
    with upper end of humerus, muscles connecting 35
    with vertebral column, muscles connecting 35
Scapular anastomosis 24
Scapular artery, circumflex 16, 24
Scapular nerve, dorsal 20
Sciatic foramina
    greater 157f
    lesser 157f
Sciatic nerve 157, 159, 165
    artery for 160
    component of 162
    tibial component of 162
Scrotal edema 429
Scrotal swelling 429
Scrotum 426, 427, 477
    blood supply 428
    clinical anatomy 429
    layers of 428, 428f
    nerve supply 429
    surface features 428
    with penis 428f
Sebaceous cysts 429
Secretomotor branches 19
Segmental arteries 372
Segmental splenic veins 320
Semilunar cartilage 201, 234
    lateral 202
Semimembranosus bursa 205
Seminal colliculus 462
Seminiferous tubules 431
Sensation, loss of 123
Sensory branches 19, 182
Sensory fibers 304, 413
Sensory loss 22, 111
Serratus anterior muscle 11, 13, 14
Serum acid phosphatase 425
Sesamoid bones 186
Shaft of radius, posterior surface of 63
Shaft of ulna, posterior surface of 62
Sheath, contents of 245
Shock absorbing function 222

Shoulder
    abduction disability of 122
    action on 28
    pain 47
    separation 40
Shoulder girdle 35, 36, 46
    movements of 38
    muscular component of 35
    skeletal framework of 35
Shoulder joint 2, 35, 40, 41f, 46, 106, 126
    abduction of 45f
    adduction 45, 45f
    arterial supply 44
    articulating surfaces 41
    circumduction 46
    clinical anatomy 46
    coracohumeral ligament of 43f
    factors maintaining stability of 44
    fibrous capsule 41
    flexion and extension 45
    glenoid labrum 41
    lateral and medial rotation 46
    movements of 45
    multiaxial 45, 125
    nerve supply 44
    rotator cuff 42
    secondary socket for 44f
    special characteristics of 40
    transverse humeral ligament of 43, 43f
Sigmoid arteries 337
Sigmoid colon 260
Sigmoid mesocolon 260, 262
Sinus 406
    tarsi 215
Sinusoids 297
Skeletal muscle fibers 400, 440
Skin 7
    puckering of 120
Slit valve mechanism 252, 467
Small bowel obstruction 329
Small intestine
    coils of 277
    jejunum and ileum of 260
    mesentery of 283, 283f
Smith's fracture of radius 102
Smooth muscle 428
    fibers 403, 422, 440
Snapping finger 79
Sole
    deep veins of 227
    pulp 227
    pump 189
Sole of foot
    interosseous muscles of 187
    muscles of second layer of 186, 186f
    nerves of 188
    parts of 218f
    veins of 189

Soleal arch 165
Soleal pump 189, 224, 227
Soleal venous
    plexus 184
    sinus 226, 228
Soleus muscle 184, 184f, 236
Somatic nerve 401
Space of Disse 297
Space of Larrey 362
Space of Mall 297, 298
Space of Parona 94
Spaces of hand, clinical anatomy of 93
Spermatic cord 247, 248
    coverings of 249
Spermatic fascia
    external 249, 428
    internal 249, 249f, 428
Sphincter choledochus 303
Sphincter mechanism, internal 464
Sphincter of Oddi 303
Sphincter pancreaticus 303
Sphincter urethrae muscle 413, 459
Sphincter vaginae 387, 443, 464
Spinal cord injury 415
Spinal nerve roots 53
Spine 35
    of scapula, crest of 23
Spiral groove 116, 123
    injury at 118
    radial nerve in 116f
Spiral valve of Heister 302f
Splanchnic nerve 345
    greater 299, 355
    lesser 362
Spleen 314, 315, 315f
    anatomical position 316
    anatomy of 315
    arterial supply 318
    clinical anatomy 318
    clinical palpation of 318
    diaphragmatic surface of 317f
    ends 316
    enlarge 315
    external features 315
    functions of 315
    left kidney 361
    ligaments of 317f, 318
    location 315
    margins 316
    normal 315
    surfaces 316
    venous drainage 318
    visceral surface of 312, 316f
Splenectomy 319
    operation 471
    tail of 314
Splenic artery 322
    pancreatic branches of 313
Splenic circulation 319, 319f

Index

Splenic cords 320
Splenic flexure 333
Splenic ligaments, supernumerary spleen in 318
Splenic macrophages 320
Splenic plexus 355
Splenic puncture 319
Splenic trauma (rupture) 319
Splenic vein 311, 313
Spongiose urethra 463
Spring ligament 215, 220
Sternoclavicular joint 35, 36, 36f
    arterial supply 37
    capsular ligament 37
    dislocation 40
    intra-articular disk 37
    nerve supply 37
Sternocleidomastoid muscle 40
Sternocostal head 1, 2
Sternum, body of 1
Stomach 268
    anatomical position of 269
    and liver, relationship between 257
    anterosuperior surface 272
    arterial supply of 273, 273f
    bare area of 271
    blood supply of 273
    body of 271
    cardiac part 271
    changes in borders of 257
    external features 270
    features of 268
    functions 268
    fundus of 271, 361
    greater omentum of 469
    lesser curvature of 469
    lesser omentum of 294f
    lower part of 274
    lymphatic drainage of 274, 274f
    margins 269
    mucosal surface of empty 272
    muscular coat 272
    orifices 268
    parts of 271
    peritoneal relations 271
    posteroinferior surface 272
    pyloric part 271
    pylorus of 296, 310
    serous coat 272
    shape and size 269
    structures of 272
    submucous coat 272
    surfaces 269
    venous drainage of 273, 273f
    visceral and parietal relations 272
Striated muscle fibers 279
Student's elbow 70
Subacromial bursa 44
Subaponeurotic space, dorsal 93

Subareolar lymphatic plexus of Sappey 8
Subcervical mucous glands 420
Subclavian artery 14
Subclavius muscle 11
Subcostal nerve 363
    lower five 243
Subcutaneous fatty tissue 89
Subcutaneous infrapatellar
    bursa 204
    bursitis 208
Subcutaneous prepatellar bursa 204
Sub-lobular veins 298
Submucosal glands 423f
Submucous coat 281
Subperitoneal lymph plexus 9
Subphrenic peritoneal spaces, right-sided 265f
Subpsoas bursa 194
Subsartorial canal 142
Subsartorial plexus 143, 148
Subscapular artery 16
    branch of 24
Subscapular bursa 44
Subscapular nerve 21
Subscapularis muscle 14, 126
Substance of fibularis 236
Subtalar joint 214, 216
Sulcus intermedius 271
Supinator muscle 65, 72, 123
Supracolic compartment, horizontal disposition at 263
Supraduodenal artery 322
Suprapatellar bursa 142, 198, 198f, 203, 209
    large 204
Suprapatellar bursitis 208
Suprapubic cystostomy 414
Suprarenal arteries 377
Suprarenal artery, middle 348
Suprarenal cortex, tumors of 378
Suprarenal gland 374, 375f, 376f
    arterial supply of 376, 377f
    capsules of 375f
    coverings of 375
    left 361
    lymphatic drainage 377
    nerve supply 377
    peritoneal relation of 376
    right 296, 361
    surface features 376
    venous drainage 377
Suprarenal medulla 356, 377, 378
Suprarenal plexus 356
Suprascapular nerve 21
Supratrochlear artery 29
Supravesical fossa 264
Sural communicating branch 166
Sural nerve 166, 174
Suspensory ligament of Astley cooper 6

Sweat glands 401
Sympathetic chain, lumbar part of 356
Sympathetic fibers 448
Sympathetic trunk 345, 362
Sympathetic vasomotor fibers 377
Synovial joint 99, 190, 196, 210
    ball and socket type of 215
    multiaxial 40
    pivot type of 71
    saddle shaped 36
    saddle type of 216
Synovial membrane 42, 71, 100, 191, 191f, 199, 211
    reflection of 203
    vertical reflection of 201f
Synovial sheath, common 180
Synovial tendon sheaths 96
Systemic venous system 401

T

Tabes mesenterica 284
Tail muscles, components of 385
Tailor's muscle 139
Talipes 237
    calcaneus 223, 237
    equinovarus 223, 237
    equinus 223, 237
    valgus 223, 237
    varus 223, 237
Talocalcanean joint 214, 215f
Talocalcanean ligaments, lateral and medial 214
Talocalcaneonavicular joint 214, 215, 215f
Talocrural joint 209
Talofibular ligament 237
Talus 220
    trochea of 237
Tarsal bones 219f
Tarsal joints 214
Tarsal tunnel syndrome 183
Tendinous insertion, extension of 2
Tendinous intersections 243
Tendon
    conjoint 250
    formation of 173
    slip, insertion of individual 51
    vincula of 82
Tennis elbow 70, 126
    causes of 70
Tensor fasciae latae muscle 134, 156, 159
Teratoma 434
Teres major, lower border of 14, 115
Teres minor, nerve to 106
Terminal muscular branches 88
Testicular artery 349, 427, 431f
Testicular veins 432f

Testis 429, 430, 476
  arterial supply 431
  clinical anatomy 433
  coverings 430
  descent of 248, 432
  function 429
  gubernaculum of 247f, 432
  lobules of 431
  lymphatic drainage 432
  maldescended 477
  malignant tumor of 434
  nerve supply 432
  seminoma of 434
  structure of 431, 431f
  torsion of 434
  undescended 433, 477
  venous drainage 432
  with epididymis, left 430f
Thenar muscles 79, 80
Thigh
  cutaneous nerve of 147
  front of 131
  medial cutaneous nerve of 147
  medial rotation of 156
  muscles
    of front of 138f
    of medial compartment of 149, 149f
    posterior cutaneous nerve of 157, 159
Thoracic artery
  internal 37
  lateral 15
  superior 15
Thoracic lymph nodes, internal 8
Thoracic nerve
  lesion of long 122
  long 20, 122
Thoracic spinal nerve, tenth 239
Thoracic vertebra
  eighth 362
  tenth 361
  twelfth 361
Thoracoabdominal diaphragm 358, 358f, 359f
Thoracodorsal nerve 21
Thoracolumbar fascia 345, 346f
Thoracolumbar vertebrae 473
Thumb
  distal phalanx of 63, 64
  metacarpal of 64
  movements of 103
  muscles acting on 58
Thyroid gland, isthmus of 321
Tibia
  articular surface of 197
  condyle of 199
  femoral condylar articular surface for 197f
  lateral condyle of 134, 179

lower end of 210
  medial condyle of 200
  medial malleolus of 237
  nutrient artery of 185
  shaft of 161, 200
Tibial artery
  anterior 169, 178, 178f
  posterior 169, 183, 184, 185f
Tibial articular
  areas, posteroinferior 196
  surface area 197
Tibial collateral ligament 199, 207, 234
  superficial part of 200f
Tibial condyles, articular surface of 198f
Tibial nerve 165, 183
Tibial plateau 197
Tibial recurrent artery
  anterior 179
  posterior 179
Tibial tuberosity 208
Tibial vessels, anterior 175, 212
Tibialis anterior, tendon of 175, 212
Tibialis posterior, tendon of 183
Tibiocalcaneal band, middle 211
Tibiofibular joint, superior 166, 170
Tibiofibular ligament, inferior 210
Tibiofibular mortise 210
Tibiofibular socket 236
Tibionavicular band, anterior 211
Tibiotalar ligament
  anterior 211
  posterior 211
T-lymphocytes 319
Toe, great 182
Transperitoneal metastasis 274
Transurethral resection 425
Transverse acetabular ligament 190, 191
Transverse arch, existence of 218
Transverse cervical ligament 441
Transverse colon 260, 277, 332, 332f
  course of 333
Transverse injury 208
Transverse ligament 202
Transverse mesocolon 260, 262, 277, 310, 333
Transverse metacarpal ligament
  deep 77
  superficial 77
Transverse perinei muscle
  deep 459
  superficial 458
Transversus abdominis 254
Trapezium 49, 63
Trapezius, lower fibers of 2, 39f
Tredelenberg's test, positive 238
Trendelenberg's sign, positive 156, 232

Triceps brachii muscle 32, 32f
Trigger finger 79, 127
Trimalleolar fracture 214
Triquetral bone 95
Trochanteric anastomosis 162
Trochlea 213
Trochlear surface, superior 210
Trunk
  branches from 21
  cervicothoracic junction of 18
  lesion 22
  tributaries of 339
Tubal pole 450
Tube, rupture of 449
Tuber omentale 296, 307, 312
Tubercle of talus, posterior 212
Tuberculosis 378
Tuberosity, greater 123
Tunica albuginea 430, 451
Tunica vaginalis 253
  visceral layer of 430
Tunica vasculosa 430

U

Ulna 52
  abduction of 34
  surface of shaft of 64
Ulnar artery 28, 30, 76, 112
  deep branch of 88
Ulnar bursa 81, 129
  extent 81
Ulnar claw hand 89, 114, 124
  deformities in 124
Ulnar collateral artery
  inferior 29
  middle 29
  superior 29, 57
Ulnar collateral ligament 68, 69f, 100
Ulnar head 48
Ulnar nerve 21, 53, 69, 70, 76, 111
  branches 113
  clinical anatomy 113
  course 112
  deep branch of 83, 88, 88f
  dorsal branch of 87, 95, 113
  forearm 113
  front of wrist 112
  in forearm 112
  injury at wrist 113
  origin 111
  palm of hand 113
  palmar cutaneous branch of 76
  principle of distribution 112
  superficial terminal branch of 87
Ulnar recurrent artery, posterior 57
Ulnar tunnel syndrome 88
Umbilical artery
  fetal 412
  obliterated 264, 384, 390, 411

Index

Umbilical fold, medial 264, 411
Umbilical hernia
  acquired 240, 466
  congenital 240, 466
Umbilical ligament, median 264, 410, 411, 474
Umbilical region 275
Umbilical vein, obliterated left 294
Umbilicus 239, 466, 474
  anatomical significance 239
  clinical significance of 239, 466
  embryological significance 239
Uncinate process 307
Upper limb 1, 176
  major nerves of 105
Urachal cyst 414, 414f
Urachus 240, 264, 410
  congenital anomalies of 414f
Ureter 389, 407
  pelvic part of 384, 416, 416f
  pelvis of 371
  terminal part of 412
Ureteric folds 411
Ureterourethric ridge 411
Urethra 453
  anterior 461, 463, 464
  bulbous 461
  lumen of 461
  membranous 462
    part of 459
  perineal 461
  posterior 461, 464
  prostatic part of 421
  rupture of 465
  stricture of 414
  traumatic rupture of 458
Urethral artery 464
Urethral canal 461
Urethral catheterization 465
Urethral crest 421, 462
Urethral infection 465
Urethral meatus, external 463
Urethral sphincter
  external 422, 463, 464
  internal 464
  mechanism 464
Urethritis, acute 414
Urethrovaginal sphincter 464
Urinary bladder 407, 410f, 411f
  capacity 408
  clinical anatomy 414
  disrupted motor function of 415
  false 411
  in females 409
  in males 409
  interior of 411
  ligaments of 410
  lymphatic drainage 412
  micturition 413
  musculature of 412
  neck of 408, 421
  nerve supply 413
  peritoneal relations 409
  position of 408f
  situation 407
  sources of nerves 413
  superior surface of 263
  surface features of 408f
  trigone of 411, 411f
  true ligaments 410
  vascular supply 412
  visceral relations 409
  with umbilicus 240f
Urinary continence 464
Urine
  extravasation of 477
  leakage of 240, 474
Urogenital diaphragm 418, 421, 443, 460
  clinical anatomy 461
  composition 460
  contents 460
  extent 460
  functions 460
  inferior fascia of 417
  superior fascia of 417, 460
Uterine
  artery 390, 412, 416, 444, 448, 451
  cervix 416
  contraction 445
  homologue 462
  ostium 447
  pole 450
  segment
    lower 439
    upper 439
  support 443
Uterine tube 437, 442, 446, 448f, 451
  and ovary 447f
  and vagina 439f
  blood supply 448
  clinical anatomy 448
  extent 447
  functions 447
  lymphatic drainage 448
  measurement 447
  mesentery of 447
  nerve supply 448
  parts of 447
  situation 447
Uterosacral ligament 436
  role of 443
Uterovesical folds 441
Uterovesical pouch 263, 266, 409, 438
Uterus 435, 435f, 437f, 452
  after childbirth 446
  age changes of 445
  angulated position of 436
  angulations of 437f
  arterial supply 444
  arteries supplying 444f
  at puberty 445
  bicornuate 446
  broad ligament of 438, 441, 442
  cavity of 439, 439f
  cervix of 439
  clinical anatomy 446
  communication 437
  congenital anomalies 446
  cornu of 436
  during menstruation 445
  during pregnancy 445
  false ligaments of 438
  features with relations 438
  fibromyoma of 446
  function 435
  in fetal life 445
  in old age 446
  ligament of 247, 440
  lymphatic drainage 444
  parts 436
  peritoneal relations 438
  primary supports of 442, 476
  prolapse of 437, 446, 476
  retroverted 437f
    position of 446
  round ligament of 249f, 437, 440, 443, 444, 448
  secondary supports 443
  septate 446
  shape and size 436
  situation 435
  specimen of 452
  supports of 442
  true ligaments of 440f, 441f, 443, 476
  venous drainage 444
Uvula vesicae 412, 420, 423

V

Vagina, lateral fornices of 416
Vaginal artery 391, 412
Vaginal hydrocele 429, 433, 433f
Vaginal vault 436
Vagus nerve 299, 328, 354, 448
Valve of Gerlach 328
Valve of Tulpius 327
Valves of Kerckring 278, 281
Varicose ulcer, formation of 228
Varicose veins 223, 228
Vas deferens 426, 426f, 430f
  ampulla of 427
  arterial supply 427
  artery to 427
  clinical anatomy 427
  course and relations 426
  function 426
  nerve supply 427
  venous drainage 427

Vasomotor branches 19
Vastus intermedius muscle 140
Vastus lateralis muscle 140
Vastus medialis muscle 140, 141
Vein
   anastomotic 226
   anteromedial aspect of 143
   classification of 223
   direct perforating 226*f*
   indirect perforating 226*f*
   medial marginal 224
   numerous small 226
   of Retzius 472
   pericardiophrenic 362
   posteromedial 225
   small 320
   superficial 223
Vena caval opening 362
Venous plexus 421
   dorsal 420
Venous sinusoids 320
Venous thrombosis, deep 184
Venous valves 224
Ventral mesogastrium 255, 256
Ventral sacral veins 475
Vericocele 434
Vermiform appendix 325*f*, 329, 330*f*, 450
   blood supply 331
   clinical anatomy 331
   dimension and ends 329
   lymphatic drainage 331
   morphology 329
   nerve supply 331
Vertebral bodies 475
Vertebral column
   extension of 344
   lateral flexion of 344
Vertebral origin
   lateral 359
   medial 360
   posterior 359
Vertebral venous plexus, internal 475

Vertical limb, anterior 200
Verumontanum 462
Vesical artery
   inferior 391, 412, 427
   superior 390, 412
Vesical ligaments, posterior 410
Vesical plexus 413
Vesical venous plexus 412, 422, 427, 475
Vincula brevia 82
Vincula longa 82
Vincula tendinum 82
Viral hepatitis 299
Viscera, movement of 257
Visceral impressions 317
Visceral surface, lubrication of 257
Vitellointestinal artery 285
Vitellointestinal duct 285*f*
   anomalies of 285*f*
Volar carpal ligament 75, 88, 112
Volkmann's ischemic contracture 127

W

Waddling gait 156
Waiter tips paralysis 121
Waldayer's fascia 419
Wall of axilla
   anterior 13*f*
   muscles of different 12*f*
   posterior 105
Wall of pelvis, posterior 383*f*
Water shed line 239
Wedge-shaped stones 220
White line of Hilton 401
Whitlow 90
Wider caliber 323
Wounds, healing of 257
Wrist
   and hand, joint of 99, 99*f*
   drop deformity 118
   extension of 64
   extensor tendons of 100

   forced dorsiflexion of 102
   immobilization of 102
   injured at 113
   injuries 102
   muscles acting on 58
Wrist fracture 102
   types of 102
Wrist joint 66, 99
   abductor of 63
   anterior 100
   arterial supply 101
   articulating surfaces 99
   clinical anatomy 102
   distal articular surface 99
   distal to 75
   ligaments 100
   movements of 101
   muscles producing movements 101
   nerve supply 101
   posterior 100
   proximal articular surface 99
   type of 99

X

Xiphoid 362

Y

Yolk sac 285

Z

Zinc 423
Zona
   fasciculata 378
   glomerulosa 377
   orbicularis 191
      fibers 232
   reticularis 378
Zygosis 260